1988
YEAR BOOK OF
PEDIATRICS®

The 1988 Year Book Series

Year Book of Anesthesia®: Drs. Miller, Kirby, Ostheimer, Roizen, and Stoelting

Year Book of Cancer®: Drs. Hickey and Saunders

Year Book of Cardiology®: Drs. Schlant, Collins, Engle, Frye, Kaplan, and O'Rourke

Year Book of Critical Care Medicine®: Drs. Rogers, Allo, Dean, McPherson, Michael, Miller, Traystman, and Wetzel

Year Book of Dentistry®: Drs. Cohen, Hendler, Johnson, Jordan, Moyers, Robinson, and Silverman

Year Book of Dermatology®: Drs. Sober and Fitzpatrick

Year Book of Diagnostic Radiology®: Drs. Bragg, Hendee, Keats, Kirkpatrick, Miller, Osborn, and Thompson

Year Book of Digestive Diseases®: Drs. Greenberger and Moody

Year Book of Drug Therapy®: Drs. Hollister and Lasagna

Year Book of Emergency Medicine®: Drs. Wagner, Roberts, Davidson, and Greenberg

Year Book of Endocrinology®: Drs. Bagdade, Braverman, Halter, Horton, Korenman, Kornel, Metz, Molitch, Morley, Robertson, Rogol, Ryan, and Vaitukaitis

Year Book of Family Practice®: Drs. Rakel, Avant, Driscoll, Prichard, and Smith

Year Book of Geriatrics and Gerontology: Drs. Beck, Abrass, Burton, Cummings, Makinodan, and Small

Year Book of Hand Surgery®: Drs. Dobyns, Chase, and Amadio

Year Book of Hematology: Drs. Spivak, Bell, Ness, Quesenberry, and Wiernik

Year Book of Infectious Diseases®: Drs. Wolff, Barza, Keusch, Klempner, and Snydman

Year Book of Medicine®: Drs. Rogers, Des Prez, Cline, Braunwald, Greenberger, Wilson, Epstein, and Malawista

Year Book of Neurology and Neurosurgery®: Drs. DeJong, Currier, and Crowell

Year Book of Nuclear Medicine®: Drs. Hoffer, Gore, Gottschalk, Sostman, and Zaret

Year Book of Obstetrics and Gynecology®: Drs. Mishell, Kirschbaum, and Morrow

Year Book of Ophthalmology®: Drs. Ernest and Deutsch

Year Book of Orthopedics®: Dr. Coventry

Year Book of Otolaryngology–Head and Neck Surgery®: Drs. Bailey and Paparella

Year Book of Pathology and Clinical Pathology®: Drs. Brinkhous, Dalldorf, Grisham, Langdell, and McLendon

Year Book of Pediatrics®: Drs. Oski and Stockman

Year Book of Perinatal/Neonatal Medicine: Drs. Klaus and Fanaroff

Year Book of Plastic and Reconstructive Surgery®: Drs. McCoy, Brauer, Haynes, Hoehn, Miller, and Whitaker

Year Book of Podiatric Medicine and Surgery®: Dr. Jay

Year Book of Psychiatry and Applied Mental Health®: Drs. Freedman, Lourie, Meltzer, Talbott, and Weiner

Year Book of Pulmonary Disease: Drs. Green, Ball, Menkes, Michael, Peters, Terry, Tockman, and Wise

Year Book of Rehabilitation: Drs. Kaplan and Szumski

Year Book of Sports Medicine®: Drs. Shepard and Torg, Col. Anderson, and Mr. George

Year Book of Surgery®: Drs. Schwartz, Jonasson, Peacock, Shires, Spencer, and Thompson

Year Book of Urology®: Drs. Gillenwater and Howards

Year Book of Vascular Surgery: Drs. Bergan and Yao

1988

The Year Book of PEDIATRICS®

Editors

Frank A. Oski, M.D.

Given Professor and Chairman, Department of Pediatrics, The Johns Hopkins University School of Medicine; Chairman and Pediatrician-in-Chief, The Children's Medical and Surgical Center, The Johns Hopkins Hospital

James A. Stockman III, M.D.

Professor and Chairman, Department of Pediatrics, Northwestern University School of Medicine; Physician-in-Chief, The Children's Memorial Hospital, Chicago

Year Book Medical Publishers, Inc.
Chicago • London • Boca Raton

Copyright © January 1988 by YEAR BOOK MEDICAL PUBLISHERS, INC.

All rights reserved. No part of this publication may be reproduced, stored in a retrieval system, or transmitted, in any form or by any means, electronic, mechanical, photocopying, recording, or otherwise, without prior written permission from the publisher.

Printed in U.S.A.

International Standard Book Number: 0-8151-6584-6

International Standard Serial Number: 0084-3954

Editorial Director, Year Book Publishing: Nancy Gorham
Sponsoring Editor: Cara D. Suber
Literature Surveillance Supervisor: Laura J. Shedore
Assistant Director, Manuscript Services: Frances M. Perveiler
Assistant Managing Editor, Year Book Editing Services: Elizabeth Griffith
Production Manager: H.E. Nielsen
Proofroom Supervisor: Shirley E. Taylor

Table of Contents

The material covered in this volume represents literature reviewed through May 1987.

Journals Represented

Year Book Medical Publishers subscribes to and surveys more than 700 U.S. and foreign medical and allied health journals. From these journals, the Editors select the articles to be abstracted. Journals represented in this YEAR BOOK are listed below.

Acta Dermato-Venereologica
Acta Neurochirurgica
Acta Paediatrica Scandinavica
Allergy
American Heart Journal
American Journal of Clinical Nutrition
American Journal of Clinical Pathology
American Journal of Diseases of Children
American Journal of Obstetrics and Gynecology
American Journal of Orthopsychiatry
American Journal of Pediatric Hematology/Oncology
American Journal of Perinatology
American Journal of Public Health
American Journal of Roentgenology
American Journal of Sports Medicine
American Journal of Surgery
American Review of Respiratory Disease
American Surgeon
Annales de Radiologie
Annals of Emergency Medicine
Annals of Internal Medicine
Annals of Ophthalmology
Archives of Disease in Childhood
Archives of Emergency Medicine
Archives of Ophthalmology
Archives of Pathology and Laboratory Medicine
Arthritis and Rheumatism
British Dental Journal
British Heart Journal
British Journal of Psychiatry
British Medical Journal
Canadian Journal of Psychiatry
Cancer
Chest
Child Development
Cleveland Clinic Quarterly
Clinical Pediatrics
Community Dentistry and Oral Epidemiology
Critical Care Medicine
Headache
Helvetica Paediatrica Acta
Journal of Adolescent Health Care
Journal of Allergy and Clinical Immunology
Journal of the American Academy of Child Psychiatry
Journal of the American College of Cardiology
Journal of the American Medical Association

Journal of Bone and Joint Surgery (American vol.)
Journal of Chronic Diseases
Journal of Clinical Investigation
Journal of Epidemiology and Community Health
Journal of Hypertension
Journal of Marriage and Family
Journal of Medical Genetics
Journal of Neurology, Neurosurgery and Psychiatry
Journal of Pediatric Gastroenterology and Nutrition
Journal of Pediatric Orthopedics
Journal of Pediatric Surgery
Journal of Pediatrics
Journal of Rheumatology
Journal of Speech and Hearing Disorders
Journal of Thoracic and Cardiovascular Surgery
Journal of Trauma
Journal of Urology
Kidney International
Lancet
Laryngoscope
Nature
Neurology
Neuropediatrics
Neurosurgery
New England Journal of Medicine
Ophthalmology
Otolaryngology–Head and Neck Surgery
Pediatric Cardiology
Pediatric Dentistry
Pediatric Emergency Care
Pediatric Infectious Disease
Pediatric Neurology
Pediatric Pulmonology
Pediatric Research
Pediatrics
Psychosomatic Medicine
Radiology
Science
Southern Medical Journal
Spine
Survey of Ophthalmology
Vox Sanguinis
Western Journal of Medicine

Introduction

The 1988 YEAR BOOK OF PEDIATRICS marks a milestone in the history of the YEAR BOOK, at least to these editors. It has been a decade since the editorial torch was passed from the hands of Sydney Gellis. Those were capable hands, indeed. Dr. Gellis established a reputation for writing the YEAR BOOK in a concise and incisive manner, often capturing the essence of a thought in one explosively short quip, sort of like doing in a fly with a hammer as opposed to a fly swatter.

So, what has happened to the YEAR BOOK in the last 10 years? We hope that the YEAR BOOK is still as packed with information as was true in the late 1970s, and that it is as enjoyable and interesting to read. It has certainly grown a tad corpulent—more than 50% larger in recent times. The latter reflects not so much a change in the number of articles selected for review as much as the fact that, to do justice to these articles, we frequently attempt to encapsulate related literature in our commentaries. It is the related literature that has increased logarithmically. In many instances a single article represents only a fraction of the information available on a particular topic during the course of a year.

As one looks back at the YEAR BOOK of a decade ago in comparison with the 1988 YEAR BOOK, one can easily see by the contents of the present volume that much of what was in vogue in 1978 still is "in." Nonetheless, there are topics included now that would have been unimaginable a few short years ago.

This past 12 months has shown us that there are yet uncharted waters in our quest of knowledge related to such venerable and age-old topics as otitis media, asthma, tracheobronchial foreign bodies, ophthalmia neonatorum, orbital cellulitis, cystic fibrosis, patent ductus arteriosus, circumcision, adolescent suicide, Kawasaki syndrome, and gastroesophageal reflux. The index of this volume and Dr. Gellis's last contribution both have entries for all of these subjects. A while back, however, we were talking about unusual presentations of cystic fibrosis and almost primitive concepts concerning the mucocutaneous lymph node syndrome. Herein lies descriptions of the specific DNA effect of the former and the use of gammaglobulin therapy intravenously for the latter. Lest one think that everything these days is moving to the "cutting edge," the reader will find in these pages yet another double-blind study of the management of otitis media and continued descriptions of gastroesophageal reflux. This past year is one that again purported to show that circumcision is associated with a decreased risk of urinary tract infection. We pediatricians would probably not know what to do with ourselves if a truly definitive study of otitis media, gastroesophageal reflux, or the role of circumcision were published.

As much as these topics remain with us, others have seen better days. You will find little or nothing in this YEAR BOOK that was worth commenting on regarding botulism, the value of the sed rate, or *Mycoplasma* infections. Even Reye's syndrome appears to have peaked out. The 1978 YEAR BOOK was replete with comments about all of these.

Some things are new, however. Who would have thought that the management of neonatal sepsis, Kawasaki syndrome, autoimmune hemolytic

11

anemia, idiopathic thrombocytopenia, and perhaps a dozen other disorders would be revolutionized by the development of intravenous gammaglobulin? Ten years ago, who would have thought that the editors of this year's YEAR BOOK would be discussing sensorineural hearing loss from the use of cordless telephones, the risks to a child of parental smoking, or the outcome of pregnancy in long-term survivors of Wilms' tumors? Dr. Gellis's concern over the hazards of aluminum pop-top cans seems enviably simple in this era of the human immunodeficiency virus. So, as the current editors of the YEAR BOOK complete a decade of authorship, what about the future? It is indeed difficult to predict what the next ten volumes of the YEAR BOOK will contain. Perhaps it is not worth the prediction, or as Einstein noted, ". . . never try to tell the future; it will come soon enough."

James A. Stockman III, M.D.

1 The Newborn

The Apgar Score Revisited: Influence of Gestational Age

Elizabeth A. Catlin, Marshall W. Carpenter, Benjamin S. Brann, IV, Steven R. Mayfield, Philip W. Shaul, Marshall Goldstein, and William Oh (Women and Infants Hosp. of Rhode Island, Providence)

J. Pediatr. 109:865–868, November 1986   1–1

The Apgar score has been widely accepted as means of assessing the clinical state at birth, but low scores in premature infants may be related to developmental immaturity rather than to fetal distress-related depression. The relationship between Apgar scores and gestational age was examined in infants who had an uncomplicated prenatal course. Seventy-three pregnant women with normal fetuses of 22–42 weeks' gestational age were included. Fetal well-being was assessed prospectively from the pregnancy history, labor, and birth outcome, including the cord blood pH and base deficit.

Gestational age was directly related to both 1-minute and 5-minute Apgar scores (Fig 1–1). The heart rate appeared to be the component least affected by developmental immaturity (Fig 1–2). Scores for respiratory effort and muscle tone increased with advancing gestational age. Reflex irritability also increased with gestational age. Fourteen of 22 infants of less than 31 weeks' gestational age required tracheal intubation; all weighed less than 1,000 gm at birth.

Apgar scores at 1 minute and 5 minutes are positively related to gestational age in newborn infants who have a benign prenatal course. Immature infants will have low Apgar scores despite normal cord blood pH and base excess values. Infants with low 1-minute scores related to de-

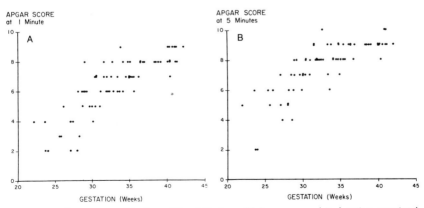

Fig 1–1.—Scattergrams of 1-minute (A) and 5-minute (B) Apgar scores plotted against gestational age. (Courtesy of Catlin, E.A., et al.: J. Pediatr. 109:865–868, November 1986.)

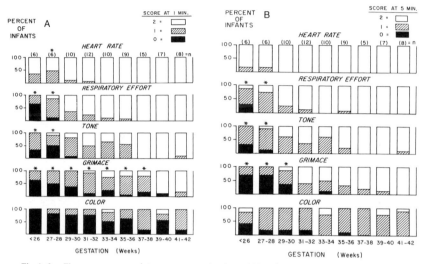

Fig 1–2.—Five components of Apgar score at 1 minute (**A**) and 5 minutes (**B**), with percentage of infants in each gestational age group scoring 0, 1, or 2. *Asterisk* denotes significantly different from older gestational age groups but not from other groups designated with asterisks. (Courtesy of Catlin, E.A., et al.: J. Pediatr. 109:865–868, November 1986.)

velopmental difficulty in initiating cardiorespiratory function at birth are logically intubated.

▶ Dr. David A. Clark, Associate Professor of Pediatrics, New York Medical College, comments.—F.A. Oski, M.D.

▶ The authors confirm the discrepancy among the various components of the Apgar score; the heart rate is least affected, and color is most unreliable at any gestational age. Respiratory effort, muscle tone, and grimace are most influenced by gestational age. Unfortunately, cord blood pH and base excess (an important inclusion criteria) were not available in 10% (7 of 73) of these infants. Although vaginal delivery is implied by the authors, it was not stated. Furthermore, no information is given regarding maternal analgesia or tocolysis (e.g., magnesium sulfate), which may have greater depressant effects on the CNS in the more immature infant.

To the chagrin of our obstetric colleagues, the data confirm how seldom an Apgar score of 10 can be awarded: 3 of 146 scores, even in "unremarkable" pregnancies with uncompromised fetuses.

The data confirm the clinical impression of many neonatologists that babies of less than 30 weeks' gestation (30% of this study) frequently require a more aggressive approach to stabilization than do more mature babies.

In general, too much importance is still being placed on the Apgar score, almost as if it is equivalent to an initial IQ test. Rather, it should be viewed as a quick screening tool to assess the need for and the intensity of resuscitation. The 5-minute score is a marker of the success of the intervention and the necessity for continued support.—D.A. Clark, M.D.

Palpable Lymph Nodes in Healthy Newborns and Infants

Mahrukh Bamji, R.K. Stone, A. Kaul, G. Usmani, F.F. Schachter, and E. Wasserman (New York Med. College, New York)

Pediatrics 78:573–575, October 1986   1–2

Several studies have investigated the etiology and management of palpable lymph nodes in children, but little has been written on palpable lymph nodes in neonates and infants. The frequency, size, and location of palpable lymph nodes at various sites were examined in 548 healthy neonates and infants up to age 1 year.

The series included 214 newborns and 334 infants who were divided into five groups on the basis of their age at the time of evaluation: Group I included newborns aged from birth to 72 hours; group II, newborns aged 4–7 days; group III, newborns aged 1–4 weeks; group IV, infants aged 1–6 months; and group V, infants aged 7–12 months. All were healthy and had been free of major or minor systemic or cutaneous infection prior to examination for the presence of cervical, inguinal, axillary, and supraclavicular lymph nodes 3 mm or larger in diameter.

Of the 214 neonates, 73 (34%) had palpable nodes at one or more sites, including 46 (37%) of 123 males and 27 (30%) of 91 females (Table 1). Uncircumcised neonates were more likely to have palpable nodes at one or more sites, but the difference was not statistically significant. The inguinal area was the most common site of palpable nodes in infants younger than age 4 weeks. Of 334 infants, 190 (57%) had palpable lymph nodes (Table 2).

TABLE 1.—Prevalence of Palpable Lymph Nodes at Various Sites From Birth to 4 Weeks of Age

	0–72 H	72 H–1 Wk	1–4 Wk	Total
No. of neonates	58	74	82	214
No. of neonates with palpable nodes	14 (24%)	26 (35%)	33 (40%)	73 (34%)
Inguinal	11 (18%)	20 (26%)	21 (25%)	52 (24%)
Cervical	7 (12%)	14 (19%)	18 (22%)	39 (17%)
Axillary	1 (1%)	5 (6%)	8 (10%)	14 (6.5%)

(Courtesy of Bamji, M., et al.: Pediatrics 78:573–575, October 1986.)

TABLE 2.—Prevalence of Palpable Lymph Nodes From 4 Weeks to 12 Months of Age

	1–6 Mo	6–12 Mo	Total
No. of infants	176	158	334
No. of infants with palpable nodes	74 (42%)	116 (73%)	190 (57%)
Inguinal	40 (22.7%)	58 (36.7%)	98 (29%)
Cervical	48 (27.2%)	88 (55%)	136 (41%)
Axillary	12 (6.8%)	22 (14%)	34 (10%)

(Courtesy of Bamji, M., et al.: Pediatrics 78:573–575, October 1986.)

Lymph nodes may be normally palpable in about a third of all normal healthy neonates and in about half of all healthy infants. However, the presence of small, palpable lymph nodes during the neonatal period does not warrant clinical investigation into its etiology.

▶ The nodes did not exceed 12 mm in diameter in newborns. Lewis Barness, in his text, *Manual of Pediatric Physical Diagnosis,* states that lymph nodes in the newborn are normally no larger than 3 mm. If he is wrong about this it will be the first time he has been wrong about anything and then it will be only by much less than an inch.—F.A. Oski, M.D.

Anterior Fontanel: Size and Closure in Term and Preterm Infants
G. Duc and R.H. Largo (Universitäts-Kinderspital Zürich, Switzerland)
Pediatrics 78:904–908, November 1986   1–3

The size of the anterior fontanelle is routinely assessed as an index of cranial development up to age 2 years, but few data on normal dimensions for age are available. The size and closure of the fontanelle from birth to age 24 months were recorded in 111 term and 128 preterm infants and related to growth measures, bone age, and gestational age. The preterm group were high-risk infants with relatively low perinatal optimality scores. Fontanelle dimensions were recorded as oblique diameters (Fig 1–3).

Closure of the fontanelle was first observed 3 months after term in about 1% of the infants. The fontanelle was closed at 12 months in 38% and at 24 months in 96%. The median age at closure in term infants was 14 months, but variability was considerable (Fig 1–4). There were no consistent differences between term and preterm infants, and age at closure was not related to fontanelle size at an early age. Low positive correlations were found between fontanelle size and infant weight and length at birth and at term. Fontanelle size was not consistently related to head circum-

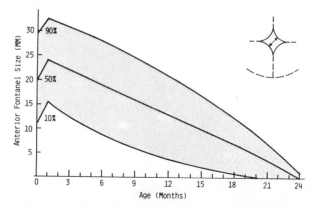

Fig 1–3.—Centiles of anterior fontanelle size from term to age 24 months for both sexes. Measurement of oblique diameter. (Courtesy of Duc, G., and Largo, R.H.: Pediatrics 78:904–908, November 1986.)

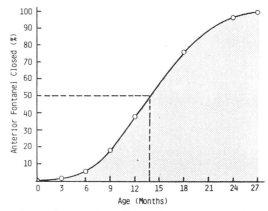

Fig 1–4.—Age of closure of anterior fontanelle (cumulative percentage). (Courtesy of Duc, G., and Largo, R.H.: Pediatrics 78:904–908, November 1986.)

ference or bone age. At birth, fontanelle size correlated with gestational age for premature infants only. Age at closure was not related to weight, length, head circumference, or bone age. The rate and timing of anterior fontanelle closure could not be related significantly to head circumference in this normal population, but under pathologic conditions, fontanelle size and closure might be related to other growth measures.

▶ Measurement of the fontanelle seems to be disappearing from the routine physical exam. This is an unfortunate omission because the size of the anterior fontanelle can be a helpful clue to the presence of a variety of conditions. For example, an unusually small fontanelle for age may reflect brain growth retardation, craniostenosis, or hyperthyroidism. Conversely, an unusually large fontanelle, without increased intracranial pressure, is seen in hypothyroidism, achondroplasia, cleidocranial dysostosis, osteogenesis imperfecta, vitamin D deficiency, and certain chromosomal abnormalities such as trisomies 9p, 13, 18, and 21. For those seeking a little culture along with their medical education, the term fontanelle is derived from the French word *fontanelle,* which is the diminutive for *fontaine,* the word for fountain. Now isn't this better than CME?—F.A. Oski, M.D.

Normal Serum Bilirubin Levels in the Newborn and the Effect of Breast-Feeding

M. Jeffrey Maisels and Kathleen Gifford (Pennsylvania State Univ., Hershey)
Pediatrics 78:837–843, November 1986   1–4

Serum bilirubin levels in newborns are determined for diagnostic and therapeutic use. Normal serum bilirubin levels were established by the National Collaborative Perinatal Project; however, the distribution of bilirubin levels is not known. The association between serum bilirubin con-

TABLE 1.—Feeding and Hyperbilirubinemia

Feeding	No. (%) of Infants With Maximum Serum Bilirubin ≤12.9 mg/dL (n = 147)	No. (%) of Infants With Maximum Serum Bilirubin >12.9 mg/dL (n = 147)		
		All Babies (n = 147)	Hyperbilirubinemia Before Discharge With No Apparent Cause (n = 81)	Hyperbilirubinemia by Day 3 With No Apparent Cause (n = 57)
Breast-fed	69 (46.9)	117 (79.6)†	67 (82.7)†	46 (80.7)†
Bottle-fed	71 (48.3)	26 (17.7)	10 (12.3)	8 (14.0)
Breast- and bottle-fed	7 (4.8)	4 (2.7)	4 (4.9)	3 (5.3)

*Apparent causes include Rh incompatibility (5 patients), ABO incompatibility (16), infant of diabetic mother (17), asphyxia (6), gestation ≤ 35 weeks (11), bruising/cephalohematoma (45), polycythemia (3), and cholestasis (1).
†$P < .00001$ vs. serum bilirubin ≤ 12.9 mg/dl.
(Courtesy of Maisels, M.J., and Gifford, K.: Pediatrics 78:837–843, November 1986.)

TABLE 2.—Percentile Ranks for White
Newborn Infants Weighing > 2,500
Grams

Percentile	Maximum Serum Bilirubin Concentration					
	Total Population* (N = 2,297)		Breast-Fed (N = 1,260)		Bottle-Fed (N = 1,026)	
	μmol/L	mg/dL	μmol/L	mg/dL	μmol/L	mg/dL
3	19	1.1	19	1.1	19	1.1
5	22	1.3	24	1.4	21	1.2
10	31	1.8	36	2.1	27	1.6
15	41	2.4	48	2.8	34	2.0
25	62	3.6	74	4.3	53	3.1
50	111	6.5	125	7.3	96	5.6
75	154	9.0	168	9.8	135	7.9
90	197	11.5	214	12.5	171	10.0
95	231	13.5	248	14.5	195	11.4
97	253	14.8	269	15.7	212	12.4
99	286	16.7	291	17.0	267	15.6

*Includes 11 infants both breast fed and bottle fed.
(Courtesy of Maisels, M.J., and Gifford, K.: Pediatrics 78:837–843, November 1986.)

centrations and breast-feeding were examined in an attempt to establish the normal distribution of serum bilirubin levels.

The serum bilirubin levels of 2,416 consecutive infants in the well-baby nursery were measured at least once by the third day and again if levels were high. When the concentration was higher than 12.9 mg/dl, several other blood tests were done. The serum bilirubin level was measured by a modified diazo method using an automatic clinical analyzer. Data on feeding, birth weight, and weight loss were obtained for every infant.

The maximum serum bilirubin level exceeded 12.9 mg/dl in 6.1% (147) of the infants. A cause for the jaundice was identified in 66 of these infants, of whom 46.9% were breast fed. Of the 81 in whom no cause for jaundice could be found, 82.7% were breast fed (Table 1). The 95th percentile for

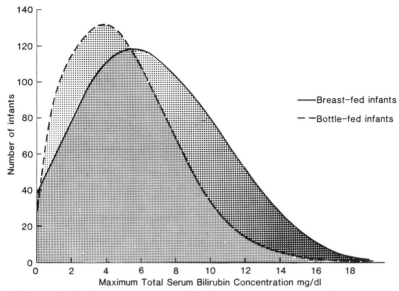

Fig 1–5.—Distribution of maximum serum bilirubin concentrations in white infants weighing more than 2,500 gm. Curves were computer generated using exponential one knot spline regression. (Courtesy of Maisels, M.J., and Gifford, K.: Pediatrics 78:837–843, November 1986.)

formula-fed infants was 11.4 mg/dl and for breast-fed infants, 14.5 mg/dl (Table 2). The distribution of serum bilirubin concentrations was shifted to significantly higher levels among healthy white infants who were breast fed compared with the formula-fed infants (Fig 1–5).

A diagnosis of jaundice may not be indicated unless the serum bilirubin level exceeds 15 mg/dl in the breast-fed infant or 12 mg/dl in the formula-fed infant. Hyperbilirubinemia might be treated by temporary cessation of breast-feeding rather than by phototherapy.

▶ The authors' suggestion that we employ a double standard for the classification of hyperbilirubinemia is a sound one. The 97th percentile for the breast-fed term infant is 15.7 mg%, while the 97th percentile for the formula-fed infant is 12.4 mg%. When the infant reaches the 97th percentile, investigation employing a hemoglobin, blood type, Coombs' test, reticulocyte count, and smear will provide an answer as to etiology in approximately half of the patients. Last year it looked as if we had a logical explanation as to why breast-fed infants became more jaundiced than infants fed artificially (1987 YEAR BOOK, p. 17). Gourley and Arend proposed that the β-glucuronidase present in human milk promoted the reabsorption of bilirubin and resulted in higher, and more protracted, bilirubin values in breast-fed infants. As might be expected, Freed and associates could not confirm this attractive explanation (*Pediatr. Res.* 21:267A, 1987). Whatever the explanation for why breast-fed infants become more jaundiced, the next article suggests that bilirubin might be good for you.—F.A. Oski, M.D.

Bilirubin Is an Antioxidant of Possible Physiological Importance

Roland Stocker, Yorihiro Yamamoto, Antony F. McDonagh, Alexander N. Glazer, and Bruce N. Ames (Univ. of California at Berkeley, and at San Francisco)

Science 235:1043–1045, Feb. 27, 1987   1–5

Bilirubin, the end product of heme metabolism in mammals, is generally regarded as a potentially cytotoxic, lipid-soluble waste product that needs to be excreted. However, bilirubin contains an extended system of conjugated double bonds and a reactive hydrogen atom, which could possess antioxidant properties. A study was conducted to determine the antioxidant activity of bilirubin. The effect of bilirubin on the rate of peroxyl radical-induced oxidation of linoleic acid in homogeneous solutions or multilamellar liposomes was examined in an in vitro system. The radical initiator 2,2′-azobis(2,4-dimethylvaleronitrile) (AMVN) was used. The relative importance of bilirubin as a possible physiologic antioxidant was also compared with that of β-carotene and α-tocopherol.

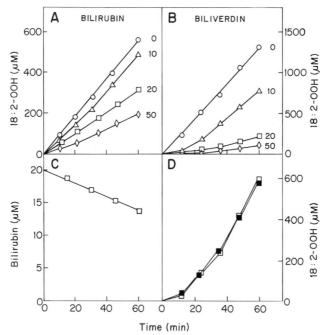

Fig 1–6.—Oxidation of purified linoleic acid initiated by AMVN in the presence and absence of heme degradation products under air. Formation of linoleic acid hydroperoxide *(18:2-OOH)* was analyzed by high-pressure liquid chromatography. Effect of recrystallized bilirubin (**A**) and biliverdin IX hydrochloride (**B**) at 0 *(circles)*, 10 *(triangles)*, 20 *(squares)*, and 50 μM *(diamonds)* on AMVN-initiated oxidation of linoleic acid is shown. Reaction solvents were chloroform in **A** and methanol in **B. C**, AMVN-induced disappearance of bilirubin in presence of linoleic acid under same conditions as in **A. D**, effects of bilirubin *(open squares)* and its two configurational photoisomers *(solid squares)* on AMVN-initiated oxidation of linoleic acid in chloroform and methanol. Data shown represent typical results for each experiment, with variance of less than 5% (*n* = 3 or 4). (Courtesy of Stocker, R., et al.: Science 235:1043–1045, Feb. 27, 1987.)

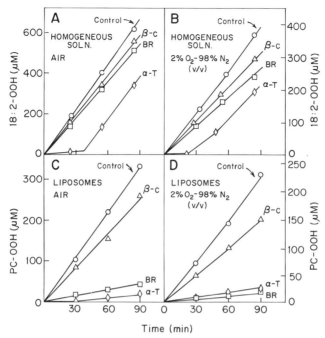

Fig 1–7.—Comparison of rates of oxidation of purified linoleic acid (**A** and **B**) in homogeneous solution and purified soybean phosphatidylcholine *(PC)* (**C** and **D**) in aqueous dispersion under air (**A** and **C**) and 2% oxygen (**B** and **D**), in absence *(circles)* or presence of trans-β-carotene *(β-C, triangles)*, recrystallized bilirubin *(BR, squares)*, or α-tocopherol *(α-T, diamonds)*. Multilamellar liposomes in water were prepared with purified soybean PC and AMVN. Formation of PC hydroperoxides *(PC-OOH)* was analyzed by high-pressure liquid chromatography. Results shown represent averages of two to four independent experiments, with variance of less than 7%. (Courtesy of Stocker, R., et al.: Science 235:1043–1045, Feb. 27, 1987.)

Bilirubin, in micromolar concentrations, significantly inhibited the oxidation of linoleic acid in a concentration-dependent manner in both homogeneous solutions and multilamellar liposomes (Fig 1–6). The data indicated that bilirubin can efficiently scavenge the peroxyl radicals generated chemically. The antioxidant activity of bilirubin increased as the experimental concentration of oxygen was decreased from 20% that of normal air to 2%, a physiologically relevant concentration. Further, in liposomes, under 2% oxygen, bilirubin significantly suppressed the oxidation of linoleic acid more than did α-tocopherol, the best antioxidant of lipid peroxidation (Fig 1–7). These findings support a "beneficial" role of bilirubin as a physiologic, chain-breaking antioxidant.

▶ What a marvelous system! During the first days of life when the infant is relatively deficient in antioxidant defenses such as vitamin E, catalase, and glutathione peroxidase, human milk feeding promotes hyperbilirubinemia and the bilirubin acts to compensate for the antioxidant deficiency. I can see it now—babies will be found to be *hypo*bilirubinemic and we will begin tc look for things to add to formulas to promote higher serum bilirubin concentrations in the bottle-fed child.—F.A. Oski, M.D.

Serum Glucose Levels in Term Neonates During the First 48 Hours of Life

Louis J. Heck and Allen Erenberg (Univ. of South Dakota and Univ. of Iowa)
J. Pediatr. 110:119–122, January 1987   1–6

An attempt was made to define normal serum glucose concentrations during the first 48 hours in healthy, term neonates; serum glucose values were compared in breast-fed and bottle-fed infants during this period. The study included 113 mothers and 114 term infants of 37–42 weeks' gestation who were examined in 1 year. None of the mothers had diabetes mellitus or hypertension, and none had been treated with any drug during the last 4 weeks of pregnancy. There was no prenatal infection or fetal distress. Of the 114 infants, 64 were breast fed and 50 were bottle fed. A single maternal serum glucose concentration was determined within 30 minutes of delivery or from the episiotomy incision immediately before delivery. Infant blood samples were obtained from the cord at birth, by heel puncture after the first feeding, and at predetermined intervals after three subsequent feedings at ages 10–18 hours, 20–28 hours, and 44–52 hours.

Although statistically significant differences were found between serum glucose concentrations in breast-fed and bottle-fed infants, the differences were not considered to be clinically significant. The fifth percentile postnatal serum glucose values did not exceed 40 mg/dl until age 24 hours in the two groups combined (table).

The small differences in mean serum glucose concentrations between breast-fed and bottle-fed infants may result from differences in intake. On the basis of these findings, hypoglycemia in full-term infants may be defined as a serum glucose concentration of less than 30 mg/dl in the first day or of less than 40 mg/dl in the second.

▶ The 30/24 and the 40/48 rule appear to be useful guidelines for the interpretation of blood glucose values during the first 2 days of life. Many babies in the recent past were labeled as hypoglycemic during the first day of life with glucose values in the 30–40 mg% range. Sexson pointed out that using a value of 40 mg% as the lower limit of normal blood sugar during the first day of life results in a 20% incidence of hypoglycemia in full-term infants (*J. Pediatr.* 105:149, 1984). This is an easy approach to the problem of neonatal hypoglycemia—make it disappear by changing the definition. I am reminded of Menck-

Percentile	Maternal	Cord	1 Hr	2 Hr	5-6 Hr	10-14 Hr	20-28 Hr	44-52 Hr
5th	73	63	36	39	34	33	46	48
50th	104	90	56	58	56	56	60	65
95th	188	158	99	89	77	74	81	79
n	97	110	113	107	105	102	101	92
Mean	112	97	60	61	56	56	61	64
SD	37	29	18	15	11	12	10	10

MATERNAL AND NEONATAL SERUM GLUCOSE VALUES (MG/DL): COMBINED GROUPS

(Courtesy of Heck, L.J., and Erenberg, A.: J. Pediatr. 110:119–122, January 1987.)

en's Rule of Unanimity: "When everyone begins to believe anything it ceases to be true; for example, the notion that the ugliest girl in the party is the safest."—F.A. Oski, M.D.

Filterability of Erythrocytes and Whole Blood in Preterm and Full-Term Neonates and Adults

Otwin Linderkamp, Bernhard J. Hammer, and Rolf Miller (Univ. of Heidelberg, West Germany)

Pediatr. Res. 20:1269–1273, December 1986   1–7

Hyperviscosity in neonates is a common and potentially serious condition that can cause circulatory failure and impaired microcirculation in vital organs. Blood viscosity is usually measured by hematocrit. Decreased red blood cell (RBC) deformability contributes to increased blood viscosity. Red blood cell deformability and flow behavior in microcirculation were examined using placental blood samples obtained from 30 newborn infants. Ten were of very low birth weight and 24–30 weeks' gestation; ten were more mature preterm infants of 31–36 weeks' gestation; and ten were full-term neonates; control blood samples were obtained from ten normal adults. Filtration rates were measured by using Nucleopore filters having pore diameters of 5μ and filtration pressures of 1, 2, 5, and 10 cm water. The influence of plasma and leukocytes on filtration rates also was studied.

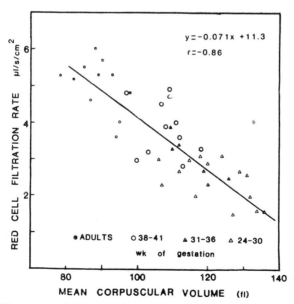

Fig 1–8.—Filtration rate of RBC (suspended in buffer at hematocrit of 10%) plotted against mean corpuscular volume. There was a highly significant inverse relationship. (Courtesy of Linderkamp, O., et al.: Pediatr. Res. 20:1269–1273, December 1986.)

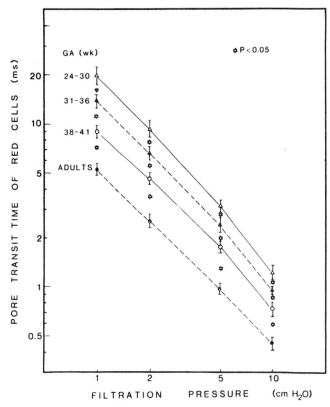

Fig 1–9.—Mean pore transit time of single RBC plotted against filtration pressure. Values are means ± SD. (Courtesy of Linderkamp, O., et al.: Pediatr. Res. 20:1269–1273, December 1986.)

At each of the four filtration pressures used, filtration rates of RBCs in buffer suspensions were significantly lower in preterm than in term neonates, and filtration rates in term neonates were lower than those in adult controls (Fig 1–8). Mean pore transit times were longer in preterm infants than in term neonates and adults (Fig 1–9). The slow RBC filtration rates in neonates were related to large cellular volumes. The filter flow resistance of RBCs obtained from preterm infants decreased more with increasing pressure than did that of RBCs from term neonates and adults. Filterability of whole blood was markedly less than that of washed RBCs, particularly in preterm infants.

▶ Several conclusions can be drawn from this work: (1) At any given pressure, RBC filtration rates through 5-μ pores are lower, and mean RBC transit times are longer in preterm infants than in term neonates and adults; (2) slow RBC filtration rates in neonates are related to their large cellular volume; and (3) the filterability of whole blood is markedly less than that of washed RBCs. The filtration of whole blood from premature and term infants may be impaired more than that of adult blood because of the higher leukocyte and nucleated

RBC counts in the babies. The resistance of leukocytes to filtration through 5-µ pores is 1,000 times greater than that of RBCs. What does this decreased filterability have to do with the problem of polycythemia? It would suggest that the viscosity of infant blood at any given hematocrit might be greater than that of adults, but this does not appear to be the case because of the higher fibrinogen concentration in the plasma of adult blood. Fibrinogen is an important determinant of whole blood viscosity. Speaking of polycythemia, Wiswell and associates (*Pediatrics* 78:26, 1986) found a 1.46% incidence of polycythemia in their institution, the Brooke Army Medical Center, over a 4-year period. Of these infants, 85% had features associated with the disorder. Frequent signs and symptoms included "feeding problems" (21.8%), lethargy (14.5%), cyanosis (14.5%), respiratory distress (9.1%), jitteriness (7.3%), and hypotonia (7.3%). In addition, 40% of the babies were hypoglycemic and 21.8% were hyperbilirubinemic. Of the polycythemic infants, 14.5% had no associated clinical symptoms or laboratory abnormalities. At the present time, nobody really knows how to best manage the baby born with a high hematocrit. It is about time we found out.—F.A. Oski, M.D.

Vitamin K Deficiency in the Newborn Infant: Prevalence and Perinatal Risk Factors

Amy D. Shapiro, Linda J. Jacobson, Mary E. Armon, Marilyn J. Manco-Johnson, Peter Hulac, Peter A. Lane, and Wm. E. Hathaway (Univ. of Colorado)
J. Pediatr. 109:675–680, October 1986   1–8

Although prophylactic administration of vitamin K at birth has been recommended since 1961, its use remains controversial because the prevalence, or even presence, of vitamin K deficiency in the newborn has not been well defined. Studies were made in a large series of infants prospectively to assess vitamin K deficiency and the influence of perinatal risk factors at birth.

The 934 infants examined were grouped by gestational age (term, pre-

TABLE 1.—INFANTS WITH POSITIVE PIVKA-II BY WEIGHT AND GESTATIONAL AGE

	Percent of study group	Percent with positive PIVKA-II
Weight		
AGA	83.4	2.7
LGA	13.7	3.1
SGA	2.9	7.4
Gestational age (wk)		
37-42	93.0	3.1
>42	1.4	0
<37	5.6	0

(Courtesy of Shapiro, A.D., et al.: J. Pediatr. 109:675–680, October, 1986.)

TABLE 2.—INFANTS* WITH POSITIVE PIVKA-II
BY PERINATAL RISK GROUP

	n	%	Positive for PIVKA-II n	%
Hypertension	93	10.0	3	3.2
Diabetes	15	1.6	1	6.7
Third-trimester antibiotics	130	13.9	5	3.8
Third-trimester bleeding	5	0.5	1	20.0
Fetal distress	119	12.7	2	1.7
Substance abuse	9	0.9	1	11.1
Respiratory distress or sepsis	54	5.8	0	0
Polyhydramnios	8	0.8	0	0
Normal	579	62.0	17	2.9

*Number: 934.
(Courtesy of Shapiro, A.D., et al.: J. Pediatr. 109:675–680, October, 1986.)

term, or postterm) and by weight (small for gestational age, appropriate for gestational age, or large for gestational age) (Table 1). Cord blood samples were assayed to detect proteins induced in the absence of vitamin K (PIVKA-II) to determine the presence of vitamin K deficiency. All infants were given vitamin K by intramuscular injection within 1 hour after birth. Maternal hypertension, diabetes, third-trimester antibiotic usage, third-trimester bleeding, substance abuse, fetal distress, respiratory distress, and suspicion of sepsis were noted (Table 2).

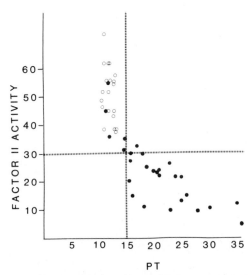

Fig 1–10.—Factor II activity and prothrombin times in infants with detectable PIVKA-II (●) and in 20 normal controls (○). *Dotted lines* represent normal limits. (Courtesy of Shapiro, A.D., et al.: J. Pediatr. 109:675–680, October, 1986.)

TABLE 3.—CORD BLOOD STUDIES FOR PIVKA-II

Author	Method	No. positive/No. studied	% Positive
Van Doorm et al, 1977	Crossed immunoelectrophoresis	0/43	0
Muntean et al, 1979	Crossed immunoelectrophoresis	15/30	50.0
Malia et al, 1980	Crossed immunoelectrophoresis	0/24	0
Meguro and Yamada, 1982	Antibody-coated beads after $BaCO_3$ absorption	2/12	16.6
Atkinson et al, 1982	Chromogenic assay (S2238) with venom	48/128	38.2
Ekelund and Hedner, 1984	Crossed immunoelectrophoresis	2/105	1.9
Motohara et al, 1985	ELISA (monoclonal antibody)	21/99	21.2
Blanchard et al, 1985	RIA (heteroantibody)	161/181	89.0
von Kries et al, 1985	Crossed immunoelectrophoresis	0/40	0
Our study 1985	Immunoelectrophoresis after $BaCO_3$ absorption	27/934	2.9

(Courtesy of Shapiro, A.D., et al.: J. Pediatr. 109:675–680, October, 1986.)

Of 934 cord blood specimens assayed, 2.9% were PIVKA-II positive (Table 3). The most infants positive for PIVKA-II were found in the smallest sized group (7.4%), followed by 3.1% in the largest infants, and 2.7% in the average size group. None of the infants with PIVKA-II in the cord sample had subsequent clinical bleeding because all had received prophylactic vitamin K injections. Analysis of perinatal risk factors showed that most of the vitamin K deficiency occurred in normal neonates (Fig 1–10). It is recommended that all infants receive prophylactic vitamin K at birth.

▶ All infants should receive vitamin K. Generally speaking, it is dangerous to generalize, but correction of vitamin K deficiency prevents classic hemorrhagic disease of the newborn and, in all probability, would prevent the late hemorrhagic disease seen in some breast-fed babies. For more on vitamin K, the reader is encouraged to see the 1987 YEAR BOOK, pp. 20–22.—F.A. Oski, M.D.

Failure of Antepartum Maternal Cultures to Predict the Infant's Risk of Exposure to Herpes Simplex Virus at Delivery

Ann M. Arvin, Paul A. Hensleigh, Charles G. Prober, Deborah S. Au, Linda L. Yasukawa, Alec E. Wittek, Paul E. Palumbo, Sharon G. Paryani, and Anne S. Yeager (Stanford Univ.)
N. Engl. J. Med. 315:796–800, Sept. 25, 1986   1–9

Neonatal infection with herpes simplex virus (HSV) is recognized as a life-threatening condition that causes severe morbidity among some infants despite antiviral therapy. Such infection in the newborn usually results from exposure to the virus in the maternal genital tract at the time of delivery. Thus, if an expectant mother has signs or symptoms of HSV infection at the onset of labor, a cesarean section is usually performed to avoid infecting the infant. Nevertheless, reactivation of genital HSV is often asymptomatic, and mothers of many infants with this infection may have no history of peripartum genital herpes. Research was conducted to test the hypothesis that cultures of specimens obtained late in gestation from women with a history of genital HSV infection predict asymptomatic shedding of HSV at delivery and therefore may be useful in planning the delivery method to prevent neonatal exposure to asymptomatic maternal herpes.

The correlation between asymptomatic viral shedding in late pregnancy

TABLE 1.—FREQUENCY OF ASYMPTOMATIC EXCRETION OF HSV DURING PREGNANCY AMONG WOMEN WITH A HISTORY OF RECURRENT GENITAL HERPES

TIME SPECIMENS WERE OBTAINED AND CLINICAL STATUS	NO. OF WOMEN	NO. OF POSITIVE CULTURES FOR HSV	NO. OF CULTURES	FREQUENCY OF POSITIVE CULTURES FOR ASYMPTOMATIC EXCRETION OF HSV
Less than 34 weeks of gestation				
Recurrences during pregnancy	116	1	216	
No recurrences during pregnancy	31	0	59	
Data incomplete	9	0	18	
Total	156	1	293	0.34%
34 weeks of gestation to 1 week before delivery				
Recurrences during pregnancy	303	10	1542	
No recurrences during pregnancy	78	2	398	
Data incomplete	14	0	74	
Total	395	12	2014	0.60%
Within 1 week of delivery				
Recurrences during pregnancy	229	3	398	
No recurrences during pregnancy	58	1	107	
Data incomplete	15	0	29	
Total	302	4	534	0.75%

(Courtesy of Arvin, A.M., et al.: N. Engl. J. Med. 315:796–800, Sept. 25, 1986.)

TABLE 2.—CLINICAL STATUS AT DELIVERY OF WOMEN
WITH A HISTORY OF GENITAL HSV INFECTION,
ACCORDING TO STATUS DURING THE LAST WEEK OF
PREGNANCY

STATUS WITHIN 1 WK OF DELIVERY		STATUS AT DELIVERY		
		ASYMPTOMATIC	LESION PRESENT	PRODROME
	total	*no. (%)*		
Asymptomatic	302	284 (94)	15 (5)	3 (1)
Lesion present	41	9 (22)	31 (76)	1 (2)
Prodrome	3	0	1 (33)	2 (67)

(Courtesy of Arvin, A.M., et al.: N. Engl. J. Med. 315:796–800, Sept. 25, 1986.)

TABLE 3.—RESULTS OF CULTURES OF SPECIMENS OBTAINED
AT DELIVERY FROM MOTHERS WITH A HISTORY OF
RECURRENT GENITAL HSV INFECTION AND FROM THEIR
INFANTS

CLINICAL STATUS OF MOTHER AT DELIVERY	NO. OF WOMEN	NO. OF WOMEN WITH CULTURES POSITIVE FOR HSV (%)	NO. OF INFANTS	NO. OF INFANTS WITH CULTURES POSITIVE FOR HSV (%)
Asymptomatic	311	3 (0.96)	316	2 (0.63)
Lesions present	41	8 (19.5)	50	0 (0)
Prodrome only	5	1 (20.0)	8	0 (0)

(Courtesy of Arvin, A.M., et al.: N. Engl. J. Med. 315:796–800, Sept. 25, 1986.)

and at delivery was evaluated in 414 pregnant women with a history of recurrent genital HSV infection. Antepartum cultures for asymptomatic reactivation of HSV registered positive in 17 of the 414 women (4.1%); none of the 17 had positive cultures at the time of delivery. Overall, 354 women (86%) were asymptomatic at delivery. Herpes simplex virus was isolated in 3 of 311 asymptomatic mothers (0.96%), a frequency similar to that of asymptomatic shedding during pregnancy (Table 1). Cultures of specimens obtained at delivery from 5 of the 354 asymptomatic mother-infant pairs (1.4%) were positive for asymptomatic excretion of HSV; none of these women had antepartum cultures demonstrating asymptomatic excretion of HSV despite the fact that culturing was performed repeatedly during the 4 weeks prior to delivery. Most women (94%) who were asymptomatic 1 week before delivery remained asymptomatic at delivery, but 18 (6%) had symptoms by the day of delivery (Table 2). Sixty women had either prodromal symptoms (8 of 414, or 1.9%) or lesions (54 of 414, or 12.6%) at onset of labor. Specimens were taken from 41 of the 52 with lesions who had recurrences of HSV at delivery; eight of these cultures (19.5%) were positive for HSV (Table 3). The asymptomatic shedding of HSV occurred with the same frequency at delivery, whether or not any episodes of symptomatic recurrence were observed during pregnancy (1.4% vs. 1.3%). Antepartum maternal cultures apparently cannot predict the infant's risk of exposure to HSV at delivery.

Low Risk of Herpes Simplex Virus Infections in Neonates Exposed to the Virus at the Time of Vaginal Delivery to Mothers With Recurrent Genital Herpes Simplex Virus Infections

Charles G. Prober, Wayne M. Sullender, Linda Lew Yasukawa, Deborah S. Au, Anne S. Yeager, and Ann M. Arvin (Stanford Univ.)
N. Engl. J. Med. 316:240–244, Jan. 29, 1987   1–10

Infants born to women with primary herpes simplex virus (HSV) infection are at high risk of contracting clinically manifest infection. The risk to infants born to mothers with recurrent genital HSV infection is much lower. To quantify this risk, 34 infants exposed to HSV at the time of vaginal delivery to mothers with recurrent genital HSV infections were monitored clinically and evaluated for immunologic evidence of subclinical HSV infection.

At a minimum follow-up of 4 months, none of the 34 infants exposed to HSV type 2 acquired an HSV infection. On the basis of this sample size, the 95% confidence limit for the theoretical maximum infection rate was 8%. All 33 samples of cord blood or blood obtained during the first 2 weeks of life from exposed, uninfected neonates had demonstrable neu-

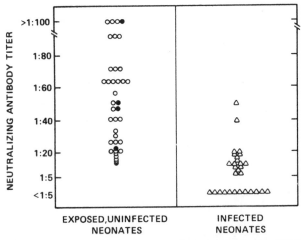

Fig 1–11.—Neutralizing antibody titers in infants exposed to herpes simplex virus (HSV) during vaginal delivery. **Left,** antibody titers in cord blood or blood obtained during the first 2 weeks of life from 33 uninfected exposed neonates whose mothers had a history of genital HSV infection *(open circles)* and from 5 uninfected exposed neonates whose mothers had no history of genital HSV infection *(filled circles).* **Right,** antibody titers in initial blood samples from 29 previously studied infected neonates who had symptoms during the first 2 weeks of life. (Courtesy of Prober, C.G., et al.: N. Engl. J. Med. 316:240–244, Jan. 29, 1987.)

tralizing antibodies to HSV type 2, and 79% had titers above 1:20 (Fig 1–11). In contrast, it was reported previously that HSV-infected neonates were significantly more likely to lack demonstrable antibody to HSV and less likely to have titers above 1:20.

Given the low attack rate, empirical antiviral therapy is not warranted in all infants exposed to HSV infection during vaginal delivery to mothers with recurrent genital HSV. The data suggest that the presence and high titers of neutralizing antibody to HSV may have contributed to the low attack rate in these neonates.

▶ Collection of facts has really challenged some previous dogma regarding the management of the pregnant woman with genital HSV infection. Neonatal infection with HSV is often life threatening and can cause severe brain injury among survivors despite antiviral therapy if therapy is not instituted promptly. In the newborn HSV infection usually results from exposure to the virus in the maternal genital tract at the time of delivery. If a pregnant woman has signs or symptoms of genital HSV at the onset of labor, it has been customary to deliver babies by cesarean section. To reduce neonatal exposure, it had been recommended that asymptomatic excretion of HSV be monitored in pregnant women at high risk for genital herpes by means of repeated cervical cultures beginning between 32 and 36 weeks of gestation so that the results of the culture obtained in the preceding week would be available when labor began. Arvin and co-workers now demonstrate, in the preceding abstract, that antepartum maternal cultures do not predict the infant's risk of exposure to HSV at delivery. Now we learn that infants delivered vaginally from mothers who have had recurrent genital herpes are at low risk of contracting herpes if the mother is asymptomatic at the time of delivery, even if exposure to the virus does occur. All bets are off if a woman is experiencing her first attack of genital HSV around the time of delivery. It still appears prudent to perform a cesarean in such women. Pediatricians are dependent on the obstetrician to alert them to the mother's history and cervical condition at the time of delivery. Any infant born of a mother with a history of herpes should be watched like a hawk. At the first sign of unusual behavior, it seems wise to culture a specimen from the infant and begin acyclovir therapy. Any vesicle is grounds for prompt action. Even though HSV infection is usually acquired at birth, some infants may be born with findings that suggest a prior intrauterine infection. Hutto and associates described 13 babies who had clinical manifestations of intrauterine HSV (*J. Pediatr.* 110:97, 1987). These manifestations included skin lesions and scars at birth (12), chorioretinitis (8), microcephaly (7), hydranencephaly (5), and microphthalmia (2). Virus, HSV-2, was isolated from each of the 13 infants. Four of these women experienced an apparent primary infection during pregnancy, one had a recurrent infection at varying times during pregnancy, and the remainder were asymptomatic. We still have a lot to learn about the best way to deal with herpes in pregnancy. By the way, which of the following does not belong in this grouping: herpes, syphilis, a condominium in Buffalo, and human immunodeficiency virus? (The answer is syphilis—you can get rid of it.).—F.A. Oski, M.D.

Intrauterine Infection With Varicella-Zoster Virus After Maternal Varicella

Sharon G. Paryani and Ann M. Arvin (Stanford Univ.)
N. Engl. J. Med. 314:1542–1546, June 12, 1986   1–11

There is limited information concerning the risks of varicella during pregnancy. A prospective study was conducted to determine the complications of primary and recurrent varicella-zoster infection in pregnant women and to evaluate the infants of these women for clinical and immunologic evidence of intrauterine varicella infection. Forty-three pregnancies complicated by varicella were compared with 14 pregnancies complicated by herpes zoster.

Varicella infection during pregnancy was associated with significant maternal morbidity in nine women and consisted of pneumonia in four (including one who died), premature labor in four, premature delivery in two, and herpes zoster in one. Possible exposure to varicella-zoster virus occurred during the first trimester in 11 infants, in the second trimester in 11, and in the third trimester in 19, including 3 in whom varicella exposure in the mother occurred less than 10 days before delivery. One infant had the congenital varicella syndrome after first-trimester exposure and three others had acute varicella at birth or herpes zoster in infancy after second-trimester or third-trimester exposure. Immunologic evidence of intrauterine varicella infection, as evidenced by immunoglobulin M antibody to varicella-zoster in the neonatal period, persistently high titers of varicella-zoster immunoglobulin G antibody at 1–2 years of age, or in vitro lymphocyte proliferation in response to varicella-zoster virus antigen, was detected in 7 of 33 (21%) patients, including 4 who were asymptomatic. Eight of 33 patients had either clinical or immunologic evidence of congenital varicella infection. In contrast, herpes zoster infection during pregnancy was not associated with serious maternal morbidity or with any evidence of intrauterine varicella infection.

Varicella during pregnancy is associated with maternal morbidity and intrauterine infection. Although its effect in preventing fetal complications remains unknown, the administration of varicella-zoster immune globulin to pregnant women who have no antibody to varicella and who had close exposure to varicella-zoster virus is justified by the significant maternal risk.

▶ This is the same virus family but a different problem. Dr. John Modlin, Associate Professor of Pediatrics, Johns Hopkins University School of Medicine, and member of the Division of Infectious Diseases, comments.—F.A. Oski, M.D.

▶ The study addresses three different, interrelated issues: (1) varicella-zoster virus (VZV) infection in the pregnant woman, (2) intrauterine infection with VZV, and (3) perinatal infection of the newborn infant when maternal varicella occurs late in gestation. Other authors have addressed each of these issues separately in retrospective studies and literature reviews. The study by Paryani and Arvin is the first attempt to examine maternal VZV infection and vertical transmission in a prospective, integrated study.

Based on their data and the data from other studies, it is reasonable to conclude that:

. 1. Pregnant women are at risk of severe, sometimes fatal infection when exposed to varicella. There are no data to prove that pregnancy enhances the already increased morbidity of varicella in adults, but there are good reasons to suspect that it does. Cell-mediated immunity is increasingly suppressed during gestation, and experimental data with other viruses clearly demonstrate that pregnancy enhances the severity of infection. The data presented by Paryani and Arvin make a compelling argument for VZIG immunoprophylaxis of exposed, seronegative pregnant women, but the efficacy of this practice is totally unknown.

2. Intrauterine infection can occur regardless of the stage of gestation, but congenital defects caused by intrauterine infection are rare. The risk of the congenital varicella syndrome following first-trimester maternal infection is about 5% (3 of 61 based on combined data from three studies). Congenital defects have been described with maternal varicella occurring as late as 14–19 weeks of gestation.

3. The risk to the fetus from maternal herpes zoster is unknown. Paryani and Arvin found no evidence of intrauterine VZV infection in 14 infants of mothers with gestational zoster. However, cataracts, microphthalmia, CNS damage, and limb abnormalities have been found in at least two infants whose mothers had zoster during the third and fourth months of pregnancy.

4. The major risk to the newborn occurs when maternal varicella appears during the last 2 weeks of gestation or shortly after delivery. Approximately 25% of infants will contract varicella under these circumstances and about 5% will die. The death rate increases to about 30% when onset of maternal illness occurs within 4 days of delivery, probably because these infants lack passively acquired maternal antibody to VZV. Prophylaxis with VZIG is recommended for infants born to women in whom the rash of varicella develops within the window of 4 days prior to delivery to 2 days afterward. However, efficacy of VZIG administration to perinatally exposed newborn infants is uncertain.—J. Modlin, M.D.

Maternal and Fetal Outcome in Neonatal Lupus Erythematosus
Ann B. McCune, William L. Weston, and Lela A. Lee (Univ. of Colorado)
Ann. Intern. Med. 106:518–523, April 1987   1–12

Neonatal lupus is associated with congenital heart block, which usually is third degree and permanent, but the prognosis for these children and their mothers is largely unknown. Follow-up study was made of 21 mothers and their children with neonatal lupus erythematosus seen from 1975 to 1986. The disease was diagnosed in infants from the dermatologic findings and positivity for anti-SSA/Ro antibody. The average follow-up was 4.5 years.

Ten mothers were symptomatic at the time of delivery of the affected infant. Most of the other women later became symptomatic if followed long enough. Twelve infants had congenital heart block without skin dis-

CLINICAL FINDINGS IN CHILDREN WITH NEONATAL LUPUS
ERYTHEMATOSUS

Child*	Sex	Clinical Findings
1	M	Heart block
2	F	Skin lesions
3	M	Heart block
4	F	Skin lesions
5†	F	Heart block, liver disease
6	M	Skin lesions
7A	F	Skin lesions
7B	F	Skin lesions
8	M	Heart block
9A	F	Heart block
9B	F	Heart block
10	F	Heart block
11	F	Skin lesions, liver disease
12	F	Heart block
13	F	Skin lesions
14	F	Skin lesions
15	F	Heart block, skin lesions
16	M	Heart block
17	M	Heart block
18	F	Skin lesions
19A†	F	Heart block, thrombocytopenia
19B	F	Heart block, skin lesions, thrombocytopenia
20	F	Skin lesions
21†	F	Heart block

*The notations A and B refer to siblings. None of these sibling pairs are twins.
†Deceased.
(Courtesy of McCune, A.B., et al.: Ann. Intern. Med. 106:518–523, April 1987.)

ease (table). Three patients with heart block died of cardiac and liver failure or of congestive heart failure. Liver disease was documented in two infants. Three children died neonatally. All surviving children have been asymptomatic, but five have pacemakers in place. No increased risk of spontaneous abortion was documented in the mothers. Three of 12 live births, however, were of another affected child.

Most mothers of children with neonatal lupus will have symptoms of connective tissue disease at some time. Mortality of these infants is significant in the first months of life, but those who survive despite congenital heart block have a good outlook. Children with skin lesions alone have an excellent prognosis. There is a significant risk of a second affected child.

Anti-SS-A Antibodies and Fetal Outcome in Maternal Systemic Lupus Erythematosus
Rosalind Ramsey-Goldman, David Hom, Jau-Shyong Deng, Gayle Casterline Ziegler, Leslie E. Kahl, Virginia D. Steen, Ronald E. LaPorte, and Thomas A. Medsger, Jr. (Univ. of Pittsburgh)
Arthritis Rheum. 29:1269–1273, October 1986   1–13

The reported fetal wastage among women with systemic lupus erythematosus (SLE) ranges from 33% to 70%, compared with an estimated 20% among normal women. Congenital heart block is a recognized manifestation of the neonatal lupus syndrome, which is associated with the serum autoantibody anti-SS-A. However, it is not known whether other adverse fetal outcomes are also linked to anti-SS-A. Studies were made of the frequency of fetal congenital heart block and of other adverse fetal outcomes in 155 women with SLE with or without anti-SS-A autoantibodies; whether the titer of anti-SS-A is a predictor of congenital heart block and/or other adverse fetal outcomes was assessed. Most of the women were white (75%); 23% were black and 2% were Asian; overall, 47 (30%) had anti-SS-A autoantibodies.

There was no difference in fertility between patients with and without anti-SS-A antibodies. Exclusive of elective abortions and ectopic pregnancies, 44 of 96 pregnancies (46%) in 47 women with anti-SS-A antibodies and 105 of 235 (45%) in 108 women without antibodies resulted in an adverse fetal outcome. There was no difference in adverse fetal outcomes according to race, age at onset or diagnosis of SLE, or history of a previous adverse fetal outcome. However, congenital heart block occurred in 6 of 96 pregnancies in women with anti-SS-A autoantibodies and in only 1 of 235 pregnancies in women without. A fetal outcome other than congenital heart block is not adversely affected by the presence of maternal anti-SS-A autoantibodies.

▶ This pair of articles (1–12 and 1–13) should provide you with a rather accurate picture of the fetal outcome of babies born to mothers with SLE. The neonatal lupus erythematosus syndrome is an uncommon, but probably underdiagnosed, disease. The following conclusions appear justified: The overall mortality of affected infants is significant during the first few months of life, largely as a result of heart failure; children with heart block who survive infancy appear to have a good prognosis, at least during early childhood; infants with manifestations only do very well in infancy and early childhood; the chances of a mother having a second affected baby is as high as 1 in 4. Maternal antibody to cardiolipin appears to be the most sensitive predictor of fetal distress or death (1987 YEAR BOOK, p. 528). For even more on neonatal lupus, please see the 1987 YEAR BOOK, p. 163.—F.A. Oski, M.D.

Hypertension in the First Month of Life

Karen F. Buchi and Richard L. Siegler (Univ. of Utah)
J. Hypertens. 4:525–528, October 1986 1–14

Although much has been written about neonatal renovascular hypertension, little information is available on other types of neonatal hypertension. A review was made of a 10-year experience with neonatal hypertension to determine its incidence, features, causes, and natural history. From the findings, a profile was developed that was intended to distinguish

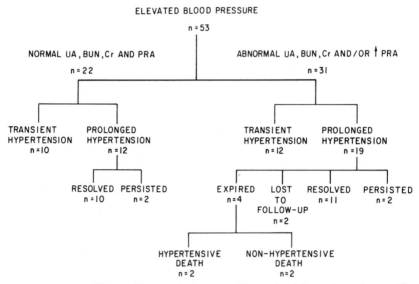

ELEVATED BLOOD PRESSURE

n = 53

NORMAL UA, BUN, Cr AND PRA

n = 22

ABNORMAL UA, BUN, Cr AND/OR ↑ PRA

n = 31

TRANSIENT HYPERTENSION n = 10

PROLONGED HYPERTENSION n = 12

TRANSIENT HYPERTENSION n = 12

PROLONGED HYPERTENSION n = 19

RESOLVED n = 10

PERSISTED n = 2

EXPIRED n = 4

LOST TO FOLLOW-UP n = 2

RESOLVED n = 11

PERSISTED n = 2

HYPERTENSIVE DEATH n = 2

NON-HYPERTENSIVE DEATH n = 2

Fig 1–12.—Natural history of hypertension in groups with normal and abnormal screening tests. The two infants with persistent hypertension and normal screening studies had aortic coarctation. (Courtesy of Buchi, K.F., and Siegler, R.L.: J. Hypertens. 4:525–528, October 1986.)

those neonates who are likely to have an identifiable cause of hypertension and who are therefore candidates for an extensive workup.

Fifty-three newborns admitted to a neonatal tertiary care hospital for treatment of prematurity with respiratory distress syndrome (30), birth asphyxia (5), aspiration syndrome (2), congestive heart failure (2), suspected sepsis (2), and other disorders (12) were found to have elevated blood pressure persisting for at least 72 hours. Hypertension was classified as transient if the newborn was normotensive and not receiving blood pressure medications at discharge from the hospital. Follow-up information was obtained from the child's private physician or from outpatient clinic records.

Causes of hypertension, identified in 23 neonates (43%), included acute tubular necrosis in renal vascular abnormalities in 8, renal structural abnormalities in 4, interstitial nephritis in 2, and coarctation of the aorta in 2. No cause for hypertension could be found in the other 30 infants.

Of the 22 infants (42%) with normal urinalysis (UA) and normal blood urea nitrogen (BUN), serum creatinine (Cr), and plasma renin activity (PRA) values, 2 had coarctation of the aorta, but no cause for hypertension was found in the other 20, all of whom were normotensive by age 30 months. However, of the 31 infants, who had abnormal UA and abnormal BUN, Cr, and PRA values, 21 (68%) had a definite cause for hypertension (Fig 1–12). Further diagnostic studies in hypertensive infants can be postponed if the UA and BUN, Cr, and PRA values are normal, because this type of hypertension appears to resolve spontaneously over time.

► Another pretty pair: If your appetite for the problem of neonatal hypertension was whetted by this one, read on.—F.A. Oski, M.D.

Epidemiology and Management of Severe Symptomatic Neonatal Hypertension

Mary Ellen Leder Skalina, Robert M. Kliegman, and Avroy A. Fanaroff (Case Western Reserve Univ.)
Am. J. Perinatol. 3:235–239, July 1986   1–15

Systemic arterial hypertension among newborns has been reported only sporadically, even though neonatal hypertension and its morbidity have serious implications for neonatal intensive care providers. The incidence, etiology, and outcome of neonatal hypertension and systemic vascular complications were reviewed.

Of 988 newborn infants admitted to the intensive and intermediate care nurseries during a 12-month period, 9 male and 11 female infants (2%)

TABLE 1.—AGE AT ONSET AND MAXIMUM MEAN ARTERIAL PRESSURE OF HYPERTENSIVE INFANTS BY BIRTH WEIGHT

	Birthweight (gm)					
	630–1000	1001–1500	1501–2000	2001–2500	2501–4000	4000
No. of patients	3	1	4	1	8	3
Age at onset (day)						
Mean	42	7	12.2	11	7.4	5
Range	25–52		1–29		1–15	5
Maximum						
Mean	93	100	96	100	95	88
Range	85–105		85–110		75–108	85–95

(Courtesy of Skalina, M.E.L., et al.: Am. J. Perinatal. 3:235–239, July 1986.)

TABLE 2.—DIAGNOSIS AT ADMISSION OF 20 INFANTS WHO BECAME HYPERTENSIVE DURING HOSPITALIZATION

Diagnosis	No. of Patients
Respiratory distress syndrome	7
Asphyxia neonatorum	3
Respiratory distress syndrome and asphyxia	2
Persistent fetal circulation	1
Phrenic nerve palsy (unilateral)	1
Vocal cord paralysis (bilateral)	1
Transposition of the great vessels	1
Multiple congenital anomalies, including coarctation of the aorta	1
Necrotizing enterocolitis	1
Group B streptococcal sepsis	1
Unilateral dysfunctional multicystic kidney	1

(Courtesy of Skalina, M.E.L., et al.: Am. J. Perinatal. 3:235–239, July 1986.)

TABLE 3.—Medications and Dosages Used
in the Treatment of Neonatal
Hypertension

Medication	Dosage
Furosemide (IV, PO)	1 mg/kg/day (1 patient required 2–3 mg/kg/day)
Hydralazine (IV, PO)	Starting: 1–2 mg/kg/day
	Maximum: 7–10 mg/kg/day
Methyldopa (IV, PO)	Starting: 10 mg/kg/day
	Maximum: 40–50 mg/kg/day
Propranolol (IV)	0.025–0.1 mg/kg/day
(PO)	Starting: 0.7–1.0 mg/kg/day
	Maximum: 3–4 mg/kg/day
Diazoxide (IV)	3–5 mg/kg/dose
Nitroprusside (IV)	Starting: 0.5 μg/kg/min
	Maximum: 3.5–4 μg/kg/min

(Courtesy of Skalina, M.E.L., et al.: Am. J. Perinatol. 3:235–239, July 1986.)

had hypertension, defined as a mean arterial blood pressure of more than 70 mm Hg on three separate determinations. Birth weights ranged from 639 gm to 4,600 gm; gestational ages ranged from 25 weeks to 41 weeks, and ages at onset of hypertension ranged from 1 day to 52 days (Table 1). Primary diagnoses at admission included respiratory distress syndrome in seven, asphyxia in three, and other disorders (Table 2). Renal dysfunction occurred in 17 (85%) infants, including increased levels of plasma renin, abnormal renal scintiscans, and evidence of renal vascular embolism or thrombus (13 infants).

Drug treatment with higher than usual doses was required in 18 of 20 infants because of a consistent mean arterial pressure of more than 80 mm Hg. Control of blood pressure elevation was achieved with one medication in only three infants; five required three medications, eight required four medications, and two required five medications before becoming normotensive (Table 3). Hydralazine was used in each of the 15 infants taking multiple drugs and was tolerated without complications. An indwelling umbilical arterial catheter had been inserted in 16 of 20 infants (80%) with the tips in the thoracic aorta rather than in the lumbar aorta; this high incidence rate suggests that the invasive procedure may have contributed to the pathogenesis of neonatal hypertension. The acute and long-term significance of neonatal hypertension is as yet unknown, but continued long-term follow-up is essential to determine future risk for these infants.

▶ Dr. Robert McLean, Associate Professor of Pediatrics, Johns Hopkins University School of Medicine, and Chief, Division of Nephrology, comments.—F.A. Oski, M.D.

▶ It is certainly helpful to find more frequent reports of the evaluation and treatment of prematures and newborns with hypertension. This particular study does employ a relatively unfamiliar definition of hypertension, that is, mean arterial blood pressure (MAP) of more than 70 mm of mercury on three separate determinations. For those of us still addicted to expressing blood pressure as systolic and diastolic blood pressures, it would be convenient to have these values available. Though this study was conducted during the calendar year of 1980, the report highlights the extremely helpful and noninvasive means of evaluating hypertension in this age group, namely, the use of ultrasonographic and radioisotopic studies of kidney function and blood flow.

This investigation included all comers with hypertension into the nursery during a 1-year period whether they were prematures or full-term infants. The overall incidence of hypertension (2%) is within the range that is generally appreciated in the perinatal age group. Not surprisingly, the most common admitting diagnosis was related to pulmonary dysfunction. The specific causes for hypertension were often unproven, but included one infant with aortic stenosis, unilateral multicystic kidney disease in one, and possible hydronephrosis in a second. Thus, only a small percentage of this group of patients had a specific etiology identified. The most pressing question raised by these investigators is how many of their patients experienced renal artery embolism from umbilical artery catheterization. Presently, the use of angiography or detailed ultrasonography may help one to pinpoint such lesions, as well as follow them sequentially (Adelman, R.D.: *Pediatr. Nephrol.* 1:35–41, 1987). The authors emphasize once again the possible role of umbilical artery catheterization in the etiology of hypertension in neonates. Eighty percent of the children in this study did receive an umbilical artery catheterization. In two autopsied patients who had received such catheterizations, there was pathologic evidence of thromboembolism in the kidney. The authors provide an important reason to look at the renal function and urinalysis in the newborn. Eighty-five percent of their patients had renal dysfunction characterized by hematuria, proteinuria, and azotemia. Their clinical findings of retinal abnormalities, including hemorrhages and nicking, is a helpful reminder of the value of using the ophthalmoscope in the newborn nursery.

The question of umbilical artery catheters in the etiology of neonatal hypertension remains an unresolved problem. Studies vary as to where they should be placed, above or below the renal arteries, and the exact role of these catheters in hypertension. These authors emphasize the high coincidence of the use of such catheters in their patients, but, unfortunately, we do not know how often such catheters were used in those patients who did not become hypertensive. Other studies (Friedman, A.L., Hustead, V.A.: *Pediatr. Nephrol.* 1:30–34, 1987) found no difference in a group of patients with hypertension in the use of umbilical artery catheters (although this study was in children in whom hypertension developed after they were discharged from the nursery). It is fair to say that there is strong circumstantial evidence of a role for these catheters in producing embolization and subsequent hypertension. Follow-up studies of the differential sizes of the kidneys and disappearance of the vascular thrombi in a number of studies indicate that thrombi and emboli do occur coincident with the recognition of hypertension. Clearly, catheters must be used with great care, but we should not limit the assessment of hypertension just to those who receive catheters in the newborn nursery.

The medical treatment of hypertension in the nursery requires high doses of the available drugs. Nevertheless, medical therapy is almost always successful and resorting to surgical treatment for hypertension is not the first line of therapy. Even patients with correctable lesions, such as coarctation of the aorta, can be treated. The use of newer drugs, such as angiotensin converting enzyme inhibitors and calcium channel blockers, are now available, though we are still operating with one hand tied behind our back because so many of these drugs are not officially released for use in infants and children.

This study provides a useful look at the problem of hypertension in the nursery and serves to point out the caution necessary in the use of umbilical artery catheters. As to how these infants fare beyond the first year of life, new data (Adelman, R.D.: *Pediatr. Nephrol.* 1:35–41, 1987) suggest that frequently they can be removed from therapy within a year. To what extent these patients contribute to the group of adults with hypertension is yet to be determined.— R.H. McLean, M.D.

Multicentre Trial of Ethamsylate for Prevention of Periventricular Haemorrhage in Very Low Birthweight Infants
John W.T. Benson, Christine Hayward, John P. Osborne, Jane F. Schulte, Mark R. Drayton, John F. Murphy, Janet M. Rennie, Brian D. Speidel, and Richard W.I. Cooke (various hospitals in England and Wales)
Lancet 2:1297–1300, Dec. 6, 1986   1–16

Periventricular hemorrhage, common in early preterm infants, is associated with an increased frequency of later neurodevelopmental disorders. Despite studies on the effect of phenobarbital, ethamsylate, vitamin E, tranexamic acid, and indomethacin, no consensus exists as to the value of drug prophylaxis for periventricular hemorrhage. Ethamsylate has been used for years to limit capillary bleeding in surgery and gynecology patients.

A multicenter, placebo-controlled, double-blind study was carried out at five centers from December 1983 to February 1986 to investigate the effectiveness of ethamsylate in the prevention of periventricular hemorrhage in 330 infants of very low birth weight without evidence of such

TABLE 1.—INCIDENCE AND SEVERITY OF PERIVENTRICULAR HEMORRHAGE IN INFANTS WITHOUT PVH ON INITIAL SCAN

	Ethamsylate group		Placebo group	
Severity of PVH	All infants (n = 162)	Survivors (n = 137)	All infants (n = 168)	Survivors (n = 146)
No PVH	123	108	108	100
PVH				
Grade 1 (subependymal)	9	9	10	9
Grade 2 (intraventricular)	22	16	33	25
Grade 3 (parenchymal)	8	4	17	12
Total PVH	39	29	60	46

Data based on fast-recorded scan grading.
(Courtesy of Benson, J.W.T., et al.: Lancet 2:1297–1300, Dec. 6, 1986.)

TABLE 2.—Infants With Periventricular Hemorrhage
on Initial Scan

—	Ethamsylate group (n = 21)	Placebo group (n = 9)
PVH on initial scan		
Grade 1 (subependymal)	10	5
Grade 2 (intraventricular)	8	4
Grade 4 (parenchymal)	3	0
PVH last scan		
Grade 1 (subependymal)	4	2
Grade 2 (intraventricular)	11 (5 died)	3 (1 died)
Grade 3 (parenchmyal)	6 (2 died)	4 (1 died)

(Courtesy of Benson, J.W.T., et al.: Lancet 2:1297–1300, Dec. 6, 1986.)

TABLE 3.—Change in Periventricular Hemorrhage
Grading From Initial Scan to Last Recorded Scan

—	Ethamsylate group (n = 183)	Placebo group (n = 177)
No change in PVH grade	135	113
Increase in PVH by 1 grade	17	12
Increase in PVH by 2 grades	23	35
Increase in PVH by 3 grades	8	17

(Courtesy of Benson, J.W.T., et al.: Lancet 2:1297–1300, Dec. 6, 1986.)

TABLE 4.—Incidence and Severity of Periventricular
Hemorrhage in Infants Without PVH on the Initial
Scan, Who Also Received Vitamin E

—	Ethamsylate group (n = 42)	Placebo group (n = 38)
No PVH	33	27
PVH grade 1 (subependymal)	1	0
PVH grade 2 (intraventricular)	7 (2 died)	5
PVH grade 3 (parenchymal)	1 (1 died)	6 (1 died)
Total PVH	9	11

(Courtesy of Benson, J.W.T., et al.: Lancet 2:1297–1300, Dec. 6, 1986.)

hemorrhage on initial cranial ultrasound examination. There were 162 infants in the ethamsylate-treated group and 168 given placebo. Thirty additional infants had evidence of periventricular hemorrhage on the initial scan. The dosage given was ethamsylate, 12.5 mg/kg, or placebo, 0.1 ml/kg. The first dose was given intravenously or intramuscularly within an hour of delivery and was followed by 6 hourly doses intravenously for 4 days.

The ethamsylate-treated survivors had fewer total and fewer major hemorrhages than did the control survivors (Table 1). Of the 30 additional infants, 21 were treated with ethamsylate and 9 were given the placebo. There were no parenchymal hemorrhages in the placebo group, but oth-

TABLE 5.—Causes of Death in Infants Dying During
the Study

Cause of death	Ethamsylate group (n = 183)	Placebo group (n = 177)
Persistent fetal circulation	0	1
Subarachnoid/subdural haemorrhage	2	2
Renal failure	1	3
"Extreme prematurity"	4	10
Septicaemia	1	2
Necrotising enterocolitis	2	0
Peritoneal/pulmonary haemorrhage	5	0
Circulatory failure	1	0
Pulmonary interstitial emphysema	3	1
Pneumothorax	5	2
Bronchopulmonary dysplasia	4	0
Respiratory distress syndrome	17	16
Birth asphyxia	1	1
PVH	13	10
Number of neontal deaths	32*(17·5%)	24*(13·6%)

*No necropsy was done on 8 infants in the ethamsylate group or 14 in the
placebo group.
(Courtesy of Benson, J.W.T., et al.: Lancet 2:1297–1300, Dec. 6, 1986.)

erwise the distribution of periventricular hemorrhage on the initial scan was similar in the two groups (Table 2). Further analysis was carried out on the total cohort of 360 infants to eliminate any bias arising from the separate analysis of two unbalanced groups of infants with periventricular hemorrhage on initial scan. The results are shown in Table 3. The difference between the groups in numbers of infants with no change and numbers of infants with an upward change in grading was significant. As to the larger increases in severity (changes in grading by two or more groups), the difference between treatments was highly significant. No infants received phenobarbital prophylactically, but three infants in each group received it for seizures at a later stage. Eighty infants without periventricular hemorrhage on the initial scan, in three units, received vitamin E, 50 mg orally twice daily, for the prophylaxis of retrolental fibroplasia. Although the numbers were small, there were fewer hemorrhages in infants treated with ethamsylate and vitamin E than in those treated with vitamin E and placebo (Table 4); the incidence of intraventricular and parenchymal hemorrhage in infants treated with vitamin E and placebo was similar to that observed in the placebo group for the trial as a whole. Similarly, the incidence of intraventricular and parenchymal hemorrhage in infants treated with vitamin E and ethamsylate (19%) was almost the same as the figure for the total ethamsylate group (18.5%). Within the 14-day study period there was no significant difference in mortality between treatment groups. The causes of death, when known, are given in Table 5.

Ethamsylate therapy reduced the incidence and severity of periventricular hemorrhage in very-low-birth-weight infants when given soon after birth and for 4 days. The effect was seen mainly in those with more extensive grades of hemorrhage, which are more likely to produce later neurologic deficit. Renal failure occurred less frequently in the ethamsylate-treated group. No unwarranted side effects were noted. Ethamsylate prophylaxis in conjunction with improved neonatal intensive care should enhance the outlook for very-low-birth-weight infants.

▶ Ethamsylate (diethylammonium 1,4 dihydroxy-3-benzene sulfonate) is a drug that has been used for years in Europe as a "hemostatic" agent. It has been shown to reduce blood loss during transurethral resection of the prostate and intrauterine device-induced menorrhagia. Two studies using ethamsylate as prophylaxis against neonatal periventricular hemorrhage have been published previously (Morgan, M. E. J., et al.: *Lancet* 2:830, 1981; Cooke, R. W. I., et al.: *Arch. Dis. Child.* 59:82, 1984) and both showed a significant reduction in frequency of hemorrhage. The present study is of much larger size than those previously reported. A small animal study using a beagle puppy model of periventricular hemorrhage also has shown that ethamsylate has prophylactic effects (Ment, L. R., et al.: *Prostaglandins* 27:245, 1984).

How does ethamsylate work? The drug has been shown in vitro to alter platelet aggregation and also to block the synthesis of 6-keto-PGF1$_\alpha$ and thromboxane B$_2$. This suggests inhibition of prostaglandin and thromboxane synthetase. Blocking prostacyclin production could prevent periventricular hemorrhage. Prostacyclin is a potent vasodilating substance and is able to disaggregate platelets. Ethamsylate has been shown to reduce the production of an immunoreactive prostacyclin metabolite in low-birth-weight infants with respiratory distress syndrome (Rennie, J. M., et al.: *Early Hum. Dev.* 14:239, 1986).

What next? I guess another clinical trial is in order. After the trial we will await a verdict from the Food and Drug Administration (FDA). Speaking of the FDA, do you remember Miazga's discovery? Miazga observed that "Death is nature's way of telling you that the Food and Drug Administration was right." The next abstract describes another potential approach to the problem of periventricular hemorrhage in the low-birth-weight infant. We may end up with more treatments than we know what to do with. By the way, intraventricular hemorrhage appears to occur less frequently in the infants of drug-addicted mothers (Cepeda, E. E., et al.: *Acta Paediatr. Scand.* 76:16, 1987).—F.A. Oski, M.D.

Vitamin E Supplementation Reduces Frequency of Periventricular Hemorrhage in Very Preterm Babies
Sunil Sinha, Jacqueline Davies, Nancy Toner, Susan Bogle, and Malcolm Chiswick (St. Mary's Hosp., Manchester, and Univ. of Manchester, England)
Lancet 1:466–471, Feb. 28, 1987   1–17

Evidence of periventricular hemorrhage is obtained in about 40% of infants born at 32 weeks' gestation or earlier, and plasma levels of vitamin E are lower in preterm infants. A randomized trial of vitamin E was carried out in a series of 231 infants born at 32 weeks' gestation or earlier. Three intramuscular doses of vitamin E, 20 mg/kg, were administered within 2 hours of randomization and again after 24 hours and 48 hours.

Supplemented infants had significantly higher mean plasma vitamin E

TABLE 1.—Distribution of Final Grade of Hemorrhage in Supplemented Infants and Controls

No (%)

	No haemorrhage	Subependymal	Intraventricular	Parenchymal
Inborn (n = 145)				
Supplemented (n = 62)	46 (74·2)*	11 (17·7)	4 (6·5)†	1 (1·6)
Control (n = 83)	40 (48·2)	11 (13·3)	29 (34·9)	3 (3·6)
Referred (n = 65)				
Supplemented (n = 40)	25 (62·5)	9 (22·5)	5 (12·5)	1 (2·5)
Control (n = 25)	10 (40·0)	3 (12·0)	8 (32·0)	4 (16·0)
All babies (n = 210)				
Supplemented (n = 102)	71 (69·6)‡	20 (19·6)	9 (8·8)*	2 (2·0)
Control (n = 108)	50 (46·3)	14 (13·0)	37 (34·3)	7 (6·5)

Significance values derived from 2 × 2 chi-square analysis: no hemorrhage vs. all types of hemorrhage; intraventricular vs. subependymal and parenchymal.
*$P < .005$; †$P < .01$; ‡$P < .001$, for differences between supplemented and control groups.
(Courtesy of Sinha, S., et al.: Lancet 1:466–471, Feb. 28, 1987.)

TABLE 2.—Distribution of Hemorrhages on First Abnormal Brain in Infants Whose Initial Scan Was Normal

No (%)

	Subependymal	Intraventricular	Parenchymal	Intraventricular or parenchymal
Supplemented (n = 31)	23 (74·2)*	8 (25·8)	0	8 (25·8)
Control (n = 58)	18 (31·0)	34 (58·6)	6 (10·3)	40 (69·0)

*$P < .001$, 2 × 2 chi-square analysis: subependymal vs. intraventricular and parenchymal.
(Courtesy of Sinha, S., et al.: Lancet 1:466–471, Feb. 28, 1987.)

levels than controls had. The proportion of study infants with abnormal hydrogen peroxide hemolysis tests declined. Excluding 18 infants with initial evidence of hemorrhage on ultrasonography, intraventricular and parenchymal hemorrhage combined was less prevalent in supplemented than in control infants (8% vs. 39%). The difference resulted largely from a much lower rate of intraventricular hemorrhage in the supplemented group (Table 1). Among infants who had hemorrhage after initial study, subependymal hemorrhage predominated in those given vitamin E and intraventricular and parenchymal hemorrhage predominated in control infants (Table 2). Survival rates were similar in the two groups.

Vitamin E may scavenge free radicals generated during ischemic injury in the subependymal region and thereby limit tissue damage as well as the extent of periventricular hemorrhage on reperfusion. The best regimen for vitamin E supplementation remains to be determined, but plasma vitamin E levels are not a reliable indicator of protection.

▶ As was the case for ethamsylate, a plausible explanation also exists for vitamin E in this condition. In this study, vitamin E appeared to be effective in rapidly limiting the extent of subependymal hemorrhage within 24 hours of its occurrence rather than preventing the initial bleed. Vitamin E, a free radical scavenger, is believed to trap the free radicals generated during ischemic injury to the tissues, thus limiting progression of tissue damage. The beagle puppy model has been used to provide support for this hypothesis, just as it did for the ethamsylate theory. The free radical scavenger superoxide dismutase protected against periventricular hemorrhage in pups exposed to hypovolemic hypotension and volume reexpansion (Ment, L. R., et al.: *J. Neurosurg.* 62:563, 1985). If vitamin E is to work it must be given promptly during the first day of life. How to best accomplish this is a problem that requires solution. For more on vitamin E and the premature infant see the 1983 YEAR BOOK, p. 38; the 1985 YEAR BOOK, p. 57; and the 1986 YEAR BOOK, p. 72. Poor vitamin E—it has promised so much. The only thing better than a lie is a true story that nobody will believe.—F.A. Oski, M.D.

Long-Term Follow-Up of Patients With Gastroschisis

Kim R. Swartz, Marvin W. Harrison, John R. Campbell, and Timothy J. Campbell (Oregon Health Sciences Univ., Portland)
Am. J. Surg. 151:546–549, May 1986   1–18

It is assumed that successful surgical reduction and closure of gastroschisis will be followed by normal growth and development. The long-term outcome of repair was examined in 104 patients with gastroschisis initially

TABLE 1.—INITIAL MANAGEMENT OF
GASTROSCHISIS FROM 1969 TO 1983

Procedure	No. Patients	Mortality n	%
Primary closure	54	3	6
Staged silo	40	7	18
Skin flaps	10	2	20
Total	104	12	12

(Courtesy of Swartz, K.R., et al.: Am. J. Surg. 151:546–549, May 1986.)

TABLE 2.—LONG-TERM BOWEL COMPLICATIONS AFTER
GASTROSCHISIS REPAIR, 1967 TO 1983

Condition	Patients (n)	PBR	PBR (n)
No problems	76	9	67
Occasional loose stools	4	3	1
Chronic diarrhea (> 5 bowel movements/day)	4	4	0
Chronic abdominal pain	3	3	0
Blind loop syndrome	1	1	0
Small bowel obstruction requiring exploration	2	2	0
Total	90	22	68

PBR: previous bowel resection.
(Courtesy of Swartz, K.R., et al.: Am. J. Surg. 151:546–549, May 1986.)

TABLE 3.—Average Percentile Values for
Height and Weight

Data	<5 Years		>5 Years	
	Height	Weight	Height	Weight
Patients with bowel resection	37	31	45	35
Patients without bowel resection	29	34	55	62
Total	32	32	51	53

(Courtesy of Swartz, K.R., et al.: Am. J. Surg. 151:546–549, May 1986.)

treated between 1967 and 1983. Ninety survivors were followed for nearly 5 years on average, and 36 of them were observed for longer than 5 years. About one fourth of the infants had associated anomalies that did not preclude operation for gastroschisis. Initial management was usually by primary closure or staged silo reduction (Table 1).

One late death resulted from lead encephalopathy in a patient with uncomplicated primary closure. Most children were doing well at follow-up. Average ranks for height and weight at follow-up were 51% and 53%, respectively. Academic performance was usually satisfactory. A few children had occasional loose stools after ingesting fruit (Table 2). Four children had chronic diarrhea, one because of short gut syndrome. All children with significant complications had undergone small bowel resection during initial management. Growth was slowed in patients who had small bowel resection (Table 3). Twelve children had secondary operations related to initial gastroschisis repair, most often ventral herniorrhaphy.

Children with isolated gastroschisis generally grow and develop normally after age 5 years, after operative repair in infancy, and have no significant bowel sequelae. Infants with bowel atresia or complications necessitating small bowel resection are at increased risk of long-term bowel problems and their growth may be slowed.

▶ Dr. Alex Haller, the Garrett Professor of Pediatric Surgery, Johns Hopkins University School of Medicine, and Surgeon-in-Chief, Johns Hopkins Children's Center, comments.—F.A. Oski, M.D.

▶ Follow-up on 90 patients who survived neonatal gastroschisis repair averages more than 5 years in this important report. During the 16-year period (1967–1983) of operative repair, a strong trend toward primary fascial closure evolved with avoidance of simple closure with skin flaps. A staged repair with a silo type expansion of the abdominal cavity was necessary initially in 40%, followed by delayed secondary closure. Of great interest is the fact that the mortality was greater in the staged group, but the numbers are small and the indication for the silo was usually a smaller baby and a much larger extrusion of abdominal contents; both of these factors contributed to the higher mortality. This series further emphasizes the intestinal dysfunction associated with gastroschisis, because the surviving babies required an average of 26 days before full enteral feedings were tolerated. This fact underlines the early growth failure and specifically focuses on the importance of central or peripheral *hyperalimentation,* which was used in all of the surviving babies. Without such nutritional support the vast majority of these babies would have expired. The prolonged bowel dysfunction further separates gastroschisis babies from those born with an intact omphalocele; in the latter, bowel function is usually normal by 4 or 5 postoperative days because the bowel itself is protected in its amniotic membrane.

Good experimental evidence (Haller, J. A., et al.: *J. Pediatr. Surg.* 9:627, 1974) indicates that the alteration in bowel function results both from changes in muscular function because of edema and inflammation as well as alterations in the intestinal mucosa, including the absence of critical enzymes. These changes result from prolonged exposure of the bowel to the amniotic fluid. The authors indicate that in those instances in which the bowel was reexamined after 5–15 days at the time of secondary removal of the silo and closure of the abdominal wall, the intestine appeared to have recovered significantly from the inflammation and edema with some peristaltic activity. Nevertheless, the fact that enteral feedings could not be reinstituted for an average of 26 days further emphasizes the tremendous damage to the bowel as a result of exposure to the amniotic fluid.

The critical observation that infants born with gastroschisis reach average percentile values for height and weight at 5 years of age is very encouraging and underlines the experience of most pediatric surgeons and pediatricians that a baby born with gastroschisis ultimately has an excellent prognosis. The small subgroup who had intestinal anomalies or extensive damage requiring resection and thus loss of intestinal length did not achieve this normal percentile height and weight. It would be interesting to follow this subgroup who had not achieved average height and weight at 5 years and see if they do so in the ensuing 5–15 years. They should be compared with the unresected gastroschisis children when all have finished their pubertal growth.

It is heartening to see that modern neonatal intensive care, including the life-saving use of intravenous hyperalimentation, has markedly decreased initial mortality from gastroschisis; now, this report adds further optimism to the outcome with normal growth and development in the majority of these babies by the time they reach 5 years of age. The absence of later bowel dysfunction or gastrointestinal complications suggests that the intestine in gastroschisis can eventually recover its full motor and mucosal function after it is returned to its intra-abdominal home.—A. Haller, M.D.

Randomized Controlled Trial of Exogenous Surfactant for the Treatment of Hyaline Membrane Disease

Jonathan D. Gitlin, Roger F. Soll, Richard B. Parad, Jeffrey D. Horbar, Henry A. Feldman, Jerold F. Lucey, and H. William Taeusch (Harvard Univ. and Univ. of Vermont, Burlington)
Pediatrics 79:31–37, January 1987   1–19

Despite improvements in the respiratory care of newborn infants with hyaline membrane disease, the disease continues to be an important cause

TABLE 1.—Respiratory Complications and
Duration of Respiratory Support

	Treated (n = 18)	Control (n = 23)
No. of infants with:		
Pulmonary interstitial emphysema	4	11
Pneumothorax	3*	13
Median duration (survivors only) of		
Days $FiO_2 \geq 0.40$	0.2*	3.0
Days in oxygen	7.0*	16.0
Days to extubation	4.0	11.0

*Significantly different from control group, $P < .05$.
(Courtesy of Gitlin, J.D., et al.: Pediatrics 79:31–37, January 1987.

TABLE 2.—Mortality and Common Morbidities
Associated With Prematurity and Hyaline
Membrane Disease

	Treated (n = 18)	Control (n = 23)
Patent ductus arteriosus		
Requiring indomethacin or surgery	8	9
Requiring surgery	3	6
Intraventricular hemorrhage		
Grade I-IV	9	11
Grade III-IV	6	6
Hydrocephalus	5	5
Necrotizing enterocolitis	2	1
Retinopathy of prematurity	3	4
Bronchopulmonary dysplasia	4	7
Mortality	3	6

There were no significant differences between the treated group and the control group ($P < .50$).
(Courtesy of Gitlin, J.D., et al.: Pediatrics 79:31–37, January 1987.)

of mortality and morbidity in low-birth-weight infants. To determine whether an organic solvent extract of beef lung surfactant (surfactant TA), given in the first 8 hours of life, would reduce the need for ventilatory support and improve oxygenation in infants with severe hyaline membrane disease, a prospective, randomized, unblinded, controlled trial was carried out. Forty-one low-birth-weight infants with the disease received saline or surfactant therapy within the first 8 hours after birth.

Surfactant TA given early in the course of the disease led to prompt and sustained improvement in oxygenation and a decreased need for ventilatory support. Improvement of the arterial/alveolar Po_2 and decreased mean airway pressure in the first 72 hours after therapy were the major effects. The surfactant-treated infants also had fewer pneumothoraces and fewer days in environments of fractional inspiratory oxygen of more than 0.4 mm Hg (Table 1). There were no problems with administration of the surfactant, and there were no significant differences in any complications between the saline-treated and surfactant-treated infants (Table 2). Exogenous surfactant administered early in the course of severe hyaline membrane disease can diminish the amount of respiratory therapy needed by low-birth-weight infants in the first 48 hours after birth.

▶ You were promised "more next year" (1987 YEAR BOOK, p. 43) and here it is. Another double-blind clinical trial of reconstituted bovine surfactant (Surfactant TA) in 30 low-birth-weight infants, 751–1,750 gm, with severe hyaline membrane disease also demonstrated early improvement in oxygenation and ventilation (Raju, T. N. K., et al.: *Lancet* 1:651, 1987). The combined incidence of death and severe bronchopulmonary dysplasia was significantly lower in the surfactant-treated group (3 of 17) than in the placebo-treated group (9 of 13). At the annual meeting of the Society for Pediatric Research it was reported that surfactant therapy did not increase the incidence of patent ductus arteriosus (Horgan, M. J., et al.: *Pediatr. Res.* 21:363A, 1987) and appeared to decrease the incidence of intraventricular hemorrhage in premature infants of less than 30 weeks' gestation (Willinger, S. M., et al.: *Pediatr. Res.* 21:381A, 1987). For more on surfactant therapy see the 1987 YEAR BOOK, pp. 40–43. Most all of the reports are positive, and surfactant therapy should soon become the standard of care for the very small baby.—F.A. Oski, M.D.

Broviac Catheterization in Low Birth Weight Infants: Incidence and Treatment of Associated Complications
H. Farouk Sadiq, Sherin Devaskar, William J. Keenan, and Thomas R. Weber (Cardinal Glennon Children's Hosp., St. Louis)
Crit. Care Med. 15:47–50, January 1987   1–20

The use of central venous catheters for parenteral alimentation in very-low-birth-weight (VLBW) infants is increasing. The pediatric Broviac catheter is commonly used. Earlier studies of these catheters reported an incidence of infectious complications of up to 26% and a rate of thrombotic complications of between 5% and 8%. The VLBW infant appears to be at higher risk for complications associated with Broviac catheters. Forty preterm and eight term infants had 52 Broviac catheters inserted for 1,733 days (Table 1). The mean birth weight of all infants was 1,731 gm. The mean birth weight and gestational age of the preterm infants only were 1,350 gm and 30.2 weeks, respectively. The mean number of catheter days per patient was 35 days.

There were 26 instances of infection and 10 of thrombosis, a complication rate of 1 per 48 catheter days. The infants who experienced complications had a statistically significant lower gestational age and lower birth weight than did infants without complications. Although the infants with complications had catheters inserted earlier, the difference was not significant. There were 26 catheter-associated infections; 69% occurred in the VLBW infants and only 20% in infants with birth weights of more than 1,500 gm. The most common organism isolated was *Staphylococcus epidermidis* (29%) (Table 2). Eighteen of the 26 catheter-associated in-

TABLE 1.—MEAN GESTATIONAL AGE, BIRTH WEIGHT, AGE AT INSERTION, AND DURATION OF CATHETER (± SEM)

	Gestational Age (wk)	Birth Weight (g)	Age at Insertion (days)	Duration Catheter (days)	Total Catheter (days)
All patients (n = 48)	31.8 ± 6.9	1730 ± 158	25 ± 3	33.5 ± 3.9	1733
Preterm (n = 40)	30.2 ± 0.6	1350 ± 109	25 ± 3	34.3 ± 4.4	1507
Patients with complications (n = 19)	30 ± 0.9*	1312 ± 180	20.7 ± 3	40.3 ± 7.7*	946
Patients without complications (n = 29)	33 ± 1.0	2006 ± 220	29.1 ± 4	27.1 ± 3.0	787

*Difference significant ($P < .05$) when compared with group without complications by Fischer's exact test. (Courtesy of Sadiq, H.F., et al.: Crit. Care Med. 15:47–50, January 1987.)

TABLE 2.—ORGANISMS ISOLATED, NUMBER OF SEPTIC EPISODES TREATED WITH ANTIBIOTICS WITHOUT CATHETER REMOVAL, AND NUMBER IN WHICH THIS TREATMENT WAS SUCCESSFUL

Organisms	No. of Isolates	No. Treated without Catheter Removal	No. Successfully Treated
S. epidermidis	8 (2)	6 (2)	5 (2)
S. aureus	8 (1)	6 (1)	3 (1)
C. albicans	4	0	—
E. coli	2	2	2
Enterobacter aeruginosa	2	0	—
Alpha-streptococcus	1	1	1
Group B beta hemolytic streptococcus	1	1	1
Group D streptococcus	1	1	1
Enterococcus	1	1	1
Total	28	18	14

Parentheses indicate number that were methicillin-sensitive.
(Courtesy of Sadiq, H.F., et al.: Crit. Care Med. 15:47–50, January 1987.)

fections were treated with antibiotics without catheter removal, with successful resolution of the infection in 14 instances. *Staphylococcus aureus* infections were the most difficult to eradicate without removal of the catheter. Methicillin-resistant, staphylococcal infections were treated with vancomycin given via the central line. Only two of five methicillin-resistant *S. aureus* infections were treated successfully without catheter removal. In contrast, three of four attempts to treat methicillin-resistant *S. epidermidis* infections were successful. Ten thrombotic episodes occurred in seven infants (Table 3). Infection coincidental with thrombosis was present in only 2 infants. Urokinase infusion was successful in causing thrombolysis in eight of nine thrombotic episodes.

The findings demonstrate a significantly higher rate of septicemia and thrombosis associated with Broviac catheter insertion in VLBW infants compared with more mature infants. These data also indicate that some complications can be managed selectively without sacrificing the venous access.

TABLE 3.—Clinical Presentation and Outcome in Seven Patients With Right Atrial Thrombosis

Patient	Signs/Symptoms	Treatment	Treatment Result	Outcome
1	None	Catheter removed; heparin	Thrombus resolved in 4 wk	Asymptomatic at 18 mo
2	Superior vena cava syndrome	Low dose urokinase (70–500 U/kg·h); catheter removed; heparin	Recurred 12 h after initial response; resolved in 3 wk	Asymptomatic at 27 mo
3	Bradycardia	Urokinase (10,000 U/kg·h for 24 h); heparin after pulmonary embolism	Pulmonary embolism	Died from complications of embolism/septicemia
4	None	Urokinase (1200 U/kg·h for 1 h)	Resolved	Died 3 wk later from RSV infection
5	Bradycardia	Urokinase (1500 U/kg·h for 1 h)	Resolved	Died 6 wk later from bronchopulmonary dysplasia
	Thrombus recurred 6 days later	Urokinase (1500 U/kg·h for 1 h) followed by catheter removal	Resolved	
6	Bradycardia	Urokinase (8000 U/kg·h for 24 h) followed by catheter removal	Resolved	(?) Sudden infant death syndrome 13 mo later
7	Bradycardia	Urokinase (3000 U/kg·h for 1 h); urokinase (3000 U/kg·h for 1 h)	Resolved	Died 3 mo later from respiratory failure

(Courtesy of Sadiq, H.F., et al.: Crit. Care Med. 15:47–50, January 1987.)

▶ We have unleashed a monster and don't know how to control it. I expect to see a wrestling match in the near future with the headline attraction being "Broviac versus Jake the Snake."—F.A. Oski, M.D.

Single-Dose Therapy of Gonococcal Ophthalmia Neonatorum With Ceftriaxone

Marie Laga, Warren Naamara, Robert C. Brunham, Lourdes J. D'Costa, Herbert Nsanze, Peter Piot, Dennis Kunimoto, J.O. Ndinya-Achola, Leslie Slaney, Allan R. Ronald, and Francis A. Plummer (Univ. of Nairobi, Kenya Med. Res. Inst., Nairobi, Nairobi City Commission Special Treatment Clinic, Univ. of Manitoba, Winnipeg, and Inst. of Tropical Medicine, Antwerp)
N. Engl. J. Med. 315:1382–1385, Nov. 27, 1986   1–21

A high incidence of maternal gonococcal infection and the discontinuation of ocular prophylaxis in neonates because of reported silver nitrate-induced chemical conjunctivitis have led to a high prevalence of gonococcal ophthalmia neonatorum in Kenya. A randomized clinical trial was conducted in Nairobi to compare the efficacy of three parenterally administered single-dose regimens in treating gonococcal ophthalmia neonatorum in 122 newborns younger than 28 days of age; all had purulent conjunc-

TABLE 1.—COMPARISON OF EFFICACY OF THREE TREATMENT
REGIMENS

	CEFTRIAXONE	KANAMYCIN PLUS GENTAMICIN	KANAMYC PLUS TETRACYCLINE
Day 0			
No. examined	61	32	29
No. positive for *N. gonorrhoeae*	61	32	29
Mean (±SD) severity score	7.4±1.4	6.5±1.7	6.7±1.3
Day 3			
No. examined	55	26	24
No. positive for *N. gonorrhoeae*	0	1	0
Mean (±SD) severity score	1.3±1.2	1.9±1.4	1.5±1.5
Day 7			
No. examined	46	19	23
No. positive for *N. gonorrhoeae*	0	1	1
Mean (±SD) severity score	0.4±1.0	1.0±1.6	0.5±1.0
Day 14			
No. examined	36	17	19
No. positive for *N. gonorrhoeae*	0	0	0
Mean (±SD) severity score	0.3±1.0	0.3±0.4	0.2±0.5

(Courtesy of Laga, M., et al.: N. Engl. J. Med. 315:1382–1385, Nov. 27, 1986.)

tivitis and positive ocular cultures for *Neisseria gonorrhoeae*. The infants were randomly assigned to treatment with single intramuscular doses of 125 mg of ceftriaxone, or 75 mg of kanamycin followed by topical gentamicin for 7 days, or 75 mg of kanamycin followed by topical tetracycline for 7 days. None of the infants had received ocular prophylaxis at birth, but 26 were treated with topical therapy before enrollment in the study.

Of the 61 infants treated with ceftriaxone, 55 returned for follow-up; all were clinically and microbiologically cured. Of the 32 infants treated with kanamycin and gentamicin, 24 returned and 22 were cured; 2 had persistent gonococcal conjunctivitis. Of the 29 infants treated with kanamycin and tetracycline, 26 returned and 25 were cured; 1 had persistent gonococcal conjunctivitis (Table 1). Of 43 strains tested for plasmid content and antimicrobial susceptibility, 12 (28%) produced β-lactamase (Table 2). Outpatient treatment with a single intramuscular dose of 125 mg of ceftriaxone appears to be effective in treating gonococcal ophthalmia neonatorum in a region with a high prevalence of penicillin-resistant *N. gonorrhoeae*.

Intravenous Immunoglobulin for Prevention of Sepsis in Preterm and Low Birth Weight Infants

Khalid N. Haque, Muzamil H. Zaidi, Shahnaz K. Haque, Hasan Bahakim, Mohsin El-Hazmi, and Mohsin El-Swailam (College of Med., Children's Hosp., and Armed Forces Hosp., Riyadh, Saudi Arabia)
Pediatr. Infect. Dis. 5:622–625, November 1986   1–22

TABLE 2.—Results of Antimicrobial Susceptibility Testing of 43 Strains of *Neisseria gonorrhoeae* That Were Isolated From Patients With Ophthalmia Neonatorum

	Minimal Inhibitory Concentration (μg/ml)*																	
	0.001	0.002	0.004	0.008	0.016	0.03	0.06	0.12	0.25	0.5	1	2	4	8	16	32	64	128
Penicillin							3	3	2	5	6	5	6 (2)	7 (2)	4 (3)	3 (3)	1 (1)	1 (1)
Ceftriaxone	2		10	11	7	7	3	3										
Tetracycline											27	3	13					
Spectinomycin															16	27		
Kanamycin															14	29		

*Figures in parentheses indicate number of penicillinase-producing *N. gonorrhoeae*. (Courtesy of Laga, M., et al.: N. Engl. J. Med. 315:1382–1385, Nov. 27, 1986.)

Newborns, particularly preterm and low-birth-weight infants, are highly susceptible to bacterial infections, especially in developing nations where mortality from infections reportedly is as high as 45%. Polyvalent immunoglobulin concentrates have been used successfully in Europe in the

NUMBER OF INFECTIONS AND CAUSATIVE ORGANISMS IN EACH
GROUP

	n	Blood	Cerebro-spinal Fluid	Stool	Organism
Group A	2 (4)*	2			Escherichia coli
					Escherichia coli
Group B	2 (4)	2			Escherichia coli
					Klebsiella
Control	8 (16)†	5	2	2	Escherichia coli
					Salmonella
					Klebsiella
					Escherichia coli
					Salmonella
					Salmonella
					Escherichia coli
					Serratia
					Salmonella

*Numbers in parentheses, mean.
†$P < .005$.
One infant had more than one positive culture and one infant had *Salmonella* enteritis.
(Courtesy of Haque, K.N., et al.: Pediatr. Infect. Dis. 5:622–625, November 1986.)

treatment of neonatal sepsis. An attempt was made to determine whether prophylactic treatment with polyvalent immunoglobulin soon after birth might reduce the incidence of sepsis in preterm and low-birth-weight infants.

The series included 150 preterm and low-birth-weight infants matched for gestational age, sex, and birth weight. They were divided at random into three groups of 50 neonates each. Group A infants were treated with an infusion of polyvalent immunoglobulin, 120 mg/kg for 10–15 minutes within the first 4 hours after birth; group B infants were treated as group A but received in addition, the same dose of immunoglobulin on the eighth day of life; group C infants served as controls. Blood was drawn for determination of serum levels of immunoglobulin on days 1, 8, and 12.

Two infants in group A (4%) had culture-positive systemic infections as did two (4%) in group B and eight (16%) in the control group (table). No infant in group A or group B died, but two infants with infections in group C died of their infection. No treated infant had any adverse effects from the immunoglobulin infusions, either during the study or at 6-month follow-up. Prophylactic polyvalent immunoglobulin administered intravenously appears to be a valuable new prophylactic measure in low-birth-weight neonates, particularly in developing countries.

▶ I hope neonatologists don't put on their fireman's hat and jump on the intravenous immunoglobulin (IVIG) bandwagon until we have more convincing data regarding its benefit. A sobering note was provided by Kim and Hong at the recent annual meeting of the Society for Pediatric Research (*Pediatr. Res.* 21:417A). These investigators used a rat model to determine the efficacy of IVIG in the treatment of group B streptococcal meningitis in newborn rats. The rat pups treated with penicillin and IVIG did worse than the group receiving penicillin alone. The investigators conclude: "Further studies are needed to completely understand the immunologic and pharmacologic characteristics of intravenous immunoglobulin before accepting IVIG as a possible therapeutic agent for neonatal infection." Amen.—F.A. Oski, M.D.

Seizures and Infarction in Neonates With Persistent Pulmonary Hypertension

Mark S. Scher, Kenneth W. Klesh, Timothy F. Murphy, and Robert Guthrie (Magee-Womens Hosp. and Children's Hosp. of Pittsburgh, and Univ. of Pittsburgh)
Pediatr. Neurol. 2:332–339, December 1986 1–23

Neonates with persistent pulmonary hypertension may experience significant asphyxia with subsequent recurrent episodes of hypoxia. Neonatal

TABLE 1.—CLINICAL PROFILES OF TEN INFANTS WITH PERSISTENT PULMONARY HYPERTENSION

Patient	Gestation (wks)	Birth Weight (kg)	Sex	Fetal Heart Tracing	Scalp, Cord or First ABG pH	Apgar Score (1/5 min)	Peripartum History and Early Clinical Course
1	43	4.7	M	Late decelerations	7.03	1/6	Decreased fetal movement, thick meconium
2	36	3.1	M	Flat baseline, fetal tachycardia	7.16	4/8	Early bilateral pneumothoraces
3	39	3.6	M	Severe bradycardia	—	2/7	Twin B, intubated at 5 hrs, early bilateral pneumothoraces, died at 4 days
4	37	2.2	M	—	7.09	3/5	Maternal Crohn disease, thick meconium, group B strep sepsis, died at 6 days
5	43	3.1	M	Variable decelerations	7.07	5/6	Mid-forceps delivery, intubated at 7 hrs, died at 3 days
6	43	3.5	M	Nonreactive stress test at 42 weeks	6.96	0/4	Meconium-stained
7	43	3.0	M	"Equivocal changes"	—	5/7	Meconium-stained, Pao2 < 50 torr for first 22 hrs before intubation, early bilateral pneumothoraces
8	36	3.3	M	Variable and late decelerations	—	1/5	Increasing respiratory distress, persistent hypoxemia first 24 hrs before intubation
9	43	4.1	M	Loss of baseline variability	7.12	1/3	Pre-eclampsia, meconium-stained, early hypoglycemia
10	41	3.0	M	Late decelerations	7.06	3/6	Thick meconium, early pneumothorax, died at 5 days

(Courtesy of Scher, M.S., et al.: Pediatr. Neurol. 2:332–339, December 1986.)

TABLE 2.—Seizures and Cerebral Infarction in Neonates with Persistent Pulmonary Hypertension

Patient	Clinical Seizures Prior to EEG	EEG Seizures	Response to Antiepileptic Drugs	Cerebral Infarction	Other EEG Findings	Outcome
1	Day 2, buccolingual staring, tonic elbow flexion	Day 2, right temporal-occipital and right central, no clinical	Yes, phenobarbital, phenytoin, diazepam	Right temporal-parietal-occipital hemorrhagic infarction; CT on day 6	Burst-suppression; attenuation right temporal-occipital	SQ at 30 mos
2	None	Day 2, right occipital (paralyzed); SE	No, phenobarbital, diazepam	Biparietal-occipital L>R; CT on day 22	Attenuation right hemisphere	Normal at 12 mos
3	None	None	—	Periventricular leukomalacia	Marked asynchrony	Died on day 4
4	None	Day 2, left temporal-occipital (paralyzed)	Yes, phenobarbital	Sagittal, bitemporal-frontal-occipital and severe cerebral necrosis and edema	Attenuation left hemisphere and midline	Died on day 6
5	Day 3, buccolingual, staring, tonic arm extension	Day 3, right temporal with lingual movements	No, phenobarbital, phenytoin, diazepam	Bitemporal occipital infants, severe cortical necrosis and edema	Isoelectric	Died on day 3
6	Day 2, clonic, hiccups	Day 2, bioccipital, left central (paralyzed); days 4 and 6, same location, no clinical; SE	No, phenobarbital, phenytoin, primidone, diazepam	Bioccipital, left parietal, right frontal, sagittal; CT on day 34	Burst-suppression, marked asynchrony	DD-HL, seizures at 24 mos
7	None	Day 3, bioccipital (paralyzed)	Yes, phenobarbital	Bioccipital; CT on day 19	Poor sleep cycling	Normal at 24 mos
8	None	Day 2, left temporal central occipital (paralyzed); SE	No, phenobarbital, phenytoin, diazepam	Periventricular leukomalacia; Sono on day 4	Bifrontal attenuation	SQ at 24 mos
9	Day 2, buccolingual	Day 2, multifocal seizures inc. left temporal-occipital (paralyzed); SE	No, phenobarbital, phenytoin, diazepam, lorazepam	Bitemporal parietal-occipital; CT on day 15	Left temporal attenuation	SQ at 36 mos
10	None	Days 2-5 left temporal-central occipital (paralyzed); SE	No, phenobarbital, phenytoin, diazepam	Autopsy denied	Attenuation left temporal central	Died on day 5

Abbreviations: CT, computed tomography; DD, developmental delay; HL, hearing loss; SE, status epilepticus; Sono, cranial ultrasound; and SQ, spastic quadriparesis.
(Courtesy of Scher, M.S., et al.: Pediatr. Neurol. 2:332–339, December 1986.)

seizures, often accompanied by cerebral infarction, may occur in the context of perinatal asphyxia. A high incidence of both seizures and cerebral infarction was noted in a group of neonates with persistent pulmonary hypertension.

Of 19 near-term neonates admitted with this diagnosis, 10, all males, had seizures and/or cerebral infarction after moderate to severe peripartum asphyxia that had required aggressive ventilatory care (Table 1). Eight patients had both seizures and infarctions, one patient had seizures, and one had infarction (Table 2). Nine patients had an EEG diagnosis of seizures. Five had status epilepticus despite antiepilepsy drug therapy. Among nine patients with cerebral infarction, the diagnosis in five was made by CT, in one by cranial ultrasound, and in three by neuropathologic examination. No infant had been treated with extracorporeal membrane oxygenation. These findings support a previous study of seizures in patients who required paralysis for ventilatory care and confirm the importance of the neonatal EEG in the diagnosis of seizures in such patients.

▶ Persistent pulmonary hypertension is clearly a serious problem in the newborn. Aggressive treatment, however, may be worse than the underlying disease. Hyperventilation, with the resultant decrease in cerebral blood flow, may cause the complications observed in the present report. Extracorporeal membrane oxygenation (ECMO) has attracted a number of advocates because of very good published results (Bartlett, R. H., et al.: *Pediatrics* 76:479, 1985). However, patients treated with ECMO require unilateral carotid ligation (UCL), and data presented by Schumacher and associates at the recent annual meeting of the Society for Pediatric Research suggest that UCL is not without risk and that hemispheric hypoxic-ischemic injury may result from UCL in infants with severe hypoxemia prior to initiation of ECMO (*Pediatr. Res.* 21:375A). Survival of infants with persistent pulmonary hypertension appears to be improving with more gentle ventilation (Dworetz, A. R., et al.: *Pediatr. Res.* 21:360A). For more on this vexing problem, see Redmond, C. R., et al.: *J. Thorac. Cardiovasc. Surg.* 93:199, 1987, and the 1984 YEAR BOOK, p. 41.—F.A. Oski, M.D.

A Prospective Comparison of Selective and Universal Electronic Fetal Monitoring in 34,995 Pregnancies

Kenneth J. Leveno, F. Gary Cunningham, Sheryl Nelson, Micki Roark, M. Lynne Williams, David Guzick, Sharon Dowling, Charles R. Rosenfeld, and Ann Buckley (Univ. of Texas at Dallas)
N. Engl. J. Med. 315:615–619, Sept. 4, 1986   1–24

Continuous intrapartum electronic monitoring of the fetal heart rate was once used only in complicated pregnancies, but it is now recommended for use in all pregnancies. A study was designed to determine whether perinatal results were improved by monitoring all pregnancies rather than only selected high-risk cases.

Patients were monitored on an alternate-month schedule, so that mon-

TABLE 1.—INDICATIONS FOR PRIMARY CESAREAN
SECTION

INDICATION	STUDY GROUP		P VALUE*
	SELECTIVE MONITORING (N = 17,409)	UNIVERSAL MONITORING (N = 17,586)	
	no. (%) of cases		
Fetal distress†	369 (2.1)	454 (2.6)	<0.01
Labor problems‡	854 (4.9)	848 (4.8)	NS
Breech	297 (1.7)	364 (2.1)	<0.02
Multiple gestation	80 (0.1)	93 (0.1)	NS
Other	177 (1)	174 (1)	NS
Total	1777 (10.2)	1933 (11)	<0.05

*NS; not significant.
†Denotes fetal distress in single fetuses with cephalic presentations.
‡Includes cephalopelvic disproportion, failure to progress, failure of forceps procedure, and failure of induction attempt.
(Courtesy of Leveno, K.J., et al.: (N. Engl. J. Med. 315:615–619, Sept. 4, 1986.)

TABLE 2.—COMPARISON OF PERINATAL MORTALITY DURING
SELECTIVE AND UNIVERSAL MONITORING

CATEGORY	SELECTIVE MONITORING	UNIVERSAL MONITORING	P VALUE*
	no. (rate)		
Total births	17,571	17,759	—
Total stillbirths	186 (10.6/1000)	148 (8.3/1000)	<0.05
Fetuses dead before arrival at labor and delivery unit	161	118	<0.01
Live births	17,385	17,611	—
Neonatal deaths	113 (6.5/1000)	114 (6.5/1000)	NS
Perinatal deaths	299 (17/1000)	262 (14.8/1000)	NS

*NS: not significant.
(Courtesy of Leveno, K.J., et al.: N. Engl. J.Med. 315:615–619, Sept. 4, 1986.)

itoring was performed for all patients (universal) or only for high-risk pregnancies (selective). High-risk pregnancies (37% of all cases) were characterized by the use of oxytocin, dysfunctional or preterm labor, abnormal fetal heart rate, meconium in the amniotic fluid, hypertension or diabetes in the mother, vaginal bleeding, prolonged pregnancy, twins, or breech presentation. Fetuses not monitored electronically were checked by intermittent auscultation with a hand-held Doppler device.

Universal monitoring was associated with an increase in the occurrence of cesarean section because of fetal distress (Table 1). The total numbers of stillbirths and perinatal deaths were equal in the universally and selectively monitored groups (Table 2). Fetal ventilation status did not differ

TABLE 3.—Comparison of Types of Outcome That
Suggested Fetal Asphyxia in Selective-Monitoring
Months and Universal-Monitoring Months

Outcome	Selective Monitoring	Universal Monitoring	P Value*
	no. of cases (% or rate)		
Fetuses alive upon admission to labor and delivery unit	17,410	17,641	—
Fetal deaths in labor and delivery (≥500 g)	25 (1.4/1000)	30 (1.7/1000)	NS
Assisted ventilation of neonate	1259 (7.2%)	1315 (7.5%)	NS
Five-minute Apgar score ≥5	293 (1.7%)	296 (1.7%)	NS
Neonates admitted to intensive care nursery	428 (2.5%)	460 (2.6%)	NS
Neonates with seizures	45 (2.6/1000)	53 (3/1000)	NS

*NS: Not significant.
(Courtesy of Leveno, K.J., et al.: N. Engl. J. Med. 315:615–619, Sept. 4, 1986.)

between groups (Table 3). Electronic fetal monitoring during labor is not useful during all pregnancies, especially those with small risks of perinatal complications.

▶ With all this monitoring, cesarean birth rates have increased from 14.1% in 1979 to 19% in 1984. (You thought it was close to 100%, didn't you?) Fetal distress, or apparent fetal distress, accounted for a larger proportion of primary cesarean deliveries in 1984 (21%) compared with 14% in 1979 (Shiono, P. H., et al.: *JAMA* 257:494, 1987). Despite this increase in the cesarean section rate, the incidence of cerebral palsy has not declined, but malpractice premiums for obstetricians have climbed astronomically. Once obstetricians realize that they are not responsible for most infants with cerebral palsy, the public will find out and stop suing them. First, however, the obstetricians have to show that they themselves believe this by keeping their knives sheathed.— F.A. Oski, M.D.

Effect of Night and Day on Preterm Infants in a Newborn Nursery: Randomised Trial

N.P. Mann, R. Haddow, L. Stokes, S. Goodley, and N. Rutter (City Hosp., Nottingham, England)
Br. Med. J. 293:1265–1267, Nov. 15, 1986   1–25

Some parents of preterm infants believe that the poor sleeping habits of their infants once they are home were learned during the time they spent in the neonatal unit where lights are left on continuously and where no attempt is made to reduce the noise level at any time. A few parents have found that the only way they could get their infant to sleep at night was by switching on bright lights and playing music, mimicking the environ-

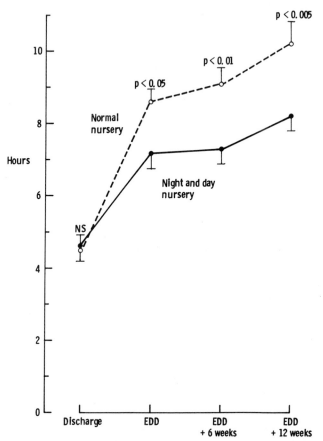

Fig 1–13.—Mean number of hours spent awake in 24 hours in each group. *Open circles* represent infants in control nursery and *filled circles,* infants in night and day nursery. *Bars* represent SE. Differences at each time point compared with Student's *t* test. Analysis of covariance shows an overall difference between groups with time ($P < .001$). (Courtesy of Mann, N.P., et al.: Br. Med. J. 293:1265–1267, Nov. 15, 1986.)

ment the infant was used to in the hospital. A 6-month study was carried out to learn whether exposure to a cyclic day and night environment before discharge would influence the subsequent sleep patterns of preterm infants.

The study included 41 healthy preterm infants who no longer needed care in a neonatal intensive care unit. The infants were randomly assigned to either a control nursery (21), where no attempt was made to control noise levels and where the lights were on around the clock, or to a study nursery (20), where light and noise were reduced between 7 PM and 7 AM. During the day both environments were identical.

After discharge from the hospital it became apparent that infants from the night and day nursery slept an average of 2 hours more per 24 hours than those who had been in the control nursery (Fig 1–13). This extra

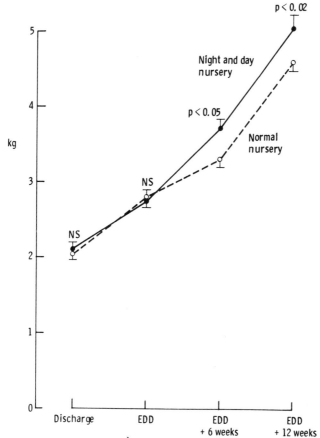

Fig 1–14.—Mean weights of infants in the two groups. *Open circles* represent infants in control nursery and *filled circles,* infants in night and day nursery. *Bars* denote SE. Differences at each time point compared with Student's *t* test. Analysis of covariance shows overall difference between groups with time ($P < .005$). (Courtesy of Mann, N.P., et al.: Br. Med. J. 293:1265–1267, Nov. 15, 1986.)

sleep was not only during the night, but was evenly distributed over the 24-hour period. Both groups had proportionately less sleep by day and more sleep by night with increasing age (table). Infants from the night and day nursery spent an average of 1 hour less each day feeding, but they had significantly greater weight gain than controls after discharge (Fig 1–14). By 3 months after the expected date of delivery, children who had been in the night and day nursery were an average of 0.5 kg heavier than those who had been in the control nursery. It is not in the best long-term interest of children, or of their parents, to leave bright lights on and not to reduce the noise level at night in a newborn nursery.

▶ Is it the light or the noise, or both, that makes the difference? Nurseries, and even hospitals, are run for the convenience of the staff and not the pa-

SLEEP DISTRIBUTION OVER 24 HOURS IN THE TWO GROUPS OF INFANTS (FIGURES ARE NUMBER OF HOURS OF SLEEP)

	Day(7am–7pm)		Night(7pm–7am)	
	Infants in control nursery	Infants in night and day nursery	Infants in control nursery	Infants in night and day nursery
On discharge	9–7	9–5	9–9	10–0
At expected date of delivery	7–5	8–0	8–0	9–0
At expected date of delivery+ six weeks	6–8	8–0	8–4	9–0
At expected date of delivery+ 12 weeks	5–3	6–5	8–6	9–6

(Courtesy of Mann, N.P., et al.: Br. Med. J. 293:1265–1267, Nov. 15, 1986.)

tients. Why can't patients realize that they are not important? Seriously, it would seem advisable, until we make reforms in nursery practices, to provide infants with eye patches and Walkman headsets. The headsets would drown out the noise with soothing music. Why not play them one of the classics such as "Night and Day"?—F.A. Oski, M.D.

2 Infectious Disease and Immunity

Viral and Bacterial Organisms Associated With Acute Pharyngitis in a School-Aged Population
Julia A. McMillan, Cathy Sandstrom, Leonard B. Weiner, Betty A. Forbes, Maureen Woods, Tom Howard, Lillian Poe, Katrine Keller, Robert M. Corwin, and James W. Winkelman (State Univ. of New York at Syracuse)
J. Pediatr. 109:747–752, November 1986   2–1

Relatively little is known of the organisms responsible for nonstreptococcal pharyngitis in children. Throat specimens from children with and without symptoms seen in a private pediatric practice were obtained in a 10-week period in early 1985 and cultured for nonstreptococcal agents. Specimens obtained from 320 patients with sore throat and 308 controls without respiratory complaints were cultured for respiratory viruses, *Mycoplasma pneumoniae*, group A streptococcus, and *Chlamydia trachomatis*. The age range was 4–18 years, and the mean age was 10 years.

Positive culture results were obtained for 60% of the patients and 26% of the controls. Viral isolates were obtained in 16% and 3% of these groups, with influenza A Philippines predominating. Further, 16% of the patients with pharyngitis and 18% of controls had cultures positive for *M. pneumoniae*. Patients with influenza A were significantly more likely to have cough, hoarseness, and abdominal pain than were those with group A streptococcal infection. Pharyngeal exudate and tender cervical adenopathy were more common in patients with group A streptococcal infection.

Means of rapidly diagnosing nonstreptococcal causes of acute pharyngitis may make timely, specific treatment possible. Detection of *M. pneumoniae* may not, however, suffice to diagnose disease caused by this organism. *Chlamydia trachomatis* was not isolated in the present series of children with acute pharyngitis.

▶ There is a great deal of useful clinical information in this study. The agents associated with a pharyngeal infection vary as a function of the time of year, age of the patient, and the population under study. This study confirms the fact that streptococcal pharyngitis cannot be diagnosed with accuracy without laboratory assistance. It has been found previously that febrile patients with a combination of symptoms of sore throat, headache and gastrointestinal tract complaints are culture positive for group A streptococcus 54% to 72% of the time. In this study, patients with streptococcal pharyngitis were significantly more likely to have pharyngeal exudate and tender cervical adenopathy than were patients with influenza A infection. The hooker was, and there is always a hooker when dealing with the diagnosis of pharyngitis, that only 34% of patients in whom cultures for group A streptococcus were positive had a pharyngeal exudate. The combined clinical findings of hoarseness, cough, and absence of pharyngeal exudate or tender cervical adenopathy were significantly associated with a positive culture for influenza A. A practical rule in the winter, if a child is so hoarse that he can't complain about his strep throat, is that it is highly likely that he doesn't have a strep throat but has influenza instead.

Other recent studies have confirmed that neither *C. trachomatis* nor *M. pneumoniae* are very common causes of acute pharyngitis in children or adolescents (Neinstein, L. S., et al.: *Pediatr. Infect. Dis.* 5:660, 1986; Gerber, M. A., et al.: *Diagn. Microbiol. Infect. Dis.* 6:263, 1987). For those who are still puzzling over the best way to diagnose streptococcal pharyngitis in the office, help is available in the review by Radetsky and associates: "Identification of streptococcal pharyngitis in the office laboratory: Reassessment of new technology," in *Pediatr. Infect. Dis. J.* 6:556, 1987).—F.A. Oski, M.D.

Once Daily Therapy for Streptococcal Pharyngitis With Cefadroxil
Michael A. Gerber, Martin F. Randolph, Julie Chanatry, Laura L. Wright, Lisa R. Anderson, and Edward L. Kaplan (Univ. of Connecticut, Farmington, and Univ. of Minnesota)
J. Pediatr 109:531–537, September 1986   2–2

Studies to date have not proved that cephalosporin therapy results in fewer bacteriologic treatment failures than oral penicillin therapy for group A β-hemolytic streptococcal (GABHS) pharyngitis. The efficacy of the oral cephalosporin cefadroxil was examined in a prospective study comparing it with conventional oral penicillin V therapy in patients with findings suggestive of GABHS pharyngitis. A total of 238 consecutive patients entered the study in the winter and spring of 1984 and 1985. Patients were assigned to receive 250 mg of penicillin V three times daily or cefadroxil in a dose of 30 mg/kg daily for 10 days and were reevaluated after 18–24 hours. The two groups were clinically comparable.

BACTERIOLOGIC RESPONSE TO ANTIBIOTIC THERAPY

| | | No. of positive throat cultures* after completion of therapy | | Cumulative no. of positive follow-up throat cultures | | | | | |
	Patients	4-6 Days	14-21 Days	Treatment failures† n	%	New acquisitions‡ n	%	Total n	%
Cefadroxil (once a day)	96	6	5	2 0§	2	9	9	11	11
Penicillin V (three times a day)	99	7	8	6 5§	6	9	9	15	15

*Only first positive culture; repeat positive not included.
†Same serotype as initial isolate.
‡Different serotype from initial isolate.
§Symptomatic.
(Courtesy of Gerber, M.A., et al.: J. Pediatr. 109:531–537, September 1986.)

Two penicillin-treated patients (2%) and no cefadroxil-treated patient had positive throat cultures at follow-up. There were no significant differences in proportions of patients with persistent symptoms. Positive cultures for GABHS were obtained in 12% of the patients followed for up to 3 weeks (table). There were six identifiable treatment failures in the penicillin group, and five of these patients were symptomatic; there were two failures in the cefadroxil group, but neither patient was symptomatic. All patients who subsequently received penicillin V for 10 days remained well during several months of follow-up.

A single daily dose of cefadroxil appears to be as effective as conventional penicillin V therapy in the treatment of GABHS pharyngitis. Treatment once daily with penicillin V is under investigation.

▶ Studies have confirmed that early treatment of streptococcal pharyngitis can reduce the duration of symptoms to less than 24 hours in most cases (1987 YEAR BOOK, pp. 77–80), decrease the incidence of suppurative complications, limit spread of the infection, and reduce the risk of rheumatic fever. Any drug that only requires once a day administration is clearly to be preferred except by those who enjoy taking medicine. Another cephalosporin, cefaclor, is at least as effective as penicillin in the treatment of group A streptococcal pharyngitis (Stillerman, M.: *Pediatr. Infect. Dis.* 5:649, 1986). Stillerman, however, prefers cephalexin over cefaclor because it costs less and the serum sickness-like illness reported with cefaclor therapy has not been seen with cephalexin. The only thing against cefadroxil at the present time is its price—we hope it will fall as the price of the company's stock rises.—F.A. Oski, M.D.

Syndrome of Periodic Fever, Pharyngitis, and Aphthous Stomatitis

Gary S. Marshall, Kathryn M. Edwards, Joseph Butler, and Alexander R. Lawton (Vanderbilt Univ. and Univ. of Alabama at Birmingham)
J. Pediatr. 110:43–46, January 1987   2–3

The term "periodic disease" encompasses a heterogeneous group of disorders of unknown origin characterized by uniform, limited periods of illness that recur regularly for many years in otherwise healthy persons. Several periodic syndromes have been identified as distinct entities with well-defined clinical and laboratory features, including human cyclic neutropenia. A syndrome of periodic fever associated with symptoms that mimic those seen during cyclic neutropenia was identified.

Twelve children had periodic febrile episodes that occurred at intervals of 4–6 weeks over periods of years. These episodes were characterized by abrupt onset of fever, malaise, chills, aphthous stomatitis, pharyngitis, headache, and tender cervical adenopathy (table). The illness resolved spontaneously within 4–5 days. In most children, onset of symptoms was before age 5 years, and the average duration of illness from onset to latest follow-up was 3.9 years. The durations of asymptomatic intervals ranged from 2 weeks to 9 weeks. No seasonal variation was found. Laboratory studies demonstrated only mild leukocytosis and elevation of the eryth-

SIGNS AND SYMPTOMS ASSOCIATED WITH SYNDROME OF PERIODIC FEVER

	Patient											
	1	2	3	4	5	6	7	8	9	10	11	12
Malaise	+	+	+	+	+	+	+	+	+	+	+	+
Chills	+	+	+	+	−	+	+	+	+*	+*	+	−
Stomatitis	+	−	+	−	+	+	−	+	+*	+*	+	+
Pharyngitis	+	+	+*	+	+	+	+	+	+	−	−	−
Headache	+	−	+	+	+	+	+	−	+	+	+	−
Cervical adenopathy	+	+	−	+	+	−	−	+	+	−	+	+
Nausea and vomiting	+	−	+	−	+	−	−	−	+	+	+	−
Abdominal pain	−	−	+	+	+	−	−	−	+	+	+*	−

*Prodromal.

(Courtesy of Marshall, G.S., et al.: J. Pediatr. 110:43–46, January 1987.)

rocyte sedimentation rate during febrile episodes. All children had normal growth and development, and all were asymptomatic between febrile episodes.

All patients had been treated with antibiotics early in the course of their illnesses, but treatment was ineffective. Two patients responded poorly to treatment with nonsteroid anti-inflammatory agents, but three experienced dramatic symptomatic relief when short courses of prednisone were given. Although the cause of this disorder remains obscure, early recognition could reduce unnecessary hospitalization and expensive investigation, because the condition is clinically benign and without long-term sequelae.

▶ This form of periodic disease could drive you periodically crazy. I agree with the authors that it is more common than currently appreciated. It is more common, in all probability, than cyclic neutropenia, which always appears on the differential diagnosis list of any patient with a low white count and in the written examinations of the American Board of Pediatrics. The recurrent aphthous stomatitis in this syndrome is reminiscent of Behçet's disease. Unlike that disease, however, these patients have no genital ulceration, uveitis, arthritis, erythema nodosum, thrombophlebitis, cardiovascular and CNS lesions, or a positive family history. What this current syndrome lacks to make it more readily diagnosable is a name—a name like "cryptogenic cankers."—F.A. Oski, M.D.

Resurgence of Acute Rheumatic Fever in the Intermountain Area of the United States
L. George Veasy, Susan E. Wiedmeier, Garth S. Orsmond, Herbert D. Ruttenberg, Mark M. Boucek, Stephen J. Roth, Vera F. Tait, Joel A. Thompson, Judy A. Daly, Edward L. Kaplan, and Harry R. Hill (Univ. of Utah and Univ. of Minnesota)
N. Engl. J. Med. 316:421–427, Feb. 19, 1987   2–4

The dramatic decline in the incidence of acute rheumatic fever during the past 30 years in the United States may justify the current concept that it has virtually disappeared. However, an outbreak of acute rheumatic

TABLE 1.—DEMOGRAPHIC DATA ON 74
PATIENTS WITH ACUTE RHEUMATIC FEVER

Age: 3–17 yr (mean, 9.7)

Sex: 44 boys (59%), 30 girls (41%)

No. of recurrences: 3 (4%)

Race: 71 whites, 2 Polynesians, 1 Asian

Average family income: $34,000*

Average no. of family members: 6.5†

*In Utah in general, the mean family income is $24,000.
†In Utah in general, the mean number of family members is 3.2.
(Courtesy of Veasy, L.G., et al.: N. Engl. J. Med. 316:421–427, Feb. 19, 1987.)

TABLE 2.—MAJOR MANIFESTATION OF ACUTE
RHEUMATIC FEVER IN 74 PATIENTS

	No. (%) OF PATIENTS
Patients with one major manifestation	
Carditis	17 (23)
Polyarthritis	3 (4)
Sydenham's chorea	4 (5)
Patients with two major manifestations	
Carditis and polyarthritis	31 (42)
Subcutaneous nodules	5 (7)
Erythema marginatum	2 (3)
Carditis and chorea	19 (26)
Subcutaneous nodules	1 (1)

(Courtesy of Veasy, L.G., et al.: N. Engl. J. Med. 316:421–427, Feb. 19, 1987.)

fever occurred recently in the intermountain area centered in Salt Lake City.

From January 1985 to June 1986, 74 children aged 3–17 years (mean, 9.7 years) had acute rheumatic fever based on the modified Jones criteria. The age-adjusted incidence of 18.10 per 100,000 in persons aged 5–17 years old represented an eightfold increase over the average annual incidence of rheumatic fever in this area during the past decade. Only three patients (4%) had recurrence of rheumatic fever. The children were predominantly from white middle class families with above-average incomes and with ready access to medical care (Table 1). Carditis, the most dominant feature of this outbreak, was confirmed by auscultation in 53 patients (72%) (Table 2). In another 14 patients mitral regurgitation was observed on Doppler ultrasound examination, raising the total incidence of carditis to 91%. Syndenham's chorea was a presenting manifestation in 23 patients (31%). Although the patients had typical antibody responses to group A β-hemolytic streptococci when tested, an outbreak of streptococcal disease or other explanations for the marked increase in acute rheumatic fever was not apparent. The only unusual feature was the prevalence of mucoid

M type 18 and M type 3 group A streptococcal strains isolated from several siblings of patients and from school children chosen at random in the area. This outbreak in the intermountain area indicates that acute rheumatic fever remains an important health problem in the United States.

▶ Rheumatic fever is back. An outbreak was also recently described in Columbus, Ohio (Hosier, D. M., et al.: *Am. J. Dis. Child* 141:730, 1987), with 40 patients seen in a period of 2 years. Twenty of the 40 patients had carditis and 5 of these patients were in heart failure. Like the report from Utah, the outbreak in Ohio did not occur primarily in a crowded inner-city area. Is it a change in the virulence of the streptococcus? Is it our failure to recognize streptococcal pharyngitis with the new quick test kits? Or is it some much more mysterious explanation? Buechner's Principle: The simplest explanation is that it doesn't make sense.—F.A. Oski, M.D.

Risk Factors for Development of Bacterial Meningitis Among Children With Occult Bacteremia
Eugene D. Shapiro, Nelson H. Aaron, Ellen R. Wald, and Darleen Chiponis (Yale Univ. and Univ. of Pittsburgh)
J. Pediatr. 109:15–19, July 1986   2–5

Serious focal infections may develop in some children with occult bacteremia. The significance of potential risk factors for the development of bacterial meningitis was evaluated in 310 children (median age, 15 months) with occult bacteremia with *Streptococcus pneumoniae, Hemophilus influenzae* type b, or *Neisseria meningitidis*. The estimates of risk were adjusted for the possible confounding effects of other characteristics by using logistic regression.

Bacterial meningitis subsequently developed in 22 (7%) of the children. Although the odds of bacterial meningitis developing in a child who had a lumbar puncture at the initial visit was 2.1 times that for children who had none, the adjusted relative risk associated with a lumbar puncture at the initial visit was not statistically significant. The type of bacteria causing the bacteremia was the only variable significantly associated with the risk of contracting bacterial meningitis. Occult bacteremia with *N. meningitidis* and *H. influenzae* type b was more likely to be associated with the subsequent development of bacterial meningitis than was occult bacteremia with *S. pneumoniae*. The development of bacterial meningitis in children with occult bacteremia is strongly associated with the species of bacteria that cause the infection, rather than other clinical variables identifiable at the initial visit.

▶ The Task Force on Diagnosis and Management of Meningitis of the American Academy of Pediatrics lists only three reasons for withholding or delaying a lumbar puncture in an infant suspected of having meningitis. They are (1) clinically important cardiorespiratory compromise in a neonate, (2) signs of increased intracranial pressure (papilledema, cranial nerve palsies, hypertension with slow pulse and respiration), and (3) infection in the area to be traversed by the needle [Task Force, AAP: *Pediatrics* 78:(Suppl):959–982, 1986].—F.A. Oski, M.D.

Sequelae of Acute Bacterial Meningitis in Children Treated for Seven Days
T. Jadavji, W.D. Biggar, R. Gold, and C.G. Prober (Hosp. for Sick Children, Toronto, and Univ. of Toronto)
Pediatrics 78:21–25, July 1986   2–6

Treatment of bacterial meningitis for 10–14 days generally is recommended in infants and children, but treatment for 1 week may be adequate. Early and late complications of meningitis were investigated in infants and children with microbiologically confirmed disease who were given antibiotic therapy intravenously for 7 days. An initial dose of ampicillin, 200–400 mg/kg daily, was given along with chloramphenicol, 100 mg/kg daily. Chloramphenicol was withdrawn if the pathogen proved sensitive to ampicillin, and the latter drug was stopped if an ampicillin-resistant strain of *Hemophilus influenzae* was isolated.

Of 235 patients in the study with meningitis caused by *H. influenzae* type b, *Streptococcus pneumoniae*, or *Neisseria meningitidis*, 55 (23%) had taken antibiotics orally before diagnosis. The case fatality rate was 6.4%; it was highest in children with pneumococcal meningitis. Hospital complications included seizures in 5.5% of the patients, motor abnormalities in 3%, and arthritis in 3%. No clinical or bacteriologic relapses occurred in the 220 survivors. Neurologic, developmental, or audiologic abnormalities were found in 20% of the 171 patients followed for at least a year after discharge. Nine patients (5%) had developmental delay.

These results are encouraging, pending a controlled clinical trial in which the duration of treatment is allocated randomly. Shorter treatment is psychologically and economically advantageous, and the incidence of nosocomial infection is reduced. These conclusions do not apply to neonatal meningitis or to meningitis caused by *Listeria monocytogenes*, *Escherichia coli*, or other unusual pathogens.

▶ The following is the current recommendation from the Report of the Task Force on the Diagnosis and Management of Meningitis regarding the duration of antibiotic therapy: "The duration of therapy is based on the causative agent, the clinical response, and the development of complications. In general, a minimum of ten days of therapy is required for meningitis caused by *H. influenzae* or *S. pneumoniae,* 14 to 21 days for that caused by group B streptococci or *L. monocytogenes,* and 21 days for disease caused by gram-negative enteric bacilli. Patients with meningococcal meningitis can usually be treated for seven to ten days." (*Pediatrics* 78(Suppl):973, 1986.)

For another view, please read "Consensus Report: Antimicrobial therapy for bacterial meningitis" (*Pediatr. Infect. Dis. J.* 6:501, 1987). Selected excerpts include the following: "On the basis of recently published studies and of general experience for many years we believe that a 7-day course of therapy is satisfactory for most infants and children with uncomplicated bacterial meningitis (George McCracken)"; "It is my belief that the recommendation that a 7 day course of therapy is satisfactory for most infants and children with uncomplicated meningitis is premature (Sheldon L. Kaplan)"; "We continue to use 10 days of therapy for *H. influenzae* and pneumococcal infections. However, I would agree that a 7-day course of therapy is adequate for most children with uncomplicated bacterial meningitis. . . (Gary Overturf)"; "I am in agreement that the total duration of antimicrobial therapy for *H. influenzae* be reduced to 7 days from previous recommendations of 10 to 14 days . . . . it is not clear whether there has been enough experience with *S. pneumoniae* to recommend therapy shorter than 14 days (Russell W. Steele)". There you have it, folks—I hope this has cleared up your indecision.—F.A. Oski, M.D.

Association Between Preadmission Oral Antibiotic Therapy and Cerebrospinal Fluid Findings and Sequelae Caused by *Haemophilus influenzae* Type b Meningitis
Sheldon L. Kaplan, E. O'Brian Smith, Cathy Wills, and Ralph D. Feigin (Baylor Univ. and Texas Children's Hosp., Houston, and Washington Univ.)
Pediatr. Infect. Dis. 5:626–632, November 1986   2–7

In children with bacterial meningitis who have been pretreated with antibiotics in standard oral doses, the chemical and morphological findings in the CSF are no different from those in children who have received no oral forms of antibiotics. Furthermore, no difference in morbidity or mortality is noted between pretreated and untreated children. Two prospective studies assessed the effect of preadmission antibiotic therapy in children with bacterial meningitis.

The first study included 151 children with a confirmed diagnosis of *Hemophilus influenzae* type b meningitis who were treated with ampicillin or chloramphenicol. The second study included 130 children with the same diagnosis treated with either ampicillin, chloramphenicol, or moxalactam. Of the 281 children studied, 187 (67%) had not received antibiotic treatment prior to admission.

Prior antibiotic therapy was associated with statistically significant decreases in the percentage of polymorphonuclear leukocytes in the CSF, protein concentrations, and the proportions of patients with positive CSF Gram stains and bacterial cultures when compared with findings in untreated children (Tables 1 and 2). However, even though these differences were statistically significant, the actual differences were minor. The duration of illness preceding admission was significantly longer in pretreated than in untreated children and was associated significantly with neurologic sequelae (Tables 3, 4, and 5, pp. 72 and 73). Administration of an antibiotic orally prior to hospital admission does not alter CSF findings in most patients with *H. influenzae* type b meningitis to such an extent that confirmation of the diagnosis would be precluded.

TABLE 1.—FINDINGS IN CSF AT ADMISSION IN CHILDREN WITH *HEMOPHILUS INFLUENZAE* TYPE B MENINGITIS

CSF Variable	Prior Antibiotics		Unadjusted* P value	Adjusted P value †		
	No	Yes		Age	Days ill preceding admission	Age and days ill preceding admission
Total white blood cells/mm³	3731‡ (1488, 6635)§ n = 186	2524 (1313, 5087) n = 92	0.13			
% of PMN	95 (87, 98) n = 181	90 (80, 98) n = 92	0.03	0.09	>0.90	>0.90
Protein (mg/dl)	191 (111, 271) n = 186	115 (60, 233) n = 94	<0.001	<0.001	<0.001	<0.001
Glucose (mg/dl)	29 (10, 49) n = 185	23 (5, 46) n = 94	0.28			
CSF:blood glucose ratio	25 (11, 41) n = 175	22 (6, 42) n = 90	0.51			
Gram stain-positive (%)	90.3 n = 186	81.9 n = 94	0.05	0.05	0.26	0.26
Culture-positive (%)	98.4 n = 187	93.6 n = 94	0.03	0.03	0.09	0.05
CIE-positive (%)	87.5 n = 176	87.6 n = 89	>0.90			
Quantitative CIE (μg/ml)	0.16 (0.04, 1.28) n = 167	0.16 (0.2, 1.28) n = 83	0.72			

Untreated versus pretreated children.

*Mann-Whitney test of medians or chi-square analysis of proportions.

†Analysis of covariance of log transformed data for continuous variables of logistic regression analysis for dichotomous variables.

‡Median value.

§Numbers in parentheses are 25th, 75th percentile values.

(Courtesy of Kaplan, S.L., et al.: Pediatr. Infect. Dis. 5:626–632, November 1986.)

TABLE 2.—LABORATORY FINDINGS FOR CHILDREN WITH *HEMOPHILUS INFLUENZAE* TYPE B MENINGITIS AND NEGATIVE CULTURES OF CSF

Age (Months)	Prior Antibiotic Therapy	CSF White Blood Cell Count/ mm³	% of PMN	CSF Glucose Concentration (mg/dl)	CSF Protein Concentration (mg/dl)	Gram Stain	CIE	Latex Agglutination	Blood Culture
4	Ampicillin	12,000	90	99	162	−	−*	ND	−
4	Ampicillin	900	46	45	68	−	+	ND	ND
5	Ampicillin	485	71	65	25	−	+	+	−
5	Ampicillin	10,800	74	62	94	−	+	ND	−
7	Ampicillin	21,000	100	19	183	+	+	ND	−
14	Ampicillin	5,700	90	20	193	+	−	+	−
17	None	100	0	81	25	ND	ND	ND	+
34	Chloramphenicol	2,730	87	67	79	−	+	ND	−
168	None	1,128	97	75	51	+	+	ND	ND

ND, not done.

*Blood specimen positive at countercurrent immunoelectrophoresis (CIE) testing.

(Courtesy of Kaplan, S.L., et al.: Pediatr. Infect. Dis. 5:626–632, November 1986.)

TABLE 3.—ASSOCIATION BETWEEN SELECTED NEUROLOGIC SEQUELAE AND ADMINISTRATION OF ORAL ANTIBIOTICS PRIOR TO ADMISSION OF CHILD WITH *HEMOPHILUS INFLUENZAE* TYPE B MENINGITIS

| Outcome Variable | Prior Antibiotics (%) | | Unadjusted* *P* value | Adjusted *P* Value† | | |
	No	Yes		Age	Days ill preceding admission	Age and days ill preceding admission
Death	3.7 n = 187	2.1 n = 94	0.37			
Paresis at discharge	5.1 n = 175	11.4 n = 88	0.07	0.08	0.24	0.25
Paresis sometime at follow-up	1.2 n = 168	6.8 n = 88	0.02	0.03	0.07	0.06
Hearing loss	3.6 n = 165	10.6 n = 85	0.03	0.03	0.09	0.08
Psychometric testing, 2-year follow-up (% CA > MA)	27.9 n = 104	36.9 n = 65	0.31			

CA > MA, chronologic age greater than mental age.
*Chi-square analysis of proportions.
†Analysis of covariance of log transformed data for continuous variables or logistic regression analysis for dichotomous variables.
(Courtesy of Kaplan, S.L., et al.: Pediatr. Infect. Dis. 5:626–632, November 1986.)

Hemophilus influenzae Type b Disease in Children Vaccinated With Type b Polysaccharide Vaccine

Dan M. Granoff, Penelope G. Shackelford, Brian K. Suarez, Moon H. Nahm, K. Lynn Cates, Trudy V. Murphy, Raymond Karasic, Michael T. Osterholm, Janardan P. Pandey, Robert S. Daum, and the Collaborative Group (Washington Univ., Minnesota Dept. of Health, Minneapolis, and other universities in the United States)
N. Engl. J. Med. 315:1584–1590, Dec. 18, 1986   2–8

Hemophilus influenzae type b polysaccharide vaccine was licensed in the United States in 1985. Because the vaccine is not 100% effective,

TABLE 4.—ASSOCIATION BETWEEN SELECTED NEUROLOGIC SEQUELAE AND ADMINISTRATION OF EFFECTIVE ANTIBIOTICS PRIOR TO ADMISSION OF CHILDREN WITH *HEMOPHILUS INFLUENZAE* TYPE B MENINGITIS

| Outcome Variable | Prior Effective Antibiotic (%) | | Unadjusted* *P* Value | Adjusted *P* Value† | | |
	No	Yes		Age	Days ill preceding admission	Age and days ill preceding admission
Paresis at discharge	5.5 n = 200	13.3 n = 60	0.04	0.06	0.15	0.16
Paresis at follow-up	2.0 n = 195	7.0 n = 57	0.08	0.10	0.19	0.22
Hearing loss	4.8 n = 188	10.2 n = 59	0.12			
Psychometric testing, 2-year follow-up (% CA > MA)	27.4 n = 124	42.9 n = 42	0.07	0.08	0.05	0.05
Death	4.2 n = 216	0.0 n = 61	0.10			

CA > MA, chronologic age greater than mental age.
*Chi-square analysis of proportions.
†Analysis of covariance of log transformed data for continuous variables or logistic regression analysis.
(Courtesy of Kaplan, S.L., et al.: Pediatr. Infect. Dis. 5:626–632, November 1986.)

TABLE 5.—DURATION OF ILLNESS AND FEVER BEFORE ADMISSION FOR CHILDREN WITH AND WITHOUT SELECTED NEUROLOGIC SEQUELAE CAUSED BY *HEMOPHILUS INFLUENZAE* TYPE B MENINGITIS

Sequelae	No. of Days Ill with or without Sequelae			No. of Days with Fever with or without Sequelae		
	No	Yes	$P*$	No	Yes	P
Paresis at admission	1.50† (1.0, 3.0)‡ $n = 246$	2.0 (1.0, 4.0) $n = 28$	0.09	1.0 (1.0, 2.0) $n = 246$	1.0 (0.7, 4.0) $n = 28$	0.26
Paresis at discharge	2.0 (1.0, 3.0) $n = 244$	3.0 (1.0, 6.0) $n = 19$	0.06	1.0 (1.0, 2.0) $n = 244$	2.0 (1.0, 6.0) $n = 19$	0.05
Paresis at follow-up	2.0 (1.0, 3.0) $n = 248$	4.0 (1.5, 6.0) $n = 18$	0.05	1.0 (1.0, 2.0) $n = 248$	4.0 (1.5, 6.0) $n = 18$	0.01
Hearing loss	1.50 (1.0, 3.0) $n = 235$	3.0 (2.0, 4.0) $n = 15$	0.01	1.0 (1.0, 2.5) $n = 235$	2.0 (2.0, 4.0) $n = 15$	0.002
Early psychometrics (CA > MA)	1.5 (1.0, 3.0) $n = 179$	2.0 (1.0, 4.0) $n = 67$	0.02	1.0 (1.0, 2.0) $n = 179$	1.0 (1.0, 4.0) $n = 67$	0.15
Psychometric testing, 2-year follow-up (CA > MA)	2.0 (1.0, 3.75) $n = 116$	2.0 (1.0, 4.0) $n = 53$	0.64	1.0 (0.75, 2.37) $n = 116$	1.0 (1.0, 3.5) $n = 53$	0.23

CA > MA, chronologic age greater than mental age.
*Mann-Whitney test.
†Median values are shown.
‡Numbers in parentheses are 25th and 75th percentiles.
(Courtesy of Kaplan, S.L., et al.: Pediatr. Infect. Dis. 5:626–632, November 1986.)

vaccine failures are to be expected. The most likely reason for development of *H. influenzae* type b disease in a vaccinated child is an inadequate serum antibody response to immunization. However, the exact cause of these vaccination failures has not been investigated. Studies were made in 55 children aged 18–47 months who contracted *H. influenzae* type b disease at least 3 weeks after vaccination with type b polysaccharide vaccine; 25 children of similar age with the disease who had never been vaccinated served as nonimmunized controls. Meningitis was diagnosed in 39 patients (71%), of whom 3 died and 6 had moderate to severe neurologic sequelae. Serum samples were available for 46 of the 55 vaccinated children.

The geometric mean concentration of antibody to type b polysaccharide in convalescent-phase serum from 31 vaccinated children with *Hemophilus* disease was significantly lower than that in serum from the 25 controls. However, only 3 of 46 patients had hypogammaglobulinemia. None of the 33 children tested had low IgG2 serum concentrations. Only 1 of 46 patients tested for IgG antibody to tetanus toxoid protein and only 1 of 20 tested for hemolytic complement activity had abnormal findings (table). Vaccine failure may be related in part to genetic factors. Most vaccinated children who contract *H. influenzae* type b disease have deficient antibody responses to the type b polysaccharide despite normal serum immunoglobulin concentrations and normal antibody responses to tetanus toxoid.

▶ It is now apparent that a child is at increased risk of contracting *H. influenzae* disease during the first several weeks after vaccination with the capsular vac-

SERUM CONCENTRATIONS OF IgG2, TETANUS TOXOID
ANTIBODY, AND *H. INFLUENZAE* TYPE b POLYSACCHARIDE
ANTIBODY IN CHILDREN WITH INVASIVE *HEMOPHILUS*
DISEASE*

	VACCINE-FAILURE GROUP		CONTROL GROUP
IgG2 (μg/ml)			
Subjects tested	33		24
Log$_{10}$ concentration	3.05±0.18	$P = NS$†	3.08±0.16
(geometric mean)	(1122)		(1202)
Tetanus IgG titer (IU/ml)			
Subjects tested	46		24
Log$_{10}$ concentration	0.53±0.09	$P = 0.052$‡	0.22±0.13
(geometric mean)	(3.4)		(1.7)
Type b antibody (μg/ml)			
Acute phase			
Subjects tested	26		17
Log$_{10}$ concentration	−0.71±0.15	$P = NS$†	−0.40±0.18
(geometric mean)	(0.19)		(0.40)
Convalescent phase			
Subjects tested	31		25
Log$_{10}$ concentration	−0.23±0.13§	$P = 0.0002$¶	0.54±0.14§
(geometric mean)	(0.59)		(3.46)

*Plus-minus values are means ± SEM.
†$P > .10$ (not significant) by analysis of covariance, with age as covariate.
‡By t test (age was not a significant covariate).
§Significantly increased from acute-phase concentrations ($P < .03$ by paired t test).
¶By analysis of covariance, with age as covariate.
(Courtesy of Granoff, D.M., et al.: N. Engl. J. Med. 315:1584–1590, Dec. 18, 1986.)

cine. Sood and co-workers presented similar data for infant rats at the annual meeting of the Society for Pediatric Research (*Pediatr. Res.* 21:335 A) and concluded that vaccination with the capsular polysaccharide vaccine may transiently reduce the anticapsular antibody concentration in the patient and thus produce a "window" of susceptibility in the early postvaccination period. Forewarned is forearmed.

The current vaccine is obviously not the final answer to our prayers. A prospective surveillance study for invasive *H. influenzae* type b disease in Texas and Minnesota revealed that the number of episodes of meningitis among children aged 24–59 months that were potentially preventable by an effective vaccine given at age 2 years was 15% in Minnesota and 11% in Texas. The remainder of the infections occurred at an earlier age. The authors calculate that the cost of vaccinating all 24-month-olds in the two regions would have been 2.4 times more than the estimated short-term and long-term costs of the disease (Murphy, T.V., et al.: *Pediatrics* 79:173, 1987). Prospects are good for a vaccine that will be immunogenic for young infants (Einhorn, M.S., et al.: *Lancet* 2:299, 1986).—F.A. Oski, M.D.

Comparative Efficacy of Ceftazidime Vs. Carbenicillin and Amikacin for Treatment of Neonatal Septicemia

Carla M. Odio, M.A. Umana, Alberto Saenz, Jose L. Salas, and George H.

McCracken, Jr. (Hospital Nacional de Ninõs, San Jose, Costa Rica, and Univ. of Texas at Dallas)
Pediatr. Infect. Dis. J. 6:371–377, April 1987   2–9

Ceftazidime is a new cephalosporin active against many of the pathogens causing neonatal sepsis, including group B streptococci, *Escherichia coli,* and other gram-negative bacilli including *Pseudomonas aeruginosa.* Conventional treatment was with intravenous age-related doses of amikacin and carbenicillin. Study patients received ceftazidime, 50 mg/kg, intravenously every 12 hours in the first week of life and then every 8 hours. Thirty-four of 69 ceftazidime-treated patients had documented infections, as did 32 of the 71 patients treated with amikacin and carbenicillin.

Six percent of the evaluable ceftazidime-treated patients and 21% of controls with documented infection died of sepsis. Treatment failures, including deaths, were significantly more frequent in the control group. Superinfections developed in five ceftazidime-treated patients and in one control. Relapse occurred in one patient in the ceftazidime group. No adverse clinical effects were noted, and transient biochemical and hematologic abnormalities were similarly frequent in the two treatment groups.

Ceftazidime may have been more effective than amikacin/carbenicillin therapy in high-risk neonates with gram-negative bacillary sepsis in this study. The effect was most evident in those with *Pseudomonas* sepsis. Ceftazidime should be considered, alone or combined with an aminoglycoside, when neonatal septicemia or meningitis frequently is caused by gram-negative enteric bacilli or *P. aeruginosa* resistant to conventional agents.

Natural Course of the Human Bite Wound: Incidence of Infection and Complications in 434 Bites and 803 Lacerations in the Same Group of Patients
Douglas Lindsey, Michael Christopher, Julene Hollenbach, James H. Boyd, and Wally E. Lindsey (Univ. of Arizona and Arizona Training Program, Coolidge)
J. Trauma 27:45–48, January 1987   2–10

Human bite wounds are frequent among some residential groups living in institutions for the developmentally disabled. The course and outcome were studied in a series of 434 bite wounds and 803 lacerations that occurred at a state training facility for persons disabled by developmental

TABLE 1.—INCIDENCE OF INFECTION

	Totals	Infected
Human bites	434	77/434 (17.7%)
Lacerations	803	108/803 (13.4%)

(Courtesy of Lindsey, D., et al.: J. Trauma 27:45–48, January 1987.)

TABLE 2.—PROPHYLACTIC ADMINISTRATION OF ANTIBIOTICS

	Instances	Proportion of Wounds	Subsequent Infection
Human bites	61	61/434 (14.0%)	18/61 (29.5%)
Lacerations	26	26/803 (3.2%)	9/26 (34.6%)

(Courtesy of Lindsey, D., et al.: J. Trauma 27:45–48, January 1987.)

TABLE 3.—THERAPEUTIC ADMINISTRATION OF ANTIBIOTICS

	Instances	Proportion of Wounds
Human bites	20	20/434 (4.6%)
Lacerations	18	18/803 (2.2%)

(Courtesy of Lindsey, D., et al.: J. Trauma 27:45–48, January 1987.)

abnormality or delay. Clients lived in small units designed to compensate maximally for limitations and allow maximum expression of capabilities for those with similar patterns of disability.

Infection developed in 13% of lacerations and in 18% of bite wounds (Table 1). No bite wound was débrided or treated operatively other than by closure, and none of these patients was admitted to the hospital. None received intravenous treatment with antibiotics, but antibiotics were used both prophylactically and therapeutically (Tables 2 and 3). No bite wound complications were recorded other than immediate loss of tissue. Proportions of definitely not affected (DNI), no observed infection (NOI), and presumptively not infected (PNI) are given in Table 4. About one fourth of the bite wounds of the hand were infected (Table 5).

Some human bite wounds become infected, but the findings of this study do not strongly support routine antimicrobial prophylaxis or aggressive surgical intervention. Prophylaxis was not highly successful in either bite wounds or lacerations in this series. The degree of increased risk of infection warrants only close observation and the oral administration of antibiotics should signs of infection develop.

▶ Two conclusions can be drawn from this study: (1) Don't bite the hand that feeds you, and (2) don't expect prophylactic antibiotics to be effective in the treatment of human bites.—F.A. Oski, M.D.

Gowers' Sign in Discitis in Childhood
Naomi Amir, Haggit Hurvitz, Isabelle Korn-Lubetzki, and Ruth S. Shalev (Bikur Cholim Hosp., Jerusalem)
Clin. Pediatr. 25:459–461, September 1986   2–11

TABLE 4.—CLASSIFICATION OF UNINFECTED WOUNDS

	Totals	Not Infected	DNI	NOI	PNI
Human bites	434	357/434	127/357 (35.6%)	45/357 (12.6%)	185/357 (51.8%)
Lacerations	803	695/803	232/695 (33.4%)	31/695 (4.4%)	432/695 (62.2%)

(Courtesy of Lindsey, D., et al.: J. Trauma 27:45–48, January 1987.)

TABLE 5.—WOUNDS OF THE HAND

	Totals	Infected
Human bites	123	33/123 (26.8%)
Lacerations	63	18/63 (28.6%)

(Courtesy of Lindsey, D., et al.: J. Trauma 27:45–48, January 1987.)

Sudden refusal to walk or a change in gait may be the presenting symptom of several diseases. Usually, when spinal or vertebral disease is suspected, survey films are made and myelography is performed. If these yield normal results, then attention is directed elsewhere. In diskitis, radiologic findings are not visualized on survey films until 4–8 weeks after onset of symptoms. However, the technetium bone scan is virtually always abnormal after 7 days of illness.

Girl, aged 2½ years, was referred for evaluation of suspected muscular dystrophy. She had refused to stand or walk for the past month. She was uncooperative and irritable. When sitting, she supported herself on extended arms, and when forced to rise from the supine position, she raised herself to a standing position by using Gowers' maneuver, flexing her legs and pushing her trunk upward by moving her hands up her thighs. Lumbosacral films, obtained 3½ weeks after onset of symptoms, indicated a narrowing of the L3–L4 interspace, with blurring and sawtoothing of the vertebral margins. A technetium bone scan revealed frank uptake at L3. Symptoms improved over several weeks without antibiotic or orthopedic treatment.

Two other children also displayed Gowers' sign and had no muscle weakness. Increased awareness of this disease and the possible significance of Gowers' maneuver as a sign of disk involvement allow early, noninvasive diagnosis and may prevent the need for traumatic procedures.

▶ Dr. Edward M. Sills, Associate Professor of Pediatrics, and Director, Division of Rheumatology, Johns Hopkins University School of Medicine, comments.—F.A. Oski, M.D.

▶ Diskitis is a poorly understood, empirically treated disorder of uncertain etiology. The most important clinical findings are related to local back pain, refusal to walk and/or sit, and disk space narrowing on x-ray study 3–4 weeks into the course. The patient is typically quite irritable when disturbed, but does not exhibit signs of systemic illness. There are multiple theories of pathogenesis, none of which entirely explains the observed phenomena. The clinical course and imaging evidence most reasonably suggest that diskitis is caused by vascular disruptions in epiphyseal endplates of (usually lumbar) vertebrae. Intervertebral disks are nurtured via vascular channels that connect between the vertebral ossification centers and the annulus fibrosus of the intervertebral disks. The natural course includes areas of bony destruction and avascular necrotic change in the disk. The bone ultimately reconstitutes completely, but the disk is left deformed and narrowed. There is insufficient evidence to support an infectious etiology. Therapy is directed toward symptom relief. The type and duration of intervention does not appear to affect the ultimate outcome in this disorder. The long-term prognosis is benign.

The predominant complaint in the child with diskitis correlates with age. Gait refusal is a striking feature in children under age 3 years, whereas there is no difficulty with walking in children older than 5 years. Abdominal pain, on the other hand, is more often the complaint in the child more than 3 years of age and is associated with hamstring muscle tenderness. These children are frequently subjected to intravenous pyelography and/or barium study of the bowel before the diagnosis of diskitis is made. Back pain is seen at all ages, usually having been present for about a month before diagnosis. In the younger child there is often abnormal posturing associated with the pain. The pain is often associated with a positive Gowers' sign without demonstrable muscle weakness, neurologic deficit, or abnormal elevation of muscle enzymes activity.

Back pain is always a significant complaint in any child. Tumor and infection must be excluded. The technetium bone scan is useful for localization. Vertebral osseous tumors usually appear as abnormalities or plain radiographs by the time pain is perceived. Signs of inflammatory stimulus, including elevated neutrophil counts, a high erythrocyte sedimentation rate, fever above 39 C, and other evidence of systemic illness should evoke suspicion of infection and lead to other investigations such as gallium scanning, blood and local tissue cultures, tuberculin testing, and the early introduction of systemic antibiotics.—E.M. Sills, M.D.

Chronic Recurrent Multifocal Osteomyelitis: A Distinct Clinical Entity
James G. Gamble and Lawrence A. Rinsky (Stanford Univ.)
J. Pediatr. Orthop. 6:579–584, September–October 1986   2–12

Chronic recurrent multifocal osteomyelitis (CRMO) is characterized by recurrent, unpredictable exacerbations and remissions that can last for several months to several years. Its etiology remains unknown and differentiation from subacute bacterial osteomyelitis is difficult. A review was made of data on 5 new patients with CRMO and findings were compared with those in 11 patients who had subacute osteomyelitis. The literature on earlier reported patients also was reviewed (Table 1).

The study included three girls and two boys aged 4–13 years with CRMO and four girls and seven boys aged 15 months to 14 years who

TABLE 1.—Distribution and Frequency
of 181 Lesions in 35 Patients

Bone	No. of lesions
Tibia	51
Clavicle	24
Fibula	18
Spine	18
Femur	16
Radius	10
Metatarsal	8
Pelvis	7
Humerus	6
Metacarpal	6
Ulna	6
Sternum	5
Mandible	2
Ribs	1
Phalanges	1
Scapula	1
Talus	1

Thirty patients are from literature and 5 are from the present series.
(Courtesy of Gamble, J.G., and Rinsky, L.A.: J. Pediatr. Orthop. 6:579–584, September–October 1986.)

TABLE 2.—SUMMARY OF FIVE NEW CASES OF CHRONIC RECURRENT MULTIFOCAL OSTEOMYELITIS

	Patient				
	1 (S.B.)	2 (A.C.)	3 (C.F.)	4 (K.R.)	5 (D.S.)
Sex	M	M	F	F	F
Age (yr) at onset	13	6	13	4	10
ESR (mm/h) at presentation	37	57	4	104	61
No. of episodes	3	5	6	3	5
No. of bones	3	6	6	3	3
No. of biopsies	2	3	1	2	2
Positive cultures	1 (ulna)	0	0	0	0
Duration of disease (mo)	12	76	14	6	14
Bones involved	L distal tibia, R ulna, T5 centrum	L proximal tibia, L distal tibia, C6 centrum, R proximal tibia, C7 centrum, L 2nd metatarsal, L 3rd metatarsal	R distal fibula, L distal fibula, R distal tibia, R innominate, R 3rd metatarsal, R 4th metatarsal	R clavicle, L proximal tibia, R ulna	L proximal tibia, R proximal tibia, R distal ulna
Total follow-up (yr)	8	6	3	3	2

ESR, erythrocyte sedimentation rate; L, left; R, right.
(Courtesy of Gamble, J.G., and Rinsky, L.A.: J. Pediatr. Orthop. 6:579–584, Sept.–Oct 1986.)

had subacute osteomyelitis. Cultures and specimens of cancellous bone were taken directly from biopsy specimens. Follow-up of patients with CRMO ranged from 2 years to 8 years (Table 2).

There were significant differences between patients with CRMO and

TABLE 3.—Characteristics of Five Cases of Chronic
Recurrent Multifocal Osteomyelitis Versus 11 Cases
of Subacute Osteomyelitis

	CRMO	Subacute osteomyelitis
Age (yr)	9.6	8.4
Age range (yr)	4–13	1¼–14
Elevated ESR (%)	80	100
WBC count >10,000/ml (%)	20	36
Positive blood cultures	0	0
Positive biopsy cultures*	1/9	4/11
Mean no. of episodes†	4.4	1
Mean no. of bones‡	3.8	1
Duration of symptoms (mo)		
Mean	22.8	8.2
Range	3–72	1–24

ESR, erythrocyte sedimentation rate.
*Significant at $P \leq .01$.
†Significant at $P \leq .005$.
‡Significant at $P \leq .01$.
(Courtesy of Gamble, J.G., and Rinsky, L.A.: J. Pediatr. Orthop. 6:579–584, Sept.–Oct. 1986.)

those with subacute osteomyelitis (Table 3). The 5 patients with CRMO had a total of 22 clinical episodes, but the 11 patients with subacute osteomyelitis had only a single clinical episode. Only 1 of 10 cultures of biopsy specimens was positive in the patients with CRMO, and the validity of this culture was suspect, whereas 4 of 11 cultures were positive for those with subacute disease. Patients with CRMO had involvement of 21 different bones, but all of those with subacute disease had involvement of only a single bone. One patient with CRMO had five clinical episodes with involvement of six bones and the centrum of the seventh cervical vertebra during a 76-month period. A radiograph of the left ankle showed a distal tibial metaphyseal lesion at the time of the second clinical episode in this patient. Although CRMO should be considered a distinct disease entity that differs from subacute osteomyelitis, it is not possible to make a differential diagnosis of CRMO during the first clinical episode because both disorders have the same initial clinical presentation.

Infant Pneumonitis Associated With Cytomegalovirus, *Chlamydia*, *Pneumocystis*, and *Ureaplasma*: Follow-Up
Dana M. Brasfield, Sergio Stagno, Richard J. Whitley, Gretchen Cloud, Gail Cassell, and Ralph E. Tiller (Univ. of Alabama at Birmingham and Children's Hosp. of Alabama, Birmingham)
Pediatrics 79:76–83, January 1987   2–13

Lower respiratory tract infections are an important cause of morbidity and mortality in infants. Mortality among hospitalized infants ranges from

PATIENT MORBIDITY AND MORTALITY

Deaths (No./total No. of patients)	7/205 (3.4%)
Wheezing	
No. of patients	86/187* (46%)
No. of episodes	202
Hospitalization	
No. of patients	29/187* (16%)
No. of episodes	47
No. of abnormal roentgenographic findings at 12 mo of age	17/109† (15%)
No. of abnormal pulmonary function tests (mean age 5 yr)	15/25‡ (60%)

*Survivors of initial episode followed from 2 weeks to 85 months.
†Patients followed for at least 12 months.
‡Patients performing pulmonary function tests.
(Courtesy of Brasfield, D.M., et al.: Pediatrics 79:76–83, January 1987.)

1% to 10%. Previous findings suggest that pneumonitis in infancy is frequently followed by a prolonged or chronic respiratory illness syndrome. In recent years, pneumonitis in young infants has been associated with a broader spectrum of infectious agents. The etiologic agents and acute clinical course of 104 of 205 infants younger than age 3 months were reported in a preliminary communication. The clinical course and long-term outcome were reviewed for the entire group.

Of the 205 infants hospitalized when younger than age 3 months because of pneumonitis, 145 (70%) had evidence of infection with one or more pathogens, most commonly *Chlamydia trachomatis* (36%), respiratory syncytial virus (23%), cytomegalovirus (20%), *Pneumocystis carinii* (17%), and *Ureaplasma urealyticum* (16%). The most common initial symptom was cough. Most infants had a normal temperature. The most frequent sign was rales (74%), but only 34% of the patients had wheezing on initial examination. Of 203 survivors, 187 (92%) were available for follow-up, which ranged from 2 weeks to 85 months.

Two patients died during the initial hospitalization, and five died during follow-up hospitalizations, for a total mortality of 3.4%. Wheezing episodes recurred in 86 (46%) of 187 patients followed. Chest x-ray films were persistently abnormal in 17 (15%) of 109 patients who were followed for at least 12 months. Abnormal pulmonary function persisted in 15 of 25 patients tested during follow-up (table). The prospective data from this study add to the evidence that respiratory infections during infancy are often predecessors of obstructive airway disease.

▶ For a review of the original report by these authors, see the 1983 YEAR BOOK, p. 88. It is obvious, and distressing, to see the serious long-term consequences of early pneumonitis in these patients. One prominent objective finding was the persistence of radiographic abnormalities. These abnormalities persisted for as long as 4 years in some patients and could not be predicted by the initial clinical course or the etiologic agent. Radiographic changes consistent with bronchiectasis have been noted previously in 25% to 60% of children after adenovirus infection (Herbert, F.A., et al.: *Can. Med. Assoc. J.* 116:274, 1977) and a 6% incidence of radiographic abnormalities as long as 7 years after respiratory syncytial virus infection (Rooney, J.C., et al.: *J. Pediatr.* 79:744, 1971). Of particular interest in this follow-up was the finding that four of the patients infected with cytomegalovirus as the cause of their initial pneumonitis died of pneumococcal meningitis, pulmonary hemosiderosis, and sudden death. These data provide further compelling evidence that respiratory infections during infancy can be the predecessors of obstructive airway disease in later life. All the more reason, if reasons are necessary, not to allow anyone to smoke in the homes of these babies.—F.A. Oski, M.D.

Can the Cost Savings of Eliminating Urine Microscopy in Biochemically Negative Urines Be Extended to the Pediatric Population?

Ayser C. Hamoudi, Sylvia C. Bubis, and Carlotta Thompson (Children's Hosp., Columbus, Oh.)
Am. J. Clin. Pathol. 86:658–660, November 1986   2–14

As early as 1979, investigators have reported on the possibility of eliminating routine microscopy on urine specimens with normal results of microscopic examination. Despite studies showing the cost of unnecessary testing, and despite the abundant evidence revealing the value of biochemical tests in predicting the significance of urine miscroscopy, laboratories remain reluctant to eliminate urine microscopy. An attempt was made to confirm the results of other studies and to determine whether or not such findings are relevant to the pediatric population.

A biochemical assay for leukocyte esterase, nitrite, pH, protein, glucose, ketones, urobilinogen, bilirubin, and blood was performed with Chemstrip-9. All urine specimens were examined without identification of the

TABLE 1.—COMPARISON OF BIOCHEMICAL RESULTS AND SIGNIFICANT SEDIMENT MICROSCOPY (1,016 URINES)

Biochemical Findings	Significant Microscopic Findings	Number (%)	Interpretation
Positive	Positive	310 (30)	TP*
Positive	Negative	11 (1)	FP
Negative	Positive	27 (3)	FN
Negative	Negative	668† (66)	TN

Sensitivity, 91%, Specificity, 98%. The predictive value of a negative result was 96.1%, and that of a positive result was 96.5%.
*TP = true positive; FP = false negative; TN = true negative.
†Includes 331 urine specimens with less than 5 WBCs/HPF.
(Courtesy of Hamoudi, A.C., et al.: Am. J. Clin. Pathol. 86:658–660, November 1986.)

TABLE 2.—DETAILS OF FALSE NEGATIVE
RESULTS (27 URINES)

Criterion	Number
5–10 WBCs	17
5–10 RBCs	3
>10 WBCs	7

(Courtesy of Hamoudi, A.C., et al.: Am. J. Clin. Pathol.
86:658–660, November 1986.)

clinical condition of the respective patients. There were 1,016 specimens studied.

The results of a comparison of biochemical findings and microscopy on the urinary sediment are presented in Table 1. The criteria for significant findings on microscopic examination are as follows: more than 5 white blood cells (WBCs) per high-power field (MPF), more than 3 red blood cells (RBCs) per HPF, renal epithelial cells, more than 1+ bacteria, and any amount or type of casts, with the exception of a rare hyaline cast. Twenty-seven urine specimens yielded false negative results; of these, 17 had 5–10 WBCs/HPF, 3 had 5–10 RBCs/HPF, and 7 had more than 10 WBCs/HPF (Table 2). Eleven urine specimens were considered to have false positive results; of these, eight had a positive leukocyte esterase test in the absence of positive microscopic results, two had positive nitrite tests, and one had occult blood that, although considered as a false positive result, could have indicated the presence of hemolysed blood or myoglobin. The sensitivity of the four parameters in predicting significant microscopy of urinary sediment was 91% and the specificity was 98%. The predictive value of a negative result was 96.1%, and that of a positive result, 96.5%. These results suggest that approximately 65% of urine microscopy procedures could be eliminated with obvious resultant savings and without risking the quality of care.

▶ Microscopic examination of the urine appears unnecessary in biochemically negative urine specimens from pediatric patients who are asymptomatic for urinary tract disease. Who has been looking anyway?—F.A. Oski, M.D.

Prevalence of Bacteriuria in Febrile Children
Howard Bauchner, Barbara Philipp, Barry Dashefsky, and Jerome O. Klein (Boston Univ. and Boston City Hosp.)
Pediatr. Infect. Dis. J. 6:239–242, March 1987   2–15

Febrile patients account for half of all those under age 5 years seen at the authors' walk-in clinic. If urinary tract infections are being missed, bacteriuria should be more prevalent than the reported occurrence of asymptomatic bacteriuria in well children. Findings in children less than 5 years old seen in a 6-month period with a temperature of at least 37.8

TABLE 1.—AGE AND TEMPERATURE OF
CHILDREN

Age (Months)	Temperature	
	<38.9°C	≥38.9°C
0–3	20	9
4–6	34	44
7–12	46	91
13–36	108	156
36–60	58	98
Total	266	398

(Courtesy of Bauchner, H., et al.: Pediatr. Infect. Dis. J. 6:239–242, March 1987.)

TABLE 2.—RESULTS OF CULTURE OF URINE

Result	CVS	BT
>10^5 colonies/ml	8*	0
10^4–10^5 colonies/ml	5	0
<10^4 colonies/ml or 2 organisms of any count	48	1†
Sterile	615	20
Total	676	21

*One culture had an organism with two antibiotic susceptibility patterns.
†A simultaneous clean voided specimen was sterile.
(Courtesy of Bauchner, H., et al.: Pediatr. Infect. Dis. J. 6:239–242, March 1987.)

TABLE 3.—PREVALENCE OF SIGNIFICANT
BACTERIURIA BY AGE AND GENDER

Age (Months)	No. with Bacteriuria/No. with Urine Obtained	
	Females	Males
0–3	2/10	3/19
4–6	1/27	2/51
7–12	1/62	0/75
13–36	0/108	0/156
37–60	2/61	0/95
Total	6/268	5/396

(Courtesy of Bauchner, H., et al.: Pediatr. Infect. Dis. J. 6:239–242, March 1987.)

C were reviewed; those whose chief complaint was dysuria were excluded. Urine cultures were obtained from 664 children.

Sixty percent of the children had temperatures of at least 38.9 C (Table 1). The results of urine culture are given in Table 2. Significant bacteriuria, defined as more than 10,000 colonies of one species per milliliter, or any growth when urine was obtained by bladder aspiration, was found in 2.2% of females and 1.3% of males (Table 3). *Escherichia coli* was the predom-

TABLE 4.—Data for Children With Significant Bacteriuria

Age (Days)	Sex	Temperature (°C)	Diagnosis	Urine Culture
19	M	37.8	Fever-suspected sepsis	Escherichia coli, >10^5 colonies/ml
66	M	38.9	Upper respiratory tract infection, impetigo	Proteus mirabilis, 30 000–50 000 colonies/ml
74	M	38.8	Fever-suspected sepsis	Escherichia coli >10^5 colonies/ml
182	M	38.5	Viral infection	Staphylococcus epidermidis, 50 000 colonies/ml
197	M	39.7	Gastroenteritis	Staphylococcus epidermidis, >10^5 colonies/ml
76	F	38.9	Otitis media, gastroenteritis	Escherichia coli >10^6 colonies/ml
103	F	39.3	Pneumonia, fever-suspected sepsis	Escherichia coli >10^5 colonies/ml
160	F	38.5	Bronchiolitis, otitis media	Escherichia coli 30 000–50 000 colonies/ml
222	F	39.5	Fever-suspected sepsis	Enterobacter cloacae, >10^5 colonies/ml
1425	F	38.9	Viral infection, scarlet fever	Escherichia coli; 30 000 colonies/ml
1790	F	39.8	Otitis media, viral infection	Escherichia coli, >10^5 colonies/ml

(Courtesy of Bauchner, H., et al.: Pediatr. Infect. Dis. J. 6:239–242, March 1987.)

inant organism (Table 4). No child with CNS infection or seizures had significant bacteriuria (Table 5).

Detection of urinary tract infection is especially important in infants and young children. In all infants admitted with fever of uncertain origin, a urine specimen should be obtained for culture by suprapubic aspiration or urethral catheterization. Urine culture also is indicated in older infants and children whose clinical features fail to suggest a source of fever, as well as in children with persistent fever.

TABLE 5.—PREVALENCE OF SIGNIFICANT BACTERIURIA BY
AGE AND DIAGNOSIS

Diagnosis	No. with Bacteriuria/No. of Urines Obtained	
	Patient <6 months old	Patient ≥7 months old
Central nervous system pleocytosis or seizure with fever	0/1	0/19
Suspected sepsis with otitis media, pneumonia, viral infection, etc.	3/33	1/27
Respiratory related infection*	4/56	2/416
Gastroenteritis	1/13	0/46
Fever alone	0/4	0/29
Miscellaneous	0/0	0/20
Total	8/107	3/557

*Includes otitis media, pneumonia, bronchiolitis, upper respiratory tract infection.

(Courtesy of Bauchner, H., et al.: Pediatr. Infect. Dis. J. 6:239–242, March 1987.)

▶ This article was accompanied by a commentary by Ronald Hogg who points out that the incidence of bacteriuria in the study described above was 7.5% in the patients less than 6 months of age. This is not a "low yield." These data in young infants are consistent with the findings of Roberts and associates (*J. Pediatr.* 103:864, 1983), who reported a frequency of 4.1% for urinary tract infections in febrile patients less than 2 years of age. It would appear that a search for a urinary tract infection is not necessary in the febrile child more than 1 year of age who has nothing to suggest a urinary tract infection, or has another obvious cause for the fever, but in the infant less than 1 year of age the urine culture should be part of the evaluation of the febrile encounter. How to collect the urine is another matter and that is discussed in the next abstract.—F.A. Oski, M.D.

Bacterial Contamination Rates For Non-Clean-Catch and Clean-Catch Midstream Urine Collections in Boys

Jacob A. Lohr, Leigh G. Donowitz, and Sharon M. Dudley (Univ. of Virginia)
J. Pediatr. 109:659–660, October 1986   2–16

Since the late 1950s the clean-catch midstream void technique has been the method of choice for collecting a urine specimen for culture. With this technique standard practice includes cleansing the urethral meatus to decrease contamination of the specimen. The influence of meatal cleansing on contamination of specimens from 102 healthy boys aged 2–14 years was evaluated. Of these, 98 were circumcised.

The first urine specimen obtained was without meatal cleansing (non clean-catch urine) and was collected in a sterile wide-mouth container with a screw lid. Twenty-four hours after collection of the first specimen, and after meatal cleansing with 2% Castile soap (clean-catch urine), a second specimen was taken using a standard clean-catch kit. Overall, 95% of the non-clean-catch urine specimens were sterile, as were 90% of the clean-catch urine specimens. The difference in the rate of urinary contamination between the cleansed and uncleansed state was not statistically significant using chi-square analysis. It was not possible to assess the impact of circumcision status because only 4% of the boys were not circumcised. Cleansing the urethral meatus prior to collecting a urine specimen for culture from circumsised boys has no demonstrable benefit.

▶ Dr. Leonard B. Weiner, Associate Professor of Pediatrics, Health Science Center at Syracuse, State University of New York, and Chief, Division of Infectious Disease, comments as follows.—F.A. Oski, M.D.

▶ The most practical and widely applicable rapid screening test for urinary tract infections (UTIs) remains the uncentrifuged urine specimen Gram stain. It appears from the data presented above that it can be used in specimens obtained without meatal cleansing from circumcised males. If at least 2 organisms per oil immersion field are visualized, then the correlation with colony counts of at least 10^5 organisms per ml is excellent; in addition, bacterial morphology and Gram stain characteristics can be observed.

Among the other nonculture screening methods the leukocyte esterase determination is quite specific and sensitive for detection of pyuria, but it does not take into account that most febrile children have pyuria that is unrelated to UTI and, conversely, that pyuria may be minimal in infants and neonates with upper tract infection. The leukocyte esterase test, when combined with the rapid test for the measurement of bacterial reduction of nitrate to nitrite, has a much higher predictive value for both positive and negative cultures but is still less reliable than an appropriately performed Gram stain of the uncentrifuged urine specimen.

Automated rapid tests that determine organism density by bioluminescence and filtration-staining techniques provide rapid information but require costly equipment and are generally not accurate enough for clinical application. The rapid methods that purport to localize the site of bacterial infection are generally not useful in pediatric patients. Antibody-coated bacteria detected by fluorescent staining defines upper tract involvement in adults but is absent in more than half of the children with renal parenchymal infection. Enzymes from infection-damaged renal tissue can also predict upper tract disease in adults, but these have not been adequately studied in children. In two studies involving pediatric patients, urinary LDH isoenzyme 5 successfully predicted upper tract infection. Urinary adenylate kinase may be a more reliable predictor of renal damage with infection, but this requires further study.

A cautionary comment is necessary concerning colony counts of 10^5 or greater as an ultimate indicator of infection. Urine culture specimens from premature and full-term infants, as well as from infants in the first few months of life, may have colony counts of only 50,000 or even 20,000 with definite infection. Furthermore, catheterized and suprapubic specimens should be considered positive with any significant quantity of organisms as long as the culture is a pure growth of a single organism. In addition, adolescents and young

TABLE 1.—Comparison of Radiologic Study Findings in 64 Children With Urinary Tract Infections

No. of Patients	Intravenous Pyelogram	Renal Ultrasound	Cystogram
52	Normal	Normal	Normal
9	Normal	Normal	Reflux
1	L calyceal dilation	Normal	Reflux grade IV left
1	Bilateral duplications	Normal	Reflux grade II
1	R renal scar	Normal	Normal

(Courtesy of Johnson, C.E., et al.: Pediatrics 78:871–878, November 1986.)

adults, especially females, often have symptomatic lower urinary tract infections with pyuria and urine cultures yielding only 10^2 bacterial colonies per milliliter.—L.B. Weiner, M.D.

Renal Ultrasound Evaluation of Urinary Tract Infections in Children
Candice E. Johnson, Boz P. DeBaz, Paul A. Shurin, and Rose DeBartolomeo (Case Western Reserve Univ.)
Pediatrics 78:871–878, November 1986   2–17

Two sets of studies were conducted to test the reliability of ultrasound as an aid in diagnosing upper and lower urinary tract infections in children. Intravenous pyelography is not longer the method of choice because of

TABLE 2.—Radiologic Study Findings in 43 Children With Urinary Tract Infection With Intravenous Pyelogram Done Only If Ultrasound or Cystogram Findings Were Abnormal

No. of Patients	Intravenous Pyelogram	Ultrasound	Cystogram
34	Not done	Normal	Normal
4	Normal	Normal	Reflux
1	L hydronephrosis	L hydronephrosis	L ureterocoele
1	Single kidney	Single kidney	Normal
1	Ectasia of pelvis and infundibula	Dilated calyces	Normal
1	Normal	Dilated calyces	Normal
1	Normal	Increased echogenicity	Normal

(Courtesy of Johnson, C.E., et al.: Pediatrics 78:871–878, November 1986.)

TABLE 3.—KIDNEY VOLUME CHANGE:
ACUTE VOLUME INCREASE COMPARED TO
BASELINE MEASUREMENT 6 WEEKS
POSTINFECTION, FOR THE KIDNEY WITH THE
LARGER VOLUME CHANGE*

% Increase in Volume	Upper Tract	Lower Tract
>30	15	4
<30	3	17

*Upper tract defined as three or four criteria present; lower tract defined as zero to one criterion present. Sensitivity of greater than 30% increase for indicating upper tract infection = 83.3%; specificity of greater than 30% increase for indicating upper tract infection = 80.9%.
(Courtesy of Johnson, C.E., et al.: Pediatrics 78:871–878, November 1986.)

TABLE 4.—ACCURACY OF A SINGLE
INITIAL RENAL ULTRASOUND FOR
IDENTIFYING THOSE KIDNEYS THAT WILL
DEMONSTRATE GREATER THAN A 30%
VOLUME INCREASE ON PAIRED STUDIES 4
TO 6 WEEKS APART

Renal Volume	Volume Increase	
	>30%	<30%
>95th percentile	18	4
<95th percentile	9	47

The 95th percentile is taken from tables based on body weight. Each kidney is counted individually. Sensitivity of single ultrasound, 66.7%; specificity of single ultrasound, 92.2%.
(Courtesy of Johnson, C.E., et al.: Pediatrics 78:871–878, November 1986.)

the pain of intravenous injection, radiation exposure to the gonads and bone marrow, and the slight risk of allergic reaction to the dye. Ultrasonography is a noninvasive, safe method.

All of the patients studied had high bacteria counts, symptoms of urinary tract infections, and no previous urologic problems. In the first series, 64 children had intravenous pyelography, renal ultrasonography, and cystography. Reflux was detected in 11 patients by cystography, but not by ultrasound. Two of the 11 children had abnormal pyelograms, one of which showed caliceal dilation, a treatable problem. The pyelogram alone picked up a renal scar. Thus ultrasound gave one false negative result, i.e., the treatable dilated calices. There were no false positive findings (Table 1).

In the second series, 43 children had ultrasound examinations and cystography; intravenous pyelography was done only if the other two test results were abnormal. Four children had reflux, which showed up in the cystogram. Ultrasound gave an incorrect diagnosis of dilated calices when pyelography showed ectasia of the pelvis and infundibulum. Dilated calices were also seen on another ultrasound scan but were determined to be falsely positive by pyelography (Table 2). Ultrasound uncovered transient increased echogenicity that required no extra treatment.

Ultrasound is useful in determining kidney volume, which, if above the 95th percentile, suggests upper tract infection. If ultrasound is done at the beginning and after 6 weeks of antibiotic therapy, the percent decrease in renal volume is a good indicator of whether the infection is in the upper or lower tract (Tables 3 and 4).

The child with a urinary tract infection should first undergo voiding cystography, followed by ultrasound examination to uncover absent or severely scarred kidneys or ureteropelvic junction obstruction. In the presence of vesicoureteral reflux or an abnormal ultrasound finding, intravenous pyelography should be done.

▶ I hope you have followed the sequence of abstracts in the preceding pages. The evaluation of the febrile patient, the positive urine culture, and now the diagnostic evaluation of the child with a presumed urinary tract infection (UTI). It would appear from this abstract and the one to follow that we have agreement on two continents as to the diagnostic evaluation. The initial studies for the child with a UTI should include ultrasonography and voiding cystography. Excretory urography is no longer the method of choice for initial evaluation. In a septic patient with a UTI voiding cystourethrography is postponed and an ultrasound scan is obtained as the initial screening procedure to determine whether medical or surgical therapy is indicated. For more on the same, see the 1987 YEAR BOOK, pp. 298–302. No more puzzling decisions to make. As Yogi Berra once said, "When you come to a fork in the road, take it."—F.A. Oski, M.D.

Ultrasonography as a Screening Procedure in Children With Urinary Tract Infection
Olli Honkinen, Olli Ruuskanen, Hellevi Rikalainen, Eero O. Mäkinen, and Ilkka Välimäki (Turku Univ., Finland)
Pediatr. Infect. Dis. 5:633–635, November 1986   2–18

It is important to diagnose vasicoureteral reflux or urinary tract anomalies, or both, in children with urinary tract infection (UTI) as early as possible, because these abnormalities can lead to permanent renal damage. It has been suggested that boys should undergo excretory urography and voiding cystourethrography after their first UTI and girls should have these procedures at least after their second infection. Ultrasonography was evaluated as a screening procedure in children with UTI.

Twenty-five of 76 children who had UTIs underwent renal ultrasonography, excretory urography, and radionuclide-voiding cystography; 51 had conventional voiding cystourethrography. Only febrile children with positive urine cultures were included. Thirty-six patients had normal findings

COMPARISON OF ULTRASONOGRAPHY AND EXCRETORY
UROGRAPHY IN 76 PATIENTS WITH UTI

Diagnosis	No. of Patients	Ultrasonography	Excretory Urography
Normal urinary tract	36	Normal in 36	Normal in 34; duplex collecting system in 2
Vesicoureteral reflux without hydronephrosis	24	Positive in 8	Positive in 7
Vesicoureteral reflux with hydronephrosis (operated)	4	Positive in 3	Positive in 4
Urinary outlet obstruction (operated)	12	Positive in 11	Positive in 12

(Courtesy of Honkinen, O., et al.: Pediatr. Infect. Dis. 5:633–635, November 1986.)

on all tests and were not tested further. The other 40 (53%) had urinary tract abnormalities that were considered to be major predisposing factors to UTI (table). These included vesicoureteral reflux with normal function in 28 patients and urinary tract obstruction in 12. Four children with reflux and all 12 with obstruction required corrective surgery. Ultrasonography as the initial procedure was capable of detecting positive findings in 14 of 16 patients. On the basis of these findings it is suggested that renal ultrasonography may be the diagnostic method of choice in children with UTI.

Lyme Arthritis in Children: An Orthopaedic Perspective
Randall W. Culp, Andrew H. Eichenfield, Richard S. Davidson, Denis S. Drummond, Mark R. Christofersen, and Donald P. Goldsmith (Children's Hosp. of Philadelphia)
J. Bone Joint Surg. [Am.] 69-A:96–99, January 1987   2–19

Typically, Lyme disease appears as a brief, intermittent attack of swelling and pain in one or more larger joints. The disease has been diagnosed in patients with oligoarticular arthritis, but no history of rash or tick bite, who had positive serologic tests. Data were reviewed on 43 children seen with clinical and serologic evidence of Lyme arthritis during a 2-year period. The mean follow-up was 20 months (range, 5–30 months).

All children had lived in or visited an endemic area for Lyme disease. In most of them symptoms developed during summer and autumn, when activity of the tick *Ixodes dammini* was maximal. More than half the patients had no history of erythema chronicum migrans, no significant prodromal illness, and no knowledge of a tick bite. Three patients had Bell's palsy, and one had a popliteal cyst in conjunction with the arthritis. All patients had oligoarticular arthritis involving the knee in all but two.

Recurrent attacks of arthritis were common before treatment and lasted from 3 days to 24 months (median, 1 week). All patients walked on the affected extremity without excessive pain. Arthritis was the first sign in most patients, and Lyme disease was diagnosed initially in only nine. Effusion was the only x-ray abnormality seen in 32 patients. The sedimentation rate was consistently abnormal; it was elevated in 30 of 36 patients tested. Immunofluorescent serologic tests for Lyme disease were uniformly positive. Thirty-three patients were given penicillin or tetracycline orally; all but two responded. The other ten patients responded to a combination of intravenous and oral antibiotic therapy. Two patients did not respond to oral antibiotic treatment but responded to the intravenous administration of penicillin.

Lyme disease should be ruled out in children who have brief, self-limited attacks of arthritis, even in the absence of the characteristic rash. Although the relapse rate in this young population is low, these patients remain at risk of exacerbation of arthritis.

Childhood Lyme Arthritis: Experience in an Endemic Area
Andrew H. Eichenfield, Donald P. Goldsmith, Jorge L. Benach, Avron H. Ross, Franklin X. Loeb, Robert A. Doughty, and Balu H. Athreya (Children's Seashore House, Children's Hosp. of Philadelphia, St. Christopher's Hosp. for Children, Philadelphia, and State Univ. of New York at Stony Brook)
J. Pediatr. 109:753–758, November 1986   2–20

Lyme disease is caused by *Borrelia burgdorferi*, a spirochete transmitted by the deer tick, whose hosts are the white-tailed deer and the white-footed mouse. The diagnosis of Lyme disease rests on clinical findings of erythema chronicum migrans and neurologic, cardiac, or articular manifestations.

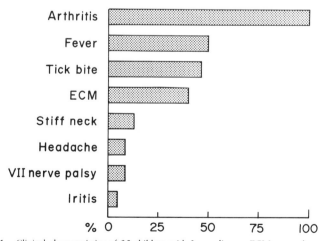

Fig 2–1.—Clinical characteristics of 25 children with Lyme disease. ECM = erythema chronicum migrans. (Courtesy of Eichenfield, A.H., et al.: J. Pediatr. 109:753–758, November 1986.)

INITIAL PRESENTATIONS IN CHILDHOOD LYME ARTHRITIS

	With rash		Without rash	
	n	%	n	%
Septic arthritis	4	16	6	24
Episodic arthritis	3	12	4	16
Pauciarticular JRA	2	8	2	8
Acute arthritis	3	12	1	4
Total	12	48	13	52

(Courtesy of Eichenfield, A.H., et al.: J. Pediatr. 109:753–758, November 1986.)

A review was made of experience with 25 young patients who had oligoarticular arthritis as the primary complaint.

Boy, 15 years, complained of left elbow stiffness, warmth, and swelling of 1 week's duration. These signs were repeated 1 month later in his right elbow, and a chest rash appeared also. Two months later the left knee was painful and swollen. Evaluation of the cloudy fluid showed 4,460 white blood cells/cu mm and a differential of 86% neutrophils and 14% mononuclear cells. Other findings were normal. To rule out juvenile rheumatoid arthritis (JRA), physical examination was carried out, as were laboratory tests later. The hemoglobin level was 14.7 gm/dl; the white blood cell count, 8,400/cu mm; platelet count, 325,000/cu mm; and Westergren sedimentation rate, 10 mm/hour. Antibody titers against the Lyme spirochete included IgM, 1:64, and IgG, 1:256, as determined by immunofluorescent assay. Treatment with tetracycline, 30 mg/kg/day, cured the joint symptoms.

All 25 patients in this series had arthritis; fever, a history of tick bite, erythema chronicum migrans, stiff neck, headache, a history of tick bite, erythema chronicum migrans, stiff neck, headache, VII nerve palsy, or iritis were present in some cases (Fig 2–1). The types of arthritis were septic, episodic, pauciarticular JRA, and acute arthritis, which were accompanied by a rash less than half of the time (table).

Lyme disease may more commonly be the cause of childhood oligoarticular arthritis than formerly thought. It should be ruled out in patients with episodic, self-limiting arthritic attacks and in patients with a current diagnosis of JRA.

▶ These two papers (2–19 and 2–20) provide a very accurate picture of the patient with Lyme disease. In any patient with arthritis, idiopathic neurologic disease, or a cardiac conduction defect, Lyme disease should be considered in the differential diagnosis. Monarticular Lyme disease is indistinguishable from acute bacterial arthritis—both have a high leukocyte count in the joint aspirate. Don't wait for the rash to appear before making the diagnosis or you may never make it. By the way, note that Bell's palsy is one of the common neurologic manifestations of the disease. Even papilledema may be observed in this disease (Wu, G., et al.: Ann. Ophthalmol. 18:252, 1986).—F.A. Oski, M.D.

Fever as a Predictor of Infection in Burned Children

Ruth Ann Parish, Alvin H. Novack, David M. Heimbach, and Loren R. Engrav (Univ. of Washington and Harborview Med. Ctr., Seattle)

J. Trauma 27:69–71, January 1987   2–21

Children with burns often have fever. To evaluate the course and duration of these fevers, the records of 223 children admitted to a regional burn center from 1979 to 1982 were reviewed and an attempt made to determine whether fever is an indicator of infection in burned children. The highest rectal temperature during each 8-hour period was recorded. Fever was defined as a rectal temperature of at least 38.2 C.

The highest mean temperature was recorded within 38–96 hours after burn injury and appeared at the same time whether or not the child had infection (Fig 2–2). All 23 children with infections and 145 of 200 uninfected children had one episode of fever during the first 2 weeks after burn, indicating that fever was not specific for the presence of infection (Table 1). Similarly, fever was not a significant predictor of infection in children younger than age 4 years (Table 2) or in those with more than 20% total body surface area burns (Table 3). The presence of infection was readily determined by physical examination alone in all but two children with infection.

Fever is not a specific indicator of infection in all burned children. Physical examination is a reliable source of information about wound infection, sepsis, or other childhood infections and should be the primary tool used in diagnosing infection in burned children.

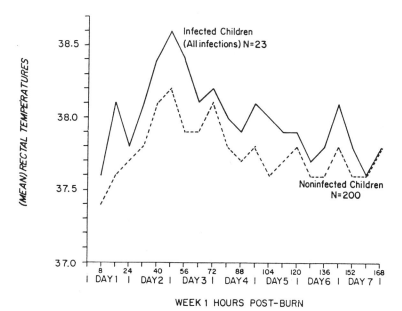

Fig 2–2.—Fever curves for infected and uninfected children, week 1. (Courtesy of Parish, R.A., et al.: J. Trauma 27:69–71, January 1987.)

TABLE 1.—Infection vs. Fever in 223
Burned Children

	Infection	No Infection
Fever	23	145
No fever	0	55

Significant difference, $P < .01$.
(Courtesy of Parish, R.A., et al.: J. Trauma 27:69–71, January 1987.)

TABLE 2.—Infection vs. Fever in 135
Burned Children Younger Than Age 4
Years

	Infection	No Infection
Fever	19	93
No fever	0	23

No significant difference, $P < .07$.
(Courtesy of Parish, R.A., et al.: J. Trauma 27:69–71, January 1987.)

TABLE 3.—Infection vs. Fever in 26
Children With More Than 20% Total Body
Surface Area Burns*

	Infection	No Infection
Fever	6	20
No fever	0	0

*No significant difference, $P < .77$.
(Courtesy of Parish, R.A., et al.: J. Trauma 27:69–71, January 1987.)

Intestinal Parasites in Pet Store Puppies in Atlanta

Jeanette K. Stehr-Green, Geneva Murray, Peter M. Schantz, and Susanne P. Wahlquist (Ctrs. for Disease Control, Atlanta)
Am. J. Public Health 77:345–346, March 1987   2–22

Certain parasites that naturally infect dogs can cause serious and potentially life-threatening illness in human beings. Pet stores can play a role in limiting infection by initiating health care of pups in their own facilities or by informing the public of appropriate measures to take. Fourteen pet stores in Atlanta were surveyed to learn if vaccinations and deworming procedures were performed on the premises and whether proper information on pet care was provided to customers at the time of sale.

Owners and/or managers of 13 of the 14 selected pet shops, when contacted by phone, agreed to participate. They were asked to complete a questionnaire concerning the store's deworming procedures and on health care information distributed to clientele. The participants were visited by an investigator who examined the pups in the store for signs of abdominal distention, diarrhea, cough, and depression. Stool samples were taken from the bottom of each pup's cage. In all, 143 pups ranging in age from 6 weeks to 28 weeks were examined.

Seventy-four pups (52%) had at least one intestinal parasite, including *Giardia* sp., *Toxocara canis,* and *Isospora* sp. Of 118 pups for which in-store deworming records were available, 14 (12%) received no anthelminthic treatment, 65 (55%) received one treatment, 17 (14%) received two treatments, and 22 (19%) received three or more treatments. Only six stores (43%) routinely provided clients with information on the need to continue deworming procedures at home. Five owners and managers (36%) did not know the zoonotic potential of canine parasites. Perhaps legislation regarding the prophylactic deworming of pups, or public health education through local health departments, should be initiated to decrease the risk of dogborne zoonoses.

▶ Most pet stores don't even advertise that they sell worms. Another good reason to drown the dog. By the way, *Campylobacter* enteritis is significantly more common among children aged less than 1 year to 5 years living in households with puppies (Salfield, N.J., et al.: *Br. Med. J.* 294:21, 1987). Relax, the cat also gets blasted a few pages from here.—F.A. Oski, M.D.

AIDS: Outcome of Children Born to HTLV-III/LAV Infected Mothers: Report of 15 Italian Cases

M. Aricò, M. Azzini, D. Caselli, R. Maccario, G. Marseglia, and G. Michelone (Università of Pavia and Università of Brescia, Italy)

Helv. Paediatr. Acta 41:477–486, 1986   2–23

Specific anti-human T cell lymphotrophic virus type III/lymphadenopathy virus (HTLV-III/LAV) seropositivity is becoming more frequent in children born to seropositive mothers in Italy. Fifteen children born to 14 seropositive, drug-addicted mothers seen at one center in the past 30 months were followed for up to 2 years. Increased levels of IgG were found in most children and of IgM in about half (Table 1). Five children had full-blown acquired immunodeficiency syndrome (AIDS) and eight had AIDS-related complex (Table 2). All but 2 of the 15 patients were hospitalized because of failure to thrive and/or recurrent infection. In four instances HTLV-III/LAV infection had been suspected. Five patients died of AIDS. Only two children in the series have remained persistently asymptomatic.

Four of 15 patients in this series had CNS involvement and 2 had liver disease. Hepatitis B virus infection occurred in two and thrombocytopenia in three children. Parental homosexual behavior was not a cause of family risk in this series. In one family a first child died of AIDS, but a younger

TABLE 1.—LABORATORY DATA

Case	AST (IU/l)	ALT (IU/l)	HBV markers patient	HBV markers mother	Platelets (count/μl)	IgG (mg/dl)	IgA (mg/dl)	IgM (mg/dl)
1	23	30	–	–	285,000	3030	509	527
2	12	8	–	–	396,000	4340	167	186
3	20	25	–	HBsAb	220,000	3758	95	122
4	22	11	HBsAb*	HBsAb	452,000	1000	51	117
5	21	18	–	–	352,000	1660	139	71
6	15	9	–	–	292,000	1200	102	190
7	42	25	–	HBsAb	310,000	5540	198	225
8	30	43	–	HBeAb	219,000	5770	167	116
9	210	180	–	–	246,000	1693	202	271
10	581	246	HBcAb	HBcAb	90,000	247	63	68
11	17	10	–	HBsAb	317,000	2340	101	280
12	24	33	HBsAb*	HBcAb	367,000	1800	184	166
13	64	50	HBcAb	HBcAb	38,000	3100	50	1000
14	76	70	–	NT	58,000	1400	135	161
15	40	15	–	NT	300,000	1980	143	67

*Vaccinated at birth.
NT, not tested; AST, aspartate aminotransferase; ALT, alanine aminotransferase; HBV, hepatitis B virus.
(Courtesy of Aricò, M., et al.: Helv. Paediatr. Acta 41:477–486, 1986.)

child had only passive, transient immunization by specific maternal IgG. One patient with AIDS-related complex appeared to heal completely when followed for longer than 3 years.

Most symptomatic infants with AIDS may be expected to present in the first 6 months of life. Widespread screening may not be justified because

TABLE 2.—CLINICAL FEATURES

Case	Sex	Birth weight	Age at onset	Clinical form and involvement	Outcome
1	M	3050	3 m	AIDS: RI, CNS	dead 15 months
2	F	3000	5 m	ARC: RI	well 33 months
3	M	3100	5 m	AIDS: RI, GI, CNS	dead 25 months
4	M	2900	–	asymptomatic	well 15 months
5	F	2800	15 m	ARC: RI	alive 21 months
6	M	2300	–	asymptomatic	well 4 months
7	F	3050	3 m	AIDS: RI, GI	dead 9 months
8	F	3000	3 m	ARC: GI	well 19 months
9	F	2450	3 m	ARC: RI, CNS	alive 21 months
10	F	3050	1 m	AIDS: RI	dead 6 months
11	M	2700	5 m	ARC: GI	alive 12 months
12	F	3050	3 m	ARC:	alive 4 months
13	M	3100	2 m	ARC: CNS	alive 8 months
14	M	2100	4 m	AIDS: RI	dead 6 months
15	M	2100	6 m	ARC: GI	alive 37 months

RI, severe lower respiratory infections; GI, gastrointestinal infections; CNS, central nervous system disease; ARC, AIDS-related complex.
(Courtesy of Aricò, M., et al.: Helv. Paediatr. Acta 41:477–486, 1986.)

of the inadequacy of present treatment approaches to AIDS and AIDS-related complex.

▶ It is dangerous to make comments regarding AIDS. Anything written in 1987 could prove to be wrong, or certainly hopelessly outdated, by the time you read this in 1988. But fools do rush in. There is now a wealth of information about clinical and immunologic dysfunction in children infected with the human immunodeficiency virus (HIV), but little is known about perinatal transmission, particularly the risk of an HIV-positive woman transferring the infection to her infant. As part of European research activities on AIDS, infants born to HIV-positive mothers are being followed from birth. A recent report (Mok, J.G., et al.: *Lancet* 1:1164, 1987) describes 71 of these infants who have been followed to a median age of 6 months (range, 1–15 months). Five of these infants had symptoms of AIDS or AIDS-related complex (ARC) and three of them died. The mean age at maternal antibody loss was 10 months, and an estimated 75% of the infants will have lost maternal antibody by 12 months. Loss of antibody, however, did not exclude infection, as confirmed by virus culture.

Unfortunately, it appears that current antibody screening techniques may be insufficient for screening infants. Borkowsky and associates reported that 9 of 85 children with HIV infections lacked antibody to HIV as measured by a commercial enzyme-linked immunoassay. All nine had antigen detected by a more sensitive antigen-capture technique (*Lancet* 1:1168, 1987). We need answers fast. James Chin, World Health Organization epidemiologist, says there may be 3,000 HIV infected newborns this year. The Centers for Disease Control (CDC) say that 504 children under 13 years of age, as well as 145 teenagers, have had AIDS and that 64% have died. Pediatric AIDS had been reported in 33 states by the late summer of 1987.

The prevalence of AIDS will increase dramatically because of a chance in the CDC definition of AIDS to include general wasting, progressive neurologic defects, and repeated bacterial infections in a HIV-positive patient. It is estimated that by 1991 there may be 10,000 children with AIDS symptoms requiring at least 30–40 days of hospitalization each year. They will need 1,000 beds, or 2% of this country's pediatric beds. It is now appreciated that clinical problems in pediatrics AIDS differ significantly from those seen in adults. The most common presenting signs are severe recurrent bacterial infections and failure to thrive. Generalized lymphadenopathy, oral candidiasis, protracted or recurrent diarrhea, otitis media, neurologic deficits, hepatosplenomegaly, and lymphoid interstitial pneumonitis are seen commonly in the pediatric patient. For an unusual neurologic complication, please see the next abstract.—F.A. Oski, M.D.

AIDS: Calcification of the Basal Ganglia in Infants and Children
Anita Lesgold Belman, George Lantos, Dikran Horoupian, Brian E. Novick, Monica H. Ultmann, Dennis W. Dickson, and Arye Rubinstein (State Univ. of New York at Stony Brook and Albert Einstein College of Med., N.Y.)
Neurology 36:1192–1199, September 1986   2–24

Neurologic involvement occurs in children with acquired immunodeficiency syndrome (AIDS). Neural calcification was found in 8 of 13 pediatric AIDS patients. Encephalopathy was prominent in 12 children. In five, CT revealed bilateral symmetric calcium densities in the region of the basal ganglia. Serial studies showed calcification and cerebral atrophy, and T2-weighted images indicated extensive hyperintensity. Computed tomography showed calcification and generalized atrophy. Neuropathologic examination of four of the five children who died revealed vessel calcification in the basal ganglia involving the putamen and the outer globus pallidus.

Calcification of the basal ganglia is not common in adults with AIDS. The present findings may indicate a greater vulnerability of the pediatric nervous system to a metabolic or infectious insult.

▶ Incidentally, a T cell lymphotropic virus has been isolated from cats in a cattery. A number of cats in one pen had died and several had an immunodeficiency-like syndrome. This virus, tentatively designated feline T-lymphotropic lentivirus, appears to be antigenically distinct from the human immunodeficiency virus. Kittens experimentally infected by way of blood or plasma from naturally infected animals had generalized lymphadenopathy several weeks later, became transiently febrile and leukopenic, and continued to show a generalized lymphadenopathy 5 months after infection (Pedersen, N.C., et al.: *Science* 235:790, 1987). Don't worry, folks; there is no evidence for cat-to-human transmission of this agent (yet). And you thought cat scratch disease was a problem! Garfield, please come here, there is something I would like to discuss with you.—F.A. Oski, M.D.

Fever in Respiratory Virus Infections
Anne Putto, Olli Ruuskanen, and Olli Meurman (Univ. of Turku, Finland)
Am. J. Dis. Child 140:1159–1163, November 1986   2–25

Many studies show a positive correlation between high fever and systemic bacterial infections. Although studies have demonstrated an asso-

TABLE 1.—THE HIGHEST TEMPERATURE AT HOME, ON ADMISSION TO THE HOSPITAL, AND DURING HOSPITALIZATION IN FEBRILE CHILDREN

	At Home		On Admission		In the Hospital	
	n	Temperature, °C	n	Temperature, °C	n	Temperature °C
Adenovirus	19	39.6 ± 0.7	20	39.0 ± 0.6	24	39.2 ± 0.6
Influenza A	35	39.4 ± 0.7	35	39.3 ± 0.8	41	39.6 ± 0.6
Influenza B	17	39.5 ± 0.6	10	38.8 ± 0.7	22	39.3 ± 0.6
Parainfluenza 1	14	39.2 ± 0.7	19	38.7 ± 0.6	22	39.0 ± 0.6
Parainfluenza 2	12	38.8 ± 0.6	15	39.0 ± 0.4	17	39.1 ± 0.5
Parainfluenza 3	26	39.2 ± 0.7	33	38.8 ± 0.6	40	39.1 ± 0.5
Respiratory syncytial virus	35	39.2 ± 0.6	41	39.0 ± 0.8	47	39.2 ± 0.7

Values are given as mean ± SD.
(Courtesy of Putto, A., et al.: Am. J. Dis. Child 140:1159–1163, November 1986.)

TABLE 2.—Duration of Fever Before Admission, During
Hospitalization, and Total Duration of Fever in Respiratory
Virus Infections

	Before Admission		In the Hospital		Total Duration	
	n	Days	n	Days	n	Days
Adenovirus	24	3.2±2.5	25	1.7±1.1	25	4.8±2.2
Influenza A	47	2.1±2.2	47	2.9±1.7	47	5.1±2.8
Influenza B	27	2.6±2.2	18	2.8±2.2	27	5.2±2.0
Parainfluenza 1	25	2.0±2.0	25	2.0±1.4	25	4.0±2.0
Parainfluenza 2	21	0.8±0.8	21	1.6±1.6	21	2.5±1.9
Parainfluenza 3	53	1.1±1.3	53	2.0±1.7	53	3.1±2.1
Respiratory syncytial virus	60	1.7±1.7	60	1.8±1.3	60	3.5±2.3

Values are given as mean ± SD.
(Courtesy of Putto, A., et al.: Am. J. Dis. Child 140:1159–1163, November 1986.)

ciation between high, prolonged fever and adenovirus infections, the role of fever in other respiratory virus infections has not been clearly defined. A retrospective study was made of the records of hospitalized children to assess the association between the degree and duration of fever and respiratory virus infections that could be diagnosed from nasopharyngeal mucus by rapid antigen detection by immunoassay.

The series included 101 girls and 157 boys aged 3 months to 13.8 years; all were hospitalized because of virus infections with adenovirus (25), influenza A or B (74), parainfluenza 1, 2, or 3 (99), or respiratory syncytial virus (60). A comparison group included 74 girls and 44 boys aged 3 months to 15 years with confirmed bacterial infections, including meningitis (43), urinary tract infections (41), epiglottitis (27), and septicemia (7).

Of children with respiratory virus infection, 91% had fever during some phase of the disease. Also, 78% of parents reported that their children had had fever before hospitalization, and 79% of these parents knew the exact degree of fever (Table 1). A temperature of at least 39 C was most frequently associated with adenovirus (68%), influenza A (84%), and influenza B (65%). The mean duration of fever ranged from 2.5 days for parainfluenza 2 infections to 5.2 days for influenza B infections (Table 2). The highest degree of fever in virus infections during hospitalization did not differ from the highest degree of fever in bacterial infections.

▶ These data convincingly demonstrate that high, prolonged fever is frequently associated with respiratory virus infections, at least in the hospitalized patient, and that the magnitude of the fever does not differ significantly from fever occurring in patients with serious bacterial infections. In a very small percentage (9%) of these patients with a viral infection a biphasic temperature curve was demonstrated, with an intercurrent afebrile period of about 24 hours. This was most typical of influenza A virus infections. Fever must be good for you or God wouldn't have made it so common.—F.A. Oski, M.D.

Aerosolized Ribavirin Treatment of Respiratory Syncytial Virus Infection in Infants Hospitalized During an Epidemic

Dennis A. Conrad, John C. Christenson, Joseph L. Waner, and Melvin I. Marks (Univ. of Oklahoma and Oklahoma Children's Mem. Hosp., Oklahoma City)

Pediatr. Infect. Dis. J. 6:152–158, February 1987   2–26

Ribavirin has known antiviral activity against respiratory syncytial virus (RSV). It also has proven efficacy when administered as a small particle aerosol in the treatment of RSV infection in adults and children, causing no significant adverse effects or apparent toxicity. Aerosolized ribavirin was evaluated in 33 high-risk and seriously ill infants with RSV infection seen during a 12-week epidemic.

All 33 infants had culture-confirmed RSV infection. There were 18 premature infants, 6 with cardiac disease, 2 with bronchopulmonary dysplasia, 2 with unspecified multiple congenital malformation complex syndromes, and 1 with Werdnig-Hoffman disease. Apnea was present in 13 infants and 11 had developing progressive pulmonary insufficiency. Findings in study patients were compared with those in a control group of 97

CLINICAL SEVERITY OF ILLNESS SCORING SYSTEM USED DAILY DURING RIBAVIRIN TREATMENT PERIOD TO ASSESS RESPONSE OF PATIENT SYMPTOMS AND SIGNS TO RIBAVIRIN THERAPY

System	Symptom or Sign	Clinical Scoring System[a]
Nose	Discharge	0 = absent or not evaluable
	Obstruction	1 = mild
		2 = moderate
Throat	Dysphagia	3 = severe
	Dysphonia	
	Exudate	
Chest	Retractions	
	Stridor	
	Rales	
	Tubular breath sounds	
	Cough	
	Rhonchi	
Gastrointestinal tract	Anorexia	
	Vomiting	
	Nausea	
	Diarrhea	
	Abdominal pain	
Other	Headache	
	Myalgias	
	Arthralgias	
	Rash	

[a]Assessed for each symptom or sign (potential maximum clinical score is 60).
(Courtesy of Conrad, D.A., et al.: Pediatr. Infect. Dis. J. 6:152–158, February 1987.)

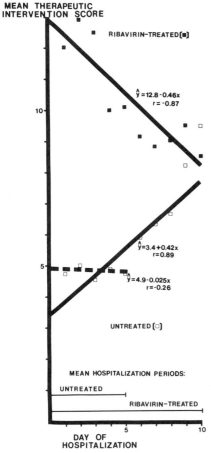

Fig 2–3.—Linear regression analysis of mean therapeutic intervention score vs. day of hospitalization for 33 ribavirin-treated patients (----) compared with linear regression analyses of 97 patient controls (——) for the mean hospitalization period. Patient control data were stratified by the mean control patient hospitalization period (5 days) and the mean ribavirin-treated patient hospitalization period (10 days), for analysis at both comparable intervals (mean hospitalization periods) and comparable absolute number of days of hospitalization. Rising slope of the line for untreated controls because of small patient numbers after day 6 ($n = 8$ for untreated controls at day 10). (Courtesy of Conrad, D.A., et al.: Pediatr. Infect. Dis. J. 6:152–158, February 1987.)

untreated hospitalized patients with RSV infection. Because of limited available supplies of aerosolized ribavirin, only seriously ill children were included in this study. A scoring system for grading the degree of illness by numerical gradation of signs pertinent to the infection was used to evaluate the response to ribavirin treatment (table).

Despite the selection of high-risk and severely ill infants for antiviral therapy, ribavirin-treated patients had a more rapid resolution of illness as determined by intervention scores than occurred in the untreated controls (Fig 2–3). The mean duration of ribavirin therapy was 5 days. The greatest clinical improvement in ribavirin-treated patients was noted between the first and second day of therapy. No adverse hematologic, hepatic, renal, or metabolic toxicities were observed in ribavirin-treated patients.

Aerosolized ribavirin is safe and effective in the treatment of RSV infection in infants and children. The optimum length of ribavirin therapy requires further study.

▶ This report and the study by Rodriguez and co-workers (*Pediatr. Infect. Dis.*

J. 6:159, 1987) serve to confirm the initial observations of Hall and associates that aerosolized ribavirin treatment is effective (see the 1985 YEAR BOOK, p. 113; 1987 YEAR BOOK, p. 103) in the treatment of respiratory syncytial virus-induced pulmonary disease. A consensus is beginning to emerge as to who needs this expensive form of treatment. Candidates for treatment include infants with bronchopulmonary dysplasia, patients with congenital heart disease, and patients with a variety of forms of chronic lung disease. Three days of therapy may be as effective, in many patients, as the 5-day course that was originally described.—F.A. Oski, M.D.

The Use of Eye-Nose Goggles to Control Nosocomial Respiratory Syncytial Virus Infection

Christine L. Gala, Caroline B. Hall, Kenneth C. Schnabel, Patricia H. Pincus, Pauline Blossom, Stephen W. Hildreth, Robert F. Betts, and R. Gordon Douglas, Jr. (Univ. of Rochester, Praxis Biologics, Rochester, and Cornell Univ., New York)
JAMA 256:2706–2708, Nov. 21, 1986   2–27

Although the nosocomial spread of respiratory syncytial virus (RSV) infection among infants in pediatric wards and nurseries has been reduced by modern infection control methods, the spread among staff remains high. Inoculation of the RSV may occur via the eye or nose but is unlikely to occur by mouth. The spread to staff members is not prevented by the use of gowns and paper face masks, because these measures only prevent the spread via the oral route. An attempt was made to determine whether disposable plastic goggles that cover the eyes and nose would help to reduce the rate of nosocomial infection during a community outbreak of RSV infection.

Infection was assessed by biweekly routine viral cultures of staff members who worked on the infant ward and in all infants admitted to that ward. Three blood samples to assess seroconversion were also obtained

TABLE 1.—FREQUENCY OF RESPIRATORY SYNCYTIAL VIRUS INFECTION IN
INFANTS WHO WERE HOSPITALIZED MORE THAN 7 DAYS AS DETECTED BY
VIRAL ISOLATION

Period	Total No. of Infants	No. of Infants Admitted With Respiratory Syncytial Virus (% of Admissions)	Total No.	Infant Contacts	
				No. (%) Hospitalized ≥7 d	No. (%) of Contacts Hospitalized ≥7 d With Nosocomial Infection
1	74	15 (20)	59	17 (29)	1 (6)†
2	77*	17 (22)	60	21 (35)	9 (43)†
Total	151	32 (21)	120	38 (32)	10 (21)

*Includes 13 children studied previously (12 in period 1, 1 in interim week) who did not acquire respiratory syncytial virus infection but were still hospitalized in period 2.
†Statistical significance, P = .04.
(Courtesy of Gala, C.L., et al.: JAMA 256:2706–08, Nov. 21, 1986.)

TABLE 2.—FREQUENCY OF RESPIRATORY SYNCYTIAL VIRUS INFECTION IN
HOSPITAL PERSONNEL AS DETECTED BY VIRAL ISOLATION AND SEROLOGY

| | | | No. (%) Infected According to | |
Period	No. of Staff Studied	No. Potentially Susceptible	Viral Isolation	Viral Isolation and Serology
1	40	40	2 (5)*	3 (8)†
2	41	39	11 (28)*	13 (34)†

*Statistical significance, P = .005.
†Statistical significance, P = .003.
(Courtesy of Gala, C.L., et al.: JAMA 256:2706–2708, Nov. 21, 1986.)

from staff members. A nosocomial infection was defined as a documented RSV infection first detected 7 or more days after admission to the ward. Clear goggles made of molded plastic were worn for 3 weeks by all staff members, but they were not used during the subsequent 3-week period.

During period 1 when goggles were worn, 2 of 40 staff members studied (5%) and 1 infant on the ward (6%) acquired nosocomial infection; during period 2 when goggles were not worn, 34% of the staff members studied and 43% of susceptible infants on the ward acquired nosocomial infection (Tables 1 and 2). Of the 13 staff members with documented RSV infection,

TABLE 3.—RATES OF NOSOCOMIAL RESPIRATORY SYNCYTIAL VIRUS (RSV)
INFECTION IN INFANTS AND STAFF AS DETERMINED BY VIRAL ISOLATION BY
YEAR AND INFECTION CONTROL TECHNIQUES USED

| | | Infants | | Staff | |
Year	Techniques	No.	No. (%) With Nosocomial RSV Infection	No.	No. (%) With RSV Infection
1975	Hand washing, gowns, open ward	44	14 (32)	24	10 (42)
1976	Hand washing, cohorting, gowns, isolation of infected infants	42	8 (19)	43	24 (56)
1977	Hand washing, cohorting, gowns	66	23 (35)	53	18 (34)
1980 (Period 1)	Hand washing, cohorting, isolation of infected infants, IFA testing*, gowns, paper face masks	25	8 (32)	30	10 (33)
1980 (Period 2)	Hand washing, cohorting, isolation of infected infants, IFA testing	27	11 (41)	26	11 (42)
1984 (Period 1)	Hand washing, cohorting, isolation of infected infants, IFA testing, eye-nose goggles	17	1 (6)	40	2 (5)
1984 (Period 2)	Hand washing, cohorting, isolation of infected infants, IFA testing	21	9 (43)	39	11 (28)

*IFA, indirect fluorescent antibody.
(Courtesy of Gala, C.L., et al.: JAMA 256:2706–2708, Nov. 21, 1986.)

31% were sick enough to miss work, 31% were sick but kept on working, and 38% had minor symptoms or were asymptomatic. For comparison, the rates of nosocomial infection in the staff and patients during the past 10 years were reviewed (Table 3).

▶ Viral spread via the eyes and nose is now being recognized more commonly. The use of goggles, in fact, has been proposed for medical personnel taking care of patients with HIV infection to prevent the inadvertent spread of virus from blood or contaminated secretions hitting the eye. The use of gogles to prevent the nosocomial spread of RSV seems like an attractive concept. The goggles will also have to be made attractive to appeal to the nursing staff and physicians who will be asked to use them. Many doctors have been accused of wearing blinders, so why not goggles?—F.A. Oski, M.D.

Clinical Features of Acute Gastroenteritis Associated With Rotavirus, Enteric Adenoviruses, and Bacteria
I. Uhnoo, E. Olding-Stenkvist, and A. Kreuger (Univ. Hosp., Uppsala, Sweden)
Arch. Dis. Child. 61:732–738, August 1986   2–28

Rotavirus has emerged as the single most important cause of pediatric diarrhea. The etiology and epidemiology of acute gastroenteritis in 416 children admitted to the hospital or treated as outpatients were studied during a year-long prospective study. A comparative analysis was undertaken of the clinical and laboratory features of diarrhea caused by rotavirus infections and those of enteric adenovirus, bacterial, mixed, and nonspecific infections.

Rotavirus was the most commonly identified agent. Rotavirus gastroenteritis was characterized by a sudden onset of vomiting, high frequency of fever and dehydration, and low occurrence of abdominal pain. The disease was milder in outpatients, because there was less pronounced vomiting. The mean duration of illness was 5.9 days. In contrast, enteric adenoviruses caused milder disease and patients predominantly had persistent diarrhea (mean, 10.8 days). Abdominal pain, bloody stools, prolonged diarrhea, leukocytosis, and a raised erythrocyte sedimentation rate strongly suggested a bacterial etiology. Compared with the others, the disease of bacterial origin caused a longer duration of fever, less prolonged vomiting, and the longest duration of diarrhea. Except for longer-lasting diarrhea (mean, 8 days), the clinical pattern of diarrhea caused by mixed infections was almost identical to that of rotavirus. The most common combination of dual pathogens was enteropathogenic *Escherichia coli* and rotavirus. Those with nonspecific gastroenteritis had symptoms similar to those of the bacterial group, although the disease was milder and only a few patients were hospitalized. There were no significant differences in the occurrence of respiratory symptoms among groups. Compared with others, patients with rotavirus and those with bacterial infections were regarded as moderately or severely ill. Hypernatremia and severe dehydration were rare. Prolonged diarrhea and temporary secondary lactose intolerance were the most common sequelae. The clinical course of acute gastroenteritis with rotavirus, enteric adenoviruses, and pathogenic bacteria is associated with features that enable the clinician to make a presumptive diagnosis.

▶ Dr. Robert Yolken, Associate Professor of Pediatrics, and Chief, Division of Pediatric Infectious Disease, Johns Hopkins University School of Medicine, comments.—F.A. Oski, M.D.

▶ It is often desirable to know the cause of acute gastroenteritis in order to institute proper epidemiologic investigations and infection control procedures. Identification of the etiologic agent of acute gastroenteritis is made more difficult by the fact that diarrheal disease in children can be caused by a number of viral, bacterial, and parasitic organisms. The work of Uhnoo and her collaborators addresses a question that is often asked about acute gastroenteritis, namely: Can a physician make an educated guess as to the causative organism of the patient's gastroenteritis on the basis of history, clinical symptoms, and common laboratory parameters such as leukocyte and sedimentation rate?

Their finding that gastroenteritis associated with rotaviruses, enteric adenoviruses, and enteric bacteria present as identifiable syndromes will be useful to physicians caring for children with these syndromes. However, it should be pointed out that the authors found a fair amount of overlap among the syndromes. For example, although elevated sedimentation rates (more than 20 mm/hour) were statistically more likely to be associated with episodes of bacterial, rather than viral, diarrheas, 16% of the episodes of gastroenteritis caused by rotaviruses were still associated with this finding. Similarly, associated respiratory symptoms, which at various times have been associated with infections with rotaviruses and other viruses, were also found to be associated with episodes of bacterial gastroenteritis. I thus think that specific diagnostic procedures (e.g., the enzyme-linked immunosorbent assay and latex agglutination assays) should be used when a specific diagnosis is required.

It should be pointed out that, despite the use of extensive microbiologic, immunologic, and electron microscopic analyses, the authors could not identify an etiologic agent in 32% of the children studied. This fact suggests that our techniques for finding exiting agents need to be improved and/or that there are still a number of agents of infantile gastroenteritis that remain to be characterized.—R. Yolken, M.D.

Plague Masquerading as Gastrointestinal Illness
Harry F. Hull, Jean M. Montes, and Jonathan M. Mann (New Mexico Health and Environment Dept., Santa Fe)
West. J. Med. 145:485–487, October 1986   2–29

The classic symptoms of plague are fever and tender lymphadenitis; gastrointestinal tract symptoms are generally not mentioned. However, a number of patients were seen with laboratory-confirmed plague who had gastrointestinal symptoms as the predominant or sole clinical manifestation of the disease. A review was made of the records of patients with plague originating in New Mexico during a 5-year period.

Of 71 reports of human plague, 65 (92%) included information on gastrointestinal symptoms. Of the 65 patients, 47 (72%) had bubonic plague and 18 (28%) had septicemic plague. All 65 patients had clinical symptoms consistent with *Yersinia pestis* infection, which was confirmed by bacterial culture, fluorescent antibody stain for *Yersinia pestis* on non-viable clinical material, and passive hemagglutination titers. Gastrointestinal tract symptoms included nausea, vomiting, diarrhea, and abdominal pain.

There were no significant differences between patients with and without gastrointestinal tract symptoms as to age, sex, race, case-fatality rate, month of onset, prevalence of secondary plague pneumonia, or time of onset to first physician visit or hospital admission. Fever was a universal symptom and 40% of all patients had malaise. Chills and headache occurred more often in those with gastrointestinal symptoms (60% and 54%, respectively) than in those without such symptoms (39% and 25%, respectively). Gastrointestinal symptoms were more common in patients with septicemic than with bubonic plague. Gastrointestinal symptoms usually occurred early in the course of the illness, sometimes preceding the appearance of lymphadenopathy or lymph node pain in patients with bubonic plague. Plague should be considered in the differential diagnosis of patients who present with fever and gastrointestinal tract symptoms if they live in rural areas in the American West, or if they have been exposed within the preceding week prior to presentation to plague vectors, e.g., wild rodents and free-roaming domestic dogs or cats.

Serum Transaminase Elevations in Infants With Rotavirus Gastroenteritis
Andrea Kovacs, Linda Chan, Chiraporn Hotrakitya, Gary Overturf, and Bernard Portnoy (Univ. of Southern California)
J. Pediatr. Gastroenterol. Nutr. 5:873–877, November–December 1986   2–30

The development of human rotavirus (HRV) antigen detection tests allows the efficient diagnosis of HRV gastroenteritis in infants with infectious diarrhea. In an evaluation of the efficacy of the Rotazyme test as a diagnostic aid, it was reported that many infants with HRV gastroenteritis had elevated serum levels of transaminase. However, this abnormality had been reported in only a few patients during earlier studies of HRV. The significance of the mild transaminase elevations seen in many hospitalized infants with HRV gastroenteritis was examined during a 6-week period.

The study included 86 infants aged from 1 month to 22 months with diarrheal illness associated with mild to severe dehydration. The presence of HRV was determined with the Rotazyme test. Concentrations of alanine aminotransferase (ALT) and aspartate aminotransferase (AST) were also determined.

Thirty-five of the 86 infants (41%) were found to have HRV gastroenteritis. On admission, disease-positive infants had higher mean and median levels of ALT and AST than did disease-negative infants (Table 1). The concentrations of ALT and AST did not correlate with the degree of de-

TABLE 1.—CONCENTRATIONS OF ALT AND AST ON ADMISSION AND DURING FIRST 3 DAYS OF HOSPITALIZATION

	On admission			Maximum*		
Parameter/Statistics	Rotazyme + (35)	Rotazyme − (51)	p Value	Rotazyme + (35)	Rotazyme − (51)	p Value
ALT (SGPT)						
Number of cases with transaminases	18	26		31	41	
Mean concentration (SE)	87.5 (20.9)	50.0 (8.45)	.07† .001‡	76.8 (13.1)	64.8 (11.9)	.50† .02‡
Median concentration	60	41	.002§	56	43	.01§
Range	39–409	9–233		24–409	21–475	
AST (SGOT)						
Number of cases with transaminases	18	25		30	41	
Mean concentration (SE)	64.3 (6.46)	44.0 (3.82)	.007† .008‡	64.1 (4.64)	55.0 (5.07)	.21† .02‡
Median concentration	67.5	42	<.05§	62.5	49	.13§
Range	22–141	19–92		33–141	19–191	

SGOT, serum glutamic oxaloacetic transaminase; *SGPT*, serum glutamic pyruvic transaminase.
Numbers.in parentheses, total number of patients.
*Highest of first three performed.
†Student's two-sample test.
‡Mann-Whitney U test.
§Median test.
(Courtesy of Kovacs, A., et al.: J. Pediatr. Gastroenterol. Nutr. 5:873–877, November–December 1986.)

hydration or electrolyte imbalance (Table 2). The findings suggest that elevated levels of serum transaminase are common in infants hospitalized with HRV gastroenteritis.

Management of Children Hospitalized for Laryngotracheobronchitis

Jeffrey S. Wagener, Louis I. Landau, Anthony Olinsky, and Peter D. Phelan (Royal Children's Hosp., Victoria, Australia)
Pediatr. Pulmonol. 2:159–162, May–June 1986   2–31

TABLE 2.—RELATIONSHIP OF CONCENTRATIONS OF ALT AND AST TO SEVERITY OF CLINICAL DEHYDRATION

	Severity of dehydration*			
Parameter/Statistics	Mild	Moderate	Severe	p Value
Max ALT†				
Number of cases (72)	23	37	8	
Mean concentration (SE)	72.2 (19.5)	62.0 (7.1)	107.1 (44.9)	.31‡ .59§
Median concentration	48	51	66	.64¶
Range	22–47ᶜ	24–233	62–409	
Max AST†				
Number of cases (71)	23	36	8	
Mean concentration (SE)	60.8 (6.5)	54.6 (3.7)	67.5 (11.8)	.41‡ .57§
Median concentration	58	50	58.5	.40¶
Range	22–191	19–141	33–120	

*Dehydration as defined by Finberg: mild = 5%, moderate = 10%, severe = 15%.
†Highest of first three performed.
‡Analysis of variance.
§Kruskal-Wallis test.
¶Median one-way analysis.
(Courtesy of Kovacs, A., et al.: J. Pediatr. Gastroenterol. Nutr. 5:873–877, November–December 1986.)

The treatment of viral laryngotracheobronchitis (LTB) in children remains controversial. In an effort to provide guidelines for future therapeutic studies, 527 consecutive admissions for 498 patients with LTB during a year-long period were evaluated to determine the epidemiology of hospitalized LTB patients and to identify those who may benefit from therapy other than close observation.

Of the 442 viral cultures, 70% were positive. Disease severity at the time of admission was unrelated to age or sex, but the duration of hospitalization was inversely related to age. Routine laboratory investigations were rarely abnormal or of therapeutic value. Patients who had stridor but no sternal or chest retractions recovered rapidly and spontaneously; 48% were discharged within 48 hours of admission, only 1% had worsening respiratory distress after admission, and none required artificial airways. Of the patients who had stridor at rest and sternal and chest wall retractions, 49% experienced progressive airway obstruction, 81% required longer hospitalization, and 6% needed artificial airways. These patients frequently received medical intervention, e.g., aqueous mist therapy or racemic epinephrine. Half of the patients with severe respiratory distress on admission and older than 6 years of age were successfully treated with a single dose of racemic epinephrine.

Children with LTB who have stridor but no sternal or chest wall retractions recover rapidly with observation only. Children with stridor and sternal and chest wall retractions, as well as the younger patient, benefit from medical intervention, e.g., aqueous mist, racemic epinephrine, or steroids. Laboratory examination rarely influences the diagnosis or management of patients with clinically typical viral LTB.

▶ Dr. Robert K. Kanter, Associate Professor of Pediatrics, College of Medicine, Health Science Center at Syracuse, State University of New York, and Director, Pediatric Intensive Care Unit, comments.—F.A. Oski, M.D.

▶ Viral laryngotracheobronchitis is an important cause of hospitalization and morbidity in otherwise healthy children. Occasionally, it results in life-threatening airway obstruction. So it is frustrating that we still have so little objective demonstration of the benefit of routine treatment. This study by Wagener et al. identifies a low-risk group—those without chest wall or sternal retractions. These children have so little chance of deterioration that they should be stratified separately or excluded in studies of therapy for LTB because they will probably recover without any special intervention.

Several issues in the management of LTB need further clarification. What is the place of x-rays in evaluating patients? Chest and lateral neck x-rays are normal in more than half of the patients with LTB. Erroneous impressions of epiglottitis in 23% of those with LTB place children at risk for unnecessary anesthesia and airway instrumentation (Stankiewicz J.A., et al.: *Laryngoscope* 95:1159, 1985). Slightly oblique views of the epiglottis may account for some of these false positive readings.

What is the role and potential mechanism of action of humidifying inhaled gas in LTB? Any benefit of breathing mist was too slight to detect in Bourchier's study of 16 children with croup (*Aust. Paediatr. J.* 20:289, 1984). Although antibiotics are of no benefit in this viral illness, their inappropriate use continues (Pianosi, P.: *Can. Med. Assoc. J.* 134:357, 1986). For the children with the most severe airway obstruction requiring an artificial airway, bacteriologic investigation of tracheal secretions may identify the few with bacterial tracheitis.

It is also worth remembering that a respiratory infection that may be caused by the influenza virus can also be complicated by the overgrowth of *Staphylococcus aureus*. Toxic shock syndrome has been recognized in some patients with this sequence of events (Dan, B.: *JAMA* 257:1094, 1987).—R.K. Kanter, M.D.

Measles Outbreak in a Fully Immunized Secondary-School Population
Tracy L. Gustafson, Alan W. Lievens, Philip A. Brunell, Ronald G. Moellenberg, Christopher M. G. Buttery, and Lynne M. Sehulster (Texas Dept. of Health, Austin, Univ. of Texas at San Antonio, and Corpus Christi-Nueces County Health Dept., Corpus Christi, Tex.)
N. Engl. J. Med. 316:771–774, March 26, 1987   2–32

Outbreaks of measles continue to occur in adolescent school populations despite school immunization requirements in all states. An outbreak occurring in Corpus Christi, Texas, in 1985, where vaccination requirements for school attendance had been enforced, was investigated. Sera were obtained from 1,806 students at two secondary schools, 8 days after the onset of the first infection. In all, 157 measles infections were reported in the county in the next 3 months, two thirds of them in children aged 10–19 years.

Only 4.1% of the students studied lacked detectable measles antibody on enzyme-linked immunosorbent assay. More than 99% had been vaccinated with live measles vaccine. The number of doses was the chief predictor of the antibody response. Seronegative rates were as high as 7% in students given only one dose of vaccine, compared with none to 3.3% in those given two doses. None of 1,732 seropositive patients contracted measles after the survey, but 14 of 74 seronegative students, all of them vaccinated previously, did so. Three seronegative students seroconverted without having symptoms.

Outbreaks of measles may occur in secondary schools despite vaccination of more than 99% of the students and the presence of immunity in more than 95% of the school population. Seronegativity was associated with receipt of only one dose of vaccine in the present study. Possible factors in these outbreaks include a decline in vaccine-induced immunity over time, immunization at too young an age, and more efficient transmission of infection than in younger populations.

▶ A quote from the *MMWR* (36:305, 1987) seems in order:
"Although the number of measles cases reported in 1986 is still only about 2% of that in the prevaccine era, the increase in the number of cases in 1986

is of concern. There may be many reasons for this large increase; however, unvaccinated preschool-aged children and vaccine failures in school-aged children are two of the major ones.... A substantial proportion of cases continue to occur in appropriately vaccinated individuals. A variety of different strategies have been suggested to decrease the number of these cases, including a routine 2-dose schedule and mass or selective revaccination either routinely or during an outbreak. Because only a small percentage of persons who were vaccinated at more than 12 months of age are susceptible and because identification of these susceptible persons is difficult, all these strategies would result in administration of a large proportion of vaccine to persons who are already immune. Some studies have demonstrated lower vaccine efficacy and higher attack rates in persons vaccinated at 12–14 months of age compared with those vaccinated at the currently recommended age of 15 months. While routine revaccination of persons vaccinated at 12–14 months of age is not recommended, revaccination during selected outbreaks, particularly those in junior and senior high schools, may be considered."

This year we learned that the vast majority of adverse reactions occurring after immunization of children with live measles-mumps-rubella (MMR) vaccine were only temporally, not causally, related to the vaccination. The true frequency of side effects was between 0.5% and 4.0%. Respiratory symptoms, nausea, and vomiting were observed more frequently in the placebo-injected group than in the MMR-vaccinated group (Peltola, H., et al.: *Lancet* 1:939, 1987). Keep children away from those placebos.—F.A. Oski, M.D.

The Treatment of Kawasaki Syndrome With Intravenous Gamma Globulin
Jane W. Newburger, Masato Takahashi, Jane C. Burns, Alexa S. Beiser, Kyung Ja Chung, C. Elise Duffy, Mary P. Glode, Wilbert H. Mason, Venudhar Reddy, Stephen P. Sanders, Stanford T. Shulman, James W. Wiggins, Raquel V. Hicks, David R. Fulton, Alan B. Lewis, Donald Y.M. Leung, Theodore Colton, Fred S. Rosen, and Marian E. Melish (Harvard Univ. and various other universities and hospitals in the United States)
N. Engl. J. Med. 315:341–347, Aug. 7, 1986   2–33

Kawasaki syndrome, an acute illness of unknown etiology seen mostly in infancy and early childhood, is associated with the development of coronary artery aneurysms or ectasia in about 15% to 25% of all patients. Treatment consists mainly of aspirin administration, but aspirin does not appear to reduce the incidence of coronary artery complications. A multicenter, randomized, clinical comparison of the frequency of coronary artery abnormalities and degree of systemic inflammation with intravenous γ-globulin therapy plus aspirin and aspirin alone was conducted.

The series included 168 children who were randomly divided into two treatment groups of 84 each. Criteria for enrollment in the trial included fever, nonexudative conjunctivitis, oropharyngeal changes, rash, and cervical adenopathy. One group was given intravenous γ-globulin therapy plus aspirin and the other was given only aspirin. The aspirin dosage for both groups was 100 mg/kg/day, administered every 6 hours through day

14. On day 15 the dosage was reduced to 3–5 mg/kg/day. The γ-globulin dosage was 400 mg/kg/day, given over 2 hours on 4 consecutive days. Echocardiography was used to assess the presence of coronary artery abnormalities.

Two weeks after enrollment in the study, 18 children (23%) in the aspirin group had coronary artery abnormalities, compared with 6 (8%) in the combination treatment group. Seven weeks into the study, 14 children (18%) in the aspirin group had coronary artery abnormalities, compared with 3 (4%) in the combination treatment group. Inflammation resolved more rapidly in children given γ-globulin. No child experienced serious side effects from γ-globulin treatment. One child had shaking chills and itching after the first γ-globulin injection, but these effects resolved after diphenhydramine administration. Intravenous γ-globulin injection is a safe, effective treatment for the reduction of coronary artery abnormalities in children with Kawasaki syndrome.

▶ What goes around, comes around. The article abstracted above confirms the original Japanese observation. Now the Japanese have confirmed our observation (Nagashima, N., et al.: *J. Pediatr.* 110:710, 1987), concluding that intravenous gammaglobulin (IVGG) therapy improves the outcome of Kawasaki syndrome. In a randomized, controlled study of 136 patients, treatment with IVGG (400 mg/kg/day for 3 days) plus aspirin (30 mg/kg/day) produced a significantly shorter febrile period and reduced significantly the incidence of coronary artery lesions when compared with treatment with aspirin alone. The incidence of coronary lesions at 30 days after onset of treatment was 15.9% in the IVGG group and 37.3% in the control group. In 16 of the 69 patients given IVGG, fever persisted for longer than 3 days, and this subgroup had a higher incidence of coronary artery lesions. Should everybody with Kawasaki syndrome get IVGG? The answer appears to be "yes" until we can identify groups at greatest risk. It has been proposed that the use of three variables—age at time of onset, platelet count at diagnosis, and serum concentration of C-reactive protein—can produce a scoring system that predicts patients at high risk for coronary lesions (Nakano, H., et al.: *Am. J. Cardiol.* 58:739, 1986). Time will tell. Meanwhile, it is reassuring to learn that while we can't duplicate Japanese cars, VCRs, and television sets, we can duplicate the findings of clinical investigation. Let the good times roll!—F.A. Oski, M.D.

Reversal of Lymphocyte Activation In Vivo in the Kawasaki Syndrome by Intravenous Gammaglobulin

Donald Y.M. Leung, Jane C. Burns, Jane W. Newburger, and Raif S. Geha (The Children's Hosp., Boston, and Harvard Univ.)

J. Clin. Invest. 79:468–472, February 1987   2–34

Aspirin is not of proved efficacy in Kawasaki syndrome, but high intravenous doses of gamma globulin reportedly reduce the occurrence of coronary artery aneurysms when given in the acute phase of the disease. Immune abnormalities of circulating lymphocytes have been described in

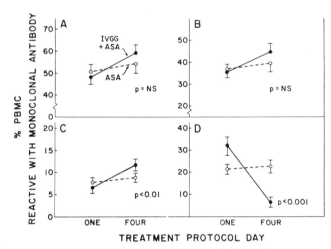

Fig 2–4.—A, Leu 4+ T cells; B, Leu 3+ T cells; C, Leu 2+ T cells; D, DR+ Leu 3+ T cells. Shown are T cell populations in 14 patients with Kawasaki syndrome treated with aspirin and 15 such patients treated with aspirin plus gamma globulin intravenously (ASA + IVGG). Values are expressed as the mean ± SEM. P values comparing the changes in monoclonal antibody binding between day 1 and day 4 of each treatment protocol are shown. (Courtesy of Leung, D.Y.M., et al.: J. Clin. Invest. 79:468–472, February 1987.)

this disease. The effects of aspirin alone and aspirin plus gamma globulin intravenously on immunoregulatory abnormalities were studied in 29 patients with Kawasaki syndrome seen without 10 days of onset of fever. Aspirin was given in a dose of 100 mg/kg daily for 2 weeks and then 3–5 mg/kg daily. Study patients also received gamma globulin, 400 mg/kg, intravenously daily for 4 consecutive days. The two treatment groups were clinically comparable.

Patients given gamma globulin had a significant reduction in helper cells and an increase in suppressor/cytotoxic T cells (Fig 2–4), as well as reduced spontaneous IgG and IgM synthesis. Secretion of T cell-derived B cell helper factors was reduced in these patients (Fig 2–5). Immune parameters did not change significantly in the patients given aspirin alone. High intravenous doses of gamma globulin suppress the activation of T and B cells in patients with acute Kawasaki syndrome. This treatment may prevent the development of coronary artery aneurysms by interrupting the immunologic events that result in vessel injury at several sites. The reduction in T cell activation and in lymphokine secretion should decrease the expression of new surface antigens on the vascular endothelium. In addition, the formation of antibodies to neoantigens on endothelial cells is inhibited. Gamma globulin also could reduce immune complex binding to reticuloendothelial cells by itself binding to Fc receptors of these cells.

▶ It always comes as a pleasant surprise to learn that seemingly empiric therapy may have a rational basis for working. It will be even better when we have some understanding of the cause of Kawasaki syndrome. It has been proposed (Burns, J. C., et al.: *Nature* 323:814) that the syndrome is caused by a lym-

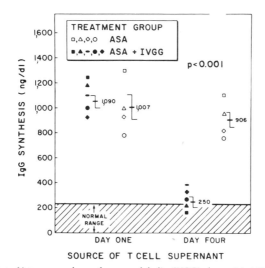

Fig 2–5.—Effect of intravenous doses of gamma globulin (IVGG) plus aspirin (ASA) and that of ASA treatment alone on the generation of B cell helper factors by T cells. Data points indicate the mean IgG production of triplicate cultures induced by T cell supernatants from individual patients with Kawasaki syndrome. The cross-hatched area represents the mean ± SD of IgG production induced by T cell supernatants from five normal donors. The mean ± SEM is shown for each group. Between enrollment and protocol day 4, T cells from patients treated with IVGG plus ASA had a significantly greater decrease in their capacity to secrete B cell helper factor ($P < .001$) than T cells from patients treated exclusively with ASA. (Courtesy of Leung, D.Y.M., et al.: J. Clin. Invest. 79:468–472, February 1987.)

photropic retrovirus. Retrovirus-associated reverse transcriptase was found in the particulate fraction from culture supernatants of peripheral blood mononuclear cells obtained from some patients with the disease. Meanwhile, it has been proposed by Moynahan (*Lancet* 1:195, 1987) that a feline retrovirus virus carried by a flea is the etiologic agent in this disease. Cats are the most popular pet in Japan. Come to think of it, I have never seen a patient with Kawasaki syndrome who didn't either have a cat or come into contact with one. We (read, I) have now linked cats to both acquired immunodeficiency syndrome and Kawasaki syndrome. Take your pick.—F.A. Oski, M.D.

Treatment of Adenosine Deaminase Deficiency With Polyethylene Glycol-Modified Adenosine Deaminase

Michael S. Hershfield, Rebecca H. Buckley, Michael L. Greenberg, Alton L. Melton, Richard Schiff, Christine Hatem, Joanne Kurtzberg, M. Louise Markert, Roger H. Kobayashi, Ai Lan Kobayashi, and Abraham Abuchowski (Duke Univ., Univ. of Nebraska, and Enzon, Inc., South Plainfield, N.J.)

N. Engl. J. Med. 316:589–596, March 5, 1987   2–35

Severe combined immunodeficiency disease associated with inherited adenosine deaminase (ADA) deficiency often is fatal, but marrow transplantation is effective in some instances. It is possible theoretically to reduce levels of toxic metabolites in ADA-deficient cells by providing exogenous

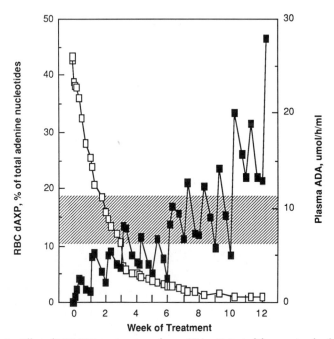

Fig 2–6.—Effect of PEG-ADA treatment on plasma ADA activity *(solid squares)* and red blood cell deoxyadenosyl nucleotides (dAXP, *open squares*). The latter is expressed as a percentage of total red blood cell adenine ribonucleotides plus deoxyribonucleotides. The *hatched area* represents the range of blood (erythrocyte) ADA activity in normal individuals. (Courtesy of Hershfield, M.S., et al.: N. Engl. J. Med. 316:589–596, March 5, 1987.)

ADA. Covalent attachment of polyethylene glycol (PEG) prevents access to sites on protein surfaces, inhibiting circulatory clearance and attack by degradative enzymes. Adding PEG to bovine ADA decreases its immunogenicity in mice and markedly prolongs its plasma half-life.

Two children with ADA deficiency and severe combined immunodeficiency disease received injections of bovine ADA modified by conjugation with PEG. The modified enzyme had a plasma half-life of 48–72 hours after intramuscular injection. Weekly doses of about 15 units per kg maintained plasma ADA activity at two to three times the level of red blood cell ADA activity in normal persons (Fig 2–6). The biochemical effects of ADA deficiency were nearly completely reversed, without apparent toxic effects or hypersensitivity. Markedly improved cellular immunity (Fig 2–7) and increases in circulating T lymphocytes were observed. The patients were not infected and they resumed gaining weight.

Injections of PEG-modified ADA appear preferable to red blood cell transfusion in treating ADA deficiency. The PEG-modified enzymes might also prove useful in treatment of purine nucleoside phosphorylase deficiency, Gaucher's disease, Fabry's disease, and disorders of amino acid and urea cycle metabolism in which accumulated metabolites equilibrate with plasma.

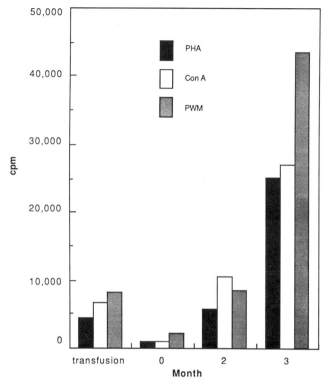

Fig 2–7.—Response of peripheral blood mononuclear cells to mitogens during treatment. "Transfusion" refers to an assay performed 10 months before the start of treatment with PEG-ADA when the patient was receiving monthly transfusions of irradiated erythrocytes. (Courtesy of Hershfield, M.S., et al.: N. Engl. J. Med. 316:589–596, March 5, 1987.)

Estimated Effects of a Delay in the Recommended Vaccination Schedule for Diphtheria and Tetanus Toxoids and Pertussis Vaccine

Ann W. Funkhouser, Steven G.F. Wassilak, Walter A. Orenstein, Alan R. Hinman, and Edward A. Mortimer, Jr. (Case-Western Reserve Univ. and Centers for Disease Control)

JAMA 257:1341–1346, March 13, 1987   2–36

The serious clinical effects occasionally noted with routine diphtheria-tetanus-pertussis (DTP) vaccination have suggested a delay in the initial schedule for immunization. Both sudden infant death syndrome and infantile spasms are less frequent in the second 6 months of life than in the first 6 months. A decision analytic model of the projected effect of delaying immunization was used to assess the effects of such delay. Recommended initial doses of DTP were delayed from 2, 4, and 6 months to 8, 10, and 12 months of age.

Analysis of the model indicated that an additional 636 cases of pertussis would occur under the proposed schedule compared with the current one.

Among these, 115 would be associated with complications, including two cases of encephalopathy. Adverse medical effects of the vaccine were assumed to be unchanged. There were 353 fewer chance associations with sudden infant death syndrome projected, but 1,311 more chance associations with seizures.

Analysis of this inferential model suggests that the current schedule of immunizing infants with DPT at ages 2, 4, and 6 months should be continued and that a delay in immunization would be expected to increase morbidity. Both complications and pertussis itself would be more frequent with delayed immunization.

▶ This is a very interesting analysis, but for those who are not reassured by numbers, help may be on the way. An acellular pertussis component diphtheria-tetanus (AC-DTP) vaccine has been found to be less reactogenic, but as immunogenic, as the standard DTP vaccine when given to 18-month-old infants in the United States as their booster shot (Lewis, K., et al.: *Am. J. Dis. Child.* 140:872, 1986). Field trials begun in Sweden in 1986, and trials here in the United States, will tell us shortly how effective and safe this preparation is when used in our current immunization schedules. There is a great deal of experience with acellular pertussis vaccine in Japan, but it has usually been given to infants between 1 and 2 years of age (see a review of subject by Noble, G.R., et al.: *JAMA* 257:1351, 1987).

For the present, we should follow the ACIP recommendations that suggest that DTP vaccine not be given to the following: (1) children who have experienced an adverse reaction to early shots—an adverse reaction is defined as a convulsion, prolonged period of unusual high-pitched crying, or collapse and a shocklike state; (2) a patient with progressive developmental delay or changing CNS findings; (3) a patient with a recent history (3 days) of convulsions or encephalopathy; (4) a patient with a CNS disorder that predisposes to progressive deterioration or convulsions, not conditions such as prematurity or cerebral palsy.—F.A. Oski, M.D.

3 Nutrition and Metabolism

Milk Consumption and Hydration Status of Exclusively Breast-Fed Infants in a Warm Climate
Kenneth H. Brown, Hilary Creed de Kanashiro, Roberto del Aguila, Guillermo Lopez de Romana, and Robert E. Black (Johns Hopkins Univ. and Instituto de Investigacion Nutricional, Lima, Peru)
J. Pediatr. 108:677–680, May 1986   3–1

The adequacy of breast-feeding as a sole source of water under extreme environmental conditions has been questioned. Theoretically, considering the renal solute load of human milk and the normal insensible losses by infants, the healthy infant free of diarrhea or other causes of fluid loss should be able to maintain water homeostasis despite extreme environmental changes. To document these theoretical calculations, the hydration status of 40 exclusively breast-fed Peruvian infants was assessed through measurements of milk intake and urinary volume and concentration during 8-hour daytime observations. Maximum home temperatures ranged from 26–33 C, and relative humidity ranged from 49% to 96%.

The mean age was 2.4 months, and all 40 infants were within normal limits of weight for length (Table 1). Milk consumption ranged from 105 gm to 528 gm during the observation period and standardized milk intakes ranged from 4.0 gm/kg/hour to 12.1 gm/kg/hour (Table 2). Urine volumes ranged from 0.9 ml/kg/hour to 6.3 ml/kg/hour (mean, 3.4 ml/kg/hour). The amount of milk consumed correlated positively with the number of voids and the total volume of urine. Maximum urinary specific gravity ranged from 1.003 to 1.017, correlated positively with age, and correlated negatively with the number of voids, total urinary volume, standardized

TABLE 1.—CHARACTERISTICS OF INFANTS IN STUDY POPULATION

	Age (completed mo) (n = 40)	Weight (kg) (n = 40)	Length* (cm) (n = 38)	L/A* (Z) (n = 38)	W/L* (Z) (n = 36)
Mean ± SD	2.4 ± 1.6	5.6 ± 1.6	59.4 ± 5.8	0.47 ± 0.98	0.04 ± 0.75
Minimum	0	2.3	46.3	−2.84	−1.58
Maximum	6	8.0	69.4	2.42	1.59

*Proportion of expected length-for-age (L/A) and weight-for-length (W/L) presented as SD (Z) scores in relation to NCHS reference data, for example, Actual length (cm) − NCHS expected length for age/NCHS SD length for age.
Length not measured in two infants, and measured lengths were below lower limits of NCHS reference data for expected weight-for-length in two others.
(Courtesy of Brown, K.H., et al.: J. Pediatr. 108:677–680, May 1986.)

TABLE 2.—Consumption of Breast Milk
by 40 Infants During 8–9 Hours
of Daytime Observation

Amount of milk consumed

	gm	gm/hr	gm/kg body weight/hr
Mean ± SD	340.3 ± 87.2	40.7 ± 10.6	7.5 ± 1.7
Minimum	105	13.1	4.0
Maximum	528	60.7	12.1

(Courtesy of Brown, K.H., et al.: J. Pediatr. 108:677–680, May 1986.)

urinary volume, and milk intake. No significant correlations were found between ambient temperature and any of the urine variables. These findings indicate that exclusively breast-fed healthy infants can maintain adequate hydration status even in hot and humid environments.

▶ Two previous studies of the urinary concentrations in limited numbers of exclusively breast-fed infants in very warm environments (*Am. J. Clin. Nutr.* 31:1154,1978; *Clin. Pediatr.* 18:424, 1979) have also demonstrated that these babies do not require supplemental water. Giving supplemental water to a breast-fed baby during the first days of life does nothing to reduce the degree of hyperbilirubinemia (1983 YEAR BOOK, p. 25). It has been said that if God wanted breast-fed babies to receive water supplements, he would have provided women with a third breast that only produced water.—F.A. Oski, M.D.

Infant Self-Regulation of Breast Milk Intake
K.G. Dewey and B. Lönnerdal (Univ. of California at Davis)
Acta Paediatr. Scand. 75:893–898, November 1986   3–2

Milk intake among normal, exclusively breast-fed infants varies widely; whether this is because of maternal supply or infant demand is unknown. A study was undertaken to determine whether breast milk production can be increased through regular expression of extra milk, and whether augmentation of the maternal milk supply affects infant intake. Eighteen mothers of exclusively breast-fed infants stimulated milk supply by daily expression of extra milk for 2 weeks. Infant milk intake was measured before, during, and after this expression phase.

Fourteen (78%) mothers increased milk production by more than 73 gm daily over the baseline value (average, 124 gm/day). Infants of these mothers significantly increased their intake immediately after the expression phase compared with the baseline intake (average, 849 gm/day vs. 732 gm/day). However, half of them returned to their baseline levels of milk intake after 1–2 weeks. Similarly, infants with relatively low milk intakes during baseline were no more likely than other infants to respond to an increased milk supply. Change in milk intake was positively correlated with weight for length and age of the infant at the end of the expression phase and was unrelated to the baseline milk intake.

The wide range in milk intake in well-nourished, exclusively breast-fed infants results from infant self-regulation of milk intake. It appears that variations in milk intake result more from infant demand than from inadequacy of milk production by mothers.

▶ We have learned from the elegant studies of Butte et al. and Dewey and co-workers (see 1985 YEAR BOOK, PP. 415–418) that the exclusively breast-fed infant requires far fewer calories and less protein for adequate growth than had been believed previously and less than the infant who is artificially fed. We now learn that the low milk volumes found in some mothers may reflect insufficient infant demand rather than insufficient maternal production capacity. The authors close with the following: "Further investigations are needed to test the idea that when a mother is strongly motivated to breast-feed, it is the infant who is the main determinant of lactation performance."

You can lead a horse to water . . . but when you can get him to jump in and float on his back you have really accomplished something.

By the way, perhaps the best pediatric anecdote of the year involves breast-feeding. It appeared in *The New Physician* and was supplied by Dr. B. B. Neu-chiller of Woodstock, Illinois. It went like this: "A young woman whom I'd never seen before entered my office and told me that the infant in her arms didn't seem to be gaining weight. I asked her what he was being fed. "He's breast-fed," she replied. I asked her to remove her blouse and bra and examined her. "The baby isn't gaining weight because you have no milk in your breasts," I told her. With a puzzled expression, she asked, "Is that important? I'm the baby's aunt. His mother couldn't come today."—F.A. Oski, M.D.

Influence of Breast-Feeding on the Restoration of the Low Serum Concentration of Vitamin E and β-Carotene in the Newborn Infant
Enrique M. Ostrea, Jr., James E. Balun, Ruth Winkler, and Thomas Porter (Hutzel Hosp., Detroit, and Wayne State Univ.)
Am. J. Obstet. Gynecol. 154:1014–1017, May 1986   3–3

Compared with such concentrations in their mothers, infants are born with significantly lower serum concentrations of vitamin E and β-carotene, important natural antioxidants. Because no information is available on the natural restoration in infants of plasma vitamin E and β-carotene concentrations in the postnatal period, the impact of breast-feeding on vitamin E and β-carotene restoration was examined in a group of newborn infants.

β-Carotene and vitamin E concentrations were determined in paired maternal venous blood and cord blood samples of 28 premature and 31 term infants. Breast milk was obtained during the first through the fifth postnatal days from 19 lactating mothers, 5 with premature and 14 with term infants. β-Carotene and vitamin E concentrations were determined in all milk samples. The effect of feeding on serum vitamin E and β-carotene

CONCENTRATIONS (MEAN ± SD) OF β-CAROTENE
AND VITAMIN E IN HUMAN MILK AND IN FORMULA

	β-Carotene (μg/dl)	Vitamin E (mg/dl)
Human milk		
Day 1 (N = 14)	213.0 ± 166.6	3.28 ± 2.93
Day 2 (N = 20)	117.0 ± 112.0	2.74 ± 2.30
Day 3 (N = 17)	120.0 ± 63.4	2.09 ± 1.44
Day 4 (N = 10)	50.4 ± 19.9	1.03 ± 0.50
Day 5 (N = 4)	39.5 ± 34.7	0.45 ± 0.33
Formula		
Similac 20 (N = 3)	Negligible*	0.91 ± 0.03
Enfamil 20 (N = 3)	Negligible	1.16 ± 0.04

*Absorbance within matching error of cuvettes.
(Courtesy of Ostrea, E.M., Jr., et al.: Am. J. Obstet. Gynecol. 154:1014–1017, May 1986.)

values was determined in 16 cesarean section-delivered term infants and 8 formula-fed infants.

The mean serum concentrations of β-carotene and vitamin E in cord blood were one eighth and one third, respectively, of maternal serum concentrations. There was a significant correlation between the cord serum concentration of β-carotene and gestational age, but not between the cord serum concentration of vitamin E and gestational age. Human milk, particularly colostrum, contained extremely high concentrations of β-carotene and vitamin E (table). Breast-fed infants attained serum concentrations of both β-carotene and vitamin E comparable with those in adults within 4–6 days of breast-feeding (Fig 3–1). Breast milk appears to play an important role in providing for a newborn infant's defense against oxygen toxicity through its high bioavailability of the antioxidants β-carotene and vitamin E.

▶ I have included this report because it is apparent that many physicians have forgotten what was known a quarter of a century ago, i.e., that the feeding of human milk to a term infant results in the infant attaining normal adult serum vitamin E values by the end of the first week of life (Wright, S. W., et al.: *Pediatrics* 7:386, 1951). Just another of the dividends.—F.A. Oski, M.D.

Bovine β-Lactoglobulin in the Human Milk: A Longitudinal Study During the Whole Lactation Period

Irene Axelsson, Irene Jakobsson, Tor Lindberg, and Birgitta Benediktsson (Univ. of Lund), Malmö, Sweden)
Acta Paediatr. Scand. 75:702–707, 1986   3–4

Food antigens can pass from the mother to the infant via breast milk, and bovine β-lactoglobulin has been identified in human milk samples. The bovine β-lactoglobulin concentration was determined in milk samples collected during lactation from 25 healthy mothers of term infants. In all,

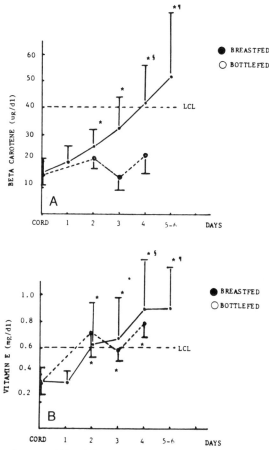

Fig 3–1.—Serum β-carotene (A) and vitamin E (B) concentrations from day 1 to day 6 in breast-fed and bottle-fed infants. Lower 95% confidence limit *(LCL)* is indicated by broken line. Asterisks denote *P* < .02 compared with cord; section marks indicate *P* < .01 compared with day 2; and paragraph marks denote *P* < .01 compared with day 3. (Courtesy of Ostrea, E.M., Jr., et al.: Am. J. Obstet. Gynecol. 154:1014–1017, May 1986.)

232 samples were obtained at 2-week intervals. Most of the infants were exclusively breast fed, but food supplements were sometimes added at age 3–4 months.

Bovine β-lactoglobulin was detected in 40% of the milk samples. Six women lacked β-lactoglobulin in all samples, but two had measurable amounts in all milk samples (Fig 3–2). Concentrations were similar throughout the time of lactation. All mothers took cow's milk, but the intake could not be related to β-lactoglobulin concentrations in breast milk. Six of seven mothers with more than 50 μg of β-lactoglobulin per L in at least one sample reported that their infants had diarrhea, vomiting, colic, or an exanthem. Twelve infants had a family history of allergy, which could not be related to the presence of β-lactoglobulin in breast milk.

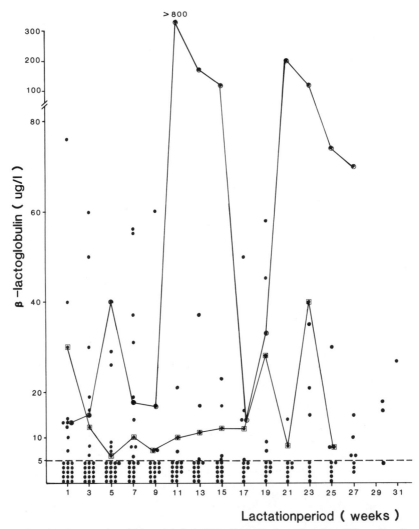

Fig 3–2.—Concentration of β-lactoglobulin in 232 milk samples from 25 mothers. Values of less than 5 μg/L were not measurable. Open squares and open circles indicate two mothers with detectable amounts in all samples. (Courtesy of Axelsson, I., et al.: Acta Paediatr. Scand. 75:702–707, 1986.)

Immunoreactive bovine β-lactoglobulin is present in human breast milk throughout lactation. Its concentration varies substantially among mothers, and higher values are related to gastrointestinal tract symptoms in the breast-feeding infant. Studies of the prophylactic effects of breast-feeding should include a dietary history and estimates of the food antigen content of the breast milk.

▶ The presence of symptoms in the infant who is being exclusively breast fed (e.g., diarrhea, vomiting, colic, and exanthema) was found to correlate significantly with high levels of β-lactoglobulin in breast milk. Having a mother re-move all milk and milk products from her diet can produce cures with 24–48 hours. If you want more convincing, please read the 1984 YEAR BOOK, P. 89–90. When things go wrong in an exclusively breast-fed infant, don't blame the mother, blame her diet.—F.A. Oski, M.D.

Metoclopramide Effect on Faltering Milk Production by Mothers of Premature Infants

Richard A. Ehrenkranz and Barbara A. Ackerman (Yale Univ. and Yale-New Haven Hosp.)

Pediatrics 78:614–620, October 1986

3–5

When mothers are separated from their premature newborn infants, they rely on milk expression until the infants can nurse. Once breast-feeding begins, milk production is adequate; however, several weeks later, milk production falters. A review was made of experience with metoclo-pramide, a drug used to stimulate milk production in women with low levels of prolactin, to stimulate milk production in mothers of premature infants.

The study included 23 mothers of premature infants whose mean gesta-tional age was 30.4 weeks. Of the 11 multiparous women, 8 had pre-viously breast fed. After delivery, each woman regularly expressed milk

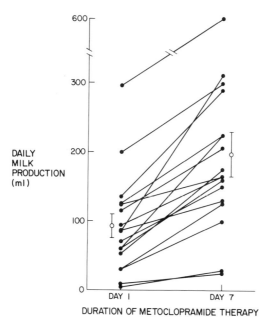

Fig 3–3.—Daily milk production (ml/day) on first and seventh day of maternal metoclopramide treatment. Milk production increased from 93.3 ± 18.0 ml/day (mean ± SEM) to 197.4 + 32.3 ml/day ($P < .001$). (Courtesy of Ehrenkranz, R.A., and Ackerman, B.A.: Pediatrics 78:614–620, October 1986.)

with a pump. In a period of weeks, milk production faltered despite appropriate diet and milk expression technique and more frequent expression of milk. Metoclopramide was initiated about 32 days post partum in a 10-mg dose taken orally three times daily for 1 week and then tapered over 2 days. During treatment women continued to pump their milk and record the volume immediately afterward. A double antibody radioimmunoassay was used to measure serum prolactin levels.

The daily volume of milk increased from an average 93.3 ml/day to 197.4 ml/day in the first 7 days (Fig 3–3). The increase in milk production correlated with the increase in serum prolactin levels from a mean of 18.1 ng/ml to 121.8 ng/ml. No serious side effects were noted by the women or in their breast-fed infants. Of the 23 women in the study, 15 successfully maintained lactation.

Increased daily milk production with metoclopramide therapy is related to a significant increase in basal prolactin concentrations. The data also establish the efficacy of metoclopramide as a stimulant of milk production in mothers who have difficulty in maintaining lactation after premature delivery.

▶ Dr. Carol E. Weichert, a member of the clinical faculty of the Department of Pediatrics, State University of New York at Syracuse, and a practicing pediatrician who specializes in problems of lactation, comments.—F.A. Oski, M.D.

▶ This is an extremely interesting study because it presents data on prolactin function in relation to milk insufficiency. It permits one to get a physiologic handle on the $64 question: Why do some women breast feed successfully and others do not? More particularly, despite previous breast feeding experience, why do women run into difficulty in sustaining lactation after delivering a premature infant?

Metoclopramide removes or antagonizes dopaminergic inhibitory tone, increasing prolactin levels. In this study, basal prolactin levels were increased with therapy. Most of these women, after premature delivery, had depressed basal prolactin levels. Their basal prolactin levels were closer to those in nonlactating postpartum women than to the prolactin levels of women lactating postpartum. Why?

I suspect this is a normal response. It may reflect an increased dopaminergic inhibitory tone that accompanies delivering a premature infant. In patients I have been able to study, therapies that ordinarily remove inhibition of prolactin are not effective in the presence of maternal emotional distress. What could be more stressful to a new mother than delivering a premature infant? It threatens her most primitive instinct: survival of the species.

Some of the pathways for prolactin and oxytocin release run in the limbic cortex as part of the mechanisms for sexual response and survival of the species. Despite increased motivation to breast feed, these women may be at the mercy of centuries-old mechanisms that act to conserve maternal energy, insure earlier ovulation (by depressing prolactin), and promote survival of the species, with a more viable infant. A recent study showed a confounding factor to be infant weight in women weaning early. Lighter-weight infants were weaned earlier than heavier infants. Of the 23 women in the present study, 8 discontinued breast-feeding. It would be interesting to know if there was a correlation in these cases with lower birth weight in the infant.

How you view these questions affects how you interpret these events to a patient. Cessation of lactation after premature delivery should not be viewed as failure by the mother. It may represent a normal physiologic event.—C.E. Weichert, M.D.

Acquired Zinc Deficiency in Two Breast-Fed Mature Infants
Yoko Kuramoto, Yutake Igarashi, Seiichi Kato, and Hachiro Tagami (Tohoku Univ., Sendai, Japan)
Acta Derm. Venereol. (Stockh) 66:359–361, 1986) 3–6

Acquired zinc deficiency in breast-fed infants has been reported in premature infants. Zinc deficiency developed in a breast-fed mature infant and her sister with the characteristic dermatitis appearing on the face and buttocks at 10 weeks of age. The infants' serum zinc levels were 11 μg/dl and 40 μg/dl, respectively, and the mother's serum zinc levels were 52 μg/dl and 102 μg/dl on both occasions. The mother's zinc levels in milk of 18 μg/dl and 14.3 μg/dl, respectively, could not be corrected by large doses of zinc supplements that otherwise increased the serum zinc concentration. Both infants received supplementary zinc 30–40 mg/day, for 2 weeks and lesions regressed within 3 days of treatment.

Mature breast-fed infants run a risk of experiencing zinc deficiency if the concentration of zinc in the breast milk is low. Maternal deficiency in the transfer process of zinc from serum to breast milk could have caused the skin changes in her infants.

▶ Well, nothing is perfect. If it looks like acrodermatitis enteropathica, it could be acrodermatitis enteropathica despite the fact that the infant was born at term and is being breast fed. For those who collect these rare occurrences, see Roberts, L. J., et al.: *J. Am. Acad. Dermatol.* 16:301, 1987.—F.A. Oski, M.D.

Bioavailability of Iron in Soy-Based Formula and Its Effect on Iron Nurture in Infancy
Eva Hertrampf, Marisol Cayazzo, Fernando Pizarro, and Abraham Stekel (Universidad de Chile, Santiago)
Pediatrics 78:640–645, October 1986 3–7

Soy-based formulas are used extensively in the United States and other countries. Soy products are known to inhibit absorption of iron; however, a large excess of iron in the formula may be expected to permit sufficient iron absorption by the infant. A study was undertaken to determine the bioavailability of iron from a soy-based formula and evaluate the iron status of infants drinking this formula.

TABLE 1.—IRON ABSORPTION FROM SOY-BASED FORMULA

Infant No.	Hemoglobin (g/dL)	Iron Concentration/ Iron-Binding Capacity (%)	Serum Ferritin* (μg/L)	Iron Absorption (% of Dose)*	
				Soy-Based Formula	Ferrous Ascorbate
1	9.9	3.9	14	6.17	98.12
2	10.0	2.7	9	4.35	76.11
3	14.8	18.9	24	1.36	71.33
4	9.8	3.0	3	3.78	58.34
5	14.5	26.1	29	1.29	50.76
6	8.2	2.0	7	5.38	46.30
7	13.8	10.0	39	3.52	36.85
8	14.2	25.6	34	0.66	36.53
9	15.8	17.3	45	2.45	36.11
10	13.1	20.7	26	1.44	35.17
11	15.0	15.6	76	1.79	27.34
12	14.0	25.9	53	0.79	25.31
13	12.9	39.4		1.02	23.67
14	15.2	32.9	501	0.47	22.49
15	14.6	27.9		0.31	15.09
16	15.6	35.8	125	2.02	11.00
Mean	13.2	19.2	31	1.7	35.9
SD	2.3	11.9	9–105	0.7–3.9	20.3–63.5

*Values are geometric means and range of 1 SD.
(Courtesy of Hertrampf, E., et al.: Pediatrics 78:640–645, October 1986.)

TABLE 2.—HEMATOLOGIC VALUES FOR INFANTS AT 9 MONTHS OF AGE

	No. of Infants	Hemoglobin* (g/dL)	Mean Corpuscular Volume* (fL)	Iron Concentration/ Iron-Binding Capacity* (%)	Free Erythrocyte Protoporphyrin* (μg/dL RBC)	Serum Ferritin† (μg/L)
Fortified milk	45	12.56 ± 0.79	72 ± 5	14.8 ± 7.0	96 ± 28	15.8 8.3–30.1
Soy-based	47	12.30 ± 0.78	74 ± 6	16.5 ± 7.0	94 ± 31	15.4 7.2–32.9
Breast milk‡	49	11.66 ± 1.03[a]	69 ± 6[a]	12.0 ± 6.4[b]	107 ± 37	10.3 4.1–25.9[c]

*Values are means ± SD.
†Values are geometric means and range of 1 SD.
‡Fortified milk and soy-based formula groups differed significantly from breast milk group: [a]$P < .001$; [b]$P < .005$; [c]$P < .05$.
(Courtesy of Hertrampf, E., et al.: Pediatrics 78:640–645, October 1986.)

Sixteen healthy multiparous women participated in the iron absorption study. On day 1 the women drank 0.24 L of formula with 1 μCi of $^{55}FeCl_3$ added. On day 2 they drank a solution containing 3 mg of ferrous sulfate labeled with 3 μCi of $^{59}FeSO_4$. On day 15 venous blood samples were taken for evaluation of hematologic characteristics and to measure radioactivity incorporated in the erythrocytes. A longitudinal study was done that included 47 infants receiving the soy-based formula, 45 infants receiving full-fat powdered milk fortified with iron and ascorbic acid, and 90 breast-fed infants. At ate 9 months, hemoglobulin, mean corpuscular volume, iron levels and iron binding capacity, free erythrocyte protoporphyrin, and serum ferritin were measured.

Maternal absorption of iron was 35.9% of the reference dose of ferrous sulfate and 1.7% of the soy-based formula (Table 1). Infants fed soy

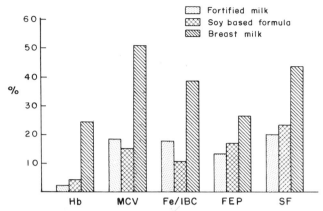

Fig 3–4.—Percentage of deficient infants at age 9 months. Hemoglobin (Hb) < gm/dL; mean corpuscular volume (MCV) < 70 fl; iron concentration/iron-binding capacity <9%; free erythrocyte protoporphyrin >120 μg/dl; RBC and serum ferritin <10 μg/L. (Courtesy of Hertrampf, E., et al.: Pediatrics 78:640–645, October 1986.)

formula and iron-fortified cow's milk had similar blood and iron profiles. In all characteristics except for free erythrocyte protoporphyrin, the breast-fed infants differed significantly from the other groups (Table 2). Anemia developed in 4.3% and 2.2% of infants given soy formula or fortified cow's milk, respectively, and in 27.3% of the breast-fed infants (Fig 3–4).

Soy formula is as effective as cow's milk in providing infants with adequate iron. This suggests that infants absorb more iron from soy formulas than what would be predicted from studies of iron absorption from soy formulas by adults.

▶ Soy formulas support adequate iron nutrition during infancy. I'm always amused by physicians who claim that milk-based, iron-fortified formulas produce gastrointestinal disturbances in their patients despite the fact that the data show otherwise. These same physicians never make this claim about soy formulas. I suspect that they don't realize that these formulas contain the same amount of iron supplementation. As stated in Iannuzzi's Universal Law of Justice, "Truth is trouble."—F.A. Oski, M.D.

Blue Sclerae: A Common Sign of Iron Deficiency?

L. Kalra, A.N. Hamlyn, and B.J.M. Jones (Wordsley Hosp., Stourbridge, and Russell's Hall Hosp., Dudley, West Midlands, England)
Lancet 2:1267–1269, Nov. 29, 1986   3–8

The association between blue sclerae and iron deficiency has been described sporadically. In all, 169 adult hospital inpatients were studied to assess this association and to define the specificity and sensitivity of this sign. Three observers independently graded the signs of blue sclerae and mucosal pallor as absent, equivocal, definite, or striking.

Definite or stiking blue sclerae, as noted by at least two observers, were evident in 47 patients (28%). Blue sclerae were significantly more common in patients with iron-deficiency anemia (40 of 46, 87%) than in those with other anemias (2 of 28, 7%) or without anemia (5 of 95, 5.3%). The frequency of blue sclerae was independent of age, sex, or color of iris. In contrast, mucosal pallor was noted in only 30% of patients with iron-deficiency anemia. Compared with mucosal pallor, the presence of blue sclerae was an equally specific (0.94 vs. 0.96) but significantly more sensitive indicator (0.87 vs. 0.20) of iron-deficiency anemia. Concordance by all three observers was achieved in more than half of the patients.

The presence of blue sclerae appears to be a good indicator of iron-deficiency anemia. Iron-deficiency may lead to impaired collagen synthesis and a thin sclera through which the choroid can be seen, making the sclerae appear blue.

▶ Sir William Osler first described this in 1908. He also probably forgot it among the myriad other things he also described for the first time. This report describes the finding in iron-deficient adults. It remains to be determined if it also occurs in children. I suspect that it does. The other physical changes that occur with iron deficiency (e.g., "spooning" of the nails, lightening of the hair, and flattening of the papillae of the tongue) are more common in children than in adults with iron deficiency. Iron deficiency remains an intriguing disease, so just keep looking. Speaking of looks, if you look like your passport photo, you're probably too ill to travel.—F.A. Oski, M.D.

Deciduous Tooth Eruption in Children Who Fail to Gain Weight
A. Shuper, M. Shohat, H. Sarnat, I. Varsano, and M. Mimouni (Beilinson Med. Ctr., Petah Tigva, and Tel Aviv Univ., Israel)
Helv. Paediatr. Acta 41:501–504, 1986   3–9

Certain studies have shown correlations between the number of erupted deciduous teeth and body measurements, whereas others studies have not. The effect of failure to gain weight after deciduous tooth eruption was studied in outpatient infants. All term infants aged 6–30 months whose weight was less than the mean for chronologic age by more than 2 SD were included, some being small-for-gestational age.

Twenty-nine infants with negative study results and 17 for whom the only explanation was intrauterine growth retardation were included. Birth weights differed significantly in the two study groups (table). The mean height and head circumference tended to be below the means for age in both groups, height by about 2 SD and head circumference by about 1.6 SD. The number of erupted deciduous teeth nevertheless was close to the normal mean, and there was no significant difference in this parameter between the two groups.

It would appear that deciduous tooth eruption should be considered a process inherent in orofacial maturation, independent of other somatic

Mean Deviations of Growth Parameters in Groups A and B, Presented as the Mean Number of SD Below the Mean for Age, in Relation to the Appropriate Growth Charts

	Total n=46	Group A n=29	Group B n=17	Significance* (P)
Boys/girls	21/25	16/13	5/12	
Age (months)†	18.0±6.4	18.8±7.01	17.1±5.0	N.S.
Birth weight (g)	2796±287	3031±279	2396±135	<0.001
Weight deviation (No. S.D.)	2.83±0.60	2.86±0.59	2.77±0.65	N.S.
Height deviation (S.D.)	1.97±1.05	1.87±1.2	2.14±0.87	N.S.
Head circumference deviation (S.D.)	1.6±1.01	1.48±0.95	1.75±1.06	N.S.
NET deviation (S.D.)	0.4±1.27	0.32±1.28	0.52±1.25	N.S.

*Significance of the difference between groups A and B.
†Numbers are mean values.
(Courtesy of Shuper, A., et al.: Helv. Paediatr. Acta 41:501–504 1986.)

developmental processes. Therefore, the number of erupted deciduous teeth is not a valid measure of body growth.

Early Growth Predicts Timing of Puberty in Boys: Results of a 14-Year Nutrition and Growth Study

James L. Mills, Patricia H. Shiono, Leona R. Shapiro, Patricia B. Crawford, and George G. Rhoads (Natl. Inst. of Child Health and Human Development, NIH, Bethesda, and Univ. of California at Berkeley)
J. Pediatr. 109:543–547, September 1986 3–10

Investigators have long been interested in the relationship between nutrition, early growth, and the onset of puberty. It is well established that malnutrition may delay puberty and that exogenous obesity may accelerate it. Studies of children in the latter part of the first decade of life suggest that height and weight are related to the onset of puberty. However, it has been difficult to determine the relationship between puberty and weight, height, and adiposity in early life because of the need for a longitudinal study of normally nourished children of documented dietary and anthropometric status. The Berkeley Nutrition and Growth Study represents an attempt to monitor the growth and nutritional status of a specific cohort of children, starting at age 6 months and continuing to age 14 years.

The study group included 78 boys, all well nourished and not grossly obese. Pubertal development was assessed at 14 years of age, and the results were then correlated with diet and early growth. No nutrients were significantly correlated with the stage of pubertal development. However, boys with more advanced pubic hair development and longer penile length were markedly heavier at ages 6 months, 2 years, and 4 years. In addition, muscle mass, as determined by the cross-sectional area of the upper arm, was substantially greater in the early maturers at the same ages. Although the more sexually mature boys also were taller and had larger skinfolds at virtually all measurements from age 6 months to 4 years, the differences were less pronounced. It would appear that, in an adequately nourished male population, body size in the first years of life is significantly correlated with the timing of puberty.

▶ A word to the wise: If your baby boy is big at 6 months of age, begin his sex education early; you have less time than you think.—F.A. Oski, M.D.

Controlled Trial of Zinc Supplementation During Recovery From Malnutrition: Effects on Growth and Immune Function
Carlos Castillo-Duran, Gloria Heresi, Mauro Fisberg, and Ricardo Uauy (Univ. of Chile, Santiago, and Univ. of Texas at Dallas)
Am. J. Clin. Nutr. 45:602–608, March 1987   3–11

Trace mineral deficiencies are being increasingly recognized in protein-energy malnutrition, but most human studies of zinc metabolism have been confounded by other specific nutritional deficits. An attempt was made to study the effects of zinc supplementation in moderately malnourished infants during recovery. Thirty-two marasmic infants with evidence of primary malnutrition were studied. In a blinded study, the infants, matched by age, birth weight, and nutritional status, were assigned to receive elemental zinc, 2 mg/kg daily, as the acetate, or a placebo solution lacking zinc. The serum zinc level was monitored to prevent reductions below 50 μg/dl.

Plasma zinc values rose in the supplemented group only in the first month (Table 1). Progress in weight for length was significantly greater in the supplemented group at 1 month and 2 months. Linear growth was similar in the two groups. More infectious illness occurred in the placebo group. Serum IgA levels increased in the zinc-supplemented group and the proportion of anergic infants declined (Table 2).

Zinc supplementation had significant effects on growth and host defenses in infants in this study recovering from protein-energy malnutrition. It is more important to evaluate the biologic effects of zinc status than the plasma level alone. Trace mineral supplementation is indicated for mar-

TABLE 1.—EFFECT OF ZINC
SUPPLEMENTATION ON PLASMA ZINC LEVELS
(μG/DL)*

Day of study	Supplemented ($n = 16$)	Placebo ($n = 16$)
0	96 ± 20	105 ± 24
30	106 ± 29	92 ± 27
60	98 ± 22	96 ± 16
90	102 ± 22	102 ± 16

*Mean ± SD.
(Courtesy of Castillo-Duran, C., et al.: Am. J. Clin. Nutr. 45:602–608, March 1987.)

TABLE 2.—EFFECT OF ZINC SUPPLEMENTATION
ON CELL-MEDIATED IMMUNITY IN
MALNOURISHED INFANTS*

	Zn supplemented	Placebo
Positive cutaneous response to PPD		
n	(15)	(12)
Day 0	5/15	4/12
90	10/15	5/12
Significance p (McNemar test)	<0.05	NS
Percent anergic to PPD and Candida		
n	(16)	(16)
Day 0	38	50
90	6	25
Significance p (McNemar test)	<0.05	NS
Blastic response to PHA		
n	(10)	(10)
Day 0	31 ± 9	59 ± 12
90	53 ± 13	58 ± 18
Significance p (paired t test)	<0.05	NS

*Mean ± SEM stimulation index, response of test case as compared with a normal control (SI, 50–100). PPD, protein purified derivative of tuberculin; PHS, phytohemagglutinin.

(Courtesy of Castillo-Duran, C., et al.: Am. J. Clin. Nutr. 45:602–608, March 1987.)

asmic infants, because cow's milk-based diets do not provide adequate amounts of zinc for optimal recovery.

▶ Marginal zinc deficiency has been found in association with chronic diarrhea, gluten enteropathy, cystic fibrosis, sickle cell anemia, cirrhosis, inflammatory bowel disease, pancreatic insufficiency, low birth weight, and protein energy malnutrition. Sensitivity of growth to zinc deficiency has been well demonstrated in both animals and man. This current report demonstrates effects of zinc on morbidity from infections and host defenses. Evidence continues to accumulate suggesting a role for zinc in the immune response as mediated via T lymphocytes. We must continually think zinc. Unfortunately, in our zeal to reduce iron deficiency we may produce marginal zinc nutrition. Excessive intake of inorganic iron appears to impair zinc bioavailability from diets (Solomons, N. W.: *J. Nutr.* 116:927, 1986). For more on zinc, read on.—F.A. Oski, M.D.

Food Consumption Patterns of Canadian Preschool Children in Relation to Zinc and Growth Status

Patricia D. Smit Vanderkooy and Rosalind S. Gibson (Univ. of Guelph, Ontario)
Am. J. Clin. Nutr. 45:609–616, March 1987
3–12

Suboptimal zinc status, with slowed physical growth, has been documented in children living in the United States. Zinc status was examined in relation to food consumption patterns and nutrient intakes in 106 Canadian preschool children aged 4–5 years; the 62 boys and 44 girls were all apparently healthy. Dietary records were obtained on three consecutive days.

The mean height, weight, and weight-for-height percentiles were 56%, 55%, and 52%, respectively. Energy and nutrient intakes (Table 1) were independent of age, parental educational level, and socioeconomic status. Grain products were a major source of energy, dietary fiber, and all nutrients. Milk and milk products were the second major source of energy and the chief source of protein, calcium, and phosphorus. These food groups, along with meat, poultry, and fish, supplied most dietary zinc (Table 2). Dietary contributions of energy, protein, and zinc are related to zinc status in Table 3.

Some of the boys in this study had evidence of a mild growth-limiting zinc deficiency syndrome, but a positive response to zinc supplementation would be required to confirm this. Suboptimal zinc nutrition in boys has been associated with lower intakes of zinc from flesh foods and greater intakes of calcium, which may inhibit zinc absorption.

TABLE 1.—Dietary Intake of Energy, Dietary Fiber, and Selected Nutrients (Mean ± SD)

Nutrient		Per day		Per kg		Per 1000 kcal
	Sex	M	F	M	F	M + F
	n	62	44	61	44	106
Energy	kcal	1494 ± 394	1292 ± 353*	80.0 ± 13.7	71.4 ± 12.7*	
Protein	g	49.4 ± 15.1	43.8 ± 15.3*	2.6 ± 0.5	2.4 ± 0.6†	33.5 ± 5.1
Dietary fiber	g	11.8 ± 5.4	10.8 ± 5.6	0.63 ± 0.21	0.59 ± 0.19	8.1 ± 2.5
Calcium	mg	760 ± 334	633 ± 287*	40.7 ± 14.0	34.8 ± 11.4†	499 ± 135
Phosphorus	mg	1054 ± 397	930 ± 442‡	56.2 ± 13.6	51.3 ± 17.3	706 ± 148
Iron	mg	11.2 ± 4.4	9.6 ± 3.4*	0.60 ± 0.18	0.53 ± 0.10‡	7.5 ± 1.6
Zinc	mg	6.9 ± 3.1	6.0 ± 2.4‡	0.36 ± 0.10	0.33 ± 0.08	4.6 ± 1.0
Copper	mg	1.1 ± 0.4	0.9 ± 0.4‡	0.06 ± 0.01	0.05 ± 0.02	0.72 ± 0.17

*$P < .001$.
†$P < .05$.
‡$P < .01$.
(Courtesy of Vanderkooy, P.D.S., and Gibson, R.S.: Am. J. Clin. Nutr. 45:609–616, March 1987.)

TABLE 2.—Percent Contributions of Energy, Dietary Fiber, and Selected Nutrients From Nine Major Food Groups for Preschool Children

Food group	Energy	Protein	Dietary fiber	Calcium	Phosphorus	Iron	Zinc	Copper
Milk and milk products	18.9	30.8	0.5	69.8	39.9	4.0	29.5	12.8
Meat, poultry, and fish	12.3	27.1	1.2	1.5	11.4	12.7	29.8	10.4
Eggs, legumes, and nuts	3.9	6.5	4.4	1.7	4.1	3.8	5.6	5.1
Grain products	33.4	27.3	51.4	18.1	27.6	55.7	25.2	39.2
Fruits	12.7	2.7	20.5	4.0	4.3	12.6	2.6	11.9
Vegetables	6.1	4.6	20.5	2.7	5.1	7.1	5.8	11.2
Fats, oils, sugar, sweets, and misc	12.6	1.1	1.6	7.5	7.6	3.9	1.1	7.3

(Courtesy of Vanderkooy, P.D.S., and Gibson, R.S.: Am. J. Clin. Nutr. 45:609–616, March 1987.)

TABLE 3.—Energy, Protein, and Zinc
Contributions From Meat, Poultry, and
Fish for Preschool Boys*

Dietary component	Group†	Per day	% of total daily intake
Energy (kcal)	A	135 ± 55	9.7 ± 3.7
	B	198 ± 120‡	13.0 ± 6.7‡
Protein (g)	A	8.7 ± 3.9	19.7 ± 9.0
	B	13.8 ± 7.7§	27.1 ± 11.7‡
Zinc (mg)	A	1.3 ± 0.7	20.6 ± 11.8
	B	2.3 ± 2.2‡	30.4 ± 15.0‖

*Mean ± SD.
†A includes boys with hair zinc concentrations of <70 µg/gm and/or height-for-age <15%, controlling for parents' heights that are at least 15% greater; B includes other boys in sample.
‡$P < .05$.
§$P < .01$.
¶$P < .10$.
(Courtesy of Vanderkooy, P.D.S., and Gibson, R.S.: Am. J. Clin. Nutr. 45:609–616, March 1987.)

▶ The hair zinc levels of the children reported here were similar in terms of absolute levels and variability to those reported by Hambidge and associates some time ago (Hambidge, K. M., et al.: *Am. J. Clin. Nutr.* 32:2532, 1979). It was Walravens and Hambidge (*Am. J. Clin. Nutr.* 29:1114, 1976) who first demonstrated that infant males given a zinc-supplemented formula grew 2.1 cm more than infants fed a conventional formula during the first 6 months of life. The relationship between zinc and growth, as described in the previous abstract as well, is something that cannot be ignored, particularly for those of us that are in the 5 ft 7 in. class.—F.A. Oski, M.D.

Calcium-Regulating Hormones and Minerals From Birth to 18 Months of Age; A Cross-Sectional Study. I. Effects of Sex, Race, Age, Season, and Diet on Vitamin D Status
P. Lichtenstein, B.L. Speckar, R.C. Tsang, F. Mimouni, and C. Gormley (Univ. of Cincinnati and Children's Hosp. Res. Found., Cincinnati)
Pediatrics 77:883–890, June 1986　　　　3–13

There is a lack of adequate normative data concerning bone metabolism and vitamin D physiology in infants younger than 18 months of age. A cross-sectional, prospective study of 198 infants was undertaken to obtain comprehensive normative data on the vitamin D status in infants younger than 18 months, particularly with regard to the influence of sex, race, age, season, and diet (cow's milk vs. human milk).

Sex did not affect any of the vitamin D metabolites measured. Black infants had significantly higher serum levels of 1,25 dihydroxyvitamin D [1,25(OH) D] than white infants had. Serum 1,25(OH) D concentrations did not change during the first 18 months of life, but serum vitamin D-binding protein concentrations increased slightly with age. Serum concentrations of 25-hydroxyvitamin D (25-OHD) and 24,25-dihydroxyvitamin D [24,25-(OH) D] were significantly lower, whereas 1,25-dihydroxyvitamin D and vitamin D-binding protein were significantly higher, in winter as compared with summer. Bottle-fed infants had significantly higher serum concentrations of all vitamin D metabolites than breast-fed infants. However, after taking into account the confounding variables of season and age, only serum 25-OHD, 24,25(OH) D, and vitamin D-binding protein concentrations were significantly higher in bottle-fed infants.

Normative values for vitamin D metabolites in infants younger than 18 months can be significantly affected by race, age, season, and diet. These factors should be considered in assessing the vitamin D status of infants.

▶ A study by Cancela and associates (*J. Endocrinol.* 110:43, 1986) clearly demonstrates the importance of the 25-OHD content of maternal milk as being primarily responsible for the vitamin D concentrations found in the serum of exclusively breast-fed infants. In contrast, serum levels of 1,25-(OH)$_2$D$_3$ measured in the breast-fed baby appear mainly related to its calcium status. Specker and Tsang have demonstrated large seasonal differences in serum 25-OHD concentrations in exclusively breast-fed infants that coincided with differences in sunshine exposure (*J. Pediatr.* 110:745, 1987). These authors conclude that white breast-fed infants may not require vitamin D supplementation if they are receiving an adequate amount of sunshine exposure. A couple of hours of facial exposure to the sun three times a week should be sufficient to remain in adequate vitamin D status. Encourage mothers to get out the infant carriage and take the baby outside. Alternatively, the mother need only "flash" a couple times a week (in the sunlight) to increase the vitamin D content of her milk (see 1986 YEAR BOOK, p. 398). The latter approach sounds like more fun.—F.A. Oski, M.D.

Fumarase Deficiency: A New Cause of Mitochondrial Encephalomyopathy
Arthur B. Zinn, Douglas S. Karr, and Charles L. Hoppel (Rainbow Babies and Children's Hosp., VA Med. Ctr., and Case Western Reserve Univ., Cleveland)
N. Engl. J. Med. 315:459–475, Aug. 21, 1986   3–14

Mitochondrial myopathies affecting both skeletal muscle and brain are termed mitochondrial encephalomyopathies. An infant was seen with progressive mitochondrial encephalomyopathy involving deficiency of both the mitochondrial and cytosolic forms of fumarase.

Infant, male, with an apparently normal perinatal period, experienced feeding difficulties, weight loss, and lethargy during the first month of life. Profound hypotonia, developmental delay, and cerebral atrophy manifested by 6 months of age, and death occurred at 8 months. Metabolic screening showed lactic and pyruvic acidemia, but no systemic acidosis, and fumaric aciduria. Oxygen uptake studies revealed selective defects in the oxidation of glutamate and of succinate, but the liver mitochondria oxidized these and other substrates normally. Fumarase activity was virtually absent in both liver and skeletal muscle mitochondria, whereas the specific activities of 7 other enzymes were normal (table). Fumarase

TRICARBOXYLIC ACID (TCA) CYCLE AND TCA CYCLE-RELATED ENZYME
ACTIVITIES IN MITOCHONDRIAL EXTRACTS

ENZYME	LIVER EXTRACTS		SKELETAL-MUSCLE EXTRACTS	
	PATIENT	CONTROLS (N = 5)	PATIENT	CONTROLS (N = 12)
	*nmol of product formed/min/mg of protein**			
Fumarase	53	2878±248 (range, 2646–3263)	23	1997±717 (range, 1187–3280)
Aspartate aminotransferase	2916	3158±361	2374	2448±1045
Citrate synthase	325	325±67	1858	1705±615
Glutamate dehydrogenase	1094	1331±504	42	19±12
Malate dehydrogenase	3075	3127±740	5656	5460±2483
Pyruvate dehydrogenase complex	8.1	9.5±4.2	50	75±34
Succinate dehydrogenase	111	114±26	65	123±88
Succinate–cytochrome *c* reductase	129	159±41	228	136±68

*Plus-minus values are means ± SD.
(Courtesy of Zinn, A.B., et al.: N. Engl. J. Med. 315:469–475, Aug. 21, 1986.)

activity was significantly reduced in both liver and skeletal muscle homogenates, indicating a deficiency of both mitochondrial and cytosolic fumarases.
These findings indicate profound combined fumarase deficiency. Organ differences in the intramitochondrial accumulation of fumarate may account for the selective oxidative defects observed in skeletal muscle mitochondria but not liver mitochondria. Contrary to the proposed biochemical classification for the mitochondrial myopathies, fumarase deficiency represents an interaction of two categories: (1) a defect of endogenous mitochondrial substrate utilization, and (2) defects of mitochondrial substrate transport. The current classification scheme should include disorders of the tricarboxylic acid cycle.

▶ Dr. David Valle, Professor of Pediatrics, Johns Hopkins University School of Medicine, comments.—F.A. Oski, M.D.

▶ This is a carefully and thoroughly performed biochemical study of a hypotonic, developmentally delayed infant who failed to thrive after birth. Detection of increased amounts of fumarase and succinate in the urine by gas chromatography/mass spectrometry provided the initial clue to the nature of this child's problem. A specific deficiency of fumarase was convincingly demonstrated in skeletal muscle and liver. As recognized by the authors, additional studies (kinetic studies of the residual fumarase activity, demonstration of the defect in cultured cells from the patient, and demonstration of reduced activity in obligate heterozygotes) are necessary before concluding with certainty that the primary defect in this patient was at the fumarase locus. Assuming that these studies do confirm a genetic fumarase deficiency, these results are interesting and provocative for several reasons: (1) This is the first description of fumarase deficiency; (2) both cytoplasmic and mitochondrial forms of the enzyme are involved; and (3) the biochemical consequences are tissue specific, depending on the metabolic functions subserved by the tricarboxylic acid cycle in the various organs.

In most instances in which an enzyme activity is localized to more than one subcellular compartment, the enzymes are separate proteins encoded by different genes. However, the demonstration of deficiency of both cytosolic and mitochondrial fumarase in this child with a presumed monogenic defect is consistent with previous biochemical, electrophoretic, and gene mapping studies, suggesting that one gene encodes both forms of fumarase, and predicts some interesting regulation of the subcellular localization of fumarase.

I concur with the authors that an improved classification scheme for monogenic defects of mitochondrial proteins is needed. I don't like the term mitochondrial myopathy because it implies that only muscle is involved. Given the complexity of mitochondria and their many functions, perhaps we should not be surprised that simple classification of these defects is difficult.—D. Valle, M.D.

4 Allergy and Dermatology

What's New In Pediatric Dermatology?

WALTER W. TUNNESSEN, JR., M.D.
Associate Professor of Pediatrics, Johns Hopkins University School of Medicine

The 12th Annual Meeting of the Society for Pediatric Dermatology was held August 6–8, 1987. A few of the highlights of the meeting have been abstracted for your interest.

Eczema in the U.K.

Dr. David Atherton, Consultant Dermatologist, The Hospital for Sick Children, Great Ormond Street, London, England, presented a stepwise approach to one of the most common skin disorders encountered in children, atopic dermatitis. Dr. Atherton's foremost message was that physicians must take the time to discuss the disorder with parents. Physicians cannot act in an indifferent or nihilistic manner toward the treatment of eczema and expect a successful therapeutic intervention.

Level I of therapy, then, begins with sympathetic listening to the parents. A good prognosis should be emphasized, but the limitations of treatment must be made clear. This is not a condition that is cured with treatment; rather, it is controlled. He points out to parents that they are suffering more than their child, because of the child's distress.

Dr. Atherton is an advocate of bathing. In fact, he advises at least two baths daily, but an emollient is applied in the bath water to lock the moisture in the skin. Bath oil is also added to the water. On the child's removal from the tub, an emollient is again applied. Emollients consisting of hydrophilic petrolatum seem to be well suited for this purpose. He points out that emollients alone are often enough to bring the skin under control. During the day emollients are applied every hour or every other hour for maximum effect until the pruritus comes under control.

The third step in level I is modification of the environment. Skin irritants such as high temperatures, radiant heat, cold winds, excessive clothing, abrasive fabrics, and detergent or enzyme residues in washed clothing all must be avoided. Many children react to foods that spill on their skin, especially salty, acidic, or spicy foods. Tobacco smoke in the air, which often triggers pruritus, also needs to be avoided. And, finally, the fingernails must be kept short and filed so there are no rough edges.

After all of the above measures are taken, corticosteroids in topical form come into the protocol. Dr. Atherton points out that topical steroids may suppress the adenopituitary axis if used inappropriately. He tries to use nothing more potent than hydrocortisone ointment, 2.5% at most, but usually 1%, applied after bathing. Hydrocortisone used in this manner is harmless in his experience.

Cotton gauze impregnated with a mixture of zinc oxide, calamine, and ichthymol (paste bandages) are occasionally wrapped around the extremities and left on for 24 hours at a time. Atherton finds these bandages particularly helpful during flare-ups of the eczema.

Attention must also be directed toward the possibility of skin infections, subclinical or overt, and appropriate antibiotic therapy instituted. For minor infections, erythromycin is usually adequate, but for more involved infections a cloxacillin, with or without penicillin, is usually required. Occasionally, antibiotics are used prophylactically, particularly erythromycin or trimethoprim, not cloxacillin, for up to 3 months.

Oral antipruritic agents are also used, but only at night to avoid soporific effects during daytime. One must be careful of paradoxical reactions to these agents, however.

Level I treatments are effective 90% of the time in Dr. Atherton's hands.

Patients in whom treatment at the first level fails are empirically started on dietary avoidance trials. Double-blind crossover studies performed in Atherton's clinic have shown that two thirds of the children with eczema improve when egg and cow milk are excluded from the diet. Sensitivity to these products was only rarely determined from the patient's history. Atherton also recommends avoidance of chicken, tartrazine and related colorings, and benzoate preservatives as well. Appropriate calcium supplements should be added to the diet. If no response occurs in 4 weeks, the diet is scrapped.

A fascinating digression on food-dependent, exercise-induced anaphylaxis was used to emphasize the intermittent exacerbation of eczema by foods. In the former syndrome, certain foods, if ingested prior to exercise, induce anaphylaxis. Exercise or the foods alone will not. Similarly, children with eczema sometimes react to certain foods and sometimes do not, perhaps dependent on exposure to stress, infections, irritants, or certain allergens.

Level II treatments work in only a minority of patients with eczema. The next level is a "few food" dietary protocol featuring turkey or rabbit, rice or potatoes, cabbage or carrots, and stewed apple. After 3 weeks, if improvement occurs, a new food is added weekly until a tolerable diet is achieved.

Level III also includes more environmental modification, including banishment of all furred and feathered pets and a reduction of house dust mite antigen exposure, a difficult task. Self-hypnosis techniques are used in older children, and beclomethasone dipropionate, a potent but short-lived steroid, is given orally four times a day. However, the latter preparation is not available in the United States at present.

Level IV includes the most aggressive therapy, not to be embarked on lightly. Dr. Atherton occasionally must resort to oral steroids, but never in children younger than age 2 years or between 10 and 16 years of age. Finally, photochemotherapy with psoralens plus ultraviolet A light (PUVA) is almost always effective, but this approach requires frequent treatments and should not be used in young children.

The message for us, as pediatricians, is that we can manage most patients with atopic dermatitis if we pay attention to details and spend time with the family explaining the nature of the disorder. Rarely will we want to progress beyond level I. Systemic steroids should not be prescribed for eczema by the pediatrician. It is interesting to see that the food allergy pendulum is swinging more prominently to the fore.

Chronic Urticaria—Still Itching for the Cause

Dr. Nicholas Soter of New York University School of Medicine reviewed the differential diagnosis and management of urticaria and angioedema. The chronic urticarias continue to plague us, because the etiology is uncovered in less than 10% of these patients. The low rate of success, however, should not prevent us from taking a careful history, performing a physical examination, and performing a few laboratory tests.

Based on current pathophysiology, urticaria/angioedema can be divided into five groups. The IgE-dependent type includes those associated with allergic diseases. Atopic patients, those reacting to specific allergens, contact allergies, and the physical urticarias, particularly cold-induced and heat-induced or cholingeric urticaria, are included in this group. Group II includes the complement-mediated types such as serum sickness, hereditary angioedema, acquired C1 inhibitor deficiency associated with malignancy or systemic lupus erythematosus, necrotizing venulitis, infection related (e.g., with hepatitis B), and reactions to blood products. The vasculitic type should be suspected if typical wheals last longer than 24 hours. Systemic symptoms are also common in this group, and laboratory abnormalities such as an increased erythrocyte sedimentation rate and decreased complement levels may be found.

Type III includes the urticarias that result from the direct degranulation of mast cells, such as occurs with opiates, radiocontrast materials, and polymyxin, or those that alter prostaglandin metabolism, such as aspirin. Agents that alter arachidonic acid metabolism comprise type IV, and, finally, idiopathic fills out the classification as type V. In a study by Harris et al. (*Ann. Allergy* 51:161, 1983) of 94 children with chronic urticaria, the disease in 8 was caused by cold urticaria, in 2 by food allergy, and in the remaining 92% the cause remained unknown.

Investigation of urticaria includes an extensive history, tests for physical urticarias, and a limited laboratory investigation consisting of a complete blood count, differential count, determination of the erythrocyte sedimentation rate, and urinalysis. Good luck in dealing with the urticarias!

News for Acyclovir Lovers

Dr. Myron Levin of the University of Colorado presented an update on and some personal impressions of acyclovir, particularly the usefulness of the oral form of this drug. Dr. Levin reminds us that acyclovir is not viricidal; rather, it inhibits the herpesviruses growing in infected cells. The concentrations of acyclovir required to inhibit herpesviruses is species specific. Herpes simplex virus (HSV) is inhibited by serum concentrations of .03–.2 µg/ml; HSV 2 by .34–.46 µg/ml; and varicella-zoster virus by .58–1.3 µg/ml. Intravenous doses of acyclovir, ranging from 5 mg/kg to 15 mg/kg, meet these requirements. Oral acyclovir is only 20% to 30% absorbed, thus high doses are required to achieve the necessary serum concentration. In addition, the half-life of the drug is 3–3.5 hours, and dosing every 4–6 hours is required.

Candidates for oral administration might include patients with severe primary herpetic gingivostomatitis, primary genital infections, eczema herpeticum, and frequent severe recurrences. Visceral involvement always requires intravenous therapy.

A suspension formulation of acyclovir for young children is currently under investigation and holds promise for extending the usefulness of this form of the drug. Keep your eyes and ears open over the next few years.

Although the efficacy of this drug in varicella zoster infections is unproven, Dr. Levin had a pearl of warning: Children with varicella who have abdominal or back pain do poorly. The reason is unclear.

The Ungracious Guest

Dr. Charles August, Clinical Director of the Transplant Unit at Children's Hospital of Philadelphia, discussed an increasingly common problem at major centers, graft vs. host reactions. Targets of this reaction include the skin, liver, gastrointestinal tract, and bone marrow. Graft vs. host disease comes in two varieties, acute and chronic. The acute form is characterized by a maculopapular skin eruption and the clinical grade of severity varies with the degree of involvement of the organ systems. Chronic graft vs. host disease is associated with a curious focal scleroderma-like rash in limited areas as well as liver fibrosis and dysfunction. The more severe the disorder, the more generalized the sclerodermatous involvement and liver fibrosis, as well as dry eyes, dry mouth, other organ fibrosis, and immune dysfunction.

Children who have received bone marrow transplants are invariably given many drugs. In the first month after transplant one cannot distinguish, clinically or by biopsy, graft vs. host disease from reactions to chemotherapy or irradiation, although rashes occurring before 21 days after transplantation are most likely to be caused by the latter.

Endocrine Disorders and the Skin

Dr. Anne Lucky of the University of Cincinnati presented a pictorial review of the dermatologic manifestations of endocrine disorders. A few "pearls" are included in lieu of pictures.

A single central incisor should always make one think of a pituitary or hypothalamic defect.

Diffuse hyperpigmentation, but accentuation in scars, creases, gums and nails, vitiligo, alopecia, and loss of pubic and axillary hair may occur in patients with hypoadrenocorticism. Don't mistake psychiatric disorders or anorexia nervosa for Addison's disease. A delay in diagnosis can prove fatal.

Secondary cutaneous features of glucocorticoid excess include tinea versicolor, candidiasis in all areas, a propensity to staphylococcal infections, and acanthosis nigricans.

Disorders with androgen excess should be considered in patients with severe acne, hirsutism, and male or female pattern alopecia.

Acanthosis nigricans finally seems to have acquired a unifying theory, insulin-resistant diabetes. All endocrinopathies with acanthosis nigricans may be associated with insulin resistance. Most patients with obesity, the most common cause of acanthosis nigricans, also have some insulin resistance.

Leiner's Disease Look-Alike

Dr. David Atherton reviewed the disorder first described by Leiner in 1908 consisting of a scaly erythroderma, diarrhea, and failure to thrive. In all probability, this was a nutritional disorder. More recently (1960s), a functional deficiency of C5 was found in patients with a similar picture. Atherton points out that most patients labeled as having Leiner's syndrome do not in fact have this defect. Drawing on his own clinic patients, he described eight children with striking erythroderma appearing in the first month of life with a universal or seborrheic distribution and large (cornflake-like) scales, failure to thrive, and diarrhea. The latter was the most variable feature, being severe in three and mild in five infants. These infants had an increased susceptibility to infection, with three deaths.

Although the picture resembles Leiner's disease, Dr. Atherton believes that this disorder is not the same. The findings do, however, represent a clinical marker of immunodeficiency, although different types were observed in this group. Increased IgE levels were found in six of the children, along with impaired neutrophil mobility, impaired response to phytohemagglutinin, and hypogammaglobulinemia in varying combinations. Two infants had severe combined immunodeficiency variations.

Diapers: Building a Better Mousetrap

Dr. James Leyden of the University of Pennsylvania School of Medicine reviewed some of his work investigating the effectiveness of diapers containing the new superabsorbing polymers (SAM) in the prevention of or reduction in severity of diaper dermatitis. Diaper dermatitis has a multifactorial etiology, but previous studies have shown that excessively hydrated stratum corneum results in skin that is more vulnerable to frictional forces, irritation by feces and urine, and the growth of microbial organisms, particularly *Candida albicans*. Diapers, while protecting us from the excrement of infants, cause the skin in the diaper area to be significantly more hydrated than other body surfaces.

The newly developed diapers impregnated with SAM create a wick effect that draws moisture away from the infant's skin. In a crossover design study involving 150 infants in which a disposable diaper with a fluff type inner liner was used for half of the period and one containing SAM for the other half, skin hydration was measured by electrical conductance as well as by a technique measuring desorption of evaporative water loss

---

from the stratum corneum. During the study period there was a 17% incidence and 26% prevalence of diaper dermatitis. At all levels of urine load in the diaper prior to measuring skin hydration, diapers containing SAM maintained a drier skin state. The average severity of diaper dermatitis was lower for the SAM diapers as well.

Perhaps a better "mousetrap" has been built. The question to be answered is: "Is it necessary?"

Brief Encounters

Dr. Robert Silverman of Case Western Reserve School of Medicine reported a burn-like dermatitis in small premature infants as an indicator of candidal sepsis. The initial case was a 900 gm premature infant who had widespread patches of erythema on the third day of life. In a prospective study, candidal sepsis in 8 of 23 infants was associated with a similar burn-like dermatitis that was KOH positive. All eight infants weighed less than 1,000 gm and were of about 30 weeks' gestation. In addition, 75% had onset of the rash in the first 3 days of life, and 75% of the mothers had cervical circlage. Another red flag to pay attention to!

Dr. Alvin Jacobs, the "Dean" of pediatric dermatologists, described six children who had innocuous looking hairy plaques on various body surfaces. Three of the six had increased pigmentation in the involved area, and some had a finely granular surface. An interesting clue to the underlying diagnosis was a puckering or thickening of the skin on rubbing. All of the sites, when biopsied, were found to be smooth-muscle hamartomas or congenital pili hamartomas. These lesions tend to persist. This disorder should get a rise out of you, or at least your patient.

Manifestations of Milk Allergy in Infancy: Clinical and Immunologic Findings
D.J. Hill, M.A. Firer, M.J. Shelton, and C.S. Hosking (Royal Children's Hosp., Parkville, Victoria, Australia)
J. Pediatr. 109:270–276, August 1986   4–1

Cow milk allergy results from an immunologic hypersensitivity to one or more milk proteins. The manifestations of cow milk allergy was analyzed in 100 children (mean age, 16.2 months) using 30 items of historical data and information relating to the effects of a standardized milk challenge that were entered into a computer data base. Clusters of patients were identified by using K means algorithm.

Group 1 consisted of 27 patients with predominantly urticarial and angioedematous eruptions that developed within 45 minutes of ingesting cow milk (Tables 1 and 2). Group 2 consisted of 53 patients who had predominantly gastrointestinal tract symptoms, i.e., pallor, vomiting, or diarrhea, which appeared between 45 minutes and 20 hours after milk challenge. The slow onset of eczema and diarrhea, and the insidious onset of bronchitic symptoms (e.g., coughing and wheezing), more than 20 hours after milk challenge, characterized the 20 patients in Group 3; failure to

TABLE 1.—INITIAL FEATURES IN COW'S MILK ALLERGY

	Group 1 (n = 27)	Group 2 (n = 53)	Group 3 (n = 20)	P* a	b	c
Median age (mo)	10[a]	10[b]	17[ab]	0.015	0.002	
Urticaria, acute	20[ab]	11[ac]	0[bc]	<0.001	<0.001	<0.001
Eczema, chronic	5	6[a]	9[a]	0.003		
Vomiting						
Episodic	10[a]	27[b]	2[ab]	0.036	0.006	
Persistent	1	10	3			
Diarrhea						
Episodic	2[a]	21[ab]	3[b]	0.002	0.04	
Persistent	9	17	9			
Wheeze, episodic	7[a]	2[a]	2	0.006		
Wheeze/bronchitis, persistent	6[a]	7[b]	11[ab]	0.02	<0.001	
Weight <3rd centile	4[a]	10	8[a]	0.05		
Height <3rd centile	1	4	1			

Frequency of symptoms at presentation in groups 1, 2, and 3. Level of difference indicated if $P < .05$ by chi-square analysis and Fisher exact test. There was no significant difference in frequency between persistent vomiting, persistent diarrhea, or height less than the third centile at presentation between groups. Differences in age at presentation analyzed by Mann Whitney U Test and two-tailed test.

P values derived by comparing two values with same superscript letter (e.g., for episodic vomiting, group 1 is significantly different from group 3, $P = .036$; group 2 is also different from group 3., $P = .006$).

(Courtesy of Hill, D.J., et al.: J. Pediatr. 109:270–276, August 1986.)

TABLE 2.—EFFECT OF MILK CHALLENGE IN COW'S MILK ALLERGY

	Group 1	Group 2	Group 3	P a	b	c
Patients	27	53	20			
Angioedema/urticaria	21[ab]	6[a]	2[b]	<0.001	<0.001	
Eczema	3	2[a]	7[b]	0.001		
Morbilli	1	4	0			
Vomiting	9[ab]	32[ac]	0[bc]	0.02	0.003	<.001
Diarrhea	4[ab]	32[a]	12[b]	<0.001	0.001	
Colic/irritable	10	24	10			
Cough/wheeze	8[a]	2[ab]	10[b]	0.002	<0.001	
Stridor	2	0	0			
Rhinitis	2	4	6			

Frequency of symptoms induced by formal milk challenge in Groups 1, 2, and 3. Level of difference indicated if $P < .05$ by chi-square analysis and Fisher exact test. There was no significant difference in frequency of morbilliform eruptions, colic, stridor, or rhinitis between each of the groups.

P values derived by comparing two values with same superscript letter (e.g., for diarrhea, group 1 is significantly different from group 2, $P < .001$, and group 3, $P = .001$).

(Courtesy of Hill, D.J., et al.: J. Pediatr. 109:270–276, August 1986.)

thrive was most common in this group. Elevated serum antimilk immunoglobulin IgE antibody levels and positive skin test reactions were significantly more frequent in patients in group 1 than in group 2 and group 3 (Tables 3 and 4). Group 2 patients were relatively IgA deficient, whereas only those with eczema in group 3 had a positive skin test reaction and elevated IgE antibodies to milk. Patients in group 3 were the most difficult to identify initially because their symptoms were chronic and often unrelated to milk ingestion.

It is unlikely that a single laboratory test will identify all patients with cow milk allergy in view of the heterogeneous clinical and immunologic findings in these patients. For the present, the diagnosis of cow milk allergy

TABLE 3.—Immunoglobulins in Cow's Milk Allergy

	Group 1	Group 2	Group 3	P a	b
IgG percentile	23	32	33		
IgA percentile	16	13[a]	40[a]	0.034	
IgM percentile	29[a]	33[b]	65[ab]	0.019	0.019
IgE I-U/ml	77[a]	12[ab]	48[b]	0.012	0.012

Median IgG, IgA, and IgM percentiles and IgE (IU/ml) levels for groups 1, 2, and 3. Differences between each group indicated only where $P \leq .05$ using Mann Whitney U test and Fisher two-tailed test for significance.

P values derived by comparing two values with same superscript letter (e.g., for IgE levels, group 1 is significantly different from group 2, $P = .012$; group 2 is different from group 3, $P = .012$.

(Courtesy of Hill, D.J., et al.: J. Pediatr. 109:270–276, August 1986.)

TABLE 4.—Milk Specific Antibodies in Cow's Milk Allergy

	Group 1	Group 2	Group 3	P a	b
Rast ≥1	18/26[ab]	19/52[a]	4/19[b]	0.006	0.002
Prick test ≥1	16/18[ab]	7/26[a]	1/7[b]	<0.001	0.001

Frequency of RAST ≥ 1 and skin prick test ≥ 1 in groups 1, 2, and 3 patients. Difference in frequencies between each group is indicated where $P < .05$ by chi-square analysis and Fisher exact test.

P values derived by comparing two values with same superscript letter (e.g., for RAST ≥ 1, group 1 is significantly different from group 2, $P = .006$, and Group 3, $P = .002$.

(Courtesy of Hill, D.J., et al.: J. Pediatr. 109:270–276, August 1986.)

relies on a reproducible adverse response to formal milk challenge after exclusion of other nonimmune forms of milk intolerance.

▶ One of my heros, a man who put milk allergy on a scientific basis, Dr. Douglas Heiner, Professor of Pediatrics, and Chief, Division of Immunology and Allergy, UCLA School of Medicine, provided the following comment.— F.A. Oski, M.D.

▶ The observations by Dr. Hill and colleagues are similar to those made in other centers where a large number of patients with intolerance to cow milk have been studied. The spectrum of clinical manifestations of allergy to cow milk is very broad and the diagnosis is not always readily evident. Challenge tests with objective documentation of adverse effects should be pursued. If only subjective symptoms are present, the challenges should be double blind, placebo controlled. Some cases go unrecognized even in centers with a particular interest in these disorders. It is important to remember that adverse reactions to cow milk are more common in infancy than in later life. About three quarters of the instances of hypersensitivity to milk in infants resolve spontaneously before the age of 3 years. In some, subclinical hypersensitivity persists, becoming clinically important when other allergies develop later in life, e.g., to inhalants such as grass pollen or house dust mite. At that time, it often can be shown that continued ingestion of milk results in worsening of inhalant allergy, whereas removal of milk from the diet results in a lessening or disappearance of symptoms. Thus, a person who has any allergy who was milk allergic as an infant should have a renewed trial on a milk-free diet to determine whether or not milk ingestion contributes to the symptoms.

Other authors have observed, as did Hill and colleagues, that certain manifestations of milk allergy tend to be associated with IgE antibodies and immediate skin test reactivity. These include urticaria, angioedema, and atopic dermatitis. It should also be noted that some patients with respiratory or gastrointestinal tract symptoms have high levels of IgE antibodies to milk proteins as well as immediate skin test reactions. Patients whose symptoms are delayed in onset often, but not always, have negative skin tests to milk. They may or may not have increased levels of IgE antibodies. Reactions that may not be manifest until 1 or more days after exposure to milk include milk-induced enteropathies (malabsorption, protein-losing enteropathy, and milk-induced gastrointestinal bleeding) and milk-related respiratory symptoms (chronic rhinitis, wheezing, pulmonary infiltrates and, rarely, milk-induced pulmonary hemosiderosis).

By choice, Hill and colleagues divided their patients into three groups on the basis of a computer-generated cluster analysis. Cluster analyses in medical research are most valuable when they have a high level of clinical relevance. A close look at the data presented by these authors shows that each patient reacts in a unique way. Indeed, we now know that each person has a unique immune response to cow milk proteins and probably each has a unique tissue susceptibility to the products of immunologic reactions.

I find the authors' tables listing their patients' initial clinical findings and those following milk challenge to be of interest. They are similar to the findings of many others. Their cluster analysis indicates one way to construct patient groupings, but the tables in their original paper illustrate many exceptions to such groupings. I find the cluster analyses as presented to be of marginal help in the management of individual patients, although they do suggest certain types of patients who may be hard to recognize. No one can argue with the statement that patients with delayed-onset hypersensitivity are more difficult to identify than patients with immediate reactions.—D.C. Heiner, M.D., Ph.D.

Prodromal Features of Asthma
S. Beer, J. Laver, J. Karpuch, S. Chabut, and M. Aladjem (Tel Aviv Univ., Israel)
Arch. Dis. Child. 62:345–348, 1987   4–2

The prodromal features of asthma were studied in a series of 134 pediatric patients presenting to a pulmonary-allergic outpatient clinic; the 90 boys and 44 girls had a mean age of 7 years. Ninety-three children had seasonal asthma and 41 had perennial bronchial asthma. Asthma had been present for 1–7 years.

Prodromal symptoms were present at least 6 hours before the asthmatic attack in 95 patients (group A); in 39 (group B) a rapid evolution of symptoms occurred, leading to an overt attack within 6 hours. The two groups were similar in age, family history of allergy, and numbers of attacks

TABLE 1.—COMPARISON OF INDIVIDUAL
CHARACTERISTICS IN PATIENTS WITH (GROUP A) OR
WITHOUT (GROUP B) PRODROMAL SYMPTOMS BEFORE
THE ATTACK OF ASTHMA

	Group A (n=95)	Group B (n=39)
Sex (M:F)	66:29	24:15
Mean (SD) age (years)	6·7 (2·8)	7·7 (3·6)
No of patients with family history of allergy	56	24
Mean No of admissions per patient during the last year	0·55	0·56
Mean (SD) No of attacks of asthma per patient during the last year	6·8 (2·6)	7·3 (2·4)
Type of asthma:		
Seasonal	68	25
Perennial	27	14

(Courtesy of Beer, S., et al.: Arch. Dis. Child. 62:345–348, 1987.)

TABLE 2.—INITIAL PRODROMAL SYMPTOM AND ITS TIME
RELATION TO THE OVERT ATTACK OF ASTHMA

Symptom	No of patients	Interval (hours) between initial symptom and onset of overt attack Mean (SD)*	Range
Rhinorrhoea	39	26·76 (12·00)	6–60
Cough	23	20·73 (0·42)	6–48
Irritability	7	28·28 (4·53)	12–36
Apathy	7	28·28 (4·13)	12–36
Anxiety	3	30	24–36
Sleep disorders	2	18	12–24
Fever (above 38°C)	5	16·2 (4·0)	6–24
Abdominal pain	2	13·5 (6·4)	6–24
Loss of appetite	2	18	12–24
Itching	3	9	6–12
Skin eruption	1	9	6–12
Toothache	1	9	6–12

*The means and standard deviations were computed according to average representative values of the appropriate time ranges.
(Courtesy of Beer, S., et al.: Arch. Dis. Child. 62:345–348, 1987.)

and hospitalizations in the preceding year (Table 1). Respiratory tract prodromal symptoms were most frequent, followed by behavioral changes (Table 2). Initial symptoms were followed by additional symptoms in all but 3% of the patients'; usually, more than one system was involved (Table 3). Most of the patients consistently had the same prodromal features before each asthmatic attack. In 75% of those without prodromal symptoms, initial features occurred 30–60 minutes before the asthmatic attack with no warning. A significant age-related rise in IgE values was noted only in group A patients.

More appropriate treatment might be possible by distinguishing patients with prodromal symptoms and those without such symptoms preceding acute attacks. Continuous prophylaxis may be indicated for children who

TABLE 3.—Relation of Initial Prodromal Symptom to Additional Ones Preceding the Overt Attack of Asthma

Initial prodromal symptom*	Additional prodromal symptoms						
	Rhinorrhoea	Cough	Behaviour changes	Fever	Gastro-intestinal symptoms	Skin eruptions	Toothache
Rhinorrhoea (39)	—	39	10	5	3	2	1
Cough (23)	11	—	6	5	1	2	1
Behavioural changes (19)	5	19	—	1	5	2	0
Fever (5)	3	5	1	—	0	0	0
Gastrointestinal symptoms (4)	2	4	2	0	—	0	0
Skin eruption (4) and itching	1	4	1	0	0	—	0
Toothache (1)	1	1	0	0	0	0	—

Numbers in parentheses refer to the number of patients presenting with the particular set of symptoms. (Courtesy of Beer, S., et al.: Arch. Dis. Child. 62:345–348, 1987.)

have an acute onset of attacks, whereas those with prodromal symptoms might be treated only at the onset of the initial prodromal features.

▶ Orr described itching as a prodrome of asthma in 81% of episodic wheezers and 38% of nonepisodic wheezers. The most common sites of itching were the tip of the chin, the mandibular rami, the suprathyroid area, the cricothyroid region, and the suprasternal notch (see the 1972 Year Book, pp. 121–123). The authors of this present report found itching, as the initial symptom, to be far less common and attribute this to the younger age of the population they studied. The most common prodromal symptoms observed by Beer and associates were rhinorrhea, cough, irritability, apathy, and fever. The less common prodromal symptoms included abdominal pain, loss of appetite, skin eruption, and toothache. In the younger patient the prodromal symptoms were more likely to be of a nonrespiratory nature. The presence of a prodrome should be sought, because it can be used to initiate therapy promptly.

Another potentially useful predictor of an asthma attack was described by Silber who observed that the peaks in temperature velocity coincided closely with the peaks in emergency room visits for asthma (*Pediatr. Emerg. Care* 3:13, 1987). The temperature velocity is derived from a plot of the rate of change in the ambient temperature. The more rapid the change, the more likely an asthma attack. Remember: "It is better to solve problems than crises" (Guinther, J., 1978).—F.A. Oski, M.D.

Early Intervention With Short Courses of Prednisone to Prevent Progression of Asthma in Ambulatory Patients Incompletely Responsive to Bronchodilators
James B. Harris, Miles M. Weinberger, Edward Nassif, Gary Smith, Gary Milavetz, and Allan Stillerman (Univ. of Iowa and McFarland Clinic, Ames, Iowa)
J. Pediatr. 110:627–633, April 1987   4–3

Prompt systemic therapy with steroids may reduce the need for emergency care of asthmatic patients who fail to respond well to inhaled β_2 agonists. A double-blind, placebo-controlled study of the effect of high doses of prednisone orally was carried out in 42 patients with chronic asthma, all but two of them less than 18 years of age. All of the patients in this prospective series had at least grade III chronic asthma; all required daily maintenance treatment with theophylline and used an inhaled β_2 agonist when necessary. Either prednisone, in daily doses of 60 mg or 80 mg, or placebo was given for one week, starting early in the course of an acute exacerbation. The treatment groups were clinically comparable.

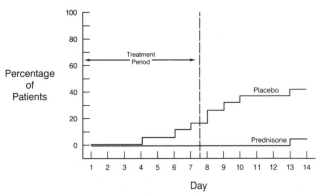

Fig 4–1.—Cumulative rate of rescue intervention during week of study medication and subsequent week because of symptoms of asthma that continued or increased despite repeated use of inhaled albuterol every 4 hours in addition to maintenance treatment with theophylline (placebo, 19 patients; prednisone, 22). Differences between groups during the 2 weeks shown were significant at the .004 confidence level. (Courtesy of Harris, J.B., et al.: J. Pediatr. 110:627–633, April 1987.)

No patient in the blinded steroid-treated group required rescue intervention with prednisone during the week of treatment, but eight patients given placebo required such intervention (Fig 4–1). Daily peak expiratory flow rate estimates followed the course of symptoms. No significant extrapulmonary effects of steroid treatment were evident.

These results support the early oral administration of prednisone when acute exacerbations of chronic asthma fail to respond completely to bronchodilator therapy. This approach is especially useful in patients who previously had a protracted course of asthma or required emergency care. Significant adverse effects did not occur in the present study.

▶ A recent study from England (Storr, J., et al.: *Lancet* 1:879, 1987) also found benefits for asthmatics from a single oral dose of prednisolone. A group of 140 children hospitalized with acute asthma entered a randomized, double-blind trial of oral prednisolone versus placebo. The dose of prednisolone was 30 mg for children under age 5 years and 60 mg for the older patients. All children also received nebulized salbutamol. On reassessment after 4 hours, 20 of 67 patients in the prednisolone group were ready for discharge, compared with only 2 of 73 in the placebo group. Children who remained in the hospital had shorter median stays and were less likely to require further steroid therapy if they had initially received prednisolone. I had assumed that everybody by now had recognized the benefit of a short course of steroids in the management of an acute asthma attack. Early use of steroids is a good example of "you can pay me now or pay me later."—F.A. Oski, M.D.

Myocardial Specific Creatine Phosphokinase Isoenzyme Elevation in Children With Asthma Treated With Intravenous Isoproterenol
James F. Maguire, Raif S. Geha, and Dale T. Umetsu (The Children's Hosp., Boston, and Harvard Univ.)
J. Allergy 78:631–636, October 1986   4–4

Intravenously administered isoproterenol is established, effective therapy for severe childhood status asthmaticus. However, ECG changes suggestive of transient myocardial ischemia have been reported in association with this treatment. Elevation of the cardiac-specific serum creatine phosphokinase MB (CPK-MB) isoenzyme was noted in 15 (group I) of 19 admissions in 14 children treated with isoproterenol intravenously in an intensive care unit setting for severe status asthmaticus unresponsive to standard emergency room therapy and intensive treatment with inhaled β_2- adrenergic agents and steroids intravenously. The results in these patients were compared with those in the 4 other patients (group II) in whom serum CPK-MB was absent.

The mean peak total serum CPK level in group I was more than twice that of group II [204 international units (IU) per L vs. 94 IU/L]. The mean peak serum CPK-MB fraction was 6.05% in group I. There was no correlation between the maximum infusion rate isoproterenol and the severity of CPK-MB elevation. The follow-up serum CPK-MB level in nine group

I patients after cessation of isoproterenol infusion was 0%. In six of these patients, a follow-up serum specimen with an undetectable CPK-MB level was obtained while the patients continued to receive aminophylline and steroids intravenously and β-adrenergic agonists by inhalation. The ST segment abnormalities were not predictive of serum CPK-MB elevation.

Elevated serum CPK-MB levels are associated with intravenously administered isoproterenol in severe childhood asthma. However, these changes are not indicative of either temporary or enduring cardiac injury in these children. Caution is therefore recommended, along with serial monitoring of serum CPK-MB levels, when isoproterenol is administered intravenously to children with severe asthma.

▶ My own serum concentration of myocardial-specific CPK isoenzyme increased as I read this report. Everyone should go slowly in jumping on the intravenous isoproterenol bandwagon. One fatality has already been reported that involved an adolescent female in whom multifocal areas of myocardial necrosis developed in association with intravenous isoproterenol therapy for status asthmaticus. We currently enjoy a low mortality rate from asthma here in the United States, with New Zealand ranked the highest (Wookcock, A. J.: *Chest* 90:40S, 1986); the differences remain unexplained, but *viva la difference*—let's keep it that way.

By the way, aerosolized metaproterenol is well tolerated in acute childhood asthma in repeated doses, and it appears to be associated with prolonged bronchodilation and improved outcome when compared with subcutaneous doses of epinephrine (Ruddy, R. M., et al.: *Pediatr. Pulmonol.* 2:231, 1986).— F.A. Oski, M.D.

The Natural History of Asthma in Childhood
H.R. Anderson, J.M. Bland, S. Patel, and C. Peckham (St. George's Hosp. Med. School and Inst. of Child Health, London)
J. Epidemiol. Community Health 40:121–129, June 1986   4–5

The National Child Development Study has followed at ages 7, 11, and 16 years nearly every child in England, Scotland, and Wales born within 1 week of March 1958 for the purpose of studying the incidence and prognosis of childhood asthma and wheezing illness. Data were collected through interviews with parents and physical examination of the child.

Complete data were available for 8,806 children who were part of a national cohort of 17,419 births occurring during the designated study week. Interviews with parents included questions concerning the occurrence and frequency of attacks of bronchitis with wheezing. In addition to the interview with parents, information was obtained from the school physician's examination made at each age.

Overall, 24.7% of the cohort had experienced asthma with wheezing at some time in their lives: 8.6% had transient asthma early in life that disappeared before age 7 years; 5.5% had asthma at age 7 years but not thereafter; 3.6% had onset of asthma between the ages of 8 and 11 years; 2.8% had onset of asthma between the ages of 12 and 16 years; and 4.2%

TABLE 1.—PREVALENCE OF ASTHMA OR WHEEZY
BRONCHITIS (AW) AT EACH INTERVIEW

Age at interview (years)

	7	11	16
Prevalence of a past history of AW at each interview			
Linked data	18·3%	12·1%	11·6%
(information at all interviews)	1608/8806	1062/8806	1019/8806
Unlinked data			
(no information at one or more interviews)	18·3%	12·7%	11·8%
	1057/5765	601/4751	308/2610
All interviewed	18·3%	12·3%	11·6
	2665/14571	1663/13557	1327/11416
Cumulative lifetime prevalence up to 16 years (linked data)	18·3%	21·9%	24·7%
	1608/8806	1927/8806	2176/8806
Prevalence of AW in past 12 months, at each interview			
Linked data	8·3%	4·7%	3·5%
	731/8806	414/8806	306/8806
Unlinked data	7·8%	5·3%	3·9%
	450/5765	250/4751	101/2610
All interviewed	8·1%	4·9%	3·6%
	1181/14571	664/13557	407/11416
Prevalence of frequent AW at each interview in linked data	0·89%	0·64%	0·5%
	78/8806	56/8806	44/8806
Cumulative prevalence of frequent AW based on 12 month period prevalences at 7, 11, and 16 years	0·89%	1·4%	1·8%
	78/8806	121/8806	155/8806

(Courtesy of Anderson, H.R., et al.: J. Epidemiol. Community Health 40:121–129, June 1986.)

had asthma with wheezing throughout their entire childhood. By age 16 years the reported life-time prevalence was 11.6%, but the life-time prevalence by age 16 years when data from all three interviews were used was 24.7% (Table 1). The prevalence of current asthma was highest at age 7 years (8.3%), followed by 4.7% at age 11 years, and 3.5% at age 16 years.

Analysis of associations between natural history and perinatal, social, environmental, and medical factors identified the following factors as predictors of onset of asthma with wheezing after age 7 years: sex of child (male), age of mother at child's birth (15–19 years), history of pneumonia, whooping cough, throat or ear infections or tonsillectomy, eczema, allergic rhinitis; and periodic vomiting or abdominal pain (Table 2).

▶ Dr. Peyton A. Eggleston, Associate Professor of Pediatrics, Johns Hopkins School of Medicine, Director of the Asthma Clinic, provided the following commentary:—F.A. Oski, M.D.

▶ Since the first descriptions of the natural history of asthma by careful, observant clinicians, our understanding has increased slowly. Even with larger prospective studies, many of the details of the natural history and its risk factors are unclear.

TABLE 2.—Association Between Eczema, Hayfever, Abdominal Pain, Vomiting, and Headaches With Natural History of Asthma or Wheezy Bronchitis

Natural history category

‑iable	Overall x^2 probability	Relative risk of: (95% confidence interval)		Never n = 6630	By 7 yr and not after n = 758	At 7 yr and not after n = 482	0–7 yr and after n = 368	8–11 yr onset n = 319
ema in first year ‑r)	<0.001	Yes:	No	0.7* (0.6–0.9)	1.2 (0.3–1.6)	1.4 (1.0–2.1)	5.4* (4.1–7.0)	1.7* (1.1–2.6)
ema after first r (7 yr)	<0.001	Yes:	No	0.8* (0.6–0.9)	1.1 (0.8–1.5)	1.3 (0.9–1.7)	4.7* (3.6–6.2)	1.3 (0.8–2.0)
ema on mination by doctor ‑r)	<0.001	Yes:	No	0.7* (0.6–1.0)	0.8 (0.5–1.4)	1.1 (0.7–2.0)	4.9* (3.5–7.0)	1.6 (0.9–2.9)
ema on mination by doctor yr)	<0.001	Yes:	No	0.7* (0.5–0.9)	1.3 (0.8–2.0)	1.4 (0.8–2.3)	4.3* (2.9–6.4)	2.5* (1.5–4.4)
ema in past year yr)	<0.001	Yes:	No	0.7* (0.6–0.9)	1.2 (0.8–1.7)	1.2 (0.8–1.9)	4.2* (3.1–5.7)	1.9* (1.3–3.0)
yfever or sneezing acks ever (7 yr)	<0.001	Yes:	No	0.6* (0.5–0.7)	1.3 (1.0–1.7)	2.0* (1.5–2.7)	7.1* (5.6–9.1)	1.5 (1.0–2.2)
yfever or allergic nitis in past year yr)	<0.001	Yes:	No	0.7* (0.6–0.9)	1.0 (0.7–1.3)	1.2 (0.9–1.6)	5.2* (4.1–6.6)	2.2* (1.6–3.1)
ema after first year s history of yfever (both asked 7 yr)	<0.001	Yes:	Neither	0.4* (0.2–0.6)	1.2 (0.6–2.4)	1.6 (0.8–3.3)	15.1* (9.9–23.0)	1.8 (0.8–4.1)
quent headaches or graine ever (7 yr)	<0.001	Yes:	No	0.9 (0.7–1.0)	1.3* (1.1–1.7)	1.5* (1.1–1.9)	2.2* (1.6–2.9)	0.8 (0.6–1.3)
current headaches migraine in past ir (11 yr)	<0.001	Yes:	No	0.9 (0.8–1.1)	1.2 (1.0–1.5)	1.1 (0.9–1.4)	1.6* (1.2–2.0)	1.2 (0.9–1.7)
riodic vomiting or ious attacks ever yr)	<0.001	Yes:	No	0.9 (0.8–1.0)	1.2* (1.0–1.5)	1.4* (1.2–1.8)	1.8* (1.4–2.3)	0.8 (0.6–1.1)
current vomiting bilious attacks past year (11 yr)	<0.091	Yes:	No	0.9 (0.7–1.2)	1.0 (0.7–1.4)	1.5* (1.0–2.2)	1.3 (0.8–2.0)	1.5 (0.9–2.3)
riodic abdominal in ever (7 yr)	<0.001	Yes:	No	0.9 (0.8–1.3)	1.4* (1.1–1.7)	1.3* (1.1–1.7)	1.5* (1.1–1.9)	0.9 (0.6–1.2)
current abdominal in in past year l yr)	<0.032	Yes:	No	1.0 (0.8–1.1)	1.3* (1.1–1.7)	1.0 (0.8–1.4)	1.1 (0.8–1.5)	1.3 (0.9–1.7)

*$P < .05$.
(Courtesy of Anderson, H.R., et al.: J. Epidemiol. Community Health 40:121–129, June 1986.)

It is agreed that the disease usually begins in the first 4–5 years of life. During this time, 14% to 18% of children will have wheezed at least once and 8% to 10% will have recurrent wheezing. By the age of 7 years, the incidence of recurrent wheezing is 5% to 7%, and this gradually decreases to 3% to 4% by adolescence. This pattern of onset in early childhood and apparent remission by adolescence has been apparent since the 1950s. It is important to emphasize that the disease is remittent in adolescents and young adults: Approximately half of these patients still have abnormally reactive airways despite their lack of symptoms, and more than half will become symptomatic again during adult life.

The onset of asthma appears to depend on the interaction of genetic and environmental factors. The strongest genetic link is with allergic disease rather than with asthma, although 30% to 40% of relatives will have demonstrable airway hyperreactivity. Approximately 60% to 70% of asthmatic patients are atopic and have another allergic disease, e.g., rhinitis or infantile eczema; 80% have first-degree relatives who are allergic. Elevated total IgE levels in umbilical cord blood are strong predictors of early and long-lasting asthma. At the same time, environmental exposure is equally important for the expression of disease. Several prospective studies show that the age of onset of asthma, and perhaps its total incidence, is lower when infants from atopic families are fed a hypoallergenic diet. Viral respiratory infections are another environmental factor important in the development of asthma. The association between the development of asthma and respiratory syncytial virus bronchiolitis in infancy has been apparent since the 1950s, and evidence has emerged recently that croup and influenza infection in infancy may also be risk factors. Air pollution is the least well-documented environmental risk factor, although it is strongly suspected. Respiratory disease in general appears to be slightly higher in children living in areas of high industrial air pollution.

Of the many factors that have been suggested as risk factors for persistent disease, only two—the severity of illness at the time the child is first seen and the presence of allergic disease—have been confirmed consistently in prospective studies. Children with frequent attacks, persistent wheezing, or abnormal pulmonary function tests between attacks have a 60% to 80% chance of persistent asthma at adolescence, a rate three to four times higher than that found in those with milder disease. The presence of other atopic illness (e.g., hay fever or eczema) or of multiple positive skin tests increases the risk of persistent disease by fivefold to sevenfold.

There has been much interest in recent years in the apparent trend toward an increased prevalence of asthma in the general population and toward more severe disease. After declining in the decade of the 1960s, hospitalizations have tripled in the last 10 years and deaths among children, especially among black children, have doubled in frequency. The reasons for this trend in the face of better drugs and more readily available medical care is not clear, but it is obviously of great concern.—P.A. Eggleston, M.D.

The Impact of Health Education on Frequency and Cost of Health Care Use by Low Income Children With Asthma
Noreen M. Clark, Charles H. Feldman, David Evans, Moshe J. Levison, Yvonne Wasilewski, and Robert B. Mellins (Univ. of Michigan and Columbia Univ.)
J. Allergy Clin. Immunol. 78:108–115, July 1986   4–6

Childhood asthma places a particularly heavy burden in terms of cost and disruption of daily life on families and communities. It is a major source of disability and the leading cause of school absenteeism. Health care costs associated with hospitalizations and emergency room visits are considerable, especially in low-income populations. A study was conducted in a large population of children with asthma to assess the effect of health education on the ability of parents and children to manage asthma and reduce the use of health services, and to determine whether such education would reduce health care costs.

The series included 310 urban children from 290 low-income families who were randomly assigned to a control group (103 children) or an experimental group (207) that received health education to improve asthma management at home. All of the families were reinterviewed 1 year after the educational intervention and hospital records were reviewed.

Although children in the experimental group had fewer hospitalizations in the follow-up year than did children in the control group, the difference

TABLE 1.—EFFECT OF THE HEALTH EDUCATION PROGRAM ON ACUTE HOSPITALIZATIONS OF CHILDREN BASED ON HISTORY OF HOSPITALIZATION

Mean No. of hospitalizations*

	No baseline hospitalizations			One or more baseline hospitalizations		
	Experimental N = 156	Control N = 65	P Value†	Experimental N = 19	Control N = 16	P Value†
Baseline year	0.00	0.00		1.21 ± 0.54	1.25 ± 0.45	NS
Follow-up year	0.10 ± 0.41	0.03 ± 0.17	NS	0.21 ± 0.54	0.94 ± 1.73	0.06
Change baseline‡ to follow-up	0.10 ± 0.41	0.03 ± 0.17	NS	−1.00 ± 0.33	−0.31 ± 1.35	0.03

*Means ± SD.
†One-tailed t tests were performed on data transformed by $\sqrt{x + 1}$.
‡Baseline to follow-up change scores were calculated from the transformed data.
NS = not significant.
(Courtesy of Clark, N.M., et al.: J. Allergy Clin. Immunol. 78:108–115, July 1986.)

TABLE 2.—EFFECT OF THE HEALTH EDUCATION PROGRAM ON EMERGENCY ROOM (ER) USE OF CHILDREN BASED ON HISTORY OF HOSPITALIZATION

Mean No. of ER visits*

	No baseline hospitalizations			One or more baseline hospitalizations		
	Experimental N = 140	Control N = 57	P Value†	Experimental N = 19	Control N = 16	P Value†
Baseline year	1.84 ± 2.91	1.49 ± 2.20	NS	7.37 ± 6.40	8.13 ± 9.08	NS
Follow-up year	1.66 ± 4.29	1.35 ± 4.00	NS	3.53 ± 5.54	8.19 ± 10.97	0.05
Change baseline‡ to follow-up	−0.18 ± 5.18	−0.14 ± 4.57	NS	−3.84 ± 8.46	0.06 ± 14.24	0.04

*Means ± SD.
†One-tailed t tests were performed on data transformed by $\sqrt{x + 1}$.
‡Baseline to follow-up change scores were calculated from the transformed data.
NS = not significant.
(Courtesy of Clark, N.M., et al.: J. Allergy Clin. Immunol. 78:108–115, July 1986.)

TABLE 3.—Effect of the Health Education Program on Emergency Room (ER) Use of Children Based on History of Baseline Hospitalization and ER Use

| | Mean No. of ER visits* | | | | Mean No. of ER visits* | | | |
| | Five or less baseline ER visits | | | | Six or more baseline ER visits | | | |
	Baseline	Follow-up	Change†	N	Baseline	Follow-up	Change	N
No baseline hospitalization								
Experimental	1.31 ± 1.53	1.21 ± 2.51	−0.10 ± 2.70	132	10.63 ± 5.53	9.13 ± 13.40	−1.50 ± 8.59	8
Control	1.11 ± 1.49	0.85 ± 1.47	−0.26 ± 1.23	54	8.33 ± 1.53	10.33 ± 16.20	2.00 ± 14.80	3
P Value‡	NS	NS	NS		NS	NS	NS	
One or more baseline hospitalizations								
Experimental	2.30 ± 1.42	1.70 ± 2.06	−0.60 ± 2.99	10	13.00 ± 4.69	5.56 ± 7.45	−7.44 ± 5.57	9
Control	2.78 ± 1.72	2.56 ± 2.56	−0.22 ± 2.64	9	15.00 ± 10.20	15.43 ± 13.55	0.43 ± 12.53	7
P Value	NS	NS	NS		NS	0.04	0.03	

*Means ± SD.
†Baseline to follow-up change scores were calculated from the transformed data.
‡One-tailed t tests were performed on data transformed by $\sqrt{x + 1}$.
NS = not significant.
(Courtesy of Clark, N.M., et al.: J. Allergy Clin. Immunol. 78:108–115, July 1986.)

was not statistically significant when findings were compared without regard to previous hospitalization (Table 1). When the comparison was restricted to children hospitalized during the baseline year, those in the experimental group experienced a statistically significant greater decrease in emergency room visits and in hospitalizations than did comparable controls (Table 2). Children who had one or more hospitalizations and six or more emergency room visits in the baseline year experienced a statistically significant greater decrease in such visits than found in comparable controls (Table 3). However, there was no significant decrease in emergency room use for those children who had a history of hospitalization and low levels of baseline emergency room use or for those children with no previous hospitalization, regardless of baseline emergency room use. The program reduced health care costs for children with one or more hospitalizations by an amount of $11.22 for every $1.00 spent on health education.

▶ An 11-fold return on the dollar! You can't expect to do better than that. Other positive outcomes of this program included improved self-management skills, school performance, and school adjustment. This type of program would be worthwhile for every child who attends an asthma clinic regardless of his financial status.

Another way of reducing emergency room visits for asthma is to eliminate exposure of children with asthma to tobacco smoke in the home. Passive smoking has been shown to correlate strongly with the number of emergency room visits. Asthmatic children from families with smokers made 63% more visits to the emergency room than did children from nonsmoking households. The extra annual cost of emergency care for children with asthma linked to passive smoking was about $92 (Evans, D., et al.: *Am. Rev. Respir. Dis.* 135:567, 1987). For more on smoking, if you really want more, see the next abstract and Chapter 9, Therapeutics and Toxicology, in this edition of the Year Book.—F.A. Oski, M.D.

Atopic Babies With Wheezy Bronchitis: Follow-Up Study Relating Prognosis to Sequential IgE Values, Type of Early Infant Feeding, Exposure to Parental Smoking and Incidence of Lower Respiratory Tract Infections

G. Geller-Bernstein, R. Kennett, L. Weisglass, S. Tsur, M. Lahav, and S. Levin (Kaplan Hosp. and Weizmann Inst. of Science, Rehovot, and Central Kupat Holim Labs., Tel-Aviv, Israel)

Allergy 42:85–91, February 1987   4–7

Transient "spastic" or "wheezy" bronchitis often is associated with upper respiratory tract viral infections in infants, but atopic patients often have wheezing as the initial sign of a hyperactive respiratory tract. A prospective study of 80 atopic wheezing infants aged 6–24 months was undertaken up to age 4–5 years to record the clinical findings and sequential IgE values. The 56 boys and 24 girls had a mean age of 13 months at the outset. Also, IgE values were determined in 60 healthy nonatopic infants living in the same area.

About two thirds of the children were symptom free for at least a year at final evaluation (Table 1). Lower respiratory tract infections correlated negatively with the recovery rate. Nearly two thirds of symptom-free patients had IgE levels of more than 2 SD above the control mean. Infections are related to parental smoking habits in Table 2. Log IgE levels at ages 2 years and 4 years were clearly related (Fig 4–2). In one third of the children a sharp rise in IgE levels occurred between ages 1 year and 2 years (Fig 4–3). The degree of rise in IgE with advancing age was not influenced by feeding or parental smoking, but a greater rise was noted in bottle-fed infants (Table 3). The course of IgE levels could not be related to the severity of asthma (Fig 4–4).

Bottle feeding and parental smoking both may lead to persistent wheezing in atopic children. Although IgE values have discriminative value in

TABLE 1.—Final Assessment of Clinical Outcome After 4 Years in 80 Wheezing Infants

	Recovered (n = 54)** %	Continued wheezing (n = 26) %	P
Male	70	69	NS
Breast feeding	72	38	< 0.01*
Parental smoking	52	77	< 0.01*
Positive skin tests	33	53	NS
IgE > mean + 2 SD	65	57	NS

*Significant at 1% level; SD, standard deviation; NS, nonsignificant; **, free of wheezing attacks for at least 1 year.
(Courtesy of Geller-Bernstein, G., et al.: Allergy 42:85–91, February 1987.)

TABLE 2.—LOWER RESPIRATORY TRACT INFECTIONS AND PARENTAL SMOKING DURING 4–YEAR STUDY OF WHEEZING ATROPIC INFANTS

Outcome (n = 80)	Lower respiratory tract infections	Parental smoking	Statistical analysis			
			a) Model of independence		b) Log linear model without 3rd order interactions	
			Expected values	Standardized residuals	Expected values	Standardized residuals
Recovered (n = 54)	a) ≥ 2 n = 14	+ 11	12.55	0.44	11.76	-0.22
		- 3	8.37	-1.86	2.23	0.51
	b) < 2 n = 40	+ 17	19.85	-0.64	16.24	0.19
		- 23	13.23	2.69*	23.77	-0.16
Persistent wheezing (n = 26)	a) ≥ 2 n = 17	+ 16	6.05	4.05*	15.24	0.19
		- 1	4.03	-1.51	1.76	-0.57
	b) > 2 n = 9	+ 4	9.56	-1.8	4.76	-0.35
		- 5	6.37	-0.54	4.25	0.37

*Statistically significant; n, number of patients.
(Courtesy of Geller-Bernstein, G., et al.: Allergy 42: 85–91, February 1987.)

diagnosing atopy, they have no prognostic value in early childhood asthma. Avoidance of certain allergens (e.g., cow's milk) and respiratory tract irritants (e.g., cigarette smoke) is important in infants at high risk of atopy.

▶ How do you treat the infant with "wheezy bronchitis"? Nebulized salbutamol was shown by Prahl et al. (*Ann. Allergy* 57:439, 1986) to have no effect in patients younger than 18 months of age, but two studies have described paradoxical deterioration in lung function after nebulized salbutamol in wheezy infants (O'Callaghan, C., et al.: *Lancet* 2:1424, 1986; Prendville, A., et al.: *Thorax* 42:86, 1987). In contrast, Lowell and associates (*Pediatrics* 79:939,

TABLE 3.—INCREASE OF IgE LEVELS FROM 1 TO 4 YEARS RELATED TO TYPE OF FEEDING AND SMOKING AT HOME

Amount of increase of IgE levels from 1–4 years	Parental smoking at home		Early feeding	
	+	–	Bottle-fed	Breast-fed (at least 3 months)
0–50 U	15	13	10	18
51–100 U	8	4	8	4
101–200 U	11	4	9	6
> 200 U	18	11	15	10
Total	52	28	42	38
P (chi-square)	NS		NS	

NS, nonsignificant.
(Courtesy of Geller-Bernstein, G., et al.: Allergy 42:85–91, February 1987.)

1987) report that subcutaneous epinephrine significantly improved the respiratory status of wheezing babies in a double-blind, randomized trial in children 24 months of age or less. Actually, 63% of patients younger than 12 months of age and 92% of those 12–24 months of age improved with epinephrine in a dosage of 0.01 ml/kg of a solution containing 1 mg/ml.

It would appear prudent to prevent the problem whenever possible. As mentioned before, nonbreast-feeding and passive smoking appear to increase the risk that an atopic infant will have a respiratory problem (McConnochie, K.M., et al.: *Pediatr. Pulmonol.* 2:260, 1986).

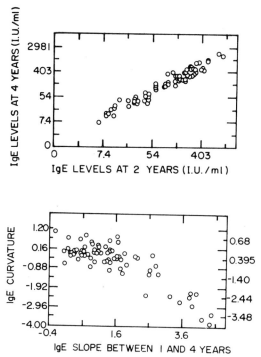

Fig 4–2 (top).—Correlation between IgE levels at ages 2 years and 4 years showing a clear linear relationship (r, .97). Regression line: IgE at 4 years, 1.447 + 1.023 × IgE at 2 years.

Fig 4–3 (bottom).—Slope and curvature of IgE levels in individual cases. Slope, IgE 4 − IgE 1. Curvature, IgE 4 − 2 IgE 2 + IgE 1.

(Courtesy of Geller-Bernstein, G., et al.: Allergy 42:85–91, February 1987.)

The magnitude of the respiratory syncytial virus (RSV)-specific IgE response at the time of an episode of RSV bronchiolitis in infants appears to predict the development of subsequent wheezing episodes (Welliver, R.C., et al.: *J. Pediatr.* 109:776, 1986).—F.A. Oski, M.D.

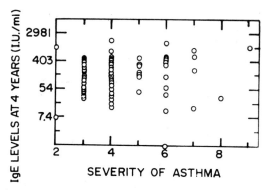

Fig 4–4.—Correlation between rise in IgE level and severity of asthma expressed as the sum of three annual clinical scores where 0 = no clinical signs or symptoms of asthma and 3 = maximal severity. (Courtesy of Geller-Bernstein, G., et al.: Allergy 42:85–91, February 1987.)

Cost-Effectiveness of Neonatal IgE-Screening for Atopic Allergy Before 7 Years of Age

K. Hjalte, S. Croner, and N.-I. Max Kjellman (Univ. Hosp., Linköping, Sweden)
Allergy 42:97–103, February 1987   4–8

The high frequency of atopic symptoms in young children who have elevated cord blood IgE levels at birth prompted a study of the cost effectiveness of neonatal IgE screening using the Phadebas IgE paper radioimmunosorbent test. The study group of 1,884 included all infants born in Linköping in a 13-month period. Families completed a questionnaire when the infant was aged 18 months, and again at ages 3 years and 6–7 years.

Obvious atopic disease developed in 18% of evaluable children before age 7 years, and occurred in more than 80% of neonates with cord blood IgE levels exceeding 0.9 kU/L. The test was only 40% sensitive; however, 94% of the patients who had severe, long-lasting atopic disease had elevated neonatal levels, and the specificity of the test was 94%. Cost calculations comparing the expense of screening with that of conventional treatment, assuming that preventive measures delay the onset of symptoms, indicated that IgE screening was cost effective both in all neonates and those with a family history of atopic disease. The cost of the screening test itself was not a very important factor.

Screening of cord blood for elevated IgE levels would seem to be worthwhile for identifying neonates to target for preventive measures against atopic disease. Actual savings are heavily dependent on patient compliance.

▶ Clinicians in the United States have been slow to accept the demonstrated predictive power of a cord blood IgE determination (see 1985 YEAR BOOK, p. 151; 1986 YEAR BOOK, p. 168; and 1987 YEAR BOOK, p. 174). I guess next year this article will be added to the list of citations with a plea that we start to identify atopic infants at birth and plan diets in a selective fashion for infants at risk.

Prolonged, exclusive breast-feeding has been shown to reduce, but not eliminate, the risk of atopic eczema. This is best observed in infants with a strong family history of atopy, elevated cord blood IgE values, and reduced numbers of suppressor T lymphocytes.

Because some breast-fed infants do become severely atopic, it became apparent that proteins could traverse the mammary barrier and appear in breast milk and thus produce a problem. It is clear that transfer of protein antigens into milk occurs after intravenous injection into lactating mice (Harmatz, P.R., et al.: *Am. J. Physiol.* 251:E227, 1986). In human beings, modification of the maternal diet can provide benefit to symptomatic infants.

Chandra and associates (*Clin. Allergy* 16:563, 1986) have performed the next logical step and demonstrated that dietary modification during pregnancy also provides benefits to the infant. Women with a history of a previous child with atopic eczema or asthma were asked to avoid cow's milk and other dairy products, eggs, fish, beef, and peanuts throughout pregnancy and for the first 6 months of lactation. When the maternal antigen avoidance group was compared with a control group it was found that infants of such mothers had less extensive and milder atopic disease. The beneficial effect was observed mainly in the breast-fed group, but the effects of maternal dietary restriction were seen also in the formula-fed infants.

Cord blood IgE anyone?—F.A. Oski, M.D.

Knuckle Pads in Children

Amy S. Paller and Adelaide A. Hebert (Rush-Presbyterian-St. Luke's Med. Ctr., Chicago; and Univ. of Texas at Houston)
Am. J. Dis. Child. 140:915–917, September 1986   4–9

Knuckle pads are asymptomatic growths that develop on the dorsal surface of digital joints, usually over the proximal interphalangeal joints. Isolated knuckle pads are benign and should therefore be distinguished from other digital lesions. Knuckle pads were identified in four children.

Case 1.—Boy, 12 years, with knuckle pads on the proximal interphalangeal joints of seven fingers (Fig 4–5), had marked thickening of the palms and soles and hyperkeratotic plaques on the elbows and knees. The lesions, which varied in size from 0.6 cm to 1.2 cm, were left untreated.

Case 2.—Girl, 14 years, had hypopigmented, smooth pads over the proximal interphalangeal joints of the fingers, thumbs, and toes. The pads developed during a 5-year period and were asymptomatic. The palms and soles were hyperkeratotic. A month of treatment with 25% urea lotion led to softening and flattening of the lesions.

Knuckle pads can be distinguished from other skin lesions by clinical and histopathologic features (table). It is important to determine the underlying cause so that it can be eliminated if possible. Patients who have knuckle pads and palmoplantar keratodermas may benefit from topical applications of keratolytic agents, e.g., lactic acid, salicylic acid, and urea.

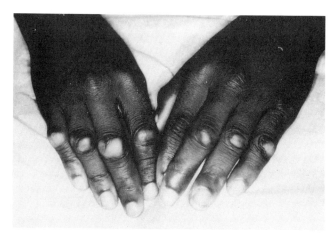

Fig 4–5.—Well-circumscribed, smooth, hypopigmented plaques overlying proximal interphalangeal joints. Patient also had palmoplantar keratoderma. (Courtesy of Paller, A.S., and Hebert, A.A.: Am. J. Dis. Child. 140:915–917, September 1986.)

DIFFERENTIAL DIAGNOSIS OF KNUCKLE PADS

Disorder	Clinical Features	Histopathologic Features	Course
Knuckle pads	Smooth fibrous thickenings, loss of skin lines, may be hypopigmented or hyperpigmented	Usually hyperkeratotic with thick epidermis; increased collagen	Often persistent
Scars, keloids	Smooth to nodular, elevated fibrous plaques at site of previous lesion	Parallel or whorled bundles of collagen; fewer capillaries and fibroblasts	Persistent
EPP	Waxy scars	Hyalin deposition	Persistent
EBA	Milia, atrophy	Atrophy, scar	Persistent
EBD	Milia, atrophy	Atrophy, scar	Persistent
Callus	Rough, fibrous, retained skin lines	Hyperkeratotic with thick epidermis	Clears if treated
GA	Subcutaneous nodule; annular plaque with papules at periphery, central clearing	Collagen degeneration surrounded by histiocytes and lymphocytes	Clears after months
Rheumatoid nodules	Subcutaneous nodules	Same as GA	Often persistent
Gottron's papules	Flat-topped violaceous papules	Variable, like dermatomyositis	Follow course

EPP: erythropoietic protoporphyria; EBA: epidermolysis bullosa acquisita; EBD: epidermolysis bullosa dystrophica; and GA: granuloma annulare.
(Courtesy of Paller, A.S., and Hebert, A.A.: Am. J. Dis. Child. 140:915–917, September 1986.)

Knuckle pads of fibrous histologic appearance may respond to corticosteroid therapy with occlusion; however, these agents should not be injected into the lesions. If the cause of the lesions is repeated trauma, moleskin bandages can protect the joints. The lesions should not be excised, as they often recur, and severe scarring or keloid formation may result.

▶ Knuckle pads were considered a real advantage in the days when children shot marbles. Now children are too busy shooting everything but marbles. I still prefer knuckle pads over knuckle heads.—F.A. Oski, M.D.

Tinea in Tiny Tots
Alvin H. Jacobs and Brigid M. O'Connell (Stanford Univ)
Am. J. Dis. Child. 140:1034–1038, October 1986   4–10

Tinea capitis infections are well recognized, but other dermatophyte infections in young children are rare and consequently often overlooked. Several patients were seen with dermatophyte infections occurring in areas other than the scalp.

Girl, aged 18 months, had a 6-month history of spreading diaper rash (Fig 4–6), with erythematous, circinate, and serpiginous patches. A potassium hydroxide (KOH) preparation showed branching hyphae, and culture yielded *Trichophyton rubrum*. Complete clearing followed application of miconazole nitrate cream twice daily for 2 weeks.

In some cases, dermatophyte infections resembled diaper rash (Figs 4–

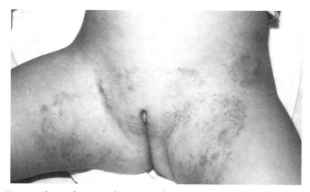

Fig 4–6.—Dermatophyte infection in diaper area of 6 months' duration caused by *T. rubrum*. Cleared with miconazole nitrate cream. (Courtesy of Jacobs, A.H., and O'Connell, B.M.: Am. J. Dis. Child. 140:1034–1038, October 1986.)

7 and 4–8). Acute, intermediate, and chronic infections had different patterns of presentation, different causative organisms, and different prognoses (table, p. 166), with the acute infections being the most responsive to treatment.

A KOH preparation should be made in all suspicious cases. The advancing border is gently scraped with a no. 15 blade, the specimen and a drop or two of KOH in 40% dimethyl sulfoxide are placed on a slide, after which a coverslip is applied; the slide is then observed within 30 minutes in dim light.

Superficial fungous infections are not rare, and suspect skin lesions should be diagnosed promptly by KOH preparations and cultures. The most effective treatments are clotrimazole, miconazole nitrate, econozole nitrate, haloprogin, and ciclopiroxolamine applied topically twice daily until the lesions disappear.

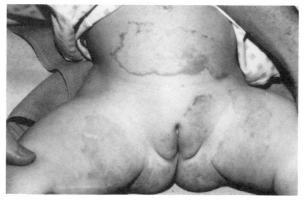

Fig 4–7.—Patient 3. Diaper eruption of 3 months' duration characterized by large annular patches. Culture yielded *T. rubrum*. Responded to topical clotrimazole treatment. (Courtesy of Jacobs, A.H., and O'Connell, B.M.: Am. J. Dis. Child. 140:1034–1038, October 1986.)

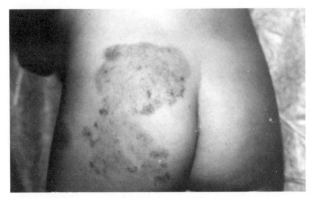

Fig 4–8.—Annular erythematous eruption in diaper area of 1 month's duration. Culture yielded *Trichophyton mentagrophytes*. The response to clotrimazole was good. (Courtesy of Jacobs, A.H., and O'Connell, B.M.: Am. J. Dis. Child. 140:1034–1038, October 1986.)

1% Permethrin Cream Rinse vs 1% Lindane Shampoo in Treating Pediculosis Capitis

Kathie Brandenburg, Amos S. Deinard, Joan DiNapoli, Steven J. Englender, Joseph Orthoefer, and Doris Wagner (Univ. of Minnesota and various city and county health departments in the United States)
Am. J. Dis. Child. 140:894–896, September 1986   4–11

Because infestation with head lice appears to be increasing in prevalence, the problem is substantial for public and private health communities. The usefulness of 1% lindane shampoo, applied for 4 minutes, was compared with that of a new ectoparasiticide, 1% permethrin cream rinse, a pyrethrin derivative, applied for 10 minutes, to treat patients with head lice infes-

PATTERNS OF PRESENTATION

Variable	Acute	Intermediate	Chronic
Pruritus	+ + +	+	0/ +
Inflammatory response	+ + +	+	0
Clinical course	Usually no recurrence	Periodic recurrence	Persistent
Immunity	Complete	Incomplete	None
Trichophyton skin test	Response in 24-48 h	Minimal response	Negative
Response to treatment	Excellent	Good	Clears but relapses
Associated organism	*Trychophyton rubrum, Trychophyton mentagrophytes*	*T mentagrophytes*	*T rubrum*

Plus signs indicate intensity; zero, absent.
(Courtesy of Jacobs, A.H., and O'Connell, B.M.: Am. J. Dis. Child. 140:1034–1038, October 1986.)

TABLE 1.—Proportion (%) of All Patients Free From Live Lice

Study Center	Day 7		Day 14	
	1% Permethrin Cream Rinse	1% Lindane Shampoo	1% Permethrin Cream Rinse	1% Lindane Shampoo
Wake County, NC	50/51 (98)	60/60 (100)	49/51 (96)	57/60 (95)
Rockford, Ill	66/66 (100)	29/31 (94)	64/64 (100)	27/30 (90)
Indianapolis	44/44 (100)	47/52 (90)	45/45* (100)	42/52 (81)
Phoenix	41/41 (100)	34/43 (79)	39/39 (100)	31/43 (72)
Nashua, NH	11/11 (100)	12/13 (92)	11/11 (100)	11/13 (85)
Minneapolis	20/20 (100)	25/27 (92)	23/23* (100)	27/32* (84)
Orange County, NC	15/15 (100)	10/10 (100)	15/15 (100)	10/10 (100)
Mecklenburg County, NC	9/9 (100)	10/11 (91)	9/9 (100)	9/11 (82)
Pooled Data†	**256/257** (99.6)	**227/247** (91.9)	**255/257** (99.2)	**214/251** (85.2)

*Includes nine patients who did not have 7-day evaluation. However, excluding these patients from analysis does not alter statistical outcome.
†These differences were statistically significant ($P < .001$) at both examinations (two-sided Cochrane-Mantel-Haenszel test).
(Courtesy of Brandenburg, K., et al.: Am. J. Dis. Child. 140:894–896, September 1986.)

tation. Preschool and school-aged children at eight centers participated in the trial after active head lice infestation was confirmed by direct visual identification. Lindane was used in 272 children and permethrin in 287. The groups were demographically similar.

Permethrin cream rinse was 99% effective at both assessments, whereas lindane shampoo was 92% effective at 7 days and 85% effective at 14 days; the differences were significant at both intervals (Table 1). Side effects were mild and transient in both groups (Table 2). Pruritus developed during treatment or became worse in about 5% of both groups; it probably reflected the infestation itself.

The 1% permethrin cream rinse tested in this study is a highly effective, safe treatment of head lice infestation and is significantly superior to 1%

TABLE 2.—Dermal Evaluation*

Reaction	No. (%) of Patients Using	
	1% Permethrin Cream Rinse (n = 287)	1% Lindane Shampoo (n = 272)
Symptoms		
Pruritus	16 (5.6)	12 (4.4)
Burning-stinging	9 (3.1)	4 (1.5)
Pain	2 (0.7)	3 (1.1)
Numbness	0 (0)	1 (0.4)
Tingling	3 (1.0)	4 (1.5)
Signs		
Edema	2 (0.7)	0 (0)
Erythema	4 (1.4)	4 (1.5)
Rash	1 (0.3)	4 (1.5)
Total	**37** (12.9)	**32** (11.8)

*Patients with signs or symptoms appearing or aggravated after treatment. Patients may have experienced a change in more than one sign or symptom.
(Courtesy of Brandenburg, K., et al.: Am. J. Dis. Child. 140:894–896, September 1986.)

lindane shampoo. A single application of the cream rinse is adequate, whereas the manufacturer recommends two applications of lindane shampoo. Nit removal is not necessary.

▶ It is good news when two groups of investigators reach the same conclusion. It looks like we can say *nix* to head lice. Both studies, this and the one that follows, conclude that 1% permethrin cream rinse is superior to 1% lindane shampoo for eradication of head lice. A single application of this synthetic pyrethroid is its chief advantage over other compounds containing pyrethrin, the naturally occurring substance from which the synthetic pyrethroids derive. This compound has photostability and thus does not require a second application, as is recommended for agents such as RID.—F.A. Oski, M.D.

Comparative Study of Permethrin 1% Creme Rinse and Lindane Shampoo for the Treatment of Head Lice
James G. Bowerman, Minerva P. Gomez, Robert D. Austin, and Diane E. Wold (Burroughs Wellcome Co., Research Triangle Park, N.C.)
Pediatr. Infect. Dis. J. 6:252–255, March 1987   4–12

Permethrin, a synthetic pyrethroid, is available as a cream rinse hair conditioner containing 1% permethrin and 20% isopropanol. It was compared with lindane shampoo because of the neurotoxicity and anemia associated with standard lindane treatment, as well as occasional resistance of head lice to lindane. A randomized single-blind investigation was carried out comparing single applications of each product in an area near Mexico City where the prevalence of head louse infestation is estimated to be between 60% and 70%. Treated patients had a mean age of 10 years.

For 296 index cases, treatment with permethrin cream rinse was at least 98% effective, whereas lindane shampoo was 90% effective at 7 days and 76% effective at 14 days (table). A safety study in more than 1,000 children showed adverse effects in 1.2% of permethrin-treated patients and in 2.6%

Day 7 and Day 14 Efficacy Results That Compared Permethrin and Lindane in Population Infested With Head Lice

	Day 7		Day 14	
	Index	All	Index	All
No. of patients evaluated				
Permethrin	195	652	195	652
Lindane	99	380	99	380
No. of patients (%) louse-free				
Permethrin	194 (99)	649 (99)	191 (98)	639 (98)
Lindane	89 (90)	339 (89)	76 (76)	283 (74)
P*	<0.001		<0.001	

*Two-sided Fisher's exact test.
(Courtesy of Bowerman, J.G., et al.: Pediatr. Infect. Dis. J. 6:252–255, March 1987.)

of patients treated with lindane. No neurologic side effects were reported, and there were no serious complications. Pruritus and erythema were the most frequent side effects.

Permethrin proved to be an effective, safe treatment for head louse infestation in this study. The substance remains on hair at considerable levels for at least 2 weeks despite repeated shampooing. This treatment is especially useful when reinfestation is likely to occur. Efficacy of 98% was achieved at 2 weeks with a single application in this high infestation community.

Gianotti-Crosti Syndrome Associated With Infections Other Than Hepatitis B
Zoe Kececioglu Draelos, Ronald C. Hansen, and William D. James (Univ. of Arizona and Walter Reed Army Med. Ctr.)
JAMA 256:2386–2388, Nov. 7, 1986   4–13

Papular acrodermatitis of childhood or Gianotti-Crosti syndrome (GCS) is characterized by nonpruritic, symmetric, flesh-colored to erythematous flat-topped papules of 3 weeks' duration that are localized to the face,

TABLE 1.—Clinical Comparison*

Symptoms	Papular Acrodermatitis of Childhood	Papulovesicular Acrolocated Syndrome	Present Study Gianotti-Crosti Syndrome
Cutaneous findings	Symmetrical, monomorphous, papular	Polymorphous, papulovesicular	Symmetrical, monomorphous, papular, rarely vesicular
Size, mm	1-5	1-2	1-5
Distribution	Face, buttocks, and limbs; absent on trunk; spares antecubital popliteal fossae	Face, buttocks, and limbs; absent on trunk; involves antecubital popliteal fossae	Face, buttocks, and limbs; occasionally trunk; variably involves antecubital fossa
Pruritus	No	Yes	Late, occasional
Duration of cutaneous findings	2-3 wk	Up to 2 mo	3-8 wk
Isomorphic response	Yes	No	Yes
Adenopathy	Yes	Yes	Variable
Hepatomegaly	Yes	No	Uncommon
Hepatitis B surface antigen	Positive	Negative	Negative
Systemic symptoms	No	No	Frequent in prodrome

*Adapted from James, W.D., et al.: J. Am. Acad. Dermatol. 6:862–866, 1982.)
(Courtesy of Draelos, Z.K., et al.: JAMA 256:2386–2388, Nov. 7, 1986.)

TABLE 2.—CLINICAL INFORMATION

Patient No./ Age/Sex	Duration, d	Distribution	Adenopathy	Hepatomegaly	HBsAg*	EBV-VCA†	Miscellaneous Laboratory Tests‡	Possible Infectious Etiology
1/2 y/M	27	Face, buttocks, and extremities	+	—	—	...	+ β-Hemolytic streptococcal throat culture; Streptozyme§ titer >1:100	β-Hemolytic streptococci
2/13 mo/M	17	Extremities	—	—	—	—	+ β-Hemolytic streptococci	β-Hemolytic streptococci
3/16 mo/M	49	Face, buttocks	—	—	—	—	+ RSV culture	RSV
4/21 mo/M	32	Extremities, trunk	—	—	—	Consistent with past infection	+ RSV titer 1:128; CMV; viral isolation	RSV
5/19 mo/F	21	Face, extremities	—	—	—	Consistent with past infection	+ Polio enterovirus status after vaccination	Enterovirus
6/14 mo/M	28	Extremities	+	+	—	—	- CMV; toxoplasmosis; viral isolation	Unknown
7/2 y/M	30	Buttocks, extremities	—	—	—	—	ALT elevated; cocci serology; viral isolation	Unknown
8/11½ y/M	60	Face, upper extremity	—	—	—	—	- Toxoplasmosis; viral isolation	Unknown
9/2⅔ y/F	21	Face, extremities, and trunk	—	—	—	Consistent with past infection	- viral isolation	Unknown

*HBsAG, hepatitis B surface antigen.
†EBV, Epstein-Barr virus; VCA, viral capsid antigen.
‡RSV, respiratory syncytial virus; CMV, cytomegalovirus; ALT, alanine aminotransferase.
§Screening test to detect presence of antibodies to five different types of streptococci.
(Courtesy of Draelos, Z.K., et al.: JAMA 256:2386–2388, Nov. 7, 1986.)

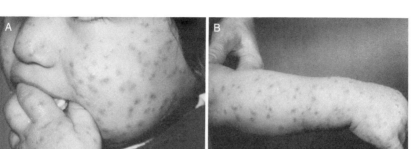

Fig 4–9.—Inflammatory, monomorphous, symmetric flat-topped papules over face (**A**) and upper extremity *(B)*. (Courtesy of Draelos, Z.K., et al.: JAMA 256:2386–2388, Nov. 7, 1986.)

buttocks, and extremities. It is also associated with lymphadenopathy, acute anicteric hepatitis of 2 months' duration that may progress to chronic liver disease, and hepatitis B surface antigenemia, subtype *ayw,* which may be persistent (Table 1). However, GCS is rarely associated with hepatitis B infection in North America. A review was made of data on nine children with GCS who had infections other than hepatitis B.

The seven boys and two girls ranged in age from 13 months to 2 years 4 months, and all had symptoms typical of GCS (Fig 4–9). Results of tests for hepatitis B surface antigen were negative, but associations with other bacterial and viral organisms were found (Table 2). Skin biopsies, taken in three patients, had findings that were consistent with those for GCS. No association was found between GCS and Epstein-Barr virus. Two patients had positive throat cultures for β-hemolytic streptococci, two had evidence of respiratory syncytial virus infection, and a polio enterovirus was isolated in one. Hepatitis B is not the causative agent of GCS in North America; rather, multiple infectious agents may be associated with this disease entity.

▶ This is a rash that is worth learning and remembering. Nobody is too old to learn, but a lot of people keep putting it off.

Gianotti-Crosti syndrome is not rare in France and also appears to be associated with a variety of viruses that are far more frequent than those that cause hepatitis B (Taieb, A., et al.: *Br. J. Dermatol.* 115:49, 1986). Of the 26 children in the report, there was serologic evidence of recent Epstein-Barr virus infection in seven, coxsackie B in three, and cytomegalovirus in one.—F.A. Oski, M.D.

Extraspinal Tendon and Ligament Calcification Associated With Long-Term Therapy With Etretinate

John J. DiGiovanna, Roberta K. Helfgott, Lynn H. Gerber, and Gary L. Peck (Natl. Cancer Inst. and Clinical Ctr., NIH, Bethesda)
N. Engl. J. Med. 315:1177–1182, Nov. 6, 1986   4–14

Synthetic vitamin A derivatives are now used in various dermatologic, oncologic, and rheumatologic disorders. Observations of tendon and ligament calcification in two etretinate-treated patients with bone and joint symptoms led to a radiographic survey of 38 patients who received etretinate, usually for Darier's disease, psoriasis, or lamellar ichthyosis. The average dose of etretinate was 0.8 mg/kg daily, and the average time of treatment was 5 years. Control radiographs were obtained from 55 patients having systemic lupus erythematosus and from other patients having pelvic radiography.

Extraspinal tendon and ligament calcification was found in 80% of the etretinate-treated patients (Table 1). The plantar ligaments and Achilles tendon were most often involved. Calcification often was symmetrical (Fig 4–10). Sixteen patients had tendon and ligament calcification in the knee region. Calcification could not be related to age or to the dose or duration of etretinate therapy. The radiographic findings correlated poorly with the presence of bone and joint symptoms (Table 2). Eleven patients had diffuse hyperostosis-like spinal involvement in addition to extraspinal calcification. Extraspinal tendon and ligament calcification was significantly more prevalent in the etretinate-treated group than in the controls with lupus (Table 3). Sequential chemotherapy with isotretinoin or vitamin A, followed by etretinate, did not significantly correlate with the occurrence of extraspinal tendon and ligament calcification.

Tendon and ligament calcification may occur without vertebral involvement in patients given long-term etretinate therapy. It also is seen as part of the spectrum of diffuse idiopathic skeletal hyperostosis, but anterior spinal ligament calcification is more closely associated with long-term isotretinoin therapy.

▶ Etretinate, a synthetic derivative of vitamin A (retinoids), has not been widely used in the United States because it has only recently been approved

TABLE 1.—Number of Patients With Radiographic Evidence of Extraspinal Tendon and Ligament Calcification in Examined Areas*

Location	No. of Affected Patients (%)
≥1 Ligament	32 (84)
Ankle	29 (76)
Pelvis	20 (53)
Knee	16 (42)
Shoulder	2 (5)
Elbow†	1

*Thirty-eight patients were examined.
†Radiographs of the elbows were obtained for this patient because of local symptoms.
(Courtesy of DiGiovanna, J.J., et al.: N. Engl. J. Med. 315:1177–1182, Nov. 6, 1986.)

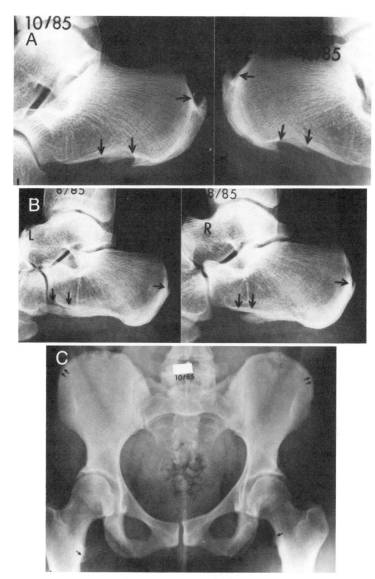

Fig 4–10.—Lateral views of the calcanei showing tendon and ligament calcification as a symmetric process. **A,** symmetric tendon and ligament calcification involving the Achilles tendons and two ligaments or tendons attaching to the plantar surfaces of the calcanei; **B,** calcaneocuboid ligaments and Achilles tendons (from a different patient) are involved, again in a bilaterally symmetric fashion. Extensive extraspinal involvement included the knees, pelvis, and shoulders but essentially normal posteroanterior and lateral radiographs of the cervical and thoracic spine; **C,** symmetric involvement of the pelvis. (Courtesy of DiGiovanna, J.J., et al.: N. Engl. J. Med. 315:1177–1182, Nov. 6, 1986.)

TABLE 2.—CORRELATION OF EXTRASPINAL TENDON
AND LIGAMENT CALCIFICATION WITH BONE
AND JOINT SYMPTOMS

X-RAY FINDINGS	SYMPTOMS IN AREA OF X-RAY FINDINGS	SYMPTOMS IN OTHER AREAS	NO. OF PATIENTS	
–	–	–	1	
–	–	+	5	21/38*
+	–	–	5	(55%)
+	–	+	10	
+	+	+	10	17/38
+	+	–	7†	(45%)

*These patients had no symptoms relevant to x-ray findings.
†Seven of the 38 patients (18%) had symptoms only in areas of x-ray findings.
(Courtesy of DiGiovanna, J.J., et al.: N. Engl. J. Med. 315:1177–1182, Nov. 6, 1986.)

TABLE 3.—PREVALENCE OF EXTRASPINAL TENDON AND
LIGAMENT CALCIFICATION IN THE TOTAL GROUP OF ETRETINATE-
TREATED PATIENTS AND IN CONTROL PATIENTS WITH SYSTEMIC
LUPUS ERYTHEMATOSUS, ACCORDING TO AGE AND SEX

SEX STUDIED	AGE AND TREATMENT GROUP					
	25–40 YR		41–68 YR		25–68 YR	
	ETRETINATE	CONTROL	ETRETINATE	CONTROL	ETRETINATE	CONTROL
	no. of affected patients/no. in group					
Male	7/10	0/6*	12/13	1/3†	19/23	1/9‡
Female	6/7	5/29§	7/8	9/17†	13/15	14/46‡
Male and female	13/17	5/35‡	19/21	10/20*	32/38	15/55‡

*.01 ≤ P < 0.05.
†P not significant.
‡P < .001.
§.001 ≤ P < .005.
(Courtesy of DiGiovanna, J.J., et al.: N. Engl. J. Med. 315:1177–1182, Nov. 6, 1986.)

by the Food and Drug Administration. It has been in use since 1975 in Europe, where it is widely prescribed. Although an ossification abnormality of the forearms (Sillevis Smitt, J.H., de Mari, F.: *Clin. Exp. Dermatol.* 9:554, 1984) and diffuse skeletal hyperostosis (Burge, S., Ryan, T.: *Lancet* 2:397, 1985) have been reported, it was not believed that this drug was associated with an increased incidence of bone toxicity. Now we know differently. I've always said that the best time to use a drug is when it is first released while it is still 100% effective and not associated with any known side effects.—F.A. Oski, M.D.

Cimetidine Treatment of Recalcitrant Acute Allergic Urticaria

Michael Rusli (The Chester County Hosp., West Chester, Penn.)
Ann. Emerg. Med. 15:1363–1365, November 1986   4–15

Although it is widely accepted that the human skin vasculature contains both H_1 and H_2 receptors, it is surprising that little is known concerning the use of H_2 receptor blockers in the treatment of acute allergic urticaria and acute allergic reactions in general. The use of H_2 receptor blockers (e.g., cimetidine) in patients with chronic idiopathic urticaria has been reported. Five consecutive patients with acute allergic urticaria caused by insect stings were treated with cimetidine. All patients were recalcitrant to treatment with epinephrine, diphenhydramine, and corticosteroids.

Each patient responded dramatically within 15 minutes to the intravenous infusion of 300 mg of cimetidine. All were discharged taking cimetidine orally, 300 mg every 6 hours, and none reported recurrences or exacerbations of urticaria on follow-up. There were no complications.

Cimetidine may be effective in patients with acute allergic urticaria recalcitrant to conventional therapies, e.g., epinephrine, H_1 receptor blockers, and corticosteroids. Controlled clinical studies are necessary to confirm these preliminary results.

▶ The five patients in this report ranged in age from 16 to 32 years, but there is no reason why cimetidine should not work equally well in children with acute allergic urticaria. Cimetidine has been studied extensively in the management of chronic idiopathic urticaria, dermographism, systemic mastocytosis, eosinophilic fasciitis, cold-induced urticaria, and the blocking of the cutaneous flushing response to intravenous doses of histamine. It is a drug that should become part of your therapeutic bag of tricks.

It seems only fitting, in view of the fact that this chapter began with an article on cow's milk allergy and ended with a report of urticaria, to close with a report of contact urticaria to cow's milk (Boso, E.B., et al.: *Allergy* 42:151, 1987). The patient, a 3½-year-old boy with a history of asthma and atopic dermatitis, as an infant would vomit cow's milk or milk products within minutes of ingestion. On two separate occasions the child spilled milk on himself and within minutes developed hives over the areas of contact. Contact sensitivity was documented to whole cow's milk, skim milk, commercial condensed milk, and even milk heated to 80 F for 30 minutes. I've heard of crying over spilt milk, but this is ridiculous. Without milk or milk products in the diet, the kid should live to be a 100.—F.A. Oski, M.D.

5 Miscellaneous Topics

Does Dress Influence How Parents First Perceive Staff Competence?
Paul G. Taylor (Univ. of Alberta, Edmonton)
Am. J. Dis. Child. 141:426–428, April 1987

It is widely assumed that, in the health care setting, the dress of the provider may help to determine the patient's or parent's initial perception of competence. An attempt was made to confirm this in a random group of parents of children admitted to pediatric inpatient services at a university teaching hospital. Two house staff physicians of each sex were photographed wearing one of three typical outfits: formal street clothes and a

TABLE 1.—15 Paired Combinations of Five
Independent Study Variables Used
in Study Cards*

| Card | Comparison | |
	Physician A	Physician B
1	FoF	FoM
2	IF	FoF
3	IM	FoF
4	FoF	OF
5	OM	FoF
6	IF	FoM
7	IM	FoM
8	FoM	OF
9	FoM	OM
10	IF	IM
11	IF	OF
12	IF	OM
13	IM	OF
14	OM	IM
15	OF	OM

*Fo, formal; F, female; M, male; I, intern;; O, operating room.
(Courtesy of Taylor, P.G.: Am. J. Dis. Child. 141:426–428, April 1987.)

TABLE 2.—DEMOGRAPHIC CHARACTERISTICS OF
STUDY PARENTS

Demographic Characteristic	Observation Level
Race, %	
White	92
Oriental	8
Age, y	
Mean	31
Range	17–51
Gender, %	
Female	72
Male	28
Education, %	
<Grade 12	22
Grade 12	45
>Grade 12	20
University degree	13
Previous hospital experience, %	
Had a child previously admitted to hospital	47
First experience with child in hospital	53

(Courtesy of Taylor, P.G.: Am. J. Dis. Child. 141:426–428, April 1987.)

long white lab coat, an operating room outfit, and an intern uniform that included a short white jacket and white or casual slacks (Table 1). Forty parents were enrolled in the study (Table 2).

More than 75% of the choices presented resulted in a positive statement of preference. Parents were twice as likely to ascribe competence to the physician wearing formal dress than to the one wearing operating room garb, and four times more likely than to the physician wearing an intern uniform. Fewer parents with a university education and fewer who had never previously had a child in the hospital made assumptions of competence.

Because relief of parental anxiety is a major goal in pediatric practice and the parent who perceives a physician as being competent will be reassured, dressing to conform to the parent's stereotype of a competent physician is an effective means of providing reassurance. The lab coat may be preferable to the intern uniform that is often issued without charge to house staff.

▶ This article does not require commentary; it only requires reading. Another issue that is worth examining is the notion that not wearing white is kinder to the children. It is my impression that being examined, and even being stuck, by some one in street clothes makes children frightened of all people in street clothes. Better to be frightened by only the men and women in white. I may be wrong about all this. Tell me, what do you prefer: plain-clothes police or the uniformed variety? Unmarked cars or the obvious state trooper's vehicle?—F.A. Oski, M.D.

Medical Students' Beliefs About Nine Different Specialties
A.F. Furnham (Univ. College, London)
Br. Med. J. 293:1607–1610, Dec. 20–27, 1986   5–2

There is yet no agreement why medical students prefer or choose one specialty over another. A study was conducted to examine the beliefs and attitudes of medical students from three London University medical schools toward nine different specialties: anesthesia, general practice, gynecology, hospital medicine, pediatrics, pathology, psychiatry, radiology, and surgery. In all, 449 preclinical and postclinical students completed one of nine versions of a 50-item questionnaire seeking their attitudes toward these specialties.

Analysis of each item yielded interesting and predictable differences: Medical students remained skeptical about the effectiveness, status, and credibility of psychiatry; were generally positive about pediatrics; believed that gynecology was one of the easiest courses and that the least intelligent persons became gynecologists; and believed that surgeons were the most materialistic. Pediatrics was conceived as the most rewarding specialty and least wasted medical education, and was considered attractive because of its intellectual comprehensiveness. Pediatricians were viewed as being the least materialistic, most emotionally stable group, as more stable than the average physician, and as the group encompassing the most intelligent physicians. The students' attitudes and beliefs, however, were multidimensional: Whereas any specialty might be seen as highly negative on one dimension, it may have been viewed as extremely positive in another. The nine specialties seemed to be discriminative on two dimensions: soft versus hard, and general versus specific. For example, psychiatry was seen as soft and specific, general practice soft and general, and surgery hard but neither general nor specific. Although these attitudes tended to differ slightly between preclinical and postclinical students, some attitudes were modified by experience.

This study establishes the current pattern of medical students' beliefs and attitudes toward nine different specialties. However, these beliefs can change over time and can be rebuffed by presentation of facts.

▶ I'd like to quote verbatim from this article because the message is good for the soul. When describing the students' attitudes about pediatricians the authors wrote: "They were perceived as the most emotionally stable group. It was also agreed that paediatrics was the least waste of the medical education; that paediatricians had time to deal with their patients' emotional problems; that fellow students will not dissuade someone from wanting to enter paediatrics; that more women than men specialised in paediatrics; that it was possibly the most rewarding specialty; that paediatricians did not spend much time seeing the wrong patients; that paediatricians were the least materialistic; that they did not talk a lot but did little; that they tended to be more stable than the average doctor; that they got most satisfaction from their work; and that paediatrics was attractive because of its intellectual comprehensiveness. The students believed that paediatrics had the most ability to show long term improvement; that paediatrics was one of the most emotionally demanding of the specialties; that paediatricians tended least to over conceptualise their subject matter; and that the most intelligent doctors become paediatricians."

Is it any wonder that pediatricians, among the medical specialties, have the lowest suicide rate, the lowest drug addiction rate, the lowest divorce rate, and the highest percentage of registered Democrats?—F.A. Oski, M.D.

Child Abuse and Recurrent Infant Apnea
Carol Lynn Rosen, James D. Frost, Jr., and Daniel G. Glaze (Baylor College of Medicine, Texas Children's Hosp., and Methodist Hosp., Houston)
J. Pediatr. 109:1065–1067, December 1986   5–3

A previous study reported mortality of 31% among 13 infants who experienced recurrent episodes of apnea that required multiple resuscitations. A retrospective study of infant apnea in 81 children found that child abuse may be a contributing factor to high mortality in infants who require multiple resuscitations.

All 81 infants were evaluated and monitored at home for apnea; 17 had experienced two or more episodes that required mouth-to-mouth resuscitation. Additional data on these 17 infants are presented in Table 1. The seven boys and ten girls were divided into three groups as follows: In group 1 patients (five) apnea had started in the presence of a parent only and was not witnessed by others; in group 2 (six) apnea had started in the presence of a parent and was witnessed by others; and in group 3 (six) apnea had started in the presence of a parent only, but was witnessed by others who were subsequently called in to help. Several parents of children

TABLE 1.—Characteristics of 17 Infants
With Apnea and Multiple Resuscitations

	Mean	Range	n	%
Sex (M/F)			7/10	
Age at presentation (wk)	9	0.12-34		
Gestational age at birth (wk)	38.8	34-40		
Birth weight (g)	3163	1960-3810		
Number of resuscitations				
2			2	12
3-10			12	70
>10			3	18
Infants needing resuscitation for initial episode			12	75
Deaths			3	18

(Courtesy of Rosen, C.L., et al.: J. Pediatr. 109:1065–1067, December 1986.)

TABLE 2.—Findings in Patients With Apnea With Multiple Resuscitations

	Group 1 (n = 5)	Group 2 (n = 6)	Group 3 (n = 6)
Onset	Parent alone	Others present	Parent alone
Resuscitation	Not witnessed	Witnessed	Witnessed
Cardiorespiratory abnormality between resuscitation episodes	1 ↑Periodic breathing	1 ↑Periodic breathing	0
Resuscitations in hospital	0	2	6
Sibling with similar history	0	0	4/5
Final diagnosis	4 Infant apnea	5 Infant apnea	3 Child abuse*
	1 ?Seizure	1 Seizure	3 ?Infant apnea
Outcome	Resolved	Resolved	3 Deaths
			3 Resolved when child removed from parent

*Video recording documented parent asphyxiating infant in two cases.
(Courtesy of Rosen, C.L., et al.: J. Pediatr. 109:1065–1067, December 1986.)

in group 3 claimed that others were present when apnea started, but investigations showed otherwise.

Analysis of the data showed that infants in group 3 had certain specific features in common that were not observed in the other two groups: No infant in group 3 had cardiorespiratory abnormalities and all six required additional resuscitation once they were in the hospital. No infant in group 1 and only two in group 2 required additional resuscitation in the hospital; in both cases apnea began in the presence of individuals other than the parents (Table 2). Three of the six children in group 3 died of apnea after their release from the hospital. The other three experienced no additional episodes of apnea after they were removed from their parents when the latter's involvement was demonstrated by hidden cameras.

The behavior of most parents of infants in group 3 is compatible with a disease entity known as Münchausen's syndrome by proxy, i.e., a form of child abuse in which a parent invents symptoms that will require the child to undergo multiple and often painful hospital procedures. The physician who suspects child abuse in an infant with apnea should obtain objective evidence and report the situation to a child welfare agency.

Death-Scene Investigation in Sudden Infant Death

Millard Bass, Richard E. Kravath, and Leonard Glass (State Univ. of New York at Brooklyn)
N. Engl. J. Med. 315:100–105, July 10, 1986   5–4

Sudden infant death syndrome (SIDS) is a diagnosis by exclusion. However, careful investigation of the death scene in suspected SIDS may provide alternative diagnoses. To prove this theory, death scene investigations were conducted in 26 consecutive infants with a presumptive diagnosis of SIDS seen in the emergency room of the Kings County Hospital Center between October 1983 and January 1985. The investigations were begun within 1 week of the infant's death.

There was strong evidence of accidental death in six instances (table).

CHARACTERISTICS OF 26 CONSECUTIVE SUDDEN INFANT DEATHS

Case No.	Infant's Age/Sex	Medical Examiners' Diagnosis*	Researchers' Death-Scene Diagnosis	Circumstances Surrounding Death
1	2 mo/M	SIDS	Overlying	An exhausted mother fell asleep nursing the infant on a soft mattress. On awakening, she found the infant dead, tucked under her breast.
2	1 mo/F	SIDS	Overlying	An obese mother fell asleep while nursing the infant. On awakening, she found the infant dead under her breasts.
3	4 wk/F	SIDS†	Suspected overlying	A teenage mother watched television until 3 a.m. and fell asleep holding her infant. The mother was suspected of drug use. The description of mother and infant positions on awakening was unclear.
4	6 wk/M	SIDS	Hyperthermia and asphyxia	The infant was sleeping near a cellar furnace with the heat on and the windows sealed. There was a gas leak; brick and soot were obstructing the flue; the mother had a headache.¶
5	3 mo/F	SIDS†	Suspected asphyxia	An infant in a body–leg cast was found face down in a loose sheet with a heavy quilt over her head; she had been unattended for 6 hr.
6	7 wk/F	SIDS	Asphyxia	The infant was face down in a bassinet, with her head sunken into a spongy, foam-rubber pillow.
7	4 mo/M‡ (triplet)	SIDS†	Suspected hyperthermia	An infant with a respiratory infection was covered with two blankets. The steam vaporizer was on, the room humidity was high, the windows were sealed, and there was an odor of fresh paint (35°C).§
8	2 mo/F	SIDS	Asphyxia	During a cold night with no heat, the infant's face was in a depression in a sagging portable crib mattress, with a playsuit hood covering the face and three blankets covering the head.
9	4 mo/M (twin)	SIDS	Hyperthermia	During a cold night, three blankets covered a colicky infant who had been treated with belladonna. A defective radiator leaked live steam near the crib. The room temperature was 41°C.§
10	3 mo/M	SIDS†	Suspected asphyxia	The infant's head was under a large pillow on an adult bed.
11	1 mo/F	Sepsis	Asphyxia	The infant was wedged between a large rubber pillow and the inside of a bassinet.
12	3 mo/M	SIDS	Undetermined	The mother had visual hallucinations for 1 wk before the infant's death and attributed the cause of death to voodoo.
13	3 mo/M	SIDS	Suspected shaken baby syndrome	A 16-year-old baby sitter shook the infant in a portable swing and then placed him on an adult bed; the baby was found dead 15 min later.
14	4 mo/M	Sepsis	Hyperthermia and asphyxia	The infant was sleeping in a bed in a converted coal bin near the furnace, with the heat on, the windows sealed, and the flue pipe disconnected. His rectal temperature was 41.5°C.¶

15	4 mo/M	SIDS	Undetermined	The infant was found dead on an adult bed in an unlicensed nursery; a retarded, violent adult was in an adjoining room.
16	4 mo/M	SIDS	Suspected hyperthermia	The infant was found dead next to a radiator; the windows were sealed, the heat was on, and two blankets covered the child.¶
17	4 mo/M	SIDS	Shaken baby syndrome	A 17-year-old baby sitter vigorously shook a hungry, crying infant to quiet him when no formula was available. The infant was found dead 10 min later on a sofa.
18	4 mo/M‡ (twin)	SIDS	Asphyxia	An 11-year-old baby sitter wedged the infant face down in a small plastic tub containing a soft pillow, sheet, and blanket.
19	1 mo/F	SIDS	Asphyxia	The infant was found in a swinging bassinet face down in loose sheets. A doubly folded blanket was wrapped around her head; she had been unattended for 6 hr.
20	2 mo/F	SIDS	Overlying and asphyxia	The infant and her mother slept on a plywood board covered with foam-rubber remnants. The infant was found dead under the mother and between the remnants.
21	4 mo/M‡ (twin)	Pneumonia	Hyperthermia	The crib was next to a radiator with a leaking steam valve. The heat came on suddenly during a mid-summer heat wave; the room temperature was 39.5°C.§
22	1 mo/F	SIDS	Asphyxia	The infant was found in a crib, face down in loose sheets with a pacifier in her mouth and a blanket over her head; she had been unattended for 6 hr.
23	3 mo/M	SIDS	Overlying	An obese 14-year-old mother shared a soft bed with the infant and an older child; the infant was found partly under the mother's breast.
24	3 mo/M	SIDS	Hyperthermia and asphyxia	An infant with a "cold" slept in a wooden drawer covered with a plastic tent attached to a steam vaporizer.¶
25	8 mo/F‡ (twin)	SIDS	Asphyxia	A large, stuffed toy animal in a thin plastic bag fell into the crib, in which the infant was found dead, face up, with the plastic bag covering her face.
26	5 mo/M	SIDS	Suspected overlying	A teenage baby sitter with a history of frequent syncopal attacks shared a bed with the infant and awoke to find the infant dead at her side.

*All autopsies were performed by the Office of the Medical Examiner, City of New York, except in cases 11 and 14, in which the autopsies were performed by the Department of Pathology of the Kings County Hospital Center. The original diagnosis of bronchopneumonia in case 1 was changed to SIDS after revaluation at the family's request.
†No autopsy was performed.
‡The infant had been born prematurely and had a low birth weight.
§Highest monitored temperature at crib mattress level.
¶Unable to monitor thermal environment.
(Courtesy of Bass, M., et al.: N. Engl. J. Med. 315:100–105, July 10, 1986.)

In 18 others, possible causes of death other than SIDS were discovered, including accidental asphyxiation by an object in the crib or bassinet, smothering by overlying while sharing a bed, hyperthermia, and shaken baby syndrome. The cause and manner of death could not be determined in 2 of 26 infants. Poor judgment of the caretaker was an important contributing factor in almost all deaths. None of the infants had a potentially fatal illness before death.

Many infant sudden deaths have a definable cause that can be revealed by careful investigation of the death scene. The extremely high rate of SIDS (4.2/1,000 live births) in the low socioeconomic area served by Kings County Medical Center may be attributed in part to accidents rather than to SIDS.

▶ I asked Dr. Bruce Beckwith, Chairman of the Department of Pathology at The Children's Hospital of Denver and a respected investigator in the SIDS field, to comment.—F.A. Oski, M.D.

▶ The central thesis of this article is that the diagnosis of SIDS requires a careful and complete examination, and that a home visit is a reasonable adjunct to investigation in any unexplained death. However, this noncontroversial view is supported by data suggesting that 24 of 26 instances of "SIDS" (92%) were attributable to defects in the environment or in standards of infant care. This allegation, if true, would return us to the attitudes of past centuries concerning these deaths.

The authors imply that those of us who developed the concept of SIDS have been uncritical in disregarding the possibility that infants might suffocate from bedclothes, be overlain by bedmates, or die from overheating by nearby radiators. Yet, they seem to be equally uncritical in accepting the opposite view on these issues. Is a pillow over the head of an infant an *a priori* cause of death? Should every infant found dead in a shared bed be assumed to have been overlain? Is the presence of a radiator near the crib proof that the dead infant died of overheating? For millenia the answer to these questions was a resounding "yes." The more humanitarian view of the past two decades has suggested that these historical attitudes are at least open to question. For the first time in history, most parents of babies found dead in their cribs are reassured that they did not kill their infants and are not treated as criminals.

My reaction at the time this article was published was the same as if it had suggested that witchcraft does exist. If a recognized advocate for the existence of witches was to "study" that issue by obtaining access through subterfuge to patients in an adolescent psychiatric clinic in Salem, Massachusetts, interviewing those patients using a skillful mixture of intimidation and leading statements, I do not doubt that histories suggestive of witchcraft might emerge! It would be surprising if so prestigious a journal as the *New England Journal of Medicine* would publish such an article. Yet, in this case, the "study" was headed by a person whose prior publications have consistently incriminated suffocation and other untoward events as major causes of SIDS. Access to the cases was by questionable means, and in fact only 22 of the cases were eventually diagnosed as SIDS (see letter from Gross, E.M., Leffers, B.: *N.*

Engl. J. Med. 315:1675, 1986, for documentation of these points). The fact that every one of the 26 families whose charts were obtained agreed to the home visits and interviews raises concern as to whether appropriate standards of informed consent were followed. The interviews were carried out by potentially biased observers, using unspecified techniques, and no control population was included. The population studied was one characterized by a notorious degree of social and economic disadvantage, where substandard home environments are the norm. Finally, all decisions concerning the cause of death were made by persons who were not free of bias.

Before the results of this study can be taken seriously, they must be confirmed by scientifically acceptable methods. Until then, it would be tragic to regress to attitudes and practices of the past. On-site investigation and interviews with caretakers are an appropriate and often mandatory part of the investigation of unexplained deaths. However, if these are not carried out by sensitive, trained, and open-minded individuals, they can do more harm than good.—J.B. Beckwith, M.D.

Preventive Screening for the Fragile X Syndrome

Gillian Turner, Hazel Robinson, Susan Laing, and Stuart Purvis-Smith (Prince of Wales Children's Hosp., Randwick, New South Wales, Australia)
N. Engl. J. Med. 315:607–609, Sept. 4, 1986   5–5

Cytogenetic screening of intellectually handicapped persons to identify those with fragile X syndrome may be an effective preventive measure, because female carriers can be identified in family studies. Affected males usually have moderate handicap and occasionally autistic features or hyperactivity. A high forehead, large jaw, long ears, and enlarged testes are

TABLE 1.—RESULTS OF SCREENING FOR FRAGILE X SYNDROME IN 1,977 INTELLECTUALLY HANDICAPPED PERSONS

	SHELTERED WORKSHOPS		SCHOOLS MODERATE TO SEVERE HANDICAP		SCHOOLS MILD HANDICAP		SUBTOTAL		TOTAL
	M	F	M	F	M	F	M	F	
Total no.	377	311	343	209	496	241	1216	761	1977
Excluded (other diagnosis)	154	113	118	108	19	15	291	236	527
Asked for permission	223	198	225	101	477	226	925	525	1450
Consented (%)	74	75	78	76	77	80	77	78	77
Karyotyped	127	119	149	60	323	143	599	322	921
Positive for fragile X	14	3	9	2	5	7	28	12	40
% of total*	3.7	1.0	2.6	1.0	1.0	2.9	2.3	1.6	2.0
% of those tested	11.0	2.5	6.0	3.3	1.5	4.9	4.7	3.7	4.3
Other chromosomal abnormalities†	3	4	4	0	6	2	13	6	19

*Assuming that prevalence of fragile X syndrome is the same for the group that did not give their consent.
†XXY, 8; XYY, 2; XO, 2; XXX, 3; autosomal aberrations, 4.
(Courtesy of Turner, G., et al.: N. Engl. J. Med. 315:607–609, Sept. 4, 1986.)

TABLE 2.—NUMBERS OF AFFECTED MALES WHO WOULD BE
BORN TO IDENTIFIED FEMALES AT RISK IF EACH HAD
TWO CHILDREN

	OBLIGATE CARRIERS	FEMALE SUBJECTS		TOTAL
		50% RISK OF BEING CARRIERS	25% RISK OF BEING CARRIERS	
No. of females	36	23	25	84
No. of children*	72	46	50	168
No. of affected males	18	5.7	3	26.7

*Assuming that each woman had two children.
(Coutesy of Turner, G., et al.: N. Engl. J. Med. 315:607–609, Sept. 4, 1986.)

usual. One third of heterozygous females may be mildly handicapped. Males are identified by the presence of a fragile site at band q27 on the X chromosome, usually in 10% to 50% of cells.

A total of 1,977 mentally handicapped persons in an Australian population of 1.2 million underwent screening for fragile X syndrome. After those with known diagnoses were excluded, 40 propositi were found among 921 study subjects (Table 1). Prevalence rates for those in public schools were 1:2,610 for males and 1:4,221 for females. Family studies identified for genetic counseling 84 obligate carriers or high-risk women younger than age 35 years with no children. If each of these women had 2 children, 27 sons with intellectual deficit would be expected (Table 2). The cost of identifying a high-risk female was $3,570.

Cytogenetic screening for fragile X syndrome is recommended in all identified intellectually handicapped persons. Children in the school system who are newly identified as handicapped should be screened routinely. The costs of screening are low compared with those of maintaining persons with intellectual handicap throughout their lives.

▶ We tend to forget that the fragile X syndrome, next to Down's syndrome, is the most common chromosomal abnormality associated with mental retardation.—F.A. Oski, M.D.

The Epidemiology of Road Accidents in Childhood

I. Barry Pless, Rene Verreault, Louise Arsenault, Jean-Yves Frappier, and Joan Stulginskas (McGill Univ.)
Am. J. Public Health 77:358–360, March 1987   5–6

A review was made of the incidence of medically attended motor vehicle accidents involving children, with emphasis on the characteristics of the mildly and the severely injured. Findings in police reports were compared with data in hospital records. The population consisted of all children living in Montreal in 1981. Eight general hospitals and two children's emergency departments supplied data. Maximum abbreviated Injury Scale (MAIS) scores ranged from 1 to 8 (1 for slight injury, 8 for near fatalities).

Scores of 2 or higher were regarded as "severe." Information from police reports describing the circumstances of the accident was linked by computer to hospital records. Rates were calculated for areas in which postal codes matched census tracts and were classified by socioeconomic strata based on a child-poverty index.

In 1981 there were 1,004 child accident victims. Of these, 57% were pedestrians, 25% were passengers, and 18% were bicyclists. Overall, 35% of the pedestrians, 27% of the cyclists, and 17% of the passengers had MAIS scores of more than 1. Of those with severe injuries, 70% were hospitalized. These most often included passengers and pedestrians with head injuries, or bicyclists with extremity fractures. Thirteen children (1.2%) were killed. Rates per 10,000 child population by sex were calculated for ages 0–4, 5–9, and 10–14 years. The total incidence was 33.6/10,000, with boys having higher rates than girls. The boy:girl ratio was highest for bicycle injuries involving children aged 10–14 years. The risk of injury to pedestrians and cyclists in low vs. high socioeconomic areas increased linearly by age for boys, from 3:1 to 9:1, but was stable (average, 6:1) for girls at all ages; no such trend was found for passengers. Drivers younger than 20 years of age, followed by those more than 60 years old, were associated with the highest rates of severe child passenger injuries; housewife drivers also had a higher rate of severely injured passengers than other occupational groups; there were more such injuries in residential than in nonresidential areas.

▶ With our focus on car safety we tend to forget that the highest rate of severe injuries occurs in the pedestrian-child. Pedestrian and bicycle injuries in low income areas were four to nine times greater than those in more affluent areas. For more on bicycle injuries and bicycle helmets, please see Chapter 7, Child Development. Unintentional injuries remain the leading cause of premature mortality in the United States (*JAMA* 257:1161, 1987). Premature mortality is measured in total years of potential life lost before age 65. The top ten, for 1985, read as follows: unintentional injuries, malignant neoplasms, diseases of the heart, suicide and homicide, congenital anomalies, prematurity, sudden infant death syndrome, chronic liver disease and cirrhosis, pneumonia, and influenza. Acquired immunodeficiency syndrome has moved into 11th place.—F.A. Oski, M.D.

A Progress Report on the Trauma Score in Predicting a Fatal Outcome
Howard R. Champion, Patricia S. Gainer, and Elizabeth Yackee (Washington Hosp. Ctr., Washington, D.C.)
J. Trauma 26:927–931, October 1986   5–7

As a result of the advances in prehospital care of trauma patients, the number who arrive in extremis in the emergency room has increased. Despite efforts to improve patient survival after major trauma, nearly 60% of trauma deaths occur immediately or within the first few hours after injury. Previous studies have shown that some massive resuscitative efforts on trauma patients in extremis are not cost effective because of low survival

TABLE 1.—Probability of Survival
Associated With Trauma Score

Trauma Score	% of Survival
16	99
15	98
14	96
13	93
12	87
11	76
10	60
9	42
8	26
7	15
6	8
5	4
4	2
3	1
2	0
1	0

(Courtesy of Champion, H.R., et al.: J. Trauma 26:927–931, October 1986.)

TABLE 2.—Resuscitation Time and Charges for Patients With Trauma Scores of Less Than or Equal to Three

Trauma	0–60 Minutes Attempted Resuscitation		>60 Minutes Attempted Resuscitation	
	CNS	CV	CNS	CV
Score				
1	12	24	1	4
2	10	15	2	4
3	2	0	0	0
Totals	24	39	3	8
Average charge per patient	$1,128.12	$1,429.33	$11,877.73	$8,851.01
Average resuscitation time	21.6 min	21.9 min	24.3 hr	5.06 hr
Total costs	$27,075.09	$55,744.00	$35,633.20	$70,808.10

(Courtesy of Champion, H.R., et al.: J. Trauma 26:927–931, October 1986.)

rates. The physiologic severity on admission and the associated costs of resuscitation efforts were evaluated in severely injured patients who died within 48 hours in an effort to identify early those patients who will benefit from intensive resuscitation efforts. Included in the study were 115 patients with major multiple injuries on whom resuscitation was started and who died in the hospital within the first 48 hours.

TABLE 3.—PREHOSPITAL CARDIOPULMONARY ARREST,
TRAUMA SCORE OF LESS THAN OR EQUAL TO THREE:
DEATHS WITHIN 1 HOUR

59	Cardiopulmonary arrest at scene or en route to hospital
14	Prehospital information unavailable
1	No prehospital arrest
74	Total TS ≤ 3

(Courtesy of Champion, H.R., et al.: J. Trauma 26:927–931, October 1986.)

TABLE 4.—SURVIVORS WITH TRAUMA SCORES OF LESS THAN
OR EQUAL TO THREE

Trauma Score	Injuries	Resuscitation Time
TS = 1	Shotgun wound to neck & face; arrived in arrest	37 minutes
TS = 3	Pedestrian struck by car; blunt injuries—head, chest, abdomen (inter-hospital transfer)	1 hour, 23 minutes
TS = 2	Gunshot wound to neck & face (interhospital transfer)	40 minutes
TS = 3	Stab wound to shoulder and arm, transecting brachial artery; cardio-pulmonary arrest; hypovolemic shock	40 minutes

(Courtesy of Champion, H.R., et al.: J. Trauma 26:927–931, October 1986.)

A Trauma Score, i.e., a measure of physiologic status associated with chance of survival (Table 1), was assigned to each patient. Seventy-four of the 115 patients (64%) had a trauma score of less than 3 and 41 patients (36%) had a trauma score of more than 5. No patient had a trauma score of 4. Total hospital charges for 63 of the 74 patients with a trauma score of 3 or less who died within 1 hour of hospital admission were $82,819 (Table 2). Fifty-nine of these 74 patients (79.7%) had cardiopulmonary arrest before arriving at the hospital (Table 3). Four patients with a trauma score of less than 3 survived (Table 4).

These results suggest that a trauma score of 3 or less is a valuable aid in identifying patients for whom prolonged resuscitation is futile. However, trauma score indices alone are insufficiently accurate for use in determining when to discontinue resuscitation.

▶ The epidemiology of pediatric prehospital care was examined recently (Tsai, A., et al.: *Ann. Emerg. Med.* 16:284, 1987). The study, performed in California, found that while the pediatric age group represented 32% of the population, they accounted for only 10% of the ambulance runs. Of the episodes involving children, 54% were in the trauma category. The largest trauma group was motor vehicle accidents involving adolescents. Medical disorders were the major reason for prehospital care in the very young. The demand for emergency medical services occurred mainly during the summer months and on weekends. Advanced life support was associated with prolonged on-scene time and had a relatively low use and success rate in the younger pediatric population. Resuscitation of 23 children with prehospital cardiac arrest produced no survivors to hospital discharge. This is all very discouraging and makes critical examination of what we are doing constantly necessary. After all is said and done, a heck of a lot more is said than done.—F.A. Oski, M.D.

Evaluation of the "Tilt Test" in Children
Susan M. Fuchs and David M. Jaffe (Northwestern Univ.)
Ann. Emerg. Med. 16:386–390, April 1987   5–8

The efficacy of the "tilt test" for acute intravascular volume loss in children was studied by comparing the orthostatic responses of volume-depleted and normally hydrated children aged 4–15 years. The former children were seen in the emergency department with vomiting and/or diarrhea. A volume depletion scoring system (Table 1) was developed for use in assessing 16 dehydrated and 21 volume-replete children. The groups were similar in age, weight, and oral temperature (Table 2).

The mean volume repletion score in dehydrated children, 5.3, was significantly greater than the score for volume-replete children (1.2). The mean orthostatic rise in heart rate was 29 beats per minute in the dehydrated group and 13 beats per minute in the normal group. Both groups had slight changes in systolic blood pressure on tilting to the supine position for 3 minutes and return to standing for 2 minutes. A heart rate change of more than 20 beats per minute was 81% specific and sensitive, and had positive and negative predictive values of 81% and 76%, respectively (Table 3). With a change of 25 beats per minute, specificity increased to 95% and sensitivity declined to 75%. The predictive value of a positive test increased to 92% (Table 4).

TABLE 1.—Volume Depletion Scoring System

Factor	Points			
	0	1	2	3
Mucous membranes	Mouth moist, lips moist	Mouth moist, lips dry	Mouth dry, lips dry	Mouth dry, lips dry, parched
Eyes	Tears	Decreased tears	No tears	No tears, sunken eyes
Urine output	Within last 3-4 hours	More than 4-6 hours	More than 6-12 hours	More than 12 hours
Urine specific gravity	1.000-1.015	1.016-1.025	1.026-1.030	$\geq$ 1.031
Extremity temperature and skin color	Warm, pink	Cool, pink	Cool, gray	Cold, mottled

(Courtesy of Fuchs, S.M., and Jaffe, D.M.: Ann. Emerg. Med. 16:386–390, April 1987.)

TABLE 2.—Sample Characteristics

	Dehydrated	Normal	P
N	16	21	
Boy	7	12	NS
Girl	9	9	
Black	2	11	< .05
White	4	8	
Hispanic	10	2	
Age (yr)*	9.8 ± 3.3	8.5 ± 3.0	NS
Oral temperature (C)	37.1 ± 1.07	36.7 ± 0.66	NS
No. patients with temperature ≥ 38 C	4	1	NS
Weight (kg)	36.2 ± 14.7	35.6 ± 16.1	NS
Mean volume depletion score	5.3 ± 2.5	1.2 ± 0.93	< .001

*Mean values ± standard deviation.

(Courtesy of Fuchs, S.M., and Jaffe, D.M.: Ann. Emerg. Med. 16:386–390, April 1987.)

TABLE 3.—Tilt Test Results Based on Criteria of a △ Heart Rate of More Than 20 Beats Per Minute

		Dehydration	Normal
	> 20	13*	4
△Heart Rate			
	≤ 20	3	17

Sensitivity, 81.3%

Specificity, 80.9%

Predictive value of a positive test — 76.4%

Predictive value of a negative test — 85.0%

*Includes two patients with near-syncope.

(Courtesy of Fuchs, S.M., and Jaffe, D.M.: Ann. Emerg. Med. 16:386–390, April 1987.)

TABLE 4.—Tilt Test Results Based on Criteria of a △ Heart Rate of More Than 25 Beats Per Minute

		Dehydration	Normal
	> 25	12*	1
△Heart Rate			
	≤ 25	4	20

Sensitivity, 75.0%

Specificity, 95.2%

Predictive value of a positive test — 92.3%

Predictive value of a negative test — 83.3%

*Includes two patients with near-syncope.

(Courtesy of Fuchs, S.M., and Jaffe, D.M.: Ann. Emerg. Med. 16:386–390, April 1987.)

Orthostatic changes in pulse, but not systolic blood pressure, distinguish clinically dehydrated and volume-replete children. An orthostatic rise of more than 25 beats per minute constitutes a positive tilt test in the appropriate clinical setting, whereas an increase in heart rate of 20 or fewer beats is a negative test.

▶ This "tilt test" is performed by having the child lie supine on the examination table for a minimum of 3 minutes prior to the onset of the test. Readings of pulse and blood pressure are recorded at 1-minute intervals in the supine position until three consecutive readings are obtained. The patient then stands erect with the arm supported at heart level, and two measurements of blood pressure and pulse are recorded at 1-minute intervals. The "tilt test" is easy to do and can be helpful when you are uncertain about the patient's status.—F.A. Oski, M.D.

High-Risk Youth and Health: The Case of Excessive School Absence
Michael Weitzman, Joel J. Alpert, Lorraine V. Klerman, Herbert Kayne, Geroge A. Lamb, Karen Roth Geromini, Karen T. Kane, and Lynda Rose (Boston Univ. and Brandeis Univ.)
Pediatrics 78:313–322, August 1986   5–9

Excessive school absenteeism is a major educational and social problem in the United States, yet little is known about its etiology or how to prevent or ameliorate it. To test the hypotheses that (1) health problems and unmet health needs are major characteristics distinguishing excessively absent students from regular attenders, and (2) a health-oriented approach using medically mediated interventions is effective in reducing absences among excessively absent students, a series of related studies was conducted in

TABLE 1.—DESIGN OF INTERVENTION STUDY

	Experimental Condition	Control Condition	
		No. 1	No. 2
Attendance monitored for all students, excessively absent students identified, 1981–1984	X	X	X
Excessively absent students and parents interviewed* (Information used by program personnel to categorize absence as either health or non-health related)	X	X	
Excessively absent students with health-related problem seen by primary care provider; program physician and primary care provider agree on health-related reasons for absence and devise intervention plan; interventions provided	X		

*Excessively absent students in experimental and control schools were interviewed with the same interview schedule, but, because of issues of confidentiality, student interviews were not available to clinical staff and were used only for research purposes. Categorization of reason for absence was based on review of parent interview by program personnel.
(Courtesy of Weitzman, M., et al.: Pediatrics 78:313–322, August 1986.)

TABLE 2.—CATEGORIES OF HEALTH-RELATED
REASONS FOR ABSENCE AMONG THE 156
EXCESSIVELY ABSENT STUDENTS ENGAGED IN THE
INTERVENTION PROGRAM

	No. (%) of Individuals With Category of Problem
Health problems among students	
Acute physical	23 (14.7)
Chronic physical†	98 (62.8)
Physical injury	5 (3.2)
Acute emotional	14 (9.0)
Chronic emotional‡	76 (48.7)
Health problems among family members	
Acute physical	2 (1.3)
Chronic physical	13 (8.3)
Physical injury	1 (0.6)
Acute emotional	0 (0)
Chronic emotional§	71 (45.5)

*Percentages do not add up to 100% because each student could have several problems.

†Asthma, specific learning disability, and dysmenorrhea accounted for approximately 50% of all diagnoses in this category.

‡Depressive disorder accounted for 54% of all diagnoses in this category, hypochondriasis 15%, drug abuse 7%.

§Family disorganization or disruption accounted for 49% of diagnoses in this category, maternal depressive symptoms 30%.

(Courtesy of Weitzman, M., et al.: Pediatrics 78:313–322, August 1986.)

seven Boston middle schools (grades 6, 7, and 8). The schools were divided into experimental and control groups (Table 1). In both groups attendance was monitored, excessively absent students were identified, and student and family interviews were conducted (Table 2). The intervention program offered in the experimental group included (1) primary care provider activities and when indicated (2) medical subspecialist activities, (3) mental health services, (4) social services, and (5) school-based activities, e.g., classroom changes, tutoring, behavior modification, and/or change of school.

In all, 298 excessively absent students and families were eligible for program participation (Table 3). Excessively absent students were older, in higher grades, white, more likely to have experienced academic failure in the past, and were bused to schools. Of the 156 students participating in the intervention program, most of the students and their parents reported health problems as the main or contributing reason for the student's excessive absences. However, compared with the regular attenders and their families, excessively absent students and their families were not confronted with greater burden of physical health problems or depressive symptoms, nor did they differ in health-related behaviors or use of health services. The intervention program, although effective in increasing enrollment of excessively absent students, was not significantly effective in reducing their absences (Table 4).

TABLE 3.—Excessively Absent Students in Experimental
and Control Schools*

	Experimental School	Control School (No. 1)
Student identified as meeting criteria for excessively absent students	1,278	1,060
Family interview completed	406 (32)	329 (31)
No indication of health-related reason for excessive absence based on clinician's review of parent interview†	46	‡
Health-related reason for excessive absence indicated based on clinician's review of parent interview	360 (89)	
Intervention not required§	62	
Intervention indicated	298 (83)	
Intervention initiated	156 (52)	
Intervention not initiated‖	142	

*Results are numbers (%) of students.
†Decision was made by program nurse and physician after review of interview with parent. Nonhealth-related reasons for absence include: dislikes school, peer pressure, laziness, misses bus, violence, suspensions, etc.
‡No further subdivisions could be made for control students because of lack of information.
§Decision was made by program nurse and physician after discussion with clinical management team and conversation with parent. Generally, no intervention was needed for self-limited illness, a condition that was no longer a problem, or a condition that was being handled by a clinician.
‖In 72 cases, parents and/or students refused to participate; in 67 cases parents and students indicated a desire to participate but never visited the students' primary care provider; in 3 cases families moved before the intervention was initiated.
(Courtesy of Weitzman, M., et al.: Pediatrics 78:313–322, August 1986.)

TABLE 4.—Effectiveness of Intervention Program at Level of the
Individual Student

Experimental Students and QFI	Days Absent (%)		
	Experimental Condition	Control Condition (No. 1)	
All phases of program operation (n = 131)			
QFI	39 ± 22 (0–100)	32 ± 17 (0–80)	NS
QFI + 4	38 ± 31 (0–100)	34 ± 28 (0–100)	
In last 4 quarters of program operation (n = 102)			
QFI	36 ± 21 (0–91)	32 ± 17 (0–100)	NS
QFI + 4	33 ± 28 (0–100)	34 ± 22 (0–100)	

QFI, Quarter of family interview; QFI + 4, same school quarter, 1 year after family interview. Results are means ± SD with actual range in parentheses.
(Courtesy of Weitzman, M., et al.: Pediatrics 78:313–322, August 1986.)

Demographic and educational characteristics of students exert a greater effect on absence behavior than does health status or receipt of health services. Consequently, a health-oriented approach alone will not have a major impact on what remains one of the most profound educational and social problems involving children in the United States today.

▶ Dr. Alain Joffe, Assistant Professor of Pediatrics, Johns Hopkins University School of Medicine, and Director, Division of Adolescent Medicine, comments.—F.A. Oski, M.D.

▶ It would be unfortunate if the results of this study dissuaded health care providers from becoming involved with the problem of excessive absenteeism. As the authors suggest, this issue has multiple and interrelated causes; to address one aspect of the complex web of causality without addressing the others will result in failure and frustration. If progress is to occur, it is likely that coordinated efforts involving school, local government, and health officials, as well as families, will be necessary. In addition, when one considers the additional problems stemming from the unique aspects of the social forces at work in Boston and its schools, it is not surprising that this intervention failed to reduce absenteeism. In a different locale and under different circumstances, the results might have been different. As such, the effect of school-based health clinics on absenteeism needs careful assessment. Nationwide, this problem is of such magnitude that even small-scale differences arising from the intervention would have a major impact. Because of the inability to enroll many eligible families, the resulting small sample size may have been inadequate to detect statistically small but meaningful results arising from this approach.

If excessive school absence is viewed as a chronic disease, it is critical that early intervention take place. For, just as in chronic disease, there comes a point when forces become irreversible and, in the case of school failure and school absenteeism, the cycle becomes self-perpetuating. Under these circumstances, intervention would most likely be beneficial at the elementary school level where 80% rather than 20% of children are grade appropriate for age. We need continually to be cognizant that a lack of enabling factors in individuals' lives may limit how effective health care-oriented interventions can be and that not all social problems can be solved by such approaches. In the latter circumstances, health care providers may be more effective on a community level as advocates for better schools.—A. Joffe, M.D.

Health Care of Poverty and Nonpoverty Children in Iowa
Linda A. Levey, N. Martin MacDowell, and Samuel Levey (Univ. of Iowa)
Am. J. Public Health 76:1000–1003, August 1986   5–10

The financing of health care services through Medicaid has had a positive impact on low-income adults and children. However, some studies have shown that Medicaid falls short in certain aspects of health care. Moreover, many children from poor families are not covered under Medicaid, and recent cutbacks and changes in the Medicaid program contribute to persistent differences in access to health care between socioeconomic groups.

The impact of Medicaid coverage on child health care was examined in 637 Iowa households with a child in the Aid to Families with Dependent Children (AFDC) program and 760 households randomly selected by random digit dial (RDD), including 17% poverty and 83% nonpoverty households. All parents were interviewed by telephone concerning access to and utilization of health services. Children included in the study ranged in age between 6 weeks and 6 years. A standardized questionnaire was used for the telephone interviews.

Most children in all groups received adequate well care. However, non-poverty children were the most likely, and AFDC children and poverty RDD children the least likely, to see a private pediatrician, see the same person at each visit, and receive immunizations and routine checkups at the same place. Random digit dial poverty children with Medicaid were the most likely, and RDD nonpoverty children the least likely, to have had a well visit in 1983. Random digit dial poverty children without Medicaid were likely not to have had a well visit in 1983 because of cost, whereas cost did not play a role in whether AFDC or RDD nonpoverty children had a well visit. However, care for illness and overnight hospitalization was affected by financial access in that RDD poverty children with some Medicaid coverage were more likely to have had at least one visit for illness or to have been hospitalized more often in the previous 12-month period than RDD poverty children with no coverage. Efforts to lower Medicaid costs by limiting eligibility or lowering reimbursement to providers can be expected to result in a reversal of progress toward equity in the provision of child health care.

▶ Dr. Catharine DeAngelis, Professor of Pediatrics, Deputy Chairman, Department of Pediatrics, Johns Hopkins University School of Medicine, and Director, Division of General Pediatrics, provided the following comment.—F.A. Oski, M.D.

▶ This study by Levey and her associates provides us with a microcosm of the status of health care utilization by poor and nonpoor children in 1983–1984. Their finding that children with AFDC and poor children in Iowa were least likely to receive continuity of care, i.e., health maintenance and illness care from a single provider or place, is very disturbing to pediatricians, but even more distressing are the indicators that inability to pay or having AFDC prevented children from receiving necessary care at any site.

These findings have been substantiated in other populations of children. For example, a study performed in Washington, D.C. (Dutton, D.: *Med. Care* 23:142, 1985) showed that income was the dominant independent influence on children's health. The fact that matters are not any better on a national scale has been shown in a recent report based on a telephone survey of a national sample. (Access to Health Care in the United States: Results of a 1986 Survey. *Spec. Report* No. 2/1987, Princeton, N.J., The Robert Wood Johnson Foundation.) The report includes all ages, but some of the data are broken down for children under 17 years of age. More than 3% of children had been hospitalized at least once in the previous year, almost 8% reported a chronic or serious illness, and 6% were in only fair or poor health. Almost 8% had no health insurance.

Fifteen percent of poor children reported no regular source of care compared with 7% of nonpoor children. Further, 27% of all children had not had an ambulatory visit in the preceding year, but 22% reported having a more expensive emergency room visit in that time. Is it possible that legislators who control the pursestrings have not considered that the long-term costs of "cutbacks" for children's care outweigh the savings, and that what is being lost is not only money but our children's health?—C. DeAngelis, M.D.

6 Neurology and Psychiatry

Recurrence Rate of Febrile Convulsion Related to the Degree of Pyrexia During the First Attack
A. Sahib El-Radhi, K. Withana, and S. Banajeh (Ahmadi Hosp., Ahmadi, Kuwait)
Clin. Pediatr. (Phila.) 26:311–313, June 1986   6–1

Certain factors are known to increase the risk of further febrile convulsions, including a history of febrile convulsions in first-degree cousins, onset under 1 year of age, and associated complications. To assess the effect of the degree of pyrexia on the likelihood of subsequent febrile convulsions, 94 children with their first febrile convulsion admitted during a 36-month period were evaluated. All children were managed according to a routine protocol of reducing body temperature. Follow-up ranged from 26 months to 62 months (mean, 44 months).

Overall, 29 of 94 children (30.9%) had recurrent febrile convulsions

RECURRENCE OF FEBRILE CONVULSIONS IN CHILDREN
WITH PYREXIA >40 DEGREES C (GROUP I) COMPARED
WITH CHILDREN WITH PYREXIA <40 DEGREES
C (GROUP II)

Age Range	Group	Children (M:F)	Children with Recurrences (%)	
6–18 months	I	38 (18:20)	4 (10.5)	
	II	25 (12:13)	19 (76.0)	$p < 0.001$
				*
19–30 months	I	14 (8:6)	2 (14.3)	
	II	10 (7:3)	4 (40.0)	NS
Over 30 months	—	7 (5:2)	0	—
Total	—	94 (50:44)	29 (30.9)	

*The difference of the recurrence rate in children aged 16–18 months and 19–30 months is also significant ($P < .01$) (Mantel-Haenszel test). [Courtesy of El-Radhi, A.S., et al.: Clin. Pediatr. (Phila.) 26:311–313, June 1986.]

(mean, 2.7) occurring between 1 month and 24 months after the original episode. For infants aged 6–18 months, the rate of recurrence was approximately seven times higher among those with fever of less than 40 C than among those with higher pyrexia (table). Age, sex, and family history of febrile convulsions did not differ between groups. Neither the presence of infections nor the limited use of antibiotics was likely to influence the findings. The degree of pyrexia may be a useful prognostic indicator of the risk of recurrence of febrile convulsions. However, further studies are needed for confirmation.

▶ Dr. John M. Freeman, Professor of Neurology and Pediatrics, Johns Hopkins University School of Medicine, commented as follows.—F.A. Oski, M.D.

▶ The message of this article is that younger infants (6–18 months of age) whose febrile seizures occurred at a lower temperature (less than 40 C) were seven times *more* likely to have recurrent febrile seizures than if their temperature was more than 40 C.

A seizure is the result of the synchronous firing of population neurons. The factors that bring about or allow this synchronized firing are incompletely understood, but among them are the multiple factors that collectively determine the threshold for firing. Genetic factors must govern components of this threshold, accounting for the genetics of particular forms of epilepsy and the genetic predisposition to both febrile seizures and epilepsy in general. Superimposed on this genetic predisposition is the gradually increasing "threshold" with age throughout childhood. Infants and toddlers are more likely to experience a seizure with any given insult—trauma, infection, or fever—than older children. Seizures can be induced with fever in kittens, but not in cats. Seventy percent of epilepsy starts in childhood. Children are also more likely to acquire infections and more likely to have higher fevers with infection.

Therefore, it is not surprising that younger infants who had seizures with a temperature less than 40 C were more likely to have recurrence of febrile seizures. They must have had a "lower threshold."

The protocol called for hospitalization of all these children, but this clearly is not necessary in general. Blood work for infection can be done on an outpatient basis, CT scans are *not* needed, and EEGs are not helpful. The inclusion of three infants with *Shigella* is disturbing because such infants are not usually considered to have "febrile seizures," but, rather, as with roseola, are considered to have seizures related to "toxins" from those specific infections. The consequences of knowing which child is more likely to have recurrence are unclear, because the current consensus appears to be that prophylactic treatment to prevent recurrence causes more morbidity than recurrence itself. Phenobarbital causes behavioral disturbance in 40% of the children, and valproate causes hepatotoxicity in 1 of 500 children in this age group. Clearly, the treatment is usually worse than the disease. However, it might be reassuring to a parent to know that their child who has a high fever (of more than 40 C) with the first febrile seizure has even less than a 30% chance of experiencing another of these frightening episodes.—J.M. Freeman, M.D.

Tourette Syndrome: An Analysis of 200 Pediatric and Adolescent Cases
Gerald Erenberg, Robert P. Cruse, and A. David Rothner (The Cleveland Clinic Found.)
Cleve. Clin. Q. 53:127–131, Summer 1986   6–2

Tourette's syndrome is characterized by the childhood onset of recurrent multiple motor tics and involuntary vocal tics. Although the incidence of reported patients was low until the 1960s, the number of those with

CHARACTERISTICS OF 200 CHILDREN
WITH TOURETTE SYNDROME

	Number	Percent
Sex		
Male	165	82
Female	35	18
Race		
White	194	97
Black	6	3
Family history of tics	74	37
Severity		
Mild	89	44
Moderate	99	50
Severe	12	6
Neurologic disorders	10	5
Febrile seizures	7	4
Afebrile seizures	3	2
Cerebral palsy	0	0
Mental retardation	6	3
Neuromuscular disorder	0	0
Learning problems	72	36
Learning disability	43	22
Repeated grade	24	12
Poor grades	35	18
Full-time special class	17	8
Part-time special class	24	12
Behavior problems	95	48
Attention deficit disorder	70	35
Adjustment reaction	20	10
Neurosis or psychosis	17	8
Abnormal neurologic examination	5	3

(Courtesy of Erenberg, G., et al.: Cleve. Clin. Q. 53:127–131, Summer 1986.)

diagnosed Tourette's syndrome has increased rapidly, largely because of increased public awareness of the disease. A review was made of the records of children and adolescents with Tourette's syndrome who were treated at The Cleveland Clinic Foundation during a 5-year period.

The series included 165 boys and 35 girls ranging in age at onset between 2 years and 15 years; the mean age at onset was 6.3 years (table). The average lag between onset of symptoms and diagnosis was 4.5 years. Most patients had been treated by several physicians before the correct diagnosis was made. About 90% were symptomatic before age 10 years. Only 15 patients (8%) had previous encephalopathic events, e.g., neonatal asphyxia or severe head trauma. Most patients were in good health, with medical disorders present in only 32 of them. However, many children (58%) had learning problems, behavioral problems, or both, which often caused more difficulties in everyday life than the tics and noises themselves.

The exact etiology of Tourette's syndrome is unknown, although an organic etiology is suspected. Because treatment with haloperidol, a dopaminergic receptor blocker, has achieved beneficial responses, it was hypothesized that excessive dopamine or increased sensitivity to dopamine action is the basis of the disorder. Other investigators have found diminished homovanillic acid in the CSF of patients with Tourette's syndrome, which was thought to indicate supersensitivity of dopamine receptors. Patients with Tourette's syndrome, and their families, require much help and understanding in dealing not only with the tics and noises, but also especially with the associated behavioral and learning difficulties.

Clinical Features and Long-Term Treatment With Pimozide in 65 Patients With Gilles de la Tourette's Syndrome
Lisbeth Regeur, Bente Pakkenberg, Rasmus Fog, and Henning Pakkenberg (Hvidovre Univ. Hosp., Denmark)
J. Neurol. Neurosurg. Psychiatry 49:791–795, July 1986   6–3

Haloperidol is the treatment of choice for patients with Gilles de la Tourette's syndrome. However, many patients experience side effects with haloperidol therapy. Because pimozide reportedly causes fewer side effects, it was used to treat 65 patients with Gilles de la Tourette's syndrome (table).

Muscular or vocal tics, or both, were present in the close family members of 38 patients (58%), including 21 (32%) who had first-degree relatives with tics. The severity of symptoms was mild in 2 (3%), moderate in 23 (35%), marked in 28 (43%), and severe in 12 (18%). Pimozide was ad-

DETAILS OF 65 PATIENTS WITH GILLES DE LA TOURETTE'S SYNDROME

Age (yr)	Age at onset (yr)	Age at diagnosis (yr)	Duration of disease	Interval from onset to diagnosis
17·8 (6–54)	5·8 (2–12)	14·8 (5–43)	11·9 (1–48)	9·0 (1–37)

(Courtesy of Regeur, L., et al.: J. Neurol. Neurosurg. Psychiatry 49:791–795, July 1986.)

ministered to patients with moderate to severe symptoms who were socially disabled, starting with low dosages that were gradually increased until an optimal clinical response was obtained or side effects occurred. Tetrabenazine or clonidine was added to the regimen if an optimal response could not be achieved with pimozide alone.

Of 59 patients treated, 50 were given pimozide alone, 5 received pimozide and tetrabenazine, and 4 received pimozide and clonidine. A good clinical response with no side effects was obtained in 48 patients (81%) and 5 (9%) had a moderate clinical response. Side effects included sedation, weight gain, depression, pseudoparkinsonism, and akathisia. No patient had tardive dyskinesia, acute dystonic reactions, blurred vision, slurred speech, or xerostomia.

Pimozide is preferred to haloperidol because it causes fewer side effects. The superiority of pimozide may result from its more specific dopamine blocking activity and the absence of norepinephrine antagonism.

▶ It is gradually becoming appreciated that Tourette's syndrome is a far more common disorder than was initially suspected and may occur in about 2.6% of the general population (Shapiro, E., et al.: *JAMA* 245:1583, 1981). Tourette's syndrome can be precipitated by the administration of psychostimulants (see 1983 YEAR BOOK, p. 385) that increase the release of epinephrine. This observation, along with the finding of a beneficial response to haloperidol, a dopaminergic receptor blocker, has led to the hypothesis that this disease is caused by excessive sensitivity to dopamine or excessive production of dopamine. Pimozide, a diphenylbutylpiperidine such as haloperidol, has a strong blocking effect on the postsynaptic dopamine receptor and, as discussed above, appears to be effective in the treatment of the disease and produces fewer side effects. As they say in the ad, "Who could ask for anything more?" For more on pimozide treatment of tic and Tourette disorders, see the excellent recent review by Shapiro and associates (*Pediatrics* 79:1032, 1987).—F.A. Oski, M.D.

Spasmus Nutans: A Benign Clinical Entity?

Robert A. King, Leonard B. Nelson, and Rudolph S. Wagner (Wills Eye Hosp., Philadelphia, and Univ. of Medicine and Dentistry of New Jersey, Newark)
Arch. Ophthalmol. 104:1501–1504, October 1986   6–4

Spasmus nutans, which appears in early childhood, consists of a triad of symptoms: small-amplitude, rapid horizontal nystagmus in one or both eyes asymmetrically; head nodding; and anomalous head position. Until 1970, spasmus nutans was considered a benign clinical condition. Since that time, reports of optic nerve or chiasmal gliomas in patients who evidently had spasmus nutans have become increasingly common. Spasmus nutans was diagnosed in eight boys and six girls aged 4–14 months at onset (average, 12.9 months) (table). There were 12 black and 2 white infants.

The fine, rapid, horizontal nystagmus was unilateral in seven infants and bilateral and asymmetric in the others. All 14 infants had head nodding

SUMMARY OF CLINICAL FINDINGS IN PATIENTS WITH SPASMUS NUTANS

Patient No./ Sex/Race	Age at Onset, mo	Age Presenting, mo	Involved Eye	Age at CT Scan, mo	Strabismus
1/F/W	11	13	OD	15	ET
2/M/B	14	15	OD	16	...
3/M/B	4	10	OD > OS	12	...
4/M/B	6	8	OS	10	...
5/M/B	7	10	OD > OS	12	...
6/M/B	6	7	OS	9†	XT
7/F/B	14	15	OD	16†	ET
8/M/B	4	7	OS	10	...
9/M/B	4	5	OS > OD	14	...
10/F/B	5	24	OD > OS	25	...
11/F/B	5	15	OS > OD	16	...
12/F/B	4	12	OD > OS	18	ET
13/F/W	6	14	OD > OS	15	ET
14/M/B	6	24	OD	25	...

CT, computed tomographic; OD, right eye; ET, esotropia; OS, left eye; and XT, exotropia.
†Magnetic resonance imaging scan was also performed.
(Courtesy of King, R.A., et al.: Arch. Ophthalmol. 104:1501–1504, October 1986.)

and anomalous head position. The head nodding was characterized by a slow-frequency, small-amplitude, horizontal or vertical oscillating movement. The anomalous head position was either of a head tilt of 5–10 degrees to the left or right or a 10-degree chin-up or chin-down posture. The head nodding and anomalous head position frequently changed character during examination. None of the infants was noted to have a tumor on CT scanning. However, one had an arachnoid cyst and an empty sella, and another had a porencephalic cyst.

The diagnosis of spasmus nutans should be reserved for the child who presents with the onset of horizontal, fine, rapid nystagmus at a young age. An anomalous head position and head nodding are needed to complete the syndrome. Strabismus is also present in many children with spasmus nutans. Asymmetric vision, afferent pupillary defect, abnormal optic nerve, vertical nystagmus, or systemic neurologic abnormality would preclude the diagnosis of spasmus nutans. Also, a history of failure to thrive or an abnormally large head circumference would suggest the diencaphalic syndrome, which may present with monocular nystagmus. Questions are raised as to who should be involved in the management of these patients and as to how they should be followed. To generate a sufficient number of patients, further study of this subject would best be carried out through a prospective multicenter approach.

▶ I always thought that infants with spasmus nutans grew up to become "yes men," but now it is clear that the entity, or a condition resembling it, is not always a joking matter.—F.A. Oski, M.D.

Personality and Behavioural Characteristics in Pediatric Migraine
S.J. Cunningham, P.J. McGrath, H.B. Ferguson, P. Humphreys, J. D'Astous, J. Latter, J.T. Goodman, and P. Firestone (Children's Hosp. of Eastern On-

tario, Ottawa, Carleton Univ., OHawa, and Univ. of OHawa)
Headache 27:16–20, January 1987   6–5

Migraine headaches in children are common, and a number of studies have outlined personality and behavioral characteristics that are believed to contribute to the occurrence of these headaches. Personality and behavioral characteristics in pediatric migraine were investigated in a comparative study of 20 boys and girls matched for age and sex with a "pain" control group of 20 children with musculoskeletal pain and with a "no pain" control group of 20 children. Common inclusion criteria for all three groups were no major medical, neurologic, or psychological problems and age 9–17 years.

When the amount of pain experienced was controlled, the only discriminating variable was that of somatic complaints, which included vomiting, nausea, and perceptual disturbances, all migraine-related phenomena. The inclusion of a "pain" control group in this study provided results indicating that the behavioral and personality features considered to be characteristic of childhood migraine are common to a chronic pain disorder, and, in fact, the manifestation of many of these features correlates directly with the amount of pain experienced. The personality and behavioral features evident in many children with migraine may result from recurrent chronic pain episodes rather than being the cause of pain.

▶ Migraineurs have classically been regarded as nervous, tense, and anxious perfectionists—good people to hire when you wanted to be sure that the job got done. Now it would appear that another myth is shattered. Migraine may not be associated with a particular personality type, but it can be associated with other problems. For example, it has been observed that 59% of the patients with complicated migraine (classic migraine complicated by sensory and/ or motor signs and symptoms) have associated mitral valve prolapse (Lanzi, G., et al.: *Headache* 26:142, 1986). Migraine may also occur in association with the dyslipoproteinemias (Glueck, C.J., et al.: *Pediatrics* 77:316, 1986). For more, much more, on migraine, see the 1985 YEAR BOOK, p. 156, p. 497, and p. 498.—F.A. Oski, M.D.

Pediatric Brain Injuries: The Nature, Clinical Course, and Early Outcomes in a Defined United States Population
Jess F. Kraus, Daniel Fife, and Carol Conroy (Univ. of California at Los Angeles)
Pediatrics 79:501–507, April 1987   6–6

Acute brain injuries lead to the hospital admission of about 100,000 children younger than 15 years of age each year in the United States. The nature and course of these injuries were studied in a series of 709 children admitted to a hospital in San Diego County, California, in 1981. All but 3% of these patients were discharged from the hospital. Nearly 25% had at least one skull or facial bone fracture. Glasgow Coma Scale scores of 3–4 were present in 2% of the children, and scores of 5–8 in another 3%.

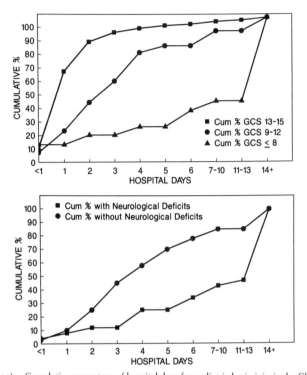

Fig 6–1 (top).—Cumulative percentage of hospital days for pediatric brain injuries by Glasgow Coma Scale (GCS), San Diego County, California, 1981. (Tabulation limited to patients discharged alive.)

Fig 6–2 (bottom).—Cumulative percentage of hospital days for pediatric brain injuries by status of neurologic deficits, San Diego County, California, 1981. (Tabulation limited to patients discharged alive.) (Courtesy of Kraus, J.F., et al.: Pediatrics 79:501–507, April 1987.)

Surgery was necessary for 23 patients, 20 of whom recovered well or with moderate disability. Of all hospital bed days, mild brain injury (Fig 6–1) accounted for 90%. The overall in-hospital case fatality rate was 3/100 children, and the rate for severely brain-injured children was 59/100. In all, 14% of children with contusion, laceration, or hemorrhage, but only one with concussion, were discharged with disability. Children with neurologic deficit had a median hospital stay of 11–12 days, compared with 3 days for those without such deficit (Fig 6–2).

Concussion was the most frequent diagnosis in this series of acutely brain-injured children. Mild injuries accounted for 93% of all cases and for about 90% of hospital bed days. Skull fracture was associated with more severe brain injuries. Children with neurologic deficit were hospitalized longer than the others, reflecting an apparent attempt to see the deficit resolve before discharge.

▶ Obviously, head injury is the major cause of disability in the adolescent and young adult and costs approximately 4 billion dollars per year in the United States. Are they really "accidents"? A study of 80 head-injured patients revealed poor premorbid academic performance in 50% of the sample (Haas,

J.F., et al.: *J. Neurol. Neurosurg. Psychiatry* 50:52, 1987). Poor academic performance, as defined by diagnosis of learning disability, multiple failed academic subjects, or school dropout during secondary education, has not been recognized previously as a risk factor for head injury except when a parent threatens to give a child "a shot in the head" when a poor report card is brought home. This finding of the premorbid prevalence of poor academic performance in patients with severe head injury is another good reason to delay the age when driver's licenses are granted.—F.A. Oski, M.D.

Cerebral Thromboembolism Due to Antithrombin III Deficiency in Two Children
P.P. Vomberg, C. Breederveld, P. Fleury, and W.F.M. Arts (Univ. of Amsterdam and Erasmus Univ., The Netherlands)
Neuropediatrics 18:42–44, 1987   6–7

A significant number of strokes in infants and children remain unexplained. Venous thromboembolism is relatively infrequent in otherwise healthy children younger than 10 years of age, but it may occur spontaneously without apparent cause. Two young children with stroke, one purely ischemic and the other ischemic with secondary hemorrhage, had antithrombin III (AT III) deficiency. One of the patients also had cyanotic congenital heart disease with right-to-left shunting, making cerebral embolism from iliac vein thrombus a possibility. One patient had a positive family history for hereditary AT III deficiency. All causes of acquired AT III deficiency were excluded.

Both children apparently had severe thromboembolic complications on the basis of congenital AT III deficiency. Primary thrombosis was venous

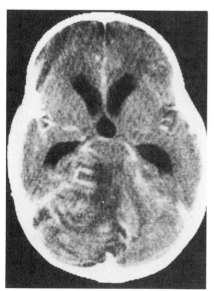

Fig 6–3.—Massive hemorrhagic infarction of both cerebellar hemispheres. (Courtesy of Vomberg, P.P., et al.: Neuropediatrics 18:42–44, 1987.)

in both cases. One patient had secondary embolism of the middle cerebral artery, and the other had sagittal sinus thrombosis with hemorrhagic cerebral and cerebellar infarcts (Fig 6–3). Primary venous thrombosis in children most often is associated with a hypercoagulable state arising from dehydration, cyanotic congenital heart disease, or nephrotic syndrome.

▶ Stroke in infancy and childhood usually ends up with no satisfactory explanation, although it is recognized that ischemic strokes may be seen in children with congenital heart disease (particularly the child with cyanotic heart disease and iron deficiency) or Moyamoya disease. Primary hemorrhagic strokes are associated with arteriovenous malformations or aneurysms. Miscellaneous causes for stroke include leukemia with a very high white blood cell count, sickle cell anemia, thrombocytopenia, hemophilia, homocystinuria, and vasculitis. Congenital AT III deficiency should now be added to the list.—F.A. Oski, M.D.

Sexual Function in Adults With Myelomeningocele

A.S. Cass, Beth Ann Bloom, and M. Luxenberg (Gillette Children's Hosp., St. Paul)

J. Urol. 136:425–426, August 1986   6–8

Advances in surgical techniques and the use of antibiotics have contributed to reduced mortality in infants born with myelomeningocele, and many such patients survive to adulthood. The sexual function and childbearing experiences of myelomeningocele patients were examined in a review of the records of 108 such patients at least 16 years of age. Interviews were conducted with 47 patients, 35 females and 12 males, including one male and 4 females aged 16–19 years, 7 males and 22 females aged

SEXUAL ACTIVITY RELATED TO FUNCTIONAL MOTOR LEVEL

	L2 and Above	L3–L5	S1 and Below	Totals
Male pts:				
No. pts.	3	5	4	12
Penile sensation	1	4	3	8
Erection (No. partial)	3 (1)	4	4	11 (1)
Ejaculation*	2 (+1)	3 (+1)	4	9 (+2)
Orgasm*	2 (+1)	3 (+1)	4	9 (+2)
Female pts.:				
No. pts.	8	15	12	35
Vulval sensation	4	14	11	29
Orgasm*	1 (+5)	6 (+4)	6 (+2)	13 (+11)
Sexual intercourse	0	8	9	17
Pregnancy	0	5	7	12

*Numbers in parentheses indicate number not known (no sexual activity).
(Courtesy of Cass, A.S., et al.: J. Urol. 136:425–426, August 1986.)

20–29 years, and 4 males and 9 females aged 30–39 years. The patients were also grouped by location of their neural tube defects, indicating whether they were wheelchair-bound (11 patients), ambulatory with extensive bracing (20), or ambulatory with minimal aids (16). Sexual activity within these groups was investigated (table).

Two of the 12 males had no sexual activity, 4 masturbated, and 6 reported sexual intercourse; 1 of these men had fathered three normal children. Eleven of 35 women had no sexual activity, 7 masturbated, and 17 had sexual intercourse, including 12 women who had a total of 20 pregnancies. Urinary diversion had been done in 10 of the 12 women who became pregnant; none of these patients required hospitalization for urinary complications after delivery. None of the 16 children born had myelomeningocele, 1 child had an undescended testis, and 1 child was born with a club foot. Most of the adults in this group had satisfactory sexual function, and the childbearing in women with ileal conduit urinary diversion did not cause major complications to mother or child.

Long-Term Renal Risk Factors in Children With Meningomyelocele
Andrew S. Brem, Diane Martin, Joseph Callaghan, and John Maynard (Rhode Island Hosp., Providence, and Brown Univ.)
J. Pediatr. 110:51–55, January 1987   6–9

Urinary drainage procedures (e.g., ileal loop diversion and clean intermittent catheterization) have significantly reduced renal morbidity in children with meningomyelocele and neurogenic bladder. However, ileal loop diversion causes some morbidity, and although intermittent catheterizaton has reduced the incidence of bacteriuria, deterioration in structure or func-

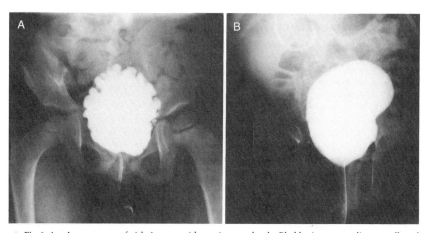

Fig 6–4.—A, cystogram of girl, 4 years, with meningomyelocele. Bladder is noncompliant, small, and trabeculated and lies within confines of pelvis. B, cystogram of girl, 2 years, with meningomyelocele. Bladder is flaccid and atonic; when filled with contrast material, it extends beyond pelvic brim. (Courtesy of Brem, A.S., et al.: J. Pediatr. 110:51–55, January 1987.)

tion occurs in about 10% of all patients so treated. A 5-year, prospective study was conducted to identify specific renal morbidity in 42 children with meningomyelocele treated for neurogenic bladder. Fourteen underwent ileal loop diversion and 28 had clean intermittent catheterization. All were observed for at least 60 months.

During the study, deterioration in three patients with ileal loop diversion was observed on x-ray examination. One of these patients died and one is undergoing hemodialysis. Nine patients who underwent intermittent catheterization had evidence of unilateral or bilateral reflux. All patients with ileal loop diversion had free ureteral reflux. Four catheterized patients experienced increased scarring and hydronephrosis during the study, requiring ileal loop diversion. In the other 24 no significant change was noted or improvement was seen on x-ray examination. Of 31 patients from both groups who were studied by voiding cystourethrography before therapy, 8 had small, noncompliant, trabeculated bladders (Fig 6–4).

Bacteriuria and reflex appeared to have little effect on renal mortality in this study. Thus, infection and reflex did not seem to be as important as might have been expected. The patients at greatest risk of renal deterioration were those who had small, noncompliant, trabeculated bladders.

Rett Syndrome: A Commonly Overlooked Progressive Encephalopathy in Girls
Majeed Al-Mateen, Michel Philippart, and W. Donald Shields (Univ. of California at Los Angeles)
Am. J. Dis. Child. 140:761–765, August 1986   6–10

Rett syndrome is a slowly progressive disorder occurring exclusively in girls and characterized by early deterioration of higher brain function with dementia and autistic behavior, ataxia, and loss of purposeful hand use. Fifteen girls with Rett syndrome were evaluated during a period of 15 months, with two new features discovered: extrapyramidal disorder and lactic acidemia.

All 15 patients had normal neurologic and mental development during their first 4–18 months of life, followed by the slowly progressive syndrome of autism, dementia, and loss of purposeful hand use (Fig 6–5, Table 1). Deceleration of head growth was evident in all cases. Seizures became apparent after the period of subacute deterioration, most occurring between the ages of 2 and 4 years. Epilepsy was either the minor motor type (nine patients) or the generalized tonic-clonic type (four patients). Electroencephalographic findings consisted of a generalized slow spike wave, independent multifocal spike and/or sharp discharges, and bursts of slow spike wave and/or generalized electrodecremental episodes. Extrapyramidal symptoms included choreoathetosis in eight patients and dystonia in four. Eight of 10 patients tested had elevated blood lactic acid levels and 5 of 11 had an increased blood pyruvic acid level (Table 2). Most of the patients had normal cranial CT scans, but in four cerebral atrophy

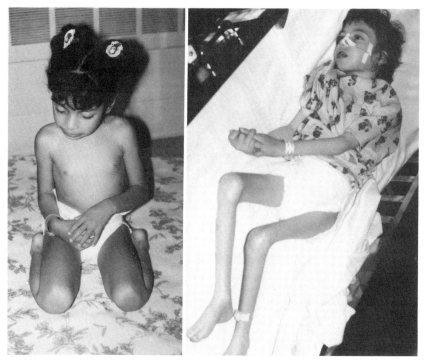

Fig 6–5.—Appearance of patients with stereotypic hand-washing movements. **Left,** patient aged 4 years 11 months, who is also grinding her teeth. **Right,** patient aged 12 years. Note diffuse muscle wasting. (Courtesy of Al-Mateen, M., et al.: Am. J. Dis. Child. 140:761–765, August 1986.)

was observed. Brain biopsy in four patients was nonspecific. Muscle wasting was diffuse and slowly progressive in 12 patients.

Rett syndrome may not be uncommon (ten additional patients have since been evaluated). The sequence of symptoms in the course of this syndrome is characteristic, starting with subacute deterioration of mental functions at 4–18 months of age, appearance of pyramidal dysfunction as the period of early deterioration comes to a halt, followed by a chronic phase of progressive muscle wasting and spasticity (Table 3). The cause remains unknown and, as yet, there is no biochemical marker for this syndrome.

▶ Dr. James Harris, Associate Professor of Psychiatry and Pediatrics, Johns Hopkins University School of Medicine, comments.—F.A. Oski, M.D.

▶ Although described in 1966 by Rett as a neurologic disorder that occurs only in girls, this syndrome was not brought to general medical attention until 1983 when Hagberg reported 35 such patients of French, Portuguese, and Swedish ancestry. The clinical course of Rett syndrome is now better established and the phases of the patient's clinical course are being clarified. The authors fur-

TABLE 1.—CLINICAL DATA ON 15 PATIENTS WITH RETT SYNDROME*

Patient	Age at Diagnosis, y	Age at End of Normal Development, mo	Age at Onset of Definite Regression, mo	Autistic Features	Stereotyped Hand-Washing Movement	Episodic Hyperventilation	Speech	Ataxia	Extrapyramidal Features	Tone	Deceleration of Head Growth (Percentile)	Growth Plateau, Height or Weight	Muscle Wasting	Vasomotor Disturbance of Lower Extremities	Sitting Without Support	Walking Independently	Age at Onset of Seizures, y
1	21	18	36	+	+	+	Lost	-	-	Spastic	+ (<2nd)	Both	+	+	+	+	11
2	20	4	18	-	+	+	Never	-	Choreoathetosis	Spastic	+ (<2nd)	Both	+	+	Lost	Never	3
3	15	15	16	+	+	+	Lost	+	Choreoathetosis, dystonia	Spastic	+ (<2nd)	Both	+	+	+	Lost	3
4	12	?	18	-	+	?	Never	?	Choreoathetosis, dystonia	Spastic	+ (<2nd)	?	+	+	+	+	6
5	12	10	12	+	+	-	Never	+	Choreoathetosis	Spastic	+ (20th)	Both	+	+	+	Lost	2.5
6	11	16	18	+	+	?	Lost	+	-	Hypotonic	+ (<2nd)	Both	+	?	Lost	Lost	3
7†	11	?	18	+	+	+	Lost	+	Choreoathetosis, dystonia	Hypotonic/ spastic	+ (<2nd)	Both	+	+	Lost	Lost	2.5
8	10	12	18	+	+	+	Lost	-	Choreoathetosis, dystonia	Spastic	+ (2nd)	-	?	+	Lost	Lost	3
9	10	10	12	+	+	+	Never	+	Choreoathetosis	Hypotonic	+ (<2nd)	Both	+	?	Lost	Lost	5
10	6	12	18	+	+	?	Lost	-	?	Hypotonic	+ (2nd)	Weight	?	?	+	+	2
11	4	18	20	+	+	?	Lost	+	?	Hypotonic	+ (<<2nd)	Both	+	?	+	+	2.5
12	4.5	6	18	+	+	+	Never	+	?	Hypotonic	+ (25th)	?	+	?	+	Never	2.25
13	4.5	10	18	+	+	?	Lost	+	?	Spastic	+ (<2nd)	Both	+	?	+	Never	None
14	3	4	24	+	+	+	Never	-	Choreoathetosis	Hypotonic/ spastic	+ (25th)	Weight	+	+	+	Never	0.33
15	3	9	15	+	+	+	Lost	+	-	Hypotonic/ spastic	+ (50th)	Weight	-	+	+	Never	None

*Plus sign, present; minute sign, absent; question mark, unknown; <, less than; <<, much less than. All patients female, with uneventful prenatal and perinatal histories.
†Patient 7 had severe combined immunodeficiency syndrome for which she received a male thymus transplant at age 5 months. Frequent infections occur, requiring monthly injections of immune human serum globulin.
(Courtesy of Al-Mateen, M., et al.: Am. J. Dis. Child. 140:761–765, August 1986.)

TABLE 2.—Lactic Acid and Pyruvic Acid Level Determinations*

Patient	Lactic Acid		Pyruvic Acid	
	Blood, mg/dL (mmol/L)	CSF, mg/dL (mmol/L)	Blood, mg/dL (μmol/L)	CSF, mg/dL (μmol/L)
2	8-44 (0.9-4.9)	...	0.3-0.7 (34-80)	...
3	5-18 (0.6-2.0)	...	0.6-1.0 (68-114)	...
4	2.7-8.5 (0.3-0.9)	...	0.6-0.7 (68-80)	...
5	6-18 (0.7-2.0)	...	0.3 (34)	...
6	25 (2.8)	...	0.3 (34)	...
7	7-20 (0.8-2.2)	17 (1.9)	1.0-1.5 (114-170)	1.1 (125)
8	4-21 (0.4-2.3)	...	1.0-3.0 (114-341)	...
9	8.4-21 (0.9-2.3)	...	0.5-1.4 (57-159)	...
10	...	...	0.5 (57)	...
14	27 (3.0)	6 (0.7)	1.2 (136)	1.5 (170)
15	3.0 (0.3)	...	0.6 (68)	...

*Values reported represent single determination or range of 2 or more determinations; CSF, cerebrospinal fluid. Normal ranges of values: blood lactic acid, 5–15 mg/dl (0.5–1.6 mmole/L); CSF lactic acid, 11–15 mg/dl (1.1–1.6 mmole/L); blood pyruvic acid 0.3–0.9 mg/dl (35–100 μmole/L); and CSF pyruvic acid, 0.8–1.1 mg/dl (90–125 μmole/L).
(Courtesy of Al-Mateen, M., et al.: Am. J. Dis. Child. 140:761–765, August 1986.)

TABLE 3.—Features of Rett Syndrome*

First phase	Second phase
Stagnation of developmental acquisitions (4 to 18 mo of age)	Minor motor seizures (onset at 2 to 4 years of age)
Insidious, occasionally acute, regression (18 to 36 mo of age)	Loss of purposeful use of extremities (apraxia)
Impairment or loss of speech	Extrapyramidal symptoms (choreoathetosis and dystonia in half of the cases)
Autistic behavior with distinctive hand movements (hand-washing automatism)	**Chronic phase**
Frequent hyperventilation	Progressive muscle wasting and spasticity
	Plateau of head circumference (as early as 1 year of age), weight, and usually height (after 10 years of age)

*All patients were female.
(Courtesy of Al-Mateen, M., et al.: Am. J. Dis. Child. 140:761–765, August 1986.)

ther highlight the manifestations of this disorder and provide certain additional features, including the extrapyramidal symptoms that may be associated. On the last page of their article, they document the natural history of the condition. The early phase has, in some instances, been confused with autism, and when autism is considered in girls during their first 3 years of life, Rett syndrome is a routine part of the differential diagnosis. However, the presentation that is referred to as autism seems more related to an encephalopathy and, on close examination, the resemblance is more superficial. The application of the new *Diagnostic and Statistical Manual of Mental Disorders,* ed. III,-R criteria for autism should help prevent misdiagnoses. The hand stereotypes in Rett syndrome are characteristic, and loss of purposeful hand movement along with midline hand wringing and mouthing suggest a behavioral phenotype, just as finger biting is in the Lesch-Nyhan syndrome.

Rett syndrome is a form of early dementia that occurs in girls and is associated with seizures as outlined by the authors. The demonstration of cerebral atrophy on CT scans and, in one instance with magnetic resonance imaging, further documents the severity of this condition.

This is a newly recognized disorder whose diagnosis is important to clarify to avoid unnecessary laboratory procedures and provide support for families.

214 / Pediatrics

There is, in addition to this paper, an issue of the *American Journal of Medical Genetics* (vol. 24, 1986) devoted to an international Rett syndrome symposium. Of interest for families is the International Rett Syndrome Association (Mrs. Cathy Hunter, 8511 Rose Marie Drive, Fort Washington, Maryland 20744), to which families may be referred for support and information regarding recent developments in the assessment, diagnosis, treatment and new research with regard to this new condition.—J. Harris, M.D.

Follow-Up Studies of Children With Fetal Alcohol Syndrome
H.-L. Spohr and H.-Chr. Steinhausen (Rittberg Hosp. of the German Red Cross, Berlin, and Free Univ. of Berlin)
Neuropediatrics 18:13–17, 1987   6–11

There is limited evidence of long-term effects from intrauterine exposure to alcohol. Data from a prospective multidisciplinary study of fetal alcohol syndrome with repeated neurologic and psychiatric assessments were reviewed. Fifty-four of 72 original patients had pediatric reevaluation after 3–4 years, and 28 of 49 patients were reassessed psychiatrically. Repeat EEG recordings were possible in 45 original patients.

The craniofacial dysmorphic features generally were significantly less evident at follow-up. Age-adapted neurologic reassessment also indicated definite improvement in performance and fewer "soft" signs, and less severe pathologic EEG patterns were seen on repeat study. Psychiatric scores were significantly lower at follow-up, and there were reductions in eating problems, concentration difficulty, problems with siblings and peers, negative mood, and phobias in individual cases. Significant improvement in IQ scores was documented, reflecting better performance by a small proportion of the children. Educational abilities were, however, quite poor. Only 17% of children of school age attended normal schools. General pediatric, neurologic, and psychiatric reevaluations all indicated improvement over time in this group of children with fetal alcohol syndrome, but hyperactivity and distractability continued to impede their educational performance.

▶ Streissguth and associates (Streissguth, A.P., et al.: *Lancet* 2:85, 1985, and 1987 Year Book, pp. 213–216) reported on the 11 children who were the first to be diagnosed as having the fetal alcohol syndrome. Two were dead and one was lost to follow-up; the remaining eight continued to be growth deficient and dysmorphic. Four of the eight were of borderline intelligence, and the other four were severely handicapped intellectually and in need of complete supervision outside the home. The picture painted here is not quite so bleak. Although the infant with the fetal alcohol syndrome may be recognized easily, the older child and adolescent, as mentioned in this paper, may not be as distinctive, making diagnosis difficult. Ask to see the baby pictures and look for the short palpebral fissures, hypoplastic philtrum, and the thin vermillion border of the upper lip. "What a cute baby" should not be your knee-jerk response after viewing the photographs.—F.A. Oski, M.D.

The Effect of Diets Rich in and Free From Additives on the Behavior of Children With Hyperkinetic and Learning Disorders

Mortimer D. Gross, Ruth A. Tofanelli, Sharyl M. Butzirus, and Earl W. Snodgrass (Chicago Med. School, North Chicago, and Summit School for Exceptional Children, Dundee, Ill.)

J. Am. Acad. Child Adolesc. Psychiatry 26:53–55, January 1987   6–12

The effects of diet on behavior remain controversial. Feingold reported that hyperkinetic children were much improved when salicylate and tartrazine were eliminated from the diet, thereby excluding preservatives and artificial flavors and colors. The Feingold diet was evaluated in 39 children aged 11–17 years with learning disorders who attended a 2-week summer camp supervised by their teachers. Eighteen children had a diagnosis of hyperkinetic syndrome/attention deficit disorder. The Feingold diet was given for the first week and a regular diet for the second week, when cookies, cakes, soft drinks, and the like were allowed.

The children much disliked the Feingold diet, but the group as a whole behaved well throughout the 2-week study period. Analysis of television tapes showed no differences in behavior between the first and second weeks (table). Motor restlessness was minimal, and disorganized behavior and misbehavior were rare. The children behaved like normal children at camp when taking a regular diet.

The strict Feingold diet is distasteful to the typical American child and it is difficult to keep children from cheating. No behavioral advantage is apparent for most children with learning disabilities, or for hyperkinetic children who have responded well to medication.

▶ Another study with disappointing results for the advocates of the Feingold study. In addition, the contention that sugar ingestion adversely affects the behavior or learning of boys with attentional deficit disorder could not be supported in a study of 16 boys (Milch, R., et al.: *J. Consult. Clin. Psychol.* 5:714, 1986). Time to take to the middle of the road on the diet-behavior hypothesis,

RATINGS OF BEHAVIOR*				
Rating	1st Rater	2nd Rater	3rd Rater	Average of All Raters
Motor restlessness				
First week	0.5 ± 0.5	1.0 ± 0.2	0.9 ± 0.3	0.8 ± 0.4
Second week	0.3 ± 0.3	1.2 ± 0.2	0.9 ± 0.4	0.8 ± 0.5
Disorganized behavior				
First week	0.3 ± 0.2	0.6 ± 0.3	0.2 ± 0.1	0.4 ± 0.4
Second week	0.2 ± 0.1	0.7 ± 0.3	0.3 ± 0.3	0.4 ± 0.4
Misbehavior				
First week	0.3 ± 0.2	0.8 ± 0.3	0.6 ± 0.2	0.6 ± 0.3
Second week	0.3 ± 0.2	0.4 ± 0.2	0.5 ± 0.1	0.4 ± 0.2
All behaviors				
First week	0.4 ± 0.3	0.8 ± 0.3	0.6 ± 0.4	0.6 ± 0.5
Second week	0.3 ± 0.2	0.8 ± 0.3	0.6 ± 0.4	0.5 ± 0.5

*Rated on a continuum of 0 to 10, the lower the number, the better the behavior. Ratings are expressed as means ± the SD. None of the differences approaches statistical significance.

(Courtesy of Gross, M.D., et al.: J. Am. Acad. Child Adolesc. Psychiatry 26:53–55, January 1987.)

remembering that the middle of the road is the best place to get run over.—
F.A. Oski, M.D.

Long-Term Follow-Up of Anorexia Nervosa
Brenda B. Toner, Paul E. Garfinkel, and David M. Garner (Clarke Inst. of Psychiatry, Toronto, and Toronto Gen. Hosp.)
Psychosom. Med. 48:520–529, September–October 1986   6–13

The outcome of anorexia nervosa varies widely using global clinical ratings. The long-term outcome of 30 restricting anorexic and 25 bulimic anorexic women (mean age, 28.2 years) was determined using standardized psychometric instruments in addition to global clinical ratings. Data were derived from a structured psychiatric interview, a battery of self-report measures, and clinical assessment. The follow-up period ranged from 5 years to 14 years.

In general, the two groups did not differ in long-term outcome according to clinical ratings and standardized assessment of anorexic symptoms, psychiatric diagnoses, and psychosocial functioning (table). The only exception was that the bulimic group had a significantly higher incidence of substance abuse disorders during the last year compared with the restricting group. Relative to a matched comparison group of 26 nonanorexic women of average weight, both bulimic and restricting anorexic women had a significantly higher life-time prevalence of affective and anxiety disorders.

▶ Given the fact that 13% to 20% of white college women are bulimic (Halmi, K., et al.: *Psychol. Med.* 11:697, 1981), it is frightening to ponder the future when we learn from this study that bulimics have a significantly higher incidence of substance abuse disorders at follow-up. Maybe it is no exaggeration to believe that there will only be two kinds of people in the United States by the year 2000: they will be the drug dependent and the drug free. For more on bulimia, see the 1984 YEAR BOOK, p. 426, and the 1987 YEAR BOOK, p. 259; for anorexia, see 1985 YEAR BOOK, p. 502, and 1987 YEAR BOOK, p. 261.—
F.A. Oski, M.D.

Autistic Children Grow Up: An Eight to Twenty-Four Year Follow-Up Study
L. Wolf and B. Goldberg (Children's Psychiatric Res. Inst., London, Ontario)
Can. J. Psychiatry 31:550–556, August 1986   6–14

Since infantile autism was first described in 1943, much controversy has surrounded the issue of diagnostic criteria for and etiology of this disorder. Numerous well-documented studies have been completed, but there are many problems of comparability of research because of a lack of consistency in the definition of study parameters. A follow-up study was made of autistic patients who met the *Diagnostic and Statistical Manual of*

COMPARISON OF RESTRICTING (R), BULIMIC ANOREXIC (B), AND CONTROL (C) GROUPS ON DSM-III DISORDERS: LIFE-TIME PREVALENCE AND INCIDENCE IN THE LAST YEAR

Percentage

Disorder	Lifetime Prevalence					Last Year				
	R	B	C	x^2	p<	R	B	C	x^2	p<
Affective Disorders	61.5[e]	52.4	11.5	15.0	0.001	38.4[b]	28.5	7.7	6.9	0.05
Major depression	46.2[b]	28.6	11.5	7.6	0.05	34.6[b]	19.0	7.7	5.8	0.05
Bipolar	3.8	9.5	0.0	2.7	NS	3.8	9.5	0.0	2.7	NS
Dysthymia	42.3[e]	33.3	0.0	13.7	0.001	—	—	—	—	—
Anxiety Disorders	57.7[e]	66.7	7.7	20.4	0.001	42.3[e]	52.4	7.7	12.1	0.01
Simple phobia	23.1	23.8	3.8	4.7	NS	19.2	23.8	3.8	4.2	NS
Social phobia	26.9	33.3	3.8	7.2	0.05	23.1	28.6	3.8	5.6	NS
Agoraphobia	11.5[e]	42.9	3.8	13.2	0.001	11.5[a]	28.5	3.8	6.2	0.05
Panic	19.2[e]	33.3	0.0	9.6	0.01	15.3[a]	33.3	3.8	10.1	0.01
Obsessive compulsive	38.5[e]	28.6	12.0	12.0	0.01	23.0[b]	9.6	0.0	7.2	0.05
Substance use disorders	23.1	42.9	15.4	4.7	NS	0.0[c]	42.9	7.7	18.4	0.001
Alcohol abuse/dependency	7.7	14.3	0.0	3.8	NS	0.0	10.0	0.0	3.8	NS
Drug abuse/dependency	11.5	9.5	7.7	0.2	NS	0.0	14.3	0.0	7.7	0.05
Tobacco	7.7[d]	28.6	11.5	4.3	NS	0.0[d]	23.8	7.7	7.8	0.05
Somatization	3.8	4.8	0.0	1.2	NS	3.8	4.8	0.0	1.2	NS
Schizophrenic disorders	0.0	4.8	0.0	—	NS	0.0	4.8	0.0	—	NS
Schizophrenia	0.0	4.8	0.0	—	NS	0.0	4.8	0.0	—	NS
Schizophreniform	0.0	0.0	0.0	—	—	0.0	0.0	0.0	—	—
Antisocial personality	0.0	0.0	0.0	—	—	0.0	0.0	0.0	—	—
Cognitive impairment	0.0	0.0	0.0	—	—	0.0	0.0	0.0	—	—

Multiple Sample Chi Square.
a, R = B = C with $P < .05$; b, B = R > C; c, c, B > R, R > C; d, C = B > R; e, B > C, R > C, R = B.
(Courtesy of Toner, B.B., et al.: Psychosom. Med. 48:520–529, September–October 1986.)

TABLE 1.—Data at Diagnosis of Original
Cases (N = 80)*

	%
Abnormal labour	18
Motor milestones delay	48
Words after 16 months	43
No useful speech	68
Intelligence quotient below 70	89
First symptoms under age 1 year	21
between 12-30 months	76
Started to talk then stopped	34
Upset by change of routine	55
Hands held in strange position	61
Walked on tip toes	15
Whirled	10
Played inappropriately with toys	65
Possible auditory dysfunction	45
Rocked back and forth	56
Not cuddly as infant	61
Made strange noises	73
Exhibited temper outbursts	76
Lacked eye contact	51
Displayed repetitive behaviour	88
Seizures present	11

*This table only reports data at diagnosis in 80 patients. All other tables report on patients who responded to the questionnaires.
(Courtesy of Wolf, L., and Goldberg, B.: Can. J. Psychiatry 31:550–556, August 1986.)

TABLE 2.—Program at Follow-Up

Program	Home (N = 20) %	Institution (N = 44) %
No Program		11
Developmental/Life Skills/ Behaviour Compliance	10	43
Trainable Class	32	16
Educable/Regular Class	15	
Vocational		14
Sheltered Workshop	20	14
Independent Work	20	2

(Courtesy of Wolf, L., and Goldberg, B.: Can. J. Psychiatry 31:550–556, August 1986.)

Mental Disorders, ed. III, criteria for infantile autism. Questionnaires were sent to 80 parents and/or caregivers of former autistic patients who were treated at the Children's Psychiatric Research Institute between 1960 and 1973 to determine the patients' present place of residence, functioning ability, language development, program involvement, and seizure activity. In addition, prenatal, perinatal, and developmental histories, as well as physical, neurologic, psychological, biochemical, EEG, and bone-age test data were extracted from casebooks.

Of 80 patients, 71 (89%) were considered mentally retarded and 9 (11%) were mentally normal or borderline (Table 1). In all, 64 replies were received and analyzed. Twenty patients were cared for at home and

TABLE 3.—INTELLIGENCE QUOTIENTS AND
PLACE OF RESIDENCE AT FOLLOW-UP

I.Q. At Diagnosis	Institution N	Institution %	Home N	Home %
Normal			1	5
Borderline	1	2	4	20
Mild	8	18	5	25
Moderate	10	23	7	35
Severe	22	50	2	10
Profound	3	7		
Retarded Unspecified			1	5

$\chi^2 = 18.863$; 7df $P = .01$.
(Courtesy of Wolf, L., and Goldberg, B.: Can. J. Psychiatry 31:550–556, August 1986.)

TABLE 4.—OUTCOME OF OTHER FOLLOW-UP STUDIES

Author	N	Outcome (Percentages) Normal	Good	Fair	Poor	Very Poor
DeMyer (1979)	69	1	9	16	24	40
Lotter (1974)	54		14	24	14	48
Rutter, Lockyer (1967)	63		13	25	13	48
DeMyer, et al (1973)	120		10	16	24	50
Rutter (1970)	63	2	17	19		64
Wolf, Goldberg (1984)	64	3	9	30		47

(Courtesy of Wolf, L., and Goldberg, B.: Can. J. Psychiatry 31:550–556, August 1986.)

44 were institutionalized (Table 2). There was a statistically significant relationship between IQ and diagnosis and place of residence in that a larger proportion of those with an IQ above 70 were living at home (Table 3). The overall prognosis at follow-up was considered from fair to very poor in 77% of the patients. These findings agree with several earlier studies and disagree with others (Table 4). There is a need for standardized psychometric measures that are tailored specifically to autistic children because of their specific cognitive and linguistic deficits.

The Personality of Children Prior to Divorce: A Prospective Study
Jeanne H. Block, Jack Block, and Per F. Gjerde (Univ. of California at Berkeley)
Child Dev. 57:827–840, August 1986   6–15

Studies on the effects of divorce on children have yielded conflicting results. Some researchers have found problems with antisocial behavior and others have reported beneficial effects. As the numbers of children of divorced parents increase, it becomes important to analyze how divorce affects their personality development.

A longitudinal study of 128 children attending nursery school was begun in 1968, with personality assessments made at ages 3, 4, and 7 years. The children were mainly of the middle and upper classes and were predom-

TABLE 1.—Relationships Between CCQ-Based Personality
Evaluations at Ages 3, 4, and 7 Years and Subsequent Parental
Divorce: Boys

CCQ Item	Age		
	3	4	7
Is considerate of other children	−.34*	−.09	−.01
Generally stretches limits	.31+	.18	.44*
Is open and straightforward	−.31+	.05	−.03
Tries to take advantage of others	.31+	.10	.07
Tends to arouse liking in adults	−.31+	−.20	−.23
Is restless and fidgety	.33+	.13	.39*
Emotionally labile	.43*	.07	.41*
Tends to exaggerate mishaps	.31+	.10	.10
Neat and orderly in dress and behavior	−.31+	−.22	−.05
Is stubborn	.36*	.19	.07
Has bodily symptoms for stress	−.04	−.31+	.21
Aggressive	.25	.29+	.34+
Helpful and cooperative	−.24	−.08	−.30+
Has transient interpersonal relationships	.15	.08	−.35*
Uses and responds to reason	−.18	−.04	−.47**
Is physically active	.16	.21	.35*
Is visibly deviant from peers	−.19	−.19	−.45**
Is resourceful in initiating activities	−.02	−.20	.32+
Tends to go to pieces under stress	−.10	.06	.32+
Shows specific mannerisms	.00	−.01	−.30+
Anxious in unpredictable environments	.16	.18	.45**
Is obedient and compliant	−.17	−.02	−.33+
Is reflective	−.29+	−.16	−.38*
Is easily victimized by other children	−.18	.00	−.34+

Note.—CCQ: California Child Q-Sort. For these analyses, there were 33 boys at age 3, 36 at age 4, and 32 at age 7. At ages 3 and 4, 8 of these boys come from families that would subsequently experience divorce. At age 7, this number is 5.
+P < .10.
*P < .05.
**P < .01.
(Courtesy of Block, J.H., et al.: Child Dev. 57:827–840, August 1986.)

inantly white. The mothers were interviewed when the child was aged 6 years or 12 years. The family status was determined when the child was aged 14 or 15 years. During the study, 60% of the families remained intact and 33% of the couples became divorced.

As early as 11 years before their parents' divorce, the behavior of boys was characterized by undercontrol of impulse, aggression, and excessive energy (Table 1). The behavior of girls in families in which the parents subsequently became divorced did not appear to be as greatly affected by predivorce familial stress (Table 2).

Friction between parents during the predivorce period has profound consequences on the personality development of their children, especially that of boys. Behavior problems often attributed to divorce may actually arise during the predivorce period.

▶ I'd like to close this chapter on a happy note, but I just could not find one. I feel like the evening network news. More than a million children each year are the victims of separation or divorce, and it is projected that, by the year 1990,

TABLE 2.—Relationships Between CCQ-Based Personality Evaluations at Ages 3, 4, and 7 Years and Subsequent Parental Divorce: Girls

CCQ Item	Age 3	Age 4	Age 7
Has unusual thought processes	.47**	.25	−.09
Is agile and well coordinated	.42**	.13	−.13
Anxious in unpredictable environments	−.31+	−.07	.04
Is planful	.35*	−.04	−.07
Responds to humor	.29+	.00	−.14
Is competent, skillful	.29+	.18	.27
Is easily victimized by other children	−.28+	−.09	.11
Prefers nonverbal communication	.05	.31*	−.20
Gets along well with other children	.02	−.28+	−.46**
Eager to please	.05	−.27+	−.18
Behaves in sex-typed manner	−.07	−.31*	−.03
Uses and responds to reason	.13	−.31*	.11
Tends to yield and give in	.07	−.28+	−.12
Indecisive and vacillating	−.26	−.30+	−.19
Emotionally labile	−.06	.26*	.07
Is calm and relaxed	.21	−.32*	−.04
Likes to be by herself	.16	.26+	−.02
Is inappropriate in emotive behavior	−.03	.29+	.19
Has transient interpersonal relationships	.03	.06	.44**
Tends to give, lend, share	.07	−.24	−.39*
High performance standards for self	.18	−.05	.33*
Is jealous and envious of others	−.21	.02	.33+
High intellectual capacity	.12	.11	.42**
Has a readiness to feel guilt	.25	−.09	.32+

Note.—CCQ: California Child Q-Sort. For these analyses, there were 37 girls at age 3, 42 at age 4, and 32 at age 7. At ages 3 and 4, 21 of these girls come from families that would subsequently experience divorce. At age 7, this number is 13.
+$P < .10$.
*$P < .05$.
**$P < .01$.
(Courtesy of Block, J.H., et al.: Child Dev. 57:827–840, August 1986.)

by the end of high school, one third of our children will have lived with a divorced parent. Just think of the impact on society if this results in children, particularly boys, being aggressive and not under control of their impulses. The only imperfect thing in nature is the human race. The lemmings may know something we don't.—F.A. Oski, M.D.

7 Child Development

Behavior in Four-Year-Olds Who Have Experienced Hospitalization and Day Care
Gunnel Elander, Alf Nilsson and Tor Lindberg (Univ. of Lund and Central Hosp., Helsingborg, Sweden)
Am. J. Orthopsychiatry 56:612–616, October 1986   7–1

Separation from parents through hospitalization has been described as a psychological upset for preschool children. Day care also entails parental separation during the daytime. The behavior of 535 four-year-old children was investigated in relation to their earlier experiences of hospitalization and day care using the Child Behavior Checklist for Ages 2–3. These items were classified into nine categories of behavior: somatic symptoms, dependency, reserved-depressive behavior, aggressiveness, anxiety, hyperactive-impulsive behavior, oral tendencies, anal-compulsive behavior, and regression.

In all, 201 (40%) of the children had been hospitalized and 323 (65%) had been attending day care. Most of the hospital stays lasted for 3 days or less. Children who had been hospitalized were significantly more hyperactive-impulsive, regressive, and aggressive than were nonhospitalized children. Children who had been in day care were more anxious than children cared for at home. However, after excluding day care, no significant difference in any behavior was noted between hospitalized and nonhospitalized children.

Unless they have been receiving day care, the behavior of children as a consequence of hospitalization does not differ from that of nonhospitalized children. Children who have experienced day care are more vulnerable and at risk for behavior problems subsequent to hospitalization.

▶ Doctor James Harris, Associate Professor of Psychiatry, Mental Hygiene and Pediatrics, Johns Hopkins University School of Medicine, Comments.— F.A. Oski, M.D.

▶ The effect of hospitalization on the behavior of children has been a topic of considerable interest since the early work of Spitz and Bowlby. In recent years, reports by Douglas (1974) and Quinton and Rutter (1975) indicated that repeated early hospitalizations, but not single hospitalizations of less than a week in duration, are associated with behavioral and emotional problems in late childhood or early adolescence.

Separation from family is considered to be a major factor related to these changes in behavior. It is made worse by social disadvantage, large families and disruptive interpersonal relationships, and/or mental illness in the parents. A particularly important factor is ongoing adversity in the child's life following hospital discharge. The current authors confirm the findings of Quinton and

224 / Pediatrics

Rutter, as well as others, that repeated hospitalization has greater effects on behavioral and emotional difficulties than does a single, short-term hospitalization. They find that hyperactivity, impulsive behavior, and aggression are most significant in children who have had multiple hospitalizations and are evaluated by their parents at 4 years of age. They found that day care was a discriminating variable in the demonstration of behavior difficulties, and noted that dependency and regression also were significant in children who were in day care and had been hospitalized, compared with those who were not. The authors rightly point out that parent/child interaction has not been addressed in their study, nor has family discord, psychiatric problems with parents, or psychosocial disadvantage. Although the study may have been conducted in a relatively homogeneous Swedish community, these variables cannot be assumed but need to be investigated directly.

The significance of the present preliminary study is to emphasize the effects of day care/hospitalization as a combined risk factor in preschool children. However, there are a number of weaknesses in the study that need to be addressed and, until done so, findings would best be considered preliminary.

1. Although statistically different, are the children here psychologically disordered? Do they also have problems in social adaptation, as well as more symptoms?

2. The lack of family psychosocial, parent/child, interpersonal, and parental interpersonal data needs to be ascertained through specific interviews with parents, such as those conducted by Quinton and Rutter.

3. The lack of specific information about entry into day care and the age of hospitalization must be taken into account. If records of hospitalization are available, they should be used to document that hospitalization did take place and discharge diagnoses and summary should be listed. The type of illness (e.g., accident and meningitis) and the reason for day care must be noted as well.

4. Cut-off points on this questionnaire need to be demonstrated to establish the incidence of disorder.

5. The quality of day care programs, in addition to parent/child home programs, needs investigation. There is considerable difference in the United States in the quality of day care and type of day care programming. Designated day care programs and family day care are different kinds of settings, and need to be determined. In the Swedish study, there apparently was a full range from family day care to day care centers.

In summary, the authors point out that prevention of behavioral problems, especially in children with repeated hospitalizations, needs ongoing attention. A long-term follow-up of these four-year-olds and more comprehensive assessment can help to answer questions about the impact of day care/family care, or their combination on children's behavior.—J. Harris, M.D.

Behavior Problems in Retarded Children With Special Reference to Down's Syndrome
Ann Gath and Dianne Gumley
Br. J. Psychiatry 149:156–161, August 1986   7–2

Behavioral problems are frequent in mentally retarded individuals, but the frequency of psychiatric disorder in children with Down's syndrome is uncertain. Data concerning behavior were collected by parent and teacher interviews, using rating scales, on 193 children with Down's syndrome and 154 children from the same schools having similar degrees of verbal and motor handicap. The Rutter A2 and B2 rating scales, the Adaptive Behaviour Scale, and the Additional Behaviour checklist were used.

Similar proportions of the two groups had high scores on the Rutter A2 scale and the Additional Behaviour checklist. Deviant behavior was much more frequent in both groups of retarded children than in their close-aged siblings. Significant behavioral disorder was found in 38% of children with Down's syndrome and 49% of the control group. Only 31% and 29%, respectively, were considered well adjusted. Conduct disorder was most frequent in the children with Down's syndrome. Psychotic disorder was the most frequent diagnosis in the control group, but also was found in Down's syndrome children. Two of the latter children and three controls met criteria for infantile autism.

A significant number of children with Down's syndrome have behavioral disorders, and in this respect they resemble non-Down's syndrome children with similar degrees of retardation. Because of the frequency of behavioral and emotional problems in retarded children, the psychiatrist clearly has a role in their management.

▶ We often lose sight of the fact that behavior problems are a common and very disturbing complication of mental retardation. The behavioral and emotional problems of the child with Down's syndrome may, in fact, be his only true handicap.

Tongue reduction surgery has been advocated as a means of improving articulation in children with Down's syndrome. However, no benefit from such surgery was observed by C. L. Parsons and associates in a group of 18 children (*Am. J. Ment. Defic.* 91:328, 1987).—F.A. Oski, M.D.

Persistence of Sleep Disturbances in Preschool Children
Sudesh Kataria, Melvin S. Swanson, and G.E. Trevathan (East Carolina Univ., Greenville, N.C.)
J. Pediatr. 110:642–646, April 1987   7–3

Sleep disturbances are among the most frequent behavioral problems in young children, and it has been suggested that persistent disorder may indicate psychological disturbance and emotional conflict. The persistence of common sleep disturbances and their relation to environmental stress and to other behavioral problems were studied in 81 children aged 15–48 months seen consecutively in well-child clinics. Sixty children remained in the study after 3 years. Sleep disturbance was defined as night waking or bedtime struggle occurring three or more nights a week and present for at least a month at the time of the initial interview.

Overall, 42% of the children had sleep disturbance initially, as did 38%

TABLE 1.—Prevalence and Persistence of
Sleep Disturbances in 60 Healthy
Study Children

	Initial interview		3-year follow-up	
	n	%	n	%
Night waking	13	22	14*	23
Bedtime struggle	8	13	8	13
Both	4	7	1	2
Total	25	42	23	38

*Includes two children with no sleep problems at initial interview.
(Courtesy of Kataria, S., et al.: J. Pediatr. 110:642–646, April 1987.)

TABLE 2.—Factors Associated With Persistent Sleep Disturbances

	Sleep disturbed (n = 23)		Non–sleep disturbed (n = 37)		
	n	%	n	%	P
Environmental stresses	14	61	7	19	<0.01
Behavior problems	7	30	7	19	NS
Working mother	11	48	22	59	NS
Mother's college education (1-7 yr)	12	52	33	89	<0.03

(Courtesy of Kataria, S., et al.: J. Pediatr. 110:642–646, April 1987.)

at follow-up after 3 years (Table 1). Night waking and bedtime struggle alone both persisted. Various environmental stresses were noted in 61% of sleep-disturbed children and in 19% of the other children (Table 2). Unaccustomed maternal absence was the most frequent stress factor, followed by child illness or accident. Seven of the 23 sleep-disturbed children had other behavior problems, as did 7 of the other 37 children. More mothers of non-sleep-disturbed children worked. Co-sleeping with one or both parents was more frequent in sleep-disturbed children, both initially and at follow-up.

Sleep disturbances are frequent in young children, and tend to persist in the preschool years. Their persistence may signify environmental stress, and other general behavior disorders also may be present. Early identification of sleep disturbance may therefore lead to timely intervention.

▶ A large number of pediatricians, as well as parents, have lost sleep over this problem. Sleep disturbances are common in early childhood and the 22% incidence of night waking, 13% for bedtime struggle, and 7% for the combination of both night waking and bedtime struggle found in this study are similar to previous reports. The most distressing aspect of this report is the very high percentage of children whose sleep disturbance was found to persist after a 3-

year follow-up. For more on this topic, see entries on "Sleeping patterns in upper-middle class families when the child awakens ill or frightened," 1984 YEAR BOOK, pp. 400–401; "Sleep behavior from 4 to 16 years," 1984, YEAR BOOK, pp. 401–403; and "Sleep and bedtime behavior in preschool-aged children," 1984 YEAR BOOK, pp. 403–405. To "sleep like a baby" may not be so wonderful after all. Looking for some guidance? Try reading "The prevention of sleep problems and colic" (Schmitt, B. D.: *Pediatr. Clin. North Am.* 33:763, 1986).—F.A. Oski, M.D.

Childhood Near-Death Experiences
Melvin Morse, Paul Castillo, David Venecia, Jerrold Milstein, and Donald C. Tyler (Univ. of Washington and Children's Orthopedic Hosp. and Med. Ctr., Seattle)
Am. J. Dis. Child. 140:1110–1114, November 1986   7–4

A near-death experience represents a unique psychological event that has been described in individuals who have survived a life-threatening illness or danger. These experiences include the following features: the sensation of seeing one's own body from a vantage point outside the physical body; panoramic life review; entering a tunnel; meeting others, including dead or living relatives; encountering a being of light; a sense of the presence of a deity; and a return to the body. Because they have a reproducible core cluster of experiences, near-death experiences can be distinguished from drug-induced psychoses and psychotic processes.

In a nonselective manner, interviews were conducted with 11 children aged 3–16 years who survived critical illnesses, including cardiac arrests and profound comas. Any memory of a time when they were unconscious was treated as a near-death experience and was recorded. Seven children had memories that included being out of the physical body (six patients), entering darkness (five), being in a tunnel (four), and deciding to return to the body (three). When 29 aged-matched survivors of illnesses that required intubation, narcotics, benzodiazepines, and admission to an intensive care unit were interviewed, none had any memories of the time when they were unconscious.

In the study population near-death experiences clearly were associated with surviving a critical illness. The elements of the near-death experiences reported are similar to those found previously in adults. No child described elements of depersonalization as part of a near-death experience. A core near-death experience triggered by the process of dying or resuscitative efforts may be a natural developmental experience.

▶ There is a mystical universal sameness to these near-death experiences described by children. See the 1985 YEAR BOOK, pp. 513–514, and the 1987 YEAR BOOK, pp. 254–255. These near-death experiences, particularly the depersonalization and the tunnel imagery, are very similar to what has been described by adults who have been "there" and back. I'm dying to find out for myself.— F.A. Oski, M.D.

Familial Bathing Patterns: Implications for Cases of Alleged Molestation and for Pediatric Practice

Alvin A. Rosenfeld, Bryna Siegel, and Robert Bailey (Columbia Univ., Stanford Univ., and Menlo Park, Calif.)
Pediatrics 79:224–229, February 1987   7-5

Reports of alleged sexual molestation in children, in which supposedly "abnormal" sexual behavior in the home was used as supporting evidence, have been increasing. To define a sexually related home behavior as nonnormative, it is important to know what is normative sexual socialization. A cross-sectional study was undertaken in 576 upper middle class children to define bathing practices in the home and their implications for reports of alleged molestation.

Families varied in their handling of bathing practices, but as a group, children bathed alone more frequently as they grew older and parents bathed less frequently with the child of the opposite sex, particularly as children grew older. It was uncommon for mothers to bathe or shower with sons older than age 8 years or for fathers to bathe or shower with daughters older than age 9 years, although most had stopped before that age. Bathing patterns were generally changed because of rules that parents made [e.g., if the child behaved in a sexual manner, at least to the parent's eye (12.3%)], or for convenience [mainly to end "splashing" or "horseplay" (23%)], but 19% of the children asked for the change.

Cross-sex aversions to cobathing are manifestations of the sex taboos in typical families. When incest is charged, and a parent's bathing with the child is used as supporting evidence, such bathing behavior should be considered abusive only if it is accompanied by more extensive and persuasive evidence of deviance.

▶ It was during family bathing that I learned that genitalia was not an Italian airline.—F.A. Oski, M.D.

Labial Fusion in Prepubescent Girls: A Marker for Sexual Abuse?

Carol D. Berkowitz, Sandra L. Elvik, and Mary K. Logan (Univ. of California at Los Angeles Med. Ctr.)
Am. J. Obstet. Gynecol. 156:16–20, January 1987   7-6

Although labial fusion is common in prepubescent girls, its precise incidence is not known. Labial fusion in young girls was studied in a retrospective review of records of children referred for evaluation of suspected sexual abuse. The medical records of 500 children (75% of them girls) yielded 10 (3%) with labial fusion. The patients ranged in age from 2 months to 5 years, and the duration of fusion ranged from 2 weeks of 2.5 years (table). Complete labial fusion was present in seven girls and partial fusion in three (Fig 7–1). Three children had urinary tract problems, including urinary incontinence in two. None of the children had vulvova-

CHARACTERISTICS OF PATIENTS WITH LABIAL FUSION

Case No.	Age	Fusion (%)	History of sexual abuse	Results of physical examination*	Urinary findings	Treatment†	Outcome
1	5 yr	Complete	+	Hymen, normal Anal, abnormal	0	+	Partial resolution
2	4 yr	Partial	+	Hymen, not visualized Anal, abnormal	+	+	Partial resolution
3	5 yr	Complete	+	Hymen, normal Anal, abnormal	0	+	Partial resolution
4	4 yr	Complete	+	Hymen, not visualized Anal, abnormal	0	+	No follow-up
5	2 yr	Complete	+	Hymen, normal Anal, normal	0	+	Complete resolution Breast hypertrophy
6	4 yr	Partial	–	Hymen, abnormal Anal, abnormal	+	+	Resolution
7	9 mo	Complete	–	Hymen, not visualized Anal, normal	0	–	No resolution
8	13 mo	Complete	–	Hymen, not visualized Anal, normal	0	+	No resolution Breast hypertrophy
9	6 mo	Partial	–	Hymen, normal Anal, normal	0	+	Complete resolution
10	12 mo	Complete	–	Hymen, not visualized Anal, normal	+	+	No follow-up

*Physical findings consistent with sexual abuse.
†Treatment with conjugated estrogen cream: + = given; – = not given.
(Courtesy of Berkowitz, C.D., et al.: Am. J. Obstet. Gynecol. 156:16–20, January 1987.)

ginitis, dermatitis, or a specific history of trauma other than related to sexual misuse. One girl had a history of maturbation.

History and/or physical findings consistent with sexual abuse were noted in six patients. Anal findings were grossly abnormal and consistent with

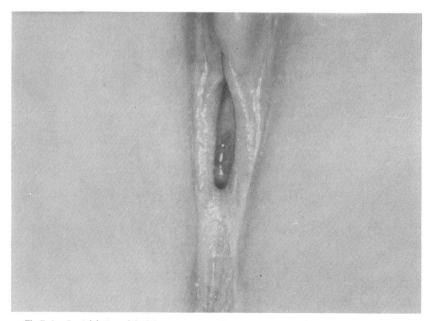

Fig 7–1.—Partial fusion of the labia minora in a child aged 4 years. (Courtesy of Berkowitz, C.D., et al.: Am. J. Obstet. Gynecol. 156:16–20, January 1987.)

anal penetration in five children. Treatment with conjugated estrogen cream in nine patients led to resolution of labial fusion in six of them. Breast hypertrophy occurred in three patients, which necessitated discontinuation of therapy. None of the patients had spontaneous resolution of the labial fusion during the study period. Although labial fusion may occur secondary to a variety of inflammatory conditions, the findings of labial fusion in older girls warrant a consideration of sexual abuse.

▶ Another useful finding to help support the diagnosis of child sexual abuse was described by White and associates at the 1987 meeting of the Ambulatory Pediatric Association (*Am. J. Dis. Child.* 141:369, 1987). These workers found that in females 1–12 years of age, a vaginal introital diameter of more than 4 mm should cause one to be highly suspicious of sexual abuse. A diameter of 4 mm or more was highly associated with a history of sexual contact (94%) compared with findings in a group with no history of sexual contact (5%). A vaginal introital diameter of less than 4 mm did not exclude the possibility of sexual abuse because these workers found that 53% of children with a history of child abuse had a vaginal introital diameter of less than 4 mm.—F.A. Oski, M.D.

Prevalence of Speech and Language Disorders in 5-Year-Old Kindergarten Children in the Ottawa-Carleton Region

Joseph H. Beitchman, Rama Nair, Marjorie Clegg, and P.G. Patel (Univ. of Toronto and Univ. of Ottawa)
J. Speech Hear. Disord. 51:98–110, May 1986 7–7

Speech and language disorders constitute a major health concern among young children because these disorders may precede academic failure and psychiatric problems. The prevalence of speech and language disorders in school children is not known, mainly because many afflicted children reside in special schools or institutions that were not included in the samples in previous studies. The prevalence of speech and language disorders was examined in kindergarten children who attended public or private English language schools and in children in nursery schools, day-care centers, and special needs centers in the Ottawa-Carleton region.

TABLE 1.—Uncorrected Percentage of Total Sample Estimated to Have Speech-Only, Speech and Language, and Language-Only Problems (SE in Parentheses)

Subjects	Number in total sample	Speech-only %	Speech & language %	Language-only %	Total %
Boys	861	4.16 (.68)	3.31 (.61)	5.76 (.79)	13.23 (1.15)
Girls	794	2.21 (.52)	2.61 (.56)	3.91 (.68)	8.73 (1.0)
Total	1,655	3.22 (.43)	2.97 (.42)	4.87 (.53)	11.08 (.77)

Standard error is standard deviation of sample distribution. This is way of indicating error in estimate caused by fluctuations in sampling.

(Courtesy of Beitchman, J.H., et al.: J. Speech Hear. Disord. 51:98–110, May 1986.)

TABLE 2.—Corrected Percentages of Total Sample
Estimated to Fail Stage II (SE in Parentheses)

Subjects	Number in total sample	Speech-only %	Speech & language %	Language-only %	Total %
Boys	861	6.58 (.85)	3.31 (.61)	8.17 (.93)	18.1 (1.3)
Girls	794	6.68 (.89)	7.06 (.91)	8.37 (.98)	22.1 (1.5)
Total	1,655	6.4 (.60)	4.56 (.51)	8.04 (.67)	19.0 (1.4)

(Courtesy of Beitchman, J.H., et al.: J. Speech Hear. Disord. 51:98–110, May 1986.)

TABLE 3.—Prevalence Estimates for Speech and Language Disorders

Source	Population	Ages	Findings
Beitchman et al. (present study)	Probability sample of Ottawa area children	5	Speech—6.4% Language—8.04% Speech and language—4.56%
Silva (1980)	Sample of all infants born at Dunedin, N.Z., hospital	3	Language—8.4%
Stevenson & Richman (1976)	Probability sample from London, England, area	3	Language—3.1%
Tuomi & Ivanoff (1977)	Probability sample of public schools near London, Ont.	5–6	Articulation—20.5% Language—6–7%
Bax & Hart (1976)	All children in Camden, London area, under 5 years on June 1, 1974	4½	Speech and language—5.0%
Fundudis et al. (1979)	Longitudinal sample of all children born in Newcastle-upon-Tyne	3 7	Speech—4.0% Speech—3.0%
Hull et al. (1971)	Probability sample of public school students in USA	6	Articulation: Moderate deviance—52.9% Extreme deviance—9.7%
Morley (1965)	All children born in Newcastle-upon-Tyne between May and June 1947	3½ 4 6½	Speech—19.0% Articulation—17.0% Articulation—3.0%
Irwin (1948)	Public school children from 10 "representative" schools in Cleveland, OH	5–11	Speech—10.0%
Mills & Streit (1942)	All public school children in Holyoke, MA	6–8	Speech—33.4%

(Courtesy of Beitchman, J.H., et al.: J. Speech Hear. Disord. 51:98–110, May 1986.)

A population sample of 861 boys and 794 girls, which represented one third of all the English-speaking children aged 5 years in the study region, participated in the first stage of a screening procedure that consisted of a 30-minute speech and language test. In the second stage, intensive tests were administered to 301 of 315 children who failed the first test and to 51 randomly selected controls who had passed it. Of the 301 children who failed the stage I test, 126 (41.9%) passed all stage II tests, but 175 (58.1%) failed at least one of these. Of 51 control children who passed the stage I test, 5 (9.8%) failed the stage II tests (Tables 1 and 2).

The overall prevalence of speech and language disorders was 19.0%. This figure corresponds to the estimate reported by other investigators (Table 3).

▶ It is troublesome to learn that a representative cross-section of 5-year-old Canadian kindergarten children demonstrated a 16% to 21% incidence of some form of impairment in speech or language, with language impairment being more common than speech impairment. Rates of nearly 25% have been reported from England and 21% in St. Louis in first graders. First we worried why Johnny couldn't read, then we learned that Johnny couldn't write, and now we find out that Johnny can't speak correctly either. Some problem, eh?—F.A. Oski, M.D.

Bicycle Helmet Use by Children: Knowledge and Behavior of Physicians

Barry D. Weiss and Burris Duncan (Univ. of Arizona)
Am. J. Public Health 76:1022–1023, August 1986   7–8

Of about 1,300 persons who die each year in the United States of injuries sustained while riding a bicycle, nearly half are children younger than age 14 years. Another 30,000 children sustain nonfatal bicycling injuries each year, of which a high percentage involve the head. Although the use of helmets would significantly reduce the bicycling accident rate, less than 2% of all school-aged children wear helmets while cycling. A survey was made of physicians in the Tucson, Arizona, area to assess their awareness of this problem.

The 161 pediatricians and family physicians listed in the Tucson telephone directory were sent a questionnaire in which they were asked to estimate the percentage of schoolchildren who use bicycle helmets, to suggest reasons why children generally do not wear them, and to state whether or not they provide information on bicycle safety to their patients. Of the 106 (65.8%) responding physicians, 16 stated that they did not provide well-child care. Of the other 90, 55 were family physicians and 35 were pediatricians. Of respondents, 55% knew that bicycle accidents are an important cause of childhood mortality, and that such accidents account for more deaths than falls, firearm injuries, and meningitis. Most respondents (92%) correctly estimated that less than 5% of children wear bicycle helmets. The most frequently suggested reason was lack of parental awareness of the importance of wearing helmets. Despite respondents' awareness of the problem, 29% reported that they never discussed bicycle safety during well-child care, and 40% reported that they almost never discussed it.

The results of this survey should be considered only preliminary, because the number of physicians queried was small. However, the problem merits further attention.

▶ Maybe you feel frustrated by many of the topics discussed in this chapter— behavioral problems in children with Down's syndrome, sleep disturbances, sexual abuse, and the high prevalence of speech and language difficulties in our youth—but this abstract should provide you with some relief. The issue of bicycle injuries and the need for advice about bicycle helmets are areas in which you can make a difference—a real difference that can save lives.—F.A. Oski, M.D.

8 Adolescent Medicine

Parental Attitudes and the Occurrence of Early Sexual Activity
Kristin A. Moore, James L. Peterson, and Frank F. Furstenberg (Child Trends, Inc., Washington, D.C., and Univ. of Pennsylvania)
J. Marriage Fam. 48:777–782, November 1986   8–1

It has been asserted that parental communication with and monitoring of adolescent children will discourage premarital sexual activity. It has been assumed that parents are uniformly negative regarding such activity, but parents' actual attitudes have not been examined directly. The hypothesis that the effects of parent-child discussion and parental supervision of teen sexual activity depend on parental attitudes was examined in a series of white adolescents aged 15 and 16 years, interviewed in the 1981 National Survey of Children. Of 461 respondents, 120 reported having had sexual intercourse.

Parental attitudes were ignored in the first set of analyses and taken into account in the next set. Little support was obtained for the hypothesis that parental communication and monitoring discourages premarital sexual activity. Only the daughters of parents holding traditional attitudes, who had communicated with them regarding sex or television, were less likely to have had intercourse. No effect of parental traditionality was observed in sons.

This analysis of adolescents aged 15 and 16 years indicated that parental discussion is associated with less frequent initiation of sexual activity only by daughters of parents holding traditional family values. The effect of family communication may depend on parental beliefs, and on whether the adolescent in question is a male or a female.

▶ Parental communication with teenage children is often recommended as a means of discouraging early sexual activity. It is disappointing, but not surprising, to learn that such communication does not guarantee that early sexual activity will not occur. One sure way to discourage early sexual activity in teenagers is to encourage them to try it. This is a variation on the adage of the late President Harry S Truman who said, "I have found that the best way to give advice to your children is to find out what they want and then advise them to do it."—F.A. Oski, M.D.

Disparities in Adolescent—Physician Views of Teen Health Information Concerns
Phyllis M. Levenson, Betty Pfefferbaum, and James R. Morrow, Jr. (Univ. of Houston and Univ. of Texas)
J. Adolesc. Health Care 8:171–176, March 1987   8–2

Information about health-related subjects is necessary for adolescents to make correct health-promoting choices. Six hundred middle-school students and 99 physicians completed written questionnaires evaluating the importance of 45 items from seven subscales: smoking, physical fitness, weight control, self-actualization, comparison with others, peer opinion, and communication. The mean student age was 12.2 years, whereas that for physicians was 44.6 years. A comparison was made based on findings from both groups. The scores for the seven scales were used as dependent variables in two multivariate analyses of variance (MANOVA).

Results of the first MANOVA suggested that the physicians and students differed significantly. Means and post hoc univariate results are presented in Table 1. A second MANOVA compared the students' perceptions of scale importance with the importance physicians estimated that adolescents would attribute to each scale. The significant MANOVA result suggests

TABLE 1.—COMPARISON OF PHYSICIAN AND
ADOLESCENT PERCEPTIONS OF THE IMPORTANCE OF
ITEMS IN THE NEED-TO-KNOW SCALES

Scale	Physician ($\bar{x} \pm$ SD)	Adolescent ($\bar{x} \pm$ SD)
Smoking (13)[a]	20.3 ± 5.1	23.2 ± 7.7[b]
Physical fitness (9)	16.5 ± 4.4	18.6 ± 4.9[b]
Weight (6)	11.2 ± 2.9	12.6 ± 4.0[b]
Self-actualization (7)	12.7 ± 3.7	12.7 ± 3.9
Comparison with others (3)	6.7 ± 1.8	7.7 ± 2.2[b]
Peer opinion (3)	6.7 ± 1.6	7.1 ± 2.4
Communication (4)	7.5 ± 2.3	8.6 ± 2.4[b]

[a]The number in parentheses represents items per scale. Items are coded 1–4; a lower score indicates a greater importance attached to the scale.
[b]$P < .001$.
(Courtesy of Levenson, P.M., et al.: J. Adolesc. Health Care 8:171–176, March 1987.)

TABLE 2.—COMPARISON OF PHYSICIAN
PERCEPTIONS OF AOLESCENT CONCERNS AND
ADOLESCENT VIEWS ABOUT ITEMS IN THE NEED-
TO-KNOW SCALES[a]

Scale	Physician mean	Adolescent mean
Smoking	34.9 ± 6.6	23.2 ± 7.7[b]
Physical fitness	26.1 ± 4.8	18.6 ± 4.9[b]
Weight	13.4 ± 3.2	12.6 ± 4.0
Self-actualization	17.3 ± 3.7	12.7 ± 3.9[b]
Comparison with others	8.8 ± 1.7	7.7 ± 2.2[b]
Peer opinion	5.7 ± 1.7	7.1 ± 2.4[b]
Communication	11.6 ± 2.3	8.6 ± 2.4[b]

[a]A lower score indicates a greater importance attached to the scale.
[b]$P < .001$.
(Courtesy of Levenson, P.M., et al.: J. Adolesc. Health Care 8:171–176, March 1987.)

TABLE 3.—THE TOP FIVE ITEMS MOST FREQUENTLY
RATED VERY IMPORTANT BY ADOLESCENTS
AND PHYSICIANS

Items adolescents most frequently rated very important	Items rated very important by physicians	Items physicians think adolescents would rate very important
How to live a long health life (70.7%)[a]	What happens to the body when a person smokes (80.6%)	How to make others think one is a special person (42.6%)
How to keep my friends from trying to make me smoke (65.8%)	Diseases that occur from smoking (71.4%)	How to change weight to look better (41.8%)
How to keep from getting diseases that result from poor nutrition (61.8%)	How to stop smoking (70.2%)	Other's opinions about them because of the physical condition they are in (38.8%)
Danger signals for telling when something is physically wrong with me (61.1%)	How they can keep friends from trying to make them smoke (64.3%)	How to avoid being teased about one's weight (37.9%)
How to stop smoking (59.8%)	How to feel good about themselves (62.5%)	How to feel good about themselves (28.9%)

[a]Percent of the group rating each item very important.
(Courtesy of Levenson, P.M., et al.: J. Adolesc. Health Care 8:171–176, March 1987.)

that physicians and adolescents differed considerably. The physicians were not able to project accurately the degree of importance that adolescents would report for a scale. Means and post hoc univariate results are given in Table 2. Physicians and adolescents differed significantly in the ratings of all scales except for weight. Physicians noticed that adolescents would place less importance on a scale than the adolescents actually reported. However, the physicians noted that the adolescents would attach more importance on peer opinion than the adolescents reported. The frequency with which individual items were rated very important by physicians and adolescents is shown in Table 3. The adolescents and physicians agreed that smoking-related items were of primary concern.

Because physicians tend to see health needs from the focus of illness, they may overestimate the importance of certain issues, whereas adolescents, whose perspectives are usually from a health focus, may be inclined to underestimate the importance of certain issues. It is hoped that the results of this study will assist in planning future health education designed to guide adolescents in present and future health needs.

▶ In the 1984 YEAR BOOK Michael Cohen wrote, "Perhaps the most important implication of this study (Walker, D. K., et al.: *J. Adolesc. Health Care* 3:82,

1982) is that it points up the value of incorporating teenagers' perceptions of their health needs with knowledge of presumed deficits based on health provider assessments. Too often, health program design is predicated on only the latter. By coupling these two approaches, a more comprehensive program of services for young people should emerge." Things haven't changed since then. For a catalogue of the health concerns and health-related behaviors of adolescents, take a look at the 1987 Year Book, pp. 262–265.—F.A. Oski, M.D.

Impaired Insulin Action in Puberty: A Contributing Factor to Poor Glycemic Control in Adolescents With Diabetes
Stephanie A. Amiel, Robert S. Sherwin, Donald C. Simonson, Albert A. Lauritano, and William V. Tamborlane (Yale Univ. and Squibb-Novo, Inc., Princeton, N.J.)
N. Engl. J. Med. 315:215–219, July 24, 1986   8–3

Adolescent patients with type I, insulin-dependent diabetes mellitus (IDDM) often have unstable metabolic control because glycemic control usually deteriorates with the onset of puberty. This metabolic deterioration is thought to be the result of adolescent psychosocial upheaval. The possibility that hormonal and physical changes of puberty contribute to diabetic hyperglycemia in adolescents was examined in 16 diabetic and 16 nondiabetic pubertal children. None was obese.

The 16 children were grouped according to stage of pubertal development and the presence or absence of diabetes; they underwent euglycemic insulin-clamp procedures after an overnight fast. Results of the clamp studies were then compared with those for 26 previously studied adults. In addition, profiles of serum growth hormone levels were obtained in 23 children before the insulin-clamp study.

Insulin-stimulated glucose metabolism was sharply lower in nondiabetic pubertal children than in nondiabetic prepubertal children and adults. Similarly, insulin-stimulated glucose metabolism was 25% to 30% lower in diabetic pubertal children than in diabetic prepubertal children and adults. At each stage of development, the stimulating effect of insulin on glucose metabolism was decreased by 33% to 42% in diabetic children, compared with healthy controls. The response to insulin correlated inversely with the mean 24-hour levels of growth hormone in all 32 children.

Insulin resistance occurs during puberty in both normal adolescents and those with IDDM. The combined adverse effects of puberty and diabetes on insulin activity may explain the problems of controlling glycemia in pubertal adolescents.

▶ As if the metabolic changes described in the abstract above and the known impact of emotional stresses experienced in adolescence (White, K., et al.: *Pediatrics* 73:749, 1984) weren't enough to make good diabetic control a real challenge for the physician, please see the next abstract for an additional confounder.—F.A. Oski, M.D.

Surreptitious Insulin Administration in Adolescents With Insulin-Dependent Diabetes Mellitus

Donald P. Orr, Thomas Eccles, Richard Lawlor, and Michael Golden (Indiana Univ. at Indianapolis)
JAMA 256:3227–3230, Dec. 19, 1986
8–4

Although most adolescents with insulin-dependent diabetes mellitus (IDDM) seem to be well adjusted psychosocially, some are at increased

DEMOGRAPHIC AND CLINICAL CHARACTERISTICS OF SIX PATIENTS WITH SURREPTITIOUS INSULIN ADMINISTRATION

Characteristic	Patient 1	Patient 2	Patient 3	Patient 4	Patient 5	Patient 6
Age at discovery of surreptitious insulin administration, y	15	15	14	15	12	15
Sex	F	M	F	F	M	F
Age at onset of insulin-dependent diabetes mellitus, y	12	14	7	6	7	$10/12$
HbA,* at discovery, %	18.0	16.6	12.2	21.5	17.1	10.6
History of declining insulin dose	Yes	Yes	Yes	Yes	Yes	Yes
DSM-III Axis I	Oppositional disorder	Adjustment disorder	Dysthymic vs major depressive disorder	Adjustment disorder, depressed mood	Adjustment disorder, depressed mood	Oppositional disorder
Axis II	Borderline traits	None	Schizoid traits	None	Mixed personality (passive aggressive and dependent traits)	None
Suicidal behavior	—	+	+	+	—	—
Duration of follow-up, y	$2^{11}/12$	$2^{1}/12$	$2^{1}/12$	$2^{4}/12$	$2^{5}/12$	$3^{4}/12$
Most recent HbA$_1$, %	16.1	12.2	NA	NA	11.7	18.7
Psychotherapy	Inpatient/outpatient	Inpatient/outpatient	Inpatient/outpatient	Episodic	Episodic	Refused

*HbA: total glycosylated hemoglobin; DSM-III: *Diagnostic and Statistical Manual of Mental Disorders*, ed. 3.
(Courtesy of Orr, D.P., et al.: JAMA 256:3227–3230, Dec. 19, 1986.)

risk of psychosocial problems, particularly those who are in poor metabolic control. The characteristics of adolescents who omit treatment and have recurrent episodes of ketoacidosis have been reported previously. However, little information is available on surreptitious insulin administration.

Two boys and four girls aged 12–15 with IDDM were seen who were secretively taking extra insulin unrelated to achieving good glycemic control. This behavior, which resulted in large discrepancies between reported and observed insulin administration, was discovered while the patients were hospitalized for poor metabolic control. Several patients had recurrent episodes of diabetic ketoacidosis and it was not possible to achieve glycemic control on an outpatient basis.

Psychological testing and psychiatric evaluation revealed a variety of psychiatric abnormalities (table). Three patients had suicidal tendencies, either when the surreptious intake of insulin was discovered or subsequently. Other patients took insulin surreptiously in attempts to manipulate their families. All patients had psychosocial problems that antedated the discovery of the surreptious use of insulin. Although the underlying psychopathologic processes varied, depression and severe personality problems were common.

▶ Julio Santiago, in an editorial that accompanied this report, writes, "Too frequently, physicians in training and specialists in diabetes exhibit considerable bravado in dealing with the short-term treatment of ketoacidosis or hypoglycemia only to prove woefully inadequate in beginning to address the root cause of the medical emergency or its prevention . . . . Evaluation and treatment of these patients is tedious, frustrating and difficult . . . . Finally, we should recall the admonition of the British physician, R. D. Lawrence, that in brittle diabetes nothing is broken except the heart of the physician caring for the patient."—F.A. Oski, M.D.

Death Due to Chronic Syrup of Ipecac Use in a Patient With Bulimia
Russell J. Schiff, Carol L. Wurzel, Sandra C. Brunson, Ilene Kasloff, Michael P. Nussbaum, and Shawn D. Frank (Long Island Jewish Med. Ctr., New Hyde Park, N.Y.)
Pediatrics 78:412–416, September 1986   8–5

Recently, there has been increased awareness of eating disorders in the pediatric population. In one study of female high school students, the incidence of bulimia was 4.9%. Another study reported the incidence of bulimia in a population of female college students to be 19%. Although many bulimic individuals induce vomiting by mechanical means, others use emetics such as syrup of ipecac. The goal of the present report was to describe a death caused by chronic ipecac use in an adolescent patient with bulimia.

Female, 17 years, presented with malaise, weakness, palpitations, dysphagia, myalgias, and weight loss of 1 month's duration. Within 24 hours of admission she experienced hypotension unresponsive to medical management, intractable congestive heart failure, and arrhythmias; she died shortly thereafter. Several empty bottles of syrup of ipecac were found among her belongings.

Syrup of ipecac is often used to induce emesis in patients who have ingested toxic substances. The major pharmacologic mechanism of this agent is attributable to the alkaloid component, emetine. Although there have been previous reports of death caused by emetine poisoning in patients taking ipecac fluid extract and in those treated for amebic dysentery, there have been only three previous reports of fatalities secondary to chronic ipecac use as a means of losing weight. The present report was the first describing death caused by chronic ipecac use in an adolescent patient with bulimia. Emetine persists in the body for long periods, and in patients who have ingested it chronically, emetine is extremely toxic to cardiac, smooth, and skeletal muscles. With the increased awareness of the importance of weight control in adolescents, the physician must carefully evaluate such patients for the use of emetics.

▶ Dr. Howard Weinberger, Professor of Pediatrics, Medical Science Center in Syracuse, S.U.N.Y., comments.—F.A. Oski, M.D.

▶ This article calls attention to the risks associated with chronic ingestion of syrup of ipecac. It is important to remember that syrup of ipecac has an excellent "track record" of safety when it is used as recommended after potentially toxic ingestions. The current packaging of the product in 30-ml amounts virtually ensures its safety in childhood accidental poisoning.

Those concerned with the management of patients with the anorexia/bulimia syndrome have proposed that access to syrup of ipecac be limited by making it available only by prescription. Those who have been in the forefront of poison prevention activities argue that such regulation would also limit access of this product to the millions of parents whose young children are at risk of accidental poisoning.

As with almost any product on the market, misuse or abuse can lead to tragedy. The question here is not just a matter of conflicting rights and responsibilities. Rumack has recommended a compromise in which pharmacists would keep syrup of ipecac behind the counter and provide it upon request (*Pediatrics* 75:1148, 1985). That would allow the pharmacist to decline to sell more than one or two bottles to any individual.

No doubt some will argue that those intent on abusing themselves by misusing syrup of ipecac will simply shop at multiple pharmacies. They may also self-induce emesis by a variety of methods, and there is no evidence that syrup of ipecac will become the method of choice.

In the balance, "free" access to syrup of ipecac should not be restricted despite its potential side effects as described in this article.—H. Weinberger, M.D.

Heterogeneity of Suicidal Adolescents
Aman U. Khan (Southern Illinois Univ.)
J. Am. Acad. Child Adolesc. Psychiatry 26:92–96, January 1987   8–6

All suicide attempters are potentially at risk of committing suicide, but the attempt is best viewed as a symptom occurring in a heterogeneous group of adolescents having different premorbid personalities and different psychological conflicts. It is not productive to regard these adolescents as a group with a unitary underlying psychopathology. Study was made of 40 hospitalized suicidal adolescents, 40 hospitalized adolescents who were not suicidal, and 40 adolescents who had never been hospitalized but who were managed at an outpatient psychiatric clinic. The first group had appeared at the emergency room after attempting suicide in a 2-year period.

The three groups were similar in age, race, and social class. Females comprised a large proportion of the suicidal group (Table 1). More than 75% of adolescents in all groups regarded their family relationships as poor. Similar proportions reported not having a close friend whom they trusted. Lower school achievement tended to be ascribed to chance. At least 70% of both hospitalized groups had lost a parent by death or divorce in the preteen years. The outpatients had more intact families. The suicidal group was heterogeneous with respect to psychopathology (Tables 2 and 3). Only 2 of 11 dexamethasone suppression tests in depressed suicidal patients were positive. The suicidal patients nearly always reported feeling overwhelmed and helpless, and most were angry and frustrated when faced with an overwhelming situation.

TABLE 1.—Characteristics of the Three Groups

Characters	Suicidal Hospitalized Group 1 (N = 40)		Nonsuicidal Hospitalized Group 2 (N = 40)		Nonsuicidal Outpatient Group 3 (N = 40)	
	N	%	N	%	N	%
Sex						
Female*	34	85	12	30	19	47.5
Male*	6	15	28	70	21	52.5
Race						
White	27	67.5	33	82.5	31	77.5
Black	13	32.5	7	17.5	9	22.5
Social Class						
Middle class	9	22.5	8	20	11	27.5
Lower middle	24	60	20	50	21	52.5
Lower class	7	17.5	12	30	8	20
Family Relations						
Good	3	7.5	8	20	11	27.5
Satisfactory	2	5	3	7.5	6	15
Poor	35	87.5	29	72.5	33	82.5
Academic Achievement						
Good	3	7.5	0	0	2	5
Satisfactory	8	20	10	25	8	20
Poor	29	72.5	30	75	30	75
Parental Loss (Death or Divorce)**						
Present	28	70	29	72.5	16	40
Absent	12	30	11	27.5	24	60
Sexual Abuse						
Present	6	15	1	2.5	3	7.5
Absent	34	85	39	97.5	37	92.5

*P < .001.
**P < .01.
(Courtesy of Khan, A.U.: J. Am. Acad. Child Adolesc. Psychiatry 26:92–96, January 1987.)

TABLE 2.—Comparison of the Three Groups for Axis I Diagnoses

AXIS I Diagnosis	Suicidal Hospitalized Group 1 (N = 40)		Nonsuicidal Hospitalized Group 2 (N = 40)		Nonsuicidal Outpatient Group 3 (N = 40)	
	N	%	N	%	N	%
Major Depressive Disorder	7	17.5	3	7.5	1	2.5
Bipolar Affective Disorder	0	0	1	2.5	1	2.5
Cylothymic Disorder	0	0	1	2.5	1	2.5
Dythymic Disorder	7	17.5	4	2.5	8	20
Schizophrenic Disorder	0	0	8	10	0	20
Conduct Disorder	10	25	19	47.5	15	37.5
Attention Deficit Disorder	0	0	0	0	2	5
Eating Disorders	0	0	1	2.5	1	2.5
Anxiety Disorders	0	0	1	2.5	2	5
Somatoform Disorders	0	0	1	2.5	3	7.5
Impulse Control Disorder	1	2.5	1	2.5	1	2.5
Functional Encopresis	0	0	0	0	1	2.5
Oppositional Disorder	0	0	0	0	1	2.5
Adjustment Disorders	15	37.5	0	0	3	7.5

(Courtesy of Khan, A.U.: J. Am. Acad. Child. Adolesc. Psychiatry 26:92–96, January 1987.)

TABLE 3.—Comparison of the Three Groups for Axis II Diagnosis

AXIS II Diagnosis	Suicidal Hospitalized Group 1 (N = 40)		Nonsuicidal Hospitalized Group 2 (N = 40)		Nonsuicidal Outpatient Group 3 (N = 40)	
	N	%	N	%	N	%
Paranoid Personality	0	0	1	2.5	0	0
Schizoid Personality	3	7.5	6	15	1	2.5
Histrionic Personality	6	15	0	0	2	5
Narcissistic Personality	9	22.5	1	2.5	3	7.5
Antisocial Personality	4	10	17	42.5	12	30
Borderline Personality	11	27.5	3	7.5	1	2.5
Avoidant Personality	0	0	1	2.5	1	2.5
Dependent Personality	5	12.5	5	12.5	7	17.5
Passive-Aggressive Personality	1	2.5	2	5	4	10
No Diagnosis	1	2.5	4	10	9	22.5

(Courtesy of Khan, A.U.: J. Am. Acad. Child Adolesc. Psychiatry 26:92–96, January 1987.)

The coping style of an adolescent under stress is important in assessing suicidal potential. Most suicidal adolescents have great difficulty in coping with anger and sadness and are less able than others to think through the results of their actions.

The Impact of Suicide in Television Movies: Evidence of Imitation

Madelyn S. Gould and David Shaffer (Columbia Univ. and New York State Psychiatric Inst., New York City)
N. Engl. J. Med. 315:690–694, Sept. 11, 1986   8–7

Suicide appears to be determined by biologic predisposition, experience, and the environment, which includes the media. Epidemics of suicides have

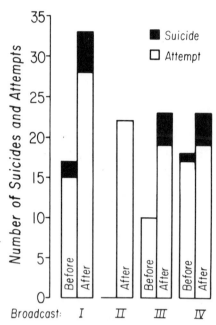

Fig 8–1.—Number of completed suicides and suicide attempts by adolescents in the greater New York area 2 weeks before and after television movies about suicide. (Courtesy of Gould, M.S., and Shaffer, D.: N. Engl. J. Med. 315:690–694, Sept. 11, 1986.)

TABLE 1.—METHOD AND DISPOSITION OF SUICIDE ATTEMPTS BEFORE AND AFTER FOUR TELEVISION MOVIES ABOUT SUICIDE

CATEGORY	BROADCAST I		BROADCAST II		BROADCAST III		BROADCAST IV	
	BEFORE	AFTER	BEFORE*	AFTER	BEFORE	AFTER	BEFORE	AFTER
No. of attempts	15	28	—	22	10	19	17	19
Method								
Overdose	15	25	—	20	9	15	15	18
Wrist laceration	0	3	—	2	1	1	1	1
Hanging	0	0	—	0	0	2	1	0
Jumping from or in front of a vehicle	0	0	—	0	0	1	0	0
								$\chi^2 = 0.95$†
Disposition								
Admitted to hospital	10	20	—	19	8	18	15	13
Released	5	8	—	2	2	1	2	5
Unknown	0	0	—	1	0	0	0	1
								$\chi^2 = 0.14$†

*There was no independent "before" period for Broadcast II because the film was shown within 2 weeks after Broadcast I.

†The four movies were pooled for this analysis. Chi-square comparisons (not significant) apply to all "before" periods vs. all "after" periods.

(Courtesy of Gould, M.S., and Shaffer, D.: N. Engl. J. Med. 315:690–694, Sept. 11, 1986.)

been noted to follow the suicides of celebrities and the publication of poems and novels about suicide. Thus, suicide appears to be a learned behavior. Suicide rates were examined after the television broadcasts of four films involving suicides that were broadcast over a 5-month period.

TABLE 2.—METHOD OF COMPLETED SUICIDES BEFORE AND AFTER FOUR TELEVISION MOVIES ABOUT SUICIDE*

METHOD	BROADCAST I		BROADCAST II		BROADCAST III		BROADCAST IV	
	BEFORE	AFTER	BEFORE†	AFTER	BEFORE	AFTER	BEFORE	AFTER
No. of suicides	2	5	—	0	0	4	1	4
Gunshot	2	2	—	0	0	1	1	0
Hanging	0	3	—	0	0	3	0	3
Carbon monoxide	0	0	—	0	0	0	0	1

*Comparison of the number of completed suicides before and after the four movies was not significant by Fisher's exact test. The four movies were pooled for this analysis.

There was no independent "before" period for Broadcast II because the film was shown within 2 weeks after Broadcast I.

(Courtesy of Gould, M.S., and Shaffer, D.: N. Engl. J. Med. 315:690–694, Sept. 11, 1986.)

Broadcast I concerned a suicide pact made by two boys, one of whom drove his car over a cliff. Broadcast II involved the suicide of a teenage boy after various interpersonal crises and depicted the suicide's effect on the family. Broadcast III dealt with a teenage boy's attempt to prevent his father's suicide. Broadcast IV was the story of a teenage couple who jointly committed suicide. The purpose of the movies was to inform the public about suicide and to encourage suicidal individuals to seek help, thus informational packets, suicide hotline telephone numbers, and other messages accompanied the programs. The study group consisted of 31 consecutive suicides by persons aged 19 years or younger in various counties in New York, New Jersey, and Connecticut. The records of 220 young people who had unsuccessfully attempted suicide also were investigated.

The average number of suicide attempts within 2 weeks after the broadcasts were significantly higher than the average number before the broadcasts (Fig 8–1). A significant excess of completed suicides over that predicted occurred after three of the broadcasts. The methods used in the suicide attempts and the severity of the injuries did not appear to differ before and after the broadcasts (Table 1). For the completed suicides, the methods did not differ before and after the broadcasts (Table 2).

Fictional television films featuring suicide may lead to imitative suicidal behavior among teenagers. It is unknown whether the suicide victims actually saw the programs, or what about the programs tended to increase the suicide rate. Further studies should be done to determine whether the film content or the accompanying educational material increased suicidal behavior.

Clustering of Teenage Suicides After Television News Stories About Suicide

David P. Phillips and Lundie L. Carstensen (Univ. of California at San Diego)
N. Engl. J. Med. 315:685–689, Sept. 11, 1986   8–8

It has been suggested that teenage suicides occur in "clusters" and that these clusters result from imitation. However, most published evidence about this suggestion has been anecdotal, and alternative explanations for the clusters have not been assessed. Scientific studies of this phenomenon are of two types: the first type is focused on a small geographic area in which evidence of clustering within that area is sought; in the second type, national suicide rates are examined after stories about suicides. Most studies of the first type have not provided evidence of clustering; however, studies of the second type have almost always found that the number of suicides reaches a peak after news stories of suicides. Because most investigations have included suicides in all age groups combined and have not provided evidence specifically about teenagers, the relationship was examined between 38 nationally televised news or feature stories about suicide from 1973 to 1979 and the fluctuation of the rate of suicide among American teenagers before and after these stories.

The observed number of suicides of teenagers from zero to 7 days after these broadcasts (1,666) was markedly greater than the number expected (1,555). The greater the number of networks that carried a story about suicide, the greater the increase in suicides thereafter. When the results were corrected for the effects of the day of the week, month, holidays, and yearly trends, these findings persisted. Teenage suicides increased more than adult suicides did after stories about suicide (6.87% vs. 0.45%). In addition, suicides increased as much after general information or feature stories about suicide as they did after news stories about a particular suicide. Although it is possible that these results could be attributed to misclassification or were statistical artifacts, the best available explanation is that television stories about suicide trigger additional suicides, perhaps because of imitation.

▶ On April 4, 1987, I opened my *New York Times* to find the following Letter to the Editor:

"Many years ago, I discovered that my country, Brazil, did not allow suicide to be mentioned in the news media. The reason was that suicide might be imitated by others who had been thinking about it.

Two weeks ago, I heard of the four teenagers who committed suicide in New Jersey, and thought it was wrong to make so much of it in the news. Then, two days later, more teenage suicides followed.

I understand why in Brazil suicide may not be mentioned in reports of the news. It is a position I now strongly support."—Maria Ferraz.

It seems strange, but have you noticed that even airline hijackings, train wrecks, and tanker oil spills appear to occur in bunches?—F.A. Oski, M.D.

9 Therapeutics and Toxicology

Public Health Service Study of Reye's Syndrome and Medications: Report of the Main Study
Eugene S. Hurwitz, Michael J. Barrett, Dennis Bregman, Walter J. Gunn, Paul Pinsky, Lawrence B. Schonberger, Joseph S. Drage, Richard A. Kaslow, D. Bruce Burlington, Gerald V. Quinnan, John R. LaMontagne, William R. Fairweather, Delbert Dayton, and Walter R. Dowdle (Public Health Service Reye Syndrome Task Force, Ctrs. for Disease Control, Atlanta, and other federal agencies)
JAMA 257:1905–1911, Apr. 10, 1987   9–1

After a pilot study showed the method to be feasible, a case-control study of the possible association between Reye's syndrome and salicylate use was undertaken. Findings in 27 patients (cases) with a confirmed diagnosis of stage II or more severe Reye's syndrome, with an appropriate antecedent illness, were compared with those in 140 controls matched for age, race, and type and timing of onset of the antecedent illness. The diagnosis of Reye's syndrome in the cases was confirmed by an expert panel; the antecedent illnesses included respiratory and gastrointestinal tract diseases and chickenpox.

A strong statistical association was found between ingestion of salicylate during the antecedent illness and the occurrence of Reye's syndrome. The odds ratio was 40, with a lower 95% confidence limit of 5.8. Only two cases were not exposed to aspirin; the odds ratio for aspirin ingestion was

EXPOSURE TO SALICYLATES DURING ANTECEDENT ILLNESSES AMONG PATIENTS NOT INCLUDED IN STUDY ANALYSES* AND AMONG ALL INCLUDED CONTROLS, BY AGE GROUP

	No. (%) of Subjects Exposed to Salicylates by Age Group, y			
	<5	5-9	10-18	Total
Patients with confirmed Reye's syndrome (cases not meeting antecedent-illness definition)†	1/1 (100)	0/0 (0)	4/4 (100)	5/5 (100)
Patients found to have other diagnoses	1/6 (17)	0/1 (0)	0/0 (0)	1/7 (14)
Patients recommended for exclusion by expert panel	5/10 (50)	0/0 (0)	3/3 (100)	8/13 (62)
All controls	3/18 (17)	8/27 (30)	42/95 (44)	53/140 (38)

*Patients who were interviewed but did not meet the study criteria.
†Excludes one patient exposed to salicylates on the day of onset of the antecedent illness, which was also the day of onset of Reye's syndrome.
(Courtesy of Hurwitz, E.W., et al.: JAMA 257:1905–1911, Apr. 10, 1987.)

26, with a lower 95% confidence limit of 6.4. The high odds ratios could not be ascribed to relevant epidemiologic issues, e.g., case-control differences in severity of antecedent illness. Experience with patients not included in the study and with all controls is shown in the table.

A strong association was found between salicylate ingestion and Reye's syndrome in this case-control study. More than 90% of cases may be attributable to salicylate. The findings emphasize the need to reduce salicylate use by children who have chickenpox and influenza-like illness.

▶ It looks like we can now pronounce Reye's syndrome officially dead or dying as a result of recognizing the relationship between aspirin usage and the appearance of the disease. The specific pathophysiologic link between salicylates and the metabolic abnormalities in this disease remains unexplained, as does the underlying variation in predisposition to the disease. Reye's syndrome has left a legacy. I think it is fair to say that the rise in the popularity of pediatric intensive care units and the development of the field of critical care medicine was largely in response to the challenge of taking care of patients with this disease. The monitoring of intracranial pressure was perfected in patients with Reye's syndrome as well. Reye's syndrome may be gone, but it won't be forgotten. Today, if you think your patient has Reye's syndrome you are probably wrong—it is much more likely to be ornithine transcarbamylase deficiency, some other urea cycle defect, or an abnormality in fatty acid oxidation. For more on Reye's syndrome or the son of Reye's (the son also Reye's), see the 1987 YEAR BOOK, pp. 551–555 and pp. 147–149.—F.A. Oski, M.D.

Poisoning Exposures and Use of Ipecac in Children Less Than 1 Year Old
Pierre Gaudreault, Mary A. McCormick, Peter G. Lacouture, and Frederick H. Lovejoy, Jr. (Children's Hosp., Boston, Massachusetts Poison Control Center, and Harvard Univ.)
Ann. Emerg. Med. 15:808–810, July 1986   9–2

Syrup of ipecac is an effective, safe emetic in the treatment of acute poisoning in children who are older than age 1 year. Until recently, however, its safety and efficacy in treating children younger than age 1 year had not been established. The frequency and severity of clinical symptoms, type of products ingested, and circumstances surrounding poisoning exposures were examined in children younger than age 1 year.

Of 38,080 calls during an 8-month period involving exposure to poison, approximately 9% concerned children who were younger than age 1 year. There were 1,344 poisoning exposures in children younger than 1 year reported during a 3-month sampling period. One hundred thirty-one infants (10%) were less than 6 months old, 473 (35%) were from 6 to 9 months old, and 740 (55%) were from 9 to 12 months old. Boys accounted for 54% of accidents in each age group. Most of the patients (94%) were asymptomatic. Of 84 symptomatic children, 58 (69%) had gastrointestinal tract symptoms, 18 (21%) had pulmonary symptoms, 4 had fever, 3 were lethargic, and 1 had a swollen tongue. One patient had a seizure after rectal administration of a promethazine suppository, and one child drowned in a bucket that contained Pine Sol.

Plants and mushrooms caused poisoning in 507 children (38%) and household products were involved in the poisoning of 404 (30%); drugs, cosmetics, cigarettes, pesticides, and other products were implicated in the remaining patients. Circumstances surrounding the ingestion were known for 699 (52%) of the patients. Syrup of ipecac was given under medical supervision to 21 children aged 9–12 months. The children vomited within 1 hour. None had significant side effects, and none was hospitalized. Syrup of ipecac appears to be safe and effective in children between the ages of 9 and 12 months.

▶ For more on ipecac, see the section on Adolescent Medicine for the report of ipecac-induced bulimia resulting in death (Abstract 8–5). For still more on ipecac, read on.—F.A. Oski, M.D.

Expired Ipecac Syrup Efficacy
Patricia A. Grbcich, Peter G. Lacouture, James J. Kresel, Margaret T. Russell, and Frederick H. Lovejoy, Jr. (Massachusetts Poison Control System, The Children's Hosp., and Harvard Univ., Boston, and New Hampshire Poison Ctr., Hanover, and Dartmouth Univ.)
Pediatrics 78:1085–1089, December 1986   9–3

Poison control centers and pediatricians recommend that parents keep ipecac syrup available for treating accidental ingestion of poison by their children. The Good Manufacturing Practice regulations require that ipecac syrup carry an expiration date, but many households have expired ipecac

COMPARISON OF EFFICACY OF EXPIRED AND UNEXPIRED IPECAC SYRUP

	Expired Ipecac Syrup (n = 200)	Unexpired Ipecac Syrup (n = 200)	Significance*
% emesis	100	99.5	NS
Time to emesis (mean min ± SEM)	24.7 ± 1.05	24.8 ± 1.42	
Time to emesis by manufacturer (mean min ± SEM): Purepac	25.3 ± 1.37	24.7 ± 1.37	NS
Successful emesis			
First dose: time to emesis (mean min ± SEM)	21.8 ± 0.8	21.0 ± 0.71	NS
Second dose: time to emesis (mean min ± SEM)	53.2 ± 4.8	65.8 ± 10.3	NS
Open bottle: time to emesis (mean min ± SEM)	23.3 ± 1.7	25.2 ± 2.7	NS
Time to emesis in patients pre-treated with milk (mean min ± SEM)	22.8 ± 3.1	22.9 ± 2.5	NS

*Significance was established by using the two-tailed Student's *t* test. All nonsignificant values of *P* were >.05.
(Courtesy of Grbcich, P.A., et al.: Pediatrics 78:1085–1089, December 1986. Reproduced by permission of Pediatrics.)

syrup on hand, because it is unlikely that expiration dates are checked routinely. The findings of two recent studies comparing the effectiveness of expired and unexpired ipecac syrup were conflicting; thus a prospective, controlled study was carried out to assess the efficacy of expired ipecac syrup.

Included in the group were 200 study patients treated with expired ipecac syrup and 200 controls treated with unexpired ipecac syrup. Ninety-seven percent of the study patients and 98% of the controls were younger than age 6 years. All parents of children who were given expired ipecac syrup were called by telephone approximately 24 hours later to determine any potential toxicity.

Over-the-counter medications were ingested in amounts sufficient to require emesis by about 75% of the children in each group. All study patients (100%) and 199 controls (99.5%) vomited. The mean time to emesis for substances with high emetic potential was 26.6 minutes in the control group and 23.5 minutes in the study group (table). Side effects for those who used expired ipecac syrup included diarrhea in 20 cases, nausea and continued vomiting in 12, and lethargy in 11. These data are comparable with the reported incidence of side effects with unexpired ipecac syrup. The findings demonstrate that expired ipecac syrup is about 100% effective in inducing emesis and can be used safely, if necessary, up to 16 years after the expiration date.

▶ Ipecac appears to be like a fine wine—it gets better with age. Speaking of ipecac, remember the old rule, "Children never vomit in the sink."—F.A. Oski, M.D.

Theophylline Toxicity in Children
M. Douglas Baker (Johns Hopkins Univ.)
J. Pediatr. 109:538–542, September 1986   9–4

Theophylline, a bronchodilator, can cause arrhythmias, seizures, and death when administered in excessive amounts. The symptoms of toxicity in 65 children were compared with their serum concentrations of theophylline in a retrospective study. All were younger than age 17 years and were seen in the emergency room for symptoms suggestive of theophylline toxicity. Serum theophylline concentrations were measured.

Acute toxicity, resulting from a single dose, was found in 44 patients. Chronic toxicity was present in 12 patients who received repeated excessive doses and in 9 who received what was normally a therapeutic dose but who showed signs of toxicity during febrile respiratory illness lasting for at least 2 days. Vomiting occurred in 97%, sinus tachycardia in 82%, tremor-agitation in 63%, and abdominal pain in 22% of both the chronic and acute groups (Table 1). The occurrence of these symptoms correlated well with the serum theophylline concentration (Table 2). Serious manifestations of toxicity (Table 3) included seizures (four patients), visual hallucinations (two), and premature ventricular contractions (three). Dos-

TABLE 1.—Signs and Symptoms of Theophylline Toxicity: Relation to Serum Concentration

Serum theophylline	n	Vomiting	Tachycardia	Tremor/agitation	Abdominal pain	Lethargy/obtundation	Headache	Seizure activity	PVC	Hypertension	Hallucination	Ataxia
<20 µg/ml												
Acute	2	2	—	—	1	—	—	—	—	—	—	—
Chronic	0	—	—	—	—	—	—	—	—	—	—	—
Total	2	2	—	—	1	—	—	—	—	—	—	—
20-29 µg/ml												
Acute	18	17	13	8	1	1	—	—	—	—	—	—
Chronic	12	10	10	6	2	2	1	—	—	—	—	—
Total	30	27	23	14	3	3	1	—	—	—	—	—
30-39 µg/ml												
Acute	15	15	14	12	5	2	1	1	—	1	2	1
Chronic	8	8	6	7	2	—	1	—	—	—	—	—
Total	23	23	20	19	7	2	2	1	—	1	2	1
>39 µg/ml												
Acute	9	9	9	7	3	4	2	3	3	1	—	—
Chronic	1	1	1	1	—	—	—	—	—	—	—	—
Total	10	10	10	8	3	4	2	3	3	1	—	—
Total	65	63	53	41	14	9	5	4	3	2	2	1
%		97	82	63	22	14	8	6	5	3	3	2

(Courtesy of Baker, M.D.: J. Pediatr. 109:538–542, September 1986.)

TABLE 2.—Symptoms at Presentation vs. Serum Theophylline Concentration

Serum theophylline	n	1	2	3	>3
<20 µg/ml					
Acute	2	1	1	—	—
Chronic	0	—	—	—	—
Total	2	1	1	—	—
20-29 µg/ml					
Acute	18	5	8	4	1
Chronic	12	2	5	4	1
Total	30	7	13	8	2
30-39 µg/ml					
Acute	15	—	4	5	6
Chronic	8	—	2	3	3
Total	23	—	6	8	9
>39 µg/ml					
Acute	9	—	—	3	6
Chronic	1	—	—	1	—
Total	10	—	—	4	6

(Courtesy of Baker, M.D.: J. Pediatr. 109:538–542, September 1986.)

ing errors accounted for 65% of the elevated theophylline concentrations, viral respiratory illness explained toxicity with appropriate doses of theophylline in 23% of the patients, and accidental overdose, suicide attempts, and concurrent erythromycin ingestion accounted for the others (Table 4). By using appropriate dosage recommendations, monitoring the patient's medication history, and measuring serum theophylline concentrations regularly, especially in patients with respiratory tract infection, the occurrence of theophylline toxicity can be reduced.

▶ Although the data in this report were collected retrospectively, certain im-

TABLE 3.—Serious Effects of Acute Theophylline Intoxication

Age (yr)	Sex	Serum theophylline* (μg/ml)	Cause	Underlying disease	Seizure activity	Premature ventricular contraction
3/12	F	46.6	Therapeutic	Bronchiolitis	+	−
11/12	M	64.3	Therapeutic	Asthma	+	+
2	M	39.0	Therapeutic	Asthma, ?Seizure disorder	+	−
15	F	101.9	Suicide	None	−	+
16	F	50.8	Suicide	None	+	+

*Measured within 45 minutes of indicated disorder.
(Courtesy of Baker, M.D.: J. Pediatr. 109:538–542, September 1986.)

TABLE 4.—Circumstances Surrounding Toxicity

Cause	Cases n	%*
Physician error	33	51
Pharmacy error	2	3
Parent error	7	11
Accidental ingestion	5	8
Suicide gesture	7	11
Respiratory tract infection	15	23
Erythromycin	1	2

*Percentages total more than 100 because of respiratory infections in five patients with other causes for toxicity.
(Courtesy of Baker, M.D.: J. Pediatr. 109:538–542, September 1986.)

plications for the management of theophylline poisoning can be found. Prior guidelines have suggested that hemodialysis or hemoperfusion be reserved for acutely toxic patients with serum theophylline concentrations of more than 80 μg/ml. The four patients in the present report who had either seizures or ventricular arrhythmias at serum concentrations of less than 80 μg/ml responded to conservative management. In chronic overdose, hemoperfusion is best reserved for patients with intractable seizures or when serum concentrations exceed 60 μg/ml. For the neonate with theophylline toxicity, administration by mouth of high-surface-area activated charcoal appears to be a promising approach (Ginoza, G. W., et al.: J. Pediatr. 111:140, 1987). Respect theophylline—it can produce serious problems.—F.A. Oski, M.D.

PCP Intoxication in Seven Young Children
Richard H. Schwartz and Arnold Einhorn (Children's Hosp. Natl. Med. Ctr., Washington, D.C., and George Washington Univ.)
Pediatr. Emerg. Care 2:238–241, December 1986   9–5

Infants and young children are highly sensitive to phencyclidine (PCP), so much so that they may become intoxicated simply from passive inhalation of PCP smoke in a small room. Their symptoms differ from those of adults. Hypertension and aggressive psychosis are rare, whereas neuro-

PHENCYCLIDINE INTOXICATION IN BABIES: PHYSICAL AND OCULAR SIGNS

Age	Sex	Physical Signs						Ocular Signs			
		Depressed sensorium, lethargy to stupor to coma	Seizure	Blunted or absent pain response	Opisthotonus	Hypotonia	Ataxia	Eyes opened, blank stare	Miosis	Nystagmus	Disconjugate gaze
5 yr	M	+	+	+	−	+	−	−	−	+	−
13 mo	F	+	−	+	+	−	+	+	+	−	−
14 mo	F	+	−	+	−	+	+	−	+	+	+
5 yr	M	+	−	+	−	+	+	+	−	+	+
2 mo	F	+	−	+	+	+	−	−	−	−	−
10 mo	F	+	−	+	−	+	+	+	+	+	−
18 mo	F	+	+	+	−	+	+	+	+	+	−
Percent		100	27	100	27	86	71	57	57	57	27

(Courtesy of Schwartz, R.H., and Einhorn, A.: Pediatr. Emerg. Care 2.:238–241, December 1986.)

logic symptoms are common. The urine of all children seen with coma, hypotonia, seizures, or a blank, uncomprehending stare should be tested for PCP by the enzyme multiplied immunoassay technique (EMIT). Physical and ocular signs in seven patients, younger than age 5 years, admitted with a diagnosis of PCP intoxication, are given in the table.

Girl, aged 2 months, had periods of irritability alternating with lethargy and feeding difficulties. Seen in the emergency department, she was irritable, lethargic, and unresponsive to tactile stimuli, with a poorly coordinated swallow and a high-pitched, irritable cry, abnormal tongue thrust, writhing movements of the arms, and opisthotonic posturing. A diphtheria-pertussis-tetanus immunization 5 days earlier raised a suspicion of pertussis vaccine encephalopathy, but a toxicology screen revealed PCP in the urine. The child slowly returned to normal during the next 4 days, and after an emergency court hearing, she was discharged to a court-appointed foster home.

Young children seen in the emergency room with serious neurologic symptoms (e.g., stupor, seizures, or coma) and a clinical history not suggestive of phenothiazine toxicity should have a urine test for PCP even when, as is often the case, parents deny any knowledge of PCP use in the home.

Emergency Gastrotomy: Treatment of Choice for Iron Bezoar

Ira Landsman, J. Timothy Bricker, Barbara S. Reid, and Robert S. Bloss (Baylor College of Medicine and Texas Children's Hosp., Houston)
J. Pediatr. Surg. 22:184–185, February 1987   9–6

Acute accidental iron poisoning is common in small children who ingest multiple brightly colored, sugar-coated iron tablets intended for adults because they look like candy. Prompt surgical treatment is indicated when partial dissolution of sugar or the gelatin coating produces a mass in the stomach that adheres tightly to the gastric mucosa.

Girl, 23 months, was admitted 6–8 hours after ingesting 60 enteric-coated ferrous sulfate tablets containing 65 mg of elemental iron per tablet, or 390 mg/kg of elemental iron, well above the lethal dose of 200–250 mg/kg. The child had been treated at a nearby center with syrup of ipecac prior to admission to Texas Children's Hospital. She had a heart rate of 130 beats per minute and a blood pressure of 114/77 mm Hg at admission, and was lethargic but arousable. She underwent immediate gastric lavage with 1 gm of deferoxamine. The gastric aspirate revealed hematest-positive fluid that was grossly bloody in appearance. An abdominal roentgenogram revealed an iron bezoar (Fig 9–1). Lavage with a French Ewald tube to dislodge the bezoar was ineffective. The child was treated with deferoxamine intramuscularly and intravenously, but emergency gastrotomy for removal of the iron bezoar was undertaken after it became evident that gastrointestinal decontamination would not be effected by conventional medical means. Hemorrhagic gastritis at points of contact with iron tablets was evident at operation. Her postoperative recovery was uneventful, and the child was discharged on the seventh postoperative day with no evidence of liver dysfunction or significant gastrointestinal tract damage.

Surgical therapy for massive iron ingestion with bezoar formation is not

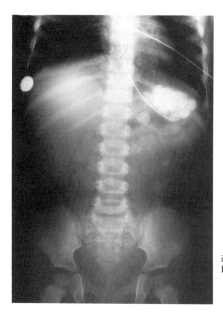

Fig 9–1.—Film of abdomen illustrating the iron bezoar. (Courtesy of Landsman, I., et al.: J. Pediatr Surg. 22:184–185, February 1987.)

emphasized in general surgical and pediatric textbooks. However, prompt operative intervention may be necessary.

▶ This is an imaginative surgical approach to a medical problem. Turnabout is fair play. Another surgical maneuver holds promise for the management of iron poisoning and other forms of poisoning as well—whole bowel irrigation (Tenenbein, M., et al.: *J. Pediatr.* 111:142, 1987). Whole bowel irrigation with polyethylene glycol electrolyte lavage solution is a widely used, safe precolonoscopy preparative procedure. It consists of the rapid administration of the material to cleanse the gut of its contents. The solution was specifically designed for this purpose because its use does not result in fluid or electrolyte absorption or secretion across the gastrointestinal tract epithelium (Davis, G. R., et al.: *Gastroenterology* 78:991, 1980). The solution, which has Food and Drug Administration approval, is marketed as Colyte (Reed and Carnick Pharmaceuticals) and as Golytely (Braintree Laboratories). Instead of washing out the mouth as a form of punishment, we can now wash out the bowel as a form of treatment.—F.A. Oski, M.D.

The Effect of Cigarette Smoke From the Mother on Bronchial Responsiveness and Severity of Symptoms in Children With Asthma

Andrew B. Murray and Brenda J. Morrison (Univ. of British Columbia, Vancouver)
J. Allergy Clin. Immunol. 77:575–581, April 1986   9–7

The results of previous epidemiologic studies of the effects of parental smoking on children have been conflicting. However, children with asthma

TABLE 1.—Differences in Indicators of Asthma Severity Among Groups
Distinguished by Smoking Habits of Parents

	History score*	FEV₁ percent predicted	FEF₂₅₋₇₅	Geometric mean PC₂₀†	
Mother					
Nonsmoker (n = 70)	6.0 ± 0.4	85.5 ± 1.8	72.3 ± 2.8	2.2	n = 31
Smoker (n = 24)	8.8 ± 0.8	74.4 ± 3.7	55.6 ± 5.6	0.46	n = 10
P Value (two-tailed)	0.001	0.004	0.005	0.002	
Father					
Nonsmoker (n = 64)	6.9 ± 0.5	81.9 ± 2.1	67.0 ± 3.1	1.7	n = 26
Smoker (n = 28)	6.4 ± 0.6	84.4 ± 2.9	70.5 ± 4.9	1.2	n = 15
p Value (two-tailed)	0.5	0.5	0.5	0.4	
Parents					
Both nonsmokers (n = 51)	6.2 ± 0.5	84.7 ± 2.1	71.6 ± 3.2	3.1	n = 21
Either smokes (n = 43)	7.4 ± 0.6	80.3 ± 2.7	63.8 ± 4.3	0.8	n = 20
p Value (two-tailed)	0.11	0.2	0.15	0.001	

Means ± standard errors are presented.
*History score available for 92 children.
†PC₂₀ was measured for all 41 children who were eligible for test. T tests were carried out on logarithm of PC₂₀ values.
(Courtesy of Murray, A.B., and Morrison, B.J.: J. Allergy Clin. Immunol. 77:575–581, April 1986.)

TABLE 2.—Correlation (R) Between Indicators of Asthma Severity and
Logarithm of Number of Cigarettes That Were Smoked in House by Parents and
Probability of R ≠ 0

	FVC (% Predicted)	FEV₁ (% Predicted)	FEF₂₅₋₇₅ (% Predicted)	Log (PC₂₀)	History score
Mother	r = 0.186	−0.300	−0.280	−0.482	0.224
	p = 0.039	0.002	0.004	0.001	0.018
Father	r = 0.036	0.028	0.001	0.075	0.084
	p = 0.367	0.395	0.495	0.319	0.218
Both parents	r = −0.081	−0.200	−0.227	−0.460	0.136
	p ± 0.228	0.031	0.017	0.001	0.107

(Courtesy of Murray, A.B., and Morrison, B.J.: J. Allergy Clin. Immunol. 77:575–581, April 1986.)

were in the minority in all of these studies. Therefore, a study was conducted exclusively of 94 asthmatic children aged 7–17 years to assess the
effects of parental smoking on wheezing and asthma severity. Parents were
interviewed concerning their child's illness during the preceding 12 months
and asthma history scores were assigned to each clinical feature. In addition, the parents were questioned about their smoking habits, the presence of gas stoves or other fume-producing kitchen appliances, and whether
they had pets. All children underwent pulmonary testing and skin prick
tests with common inhalant and pollen allergens, as well as 10% solutions
of cigarette smoke.

In all, 24 mothers and 28 fathers were smokers. There was a strong
correlation between the logarithm of the number of cigarettes smoked by
the mother and all indicators of the severity of the child's asthma. However,
there was no such relationship between the father's smoking habits and
the child's asthma severity (Table 1). There was also a strong correlation

TABLE 3.—DIFFERENCES IN INDICATORS OF ASTHMA SEVERITY BETWEEN GROUPS DISTINGUISHED BY AGE AND BY SMOKING HABITS OF MOTHER

	History score*		FEV, % predicted		FEF_{25-75} predicted		Geometric mean PC_{20}†	
	Age (>11 yr)	Age (<11 yr)	Age (>11 yr)	Age (<11 yr)	Age (>11 yr)	Age (<11 yr)	Age (>11 yr)	Age (<11 yr)
Mother Nonsmoker	6.6 ± 0.5	5.3 ± 0.6	84.5 ± 2.8	86.7 ± 2.2	73.6 ± 4.1	70.8 ± 3.7	2.3 n = 20	2.1 n = 11
Mother Smoker	10.1 ± 0.9	7.8 ± 1.2	68.7 ± 6.4	79.2 ± 4.0	52.0 ± 10.5	58.6 ± 5.6	0.4 n = 3	0.5 n = 7
p Value (two-tailed)	0.005	0.07	0.04	0.12	0.07	0.08	0.06	0.02

Forty-eight patients were aged 11 years or older and 46 were younger. Means ± standard error are presented.
*History was available for 92 children.
†PC_{20} was measured on 41 patients.
(Courtesy of Murray, A.B., and Morrison, B.J.: J. Allergy Clin. Immunol. 77:575–581, April 1986.)

between the mother's smoking habits and the child's asthma history score (Table 2). The effects of maternal cigarette smoking were greater in older than in younger children (Table 3). This finding suggests that the length of exposure to cigarette smoke also increases the severity of its adverse effects.

These results indicate that maternal smoking aggravates asthma in children. Paternal smoking was not implicated in the severity of the asthma, probably because the fathers smoked most of their cigarettes when they were away from home.

▶ This article and the two that follow are but a small sample from a very large, and growing, literature that clearly documents the hazards of passive smoking on infants and children. For example, in children aged 10–19 years, pulmonary function test results were significantly decreased if both parents smoked (*Am. Rev. Respir. Dis.* 133:966, 1986). Another study revealed a significant difference in parental smoking habits between children with and without episodes of wheezing at their fifth birthday (*Arch. Dis. Child.* 62:338, 1987). A pregnant women who smokes, smokes for two. It is well recognized that smoking during pregnancy results in growth retardation in term newborns (*Am. J. Epidemiol.* 124:633, 1986; *Pediatr. Res.* 20:716, 1986). Infants of mothers who smoke are born with increased carboxyhemoglobin values and the infant's carboxyhemoglobin concentration is nearly one third higher than that of its mother (*Hum. Toxicol.* 5:175, 1986). Maternal smoking leads to increased cord serum IgG3 values (*Allergy* 41:302, 1986), a greater frequency of fetal bradycardia, and an increased frequency of abnormal placentas, and is associated with an increased incidence of toxemia (*Obstet. Gynecol.* 68:317, 1986).

For those who still need convincing, please read "The health consequences of involuntary smoking: a report of the Surgeon General." Get it from the Office on Smoking and Health, Rockville, Maryland, Public Health Service. Smoking is a form of self-abuse; smoking around children is a form of child abuse. This form of child abuse should also be reportable.—F.A. Oski, M.D.

Influence of Passive Smoking on Admissions for Respiratory Illness in Early Childhood

Yue Chen, Wanxian Li, and Shunzhang Yu (Shanghai Med. Univ.)
Br. Med. J. 293:303–306, Aug. 2, 1986   9–8

Children exposed to parental cigarette smoking have been said to have increased risks of pneumonia, bronchitis, and other respiratory illnesses. The risk of hospital admission for respiratory illness was related to passive smoking in infants in the first 18 months of life, independent of maternal antenatal smoking effects. Evaluations were made of 1,058 Chinese infants.

Overall, 17% of the children in this survey were admitted to the hospital in the first 18 months, most for respiratory illnesses. More than two thirds of the children lived in families that included smokers. The risk of hospital admission for first respiratory illness increased with the number of cigarettes smoked daily by family members. Smoking in families was associated with a lower paternal educational level and with the presence of any adult having chronic respiratory disease. The odds ratio for admission with respiratory illness was significant for children in families smoking ten or more cigarettes a day. Passive smoking could not be related to hospital admission for all other conditions.

Household exposure of young infants to cigarette smoke was related to admission for a first episode of respiratory illness in this study. The findings support a general relationship between adult smoking and adverse health effects on children in the home.

Parental Smoking, Presence of Older Siblings, and Family History of Asthma Increase Risk of Bronchiolitis

Kenneth M. McConnochie and Klaus J. Roghmann (Rochester Gen. Hosp. and Univ. of Rochester, N.Y.)
Am. J. Dis. Child. 140:806–812, August 1986   9–9

Bronchiolitis is common in infants, causing substantial acute morbidity and sequelae. A case-control study was undertaken to identify risk factors for bronchiolitis. Fifty-three cases with bronchiolitis were each matched with two controls who had no bronchiolitis in infancy.

Passive smoking and the presence of older siblings were significant predictors of bronchiolitis (Tables 1 and 2). A family history of asthma and the presence of older siblings interacted in predicting bronchiolitis. Among cases without a family history of asthma, odds ratios for passive smoking and older siblings were 3.87 and 2.31, respectively. The odds ratio increased to 8.94 when both risk factors were present. Among cases with a family history of asthma, passive smoking was about equally strong, with an odds ratio of 4.03, but an older sibling proved to be a stronger predictor, with an odds ratio of 6.81. The risk of bronchiolitis increased linearly with the number and age of older siblings.

Children at high risk of bronchiolitis can be identified on the basis of a family history of asthma, the presence of older siblings, and passive

TABLE 1.—PREDICTORS OF BRONCHIOLITIS: BIVARIATE ANALYSIS

Predictors		No. of Subjects	Bronchiolitis Developed, No. (%)	Significance of Difference, P*	Strength of Relationship, Odds Ratio (Confidence Interval)†
Breast-fed	No	103	38 (36.9)	.20	1.50 (0.78-3.26)
	Yes	56	15 (26.8)		
Crowding index, No. of persons/No. of rooms	>0.6	76	33 (43.4)	.01	2.42 (1.23-4.76)
	≤0.6	83	20 (24.1)		
Family history of allergy	Yes	83	28 (33.7)	NS	1.01 (0.76-1.32)
	No	76	25 (32.9)		
Family history of asthma	Yes	34	16 (47.1)	.06	2.11 (0.97-4.59)
	No	125	37 (29.6)		
Older siblings	Any	99	43 (43.4)	<.001	3.84 (1.75-8.43)
	None	60	10 (16.7)		
Smoking in household					
Any	Yes	108	44 (40.7)	.004	3.21 (1.42-7.25)
	No	51	9 (17.6)		
Mother	Yes	68	30 (44.1)	.01	2.33 (1.19-4.57)
	No	91	23 (25.3)		
Father	Yes	82	32 (39.0)	.12	1.71 (0.87-3.33)
	No	77	21 (27.3)		
Socioeconomic index	Low	86	34 (39.5)	.07	1.86 (0.94-3.66)
	High	73	19 (26.0)		

*Determined by χ^2 method.
†Odds ratio was computed as ratio of cross products. Lower and upper 95% confidence intervals were computed by Woolf's method.
(Courtesy of McConnochie, K.M., and Roghmann, K.J.: Am. J. Dis. Child. 140:806–812, August 1986.)

TABLE 2.—MULTIVARIATE MODEL: BRONCHIOLITIS PREDICTED BY FAMILY HISTORY OF ASTHMA, PASSIVE SMOKING, AND OLDER SIBLINGS*

	A	B	C	D	E	F	G	H	Total
Risk factor†									
Family history	0	0	0	0	1	1	1	1	...
Passive smoking	0	0	1	1	0	0	1	1	...
Older siblings	0	1	0	1	0	1	0	1	...
Observed data									
Bronchiolitis‡	2	3	6	26	0	4	2	10	53
No bronchiolitis‡	14	20	23	31	5	3	8	2	106
Total‡	16	23	29	57	5	7	10	12	159
Odds for bronchiolitis	0.14	0.15	0.26	0.84	0.0	1.33	0.25	5.00	0.50
Modeled data									
Bronchiolitis	1.38	4.10	7.75	26.03	0.10	3.42	0.76	9.45	53
No bronchiolitis	14.62	18.90	21.25	30.97	4.90	3.58	9.24	2.55	106
Odds for bronchiolitis	0.094	0.217	0.364	0.840	0.020	0.955	0.082	3.71	0.50
Odds ratio	1.00	2.31	3.87	8.94	1.00	46.81	4.03	181.67	...
Proportion with bronchiolitis, %	8.6	17.8	26.7	45.7	2.0	48.9	7.6	78.8	...

*Goodness of fit: Pearson's χ^2 = 3.82; df = 4; and P = .43. Statistically significant predictors in best-fitting model based on one-tailed t test were as follows: intercept, λ = .6342, t = 5.04, and P <.001; passive smoking, λ = .3387, t = 2.96, and P <.005; older siblings, λ = .5794, t = 4.08, and P <.001; and the interaction term (siblings-family), λ = .3708, t = 2.83, and P <.005. Odds ratios (relative odds) may be calculated for any two cells to provide index of relative likelihood of bronchiolitis. For cells A through D, odds ratios were calculated by dividing odds for bronchiolitis (modeled data) in each cell by 0.094, the odds for bronchiolitis among subjects with no risk factors present. For cells E through H, odds ratios were calculated by dividing odds for bronchiolitis (modeled data) in each cell by 0.0204, the odds for bronchiolitis among subjects with family history of asthma but no other risk factors. This is justified on basis of failure of direct effects of family history to achieve statistical significance.
†1, Risk factor present; 0, risk factor absent.
‡Number of subjects per cell.
(Courtesy of McConnochie, K.M., and Roghmann, K.J.: Am. J. Dis. Child. 140:806–812, August 1986.)

smoking. For children with a family history of asthma, the risk of bronchiolitis developing is almost 50% and increases to about 80% when the children are exposed to cigarette smoke. Among infants without a family history of asthma, bronchiolitis may develop in 46% of those with both older siblings and passive exposure to smoke. For infants without a family history of asthma, no passive smoking, and no older siblings, the risk of bronchiolitis is only 8.6%. Hence, efforts to reduce morbidity from bronchiolitis in infants should be directed at reduction of smoking in families with previous children, particularly if there is a history of asthma. Further, contact between infants and older siblings should be eliminated during the short period when respiratory virus infection is prevalent or siblings have a respiratory illness.

Predicting Experimentation With Cigarettes: The Childhood Antecedents of Smoking Study (CASS)

Maurice B. Mittelmark, David M. Murray, Russell V. Luepker, Terry F. Pechacek, Phyllis L. Pirie, and Unto E. Pallonen (Univ. of Minnesota)
Am. J. Public Health 77:206–208, February 1987   9–10

There is much to be learned about the relationship between adolescent smoking and a host of sociodemographic and psychosocial factors. The Childhood Antecedents of Smoking Study (CASS) was undertaken to determine factors predictive of smoking onset. Students in grades 7 through 11 participated in four surveys conducted at 6-month intervals. The surveys included biochemical measures of smoking, i.e., thiocynate analysis of saliva and carbon monoxide analysis of expired air, and questionnaires about the adolescent's smoking behavior, home and school environment, the smoking behavior of significant others, and the student's values, attitudes, and beliefs about smoking.

A total of 2,209 of 2,284 participants completed the surveys. The most pervasive predictor of experimentation with cigarettes was the perceived smoking behavior of friends at baseline. The influence of smoking by siblings was exerted mainly on females and younger students. Males who smoked were more independent, less concerned with the health consequences of smoking, and lived in an egalitarian home environment. Females who smoked viewed the smoker's image positively, placed less emphasis on the positive role of adults regarding smoking, and had less educated parents. Compared with noncontinuing smokers, beginning smokers among younger students were far more likely to be less concerned with the health consequences of smoking.

Smoking prevention strategies that teach youth to cope with social influences are well founded. Younger students may be dissuaded from beginning to smoke by teaching them the health consequences of smoking.

▶ Dr. Alain Joffe, Assistant Professor of Pediatrics, Johns Hopkins University School of Medicine, and Director, Adolescent Clinic, comments.—F.A. Oski, M.D.

▶ Currently, 12.8% of senior high school girls and 11.0% of boys smoke at least half a pack per day. The Surgeon General has labeled this habit as the "chief, single, avoidable cause of [adult—my addition] death in our society and the most important public health issue of our time." Because most smokers initiate this addiction during adolescence, particularly between ages 12 and 16, pediatricians are in an optimal position to deter their young patients from adopting this life-style. As does this article, research on adolescent smoking highlights the influential aspects of peer pressure, parental modeling, and media influence, the latter through portrayal of smokers as being glamorous, sexy, and more numerous (in the eyes of adolescents) than they really are. Personal factors also play a role: Smokers know less about the health consequences of smoking than nonsmokers do and view smoking as enhancing their self-esteem and maturity. Adults may view this behavior as risky, but for teenagers it serves the useful purpose of enhancing social competence. Of course, once a teenager initiates smoking, the addictive properties of nicotine are reinforcing.

Prevention strategies must address all of these issues. Given the pervasiveness of smoking cues in our culture, individual efforts on the part of the pediatrician need to be coupled with efforts by parents and schools. Because it is easier to prevent initiation of smoking than getting a smoker to stop, pediatricians should encourage smoking parents to quit and should work with their teenage patients to develop the knowledge base and social skills to resist peer pressure to smoke (Schenke, A.: *Am. J. Public Health* 75:665–667, 1985).

Alternative strategies to enhance self-esteem should also be developed. Because adolescents respond better to information about the short-term rather than long-term health consequences of smoking, the focus of counseling should be on the immediate effects, e.g., cost, stained teeth, decrease in athletic performance, increased heart rate [as exemplified by the American Cancer Society's "Draggin Lady" (sic) campaign].

Pediatricians should also be aware of the increased use of "smokeless tobacco" by teenagers. Although perceived as less harmful by teenagers and marketed as such, this habit shares many of smoking's adverse consequences and increases the risk for oral cancers.—A. Joffe, M.D.

Accidental Ingestion of a Toothbrush!
M. Mughal (Univ. of Manchester, England)
Arch. Emerg. Med. 3:119–123, June 1986   9–11

The flexible endoscope may be used to remove foreign bodies from the stomach when these do not pass spontaneously, but some of the methods described are potentially more dangerous than operative removal. An accidentally swallowed toothbrush was removed safely from the stomach using a flexible endoscope.

Girl, 16 years, accidentally swallowed a toothbrush when she collided with her sister on running downstairs while brushing her teeth. Symptoms were absent 2 hours later. The parents had brought an identical toothbrush to the emergency room, making it possible to rehearse the proposed endoscopy procedure (Fig 9–

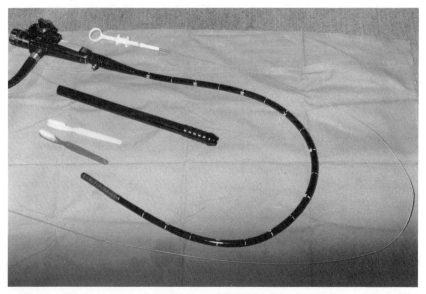

Fig 9–2.—Endoscope, sheath, and biopsy forceps. Shown are the toothbrush that was extracted and an identical brush used for rehearsal. (Courtesy of Mughal, M.: Arch. Emerg. Med. 3:119–123, June 1986.)

2). After the biopsy forceps were passed through the hole in the end of the brush handle, the brush was grasped successfully and pulled up to the scope; the sheath was then advanced over the scope. The entire assembly was removed with the head extended. No mucosal trauma was evident.

If an object identical to that swallowed is available, the removal procedure can be planned in advance. Endoscopic removal is well tolerated when local anesthesia and sedation are administered. The protective sheath must be used to avoid injuring the esophagus. Only an experienced endoscopist should attempt removal in these difficult cases.

▶ This is one good argument for flossing instead of brushing. If you think swallowing your toothbrush is a problem, how about "chopsticks dysphagia" (Myszor, M.F., et al.: *Lancet* 2:866, 1986)? It is characterized by sudden and absolute dysphagia. An illustrative case is as follows:

"A 38-year-old man presented as an emergency with absolute dysphagia. Two days previously he had noticed sudden onset of severe chest pain whilst eating. The pain subsided but he could not swallow liquids or solids. His wife noticed unusual and severe halitosis. Chest x-rays, including lateral views, were normal. Endoscopy revealed abundant putrifying food debris from the mid-esophagus downwards. . . . . At the time of the acute onset, the patient had been hurriedly eating a Chinese meal with chopsticks, and he recalled having had difficulty in swallowing a leathery piece of liver."

One of the largest studies of foreign bodies within the esophagus has been reported from Hong Kong (*Br. J. Surg.* 65:5, 1978). The moral of all this? Caution when you are eating meat with either chopsticks or a toothbrush.—F.A. Oski, M.D.

10 The Genitourinary Tract

Outpatient Pediatric Urological Surgery: Techniques for a Successful and Cost-Effective Practice
Andrew L.Siegel, Howard McC. Snyder, and John W. Duckett (Univ. of Pennsylvania)
J. Urol. 136:879–881, October 1986   10–1

With the ever-increasing regulations and cost-containment measures that have resulted from escalating hospital costs, the number of outpatient and one-night-stay operations has increased significantly. Data were reviewed concerning operations performed on an outpatient and one-night-day basis during a 10-month period in a pediatric urology division.

Of 674 pediatric urologic procedures, 62.3% were done on an outpatient basis, 12.5% were done on a one-night-stay basis, and 25.2% were done on an inpatient basis (Table 1). The outpatient and one-night-stay procedures included endoscopic, groin, scrotal, and penile procedures, as well

TABLE 1.—PATIENT DISTRIBUTION FROM JANUARY TO OCTOBER 1984

Procedure	No. Pts. (%)
Outpatient	420 (62.3)
1-night stay	84 (12.5)
Inpatient	170 (25.2)
Total	674 (100.0)

(Courtesy of Siegel, A.L., et al.: J. Urol. 136:879–881, October 1986.)

TABLE 2.—COMPLICATIONS

	No. (%)
Anesthesia:	
Nausea/vomiting	— (20)
Minor fever	— (5)
Sore throat/cough	— (5)
Urological:	
Stent problems	8 (2)
Minor hemorrhage	2 (0.5)
Urinary retention	1 (0.25)
Wound hematoma	1 (0.25)

No patient required rehospitalization.
(Courtesy of Siegel, A.L., et al.: J. Urol. 136:879–881, October 1986.)

261

as major hypospadias repairs and intra-abdominal orchiopexy. None of the children required further hospitalization.

Complications could be classified as anesthesia-related or urologic. Anesthesia-related complications included nausea with emesis, minor fever, sore throat, and cough. Urologic complications included stent problems, minor hemorrhage, retention of urine, and wound hematoma (Table 2).

Savings on two commonly performed pediatric urologic procedures, orchiopexy and hypospadias repairs, amounted to $952 and $1,435 per procedure, respectively. During the 10-month reference period the total savings amounted to $19,000 (9.2%) and $165,000 (33.8%), respectively.

Ambulatory pediatric urologic surgery is safe, convenient, readily accepted, and often preferred by parents. It is cost effective, decreases transmission of nosocomial diseases, minimizes psychological trauma, and conserves hospital beds.

Declining Frequency of Circumcision: Implications for Changes in the Absolute Incidence and Male to Female Sex Ratio of Urinary Tract Infections in Early Infancy

Thomas E. Wiswell, Robert W. Enzenauer, Mark E. Holton, J. Devn Cornish, and Charles T. Hankins (Brooke Army Med. Ctr., Ft. Sam Houston, Tex.)
Pediatrics 79:338–342, March 1987   10–2

A report in 1975 by the American Academy of Pediatrics Ad Hoc Task Force on Circumcision stated: "There is no absolute medical indication for routine circumcision of the newborn." However, most studies have been unable to show any substantial decline in the number of males who have been circumcised since this report appeared. A recent study demonstrated an increased risk of urinary tract infection in uncircumcised compared with circumcised boys. The circumcision frequency rate and its effect on urinary tract infections were examined in 427,698 infants born in all United States Army hospitals, worldwide, from 1975 to 1984.

There was an initial plateau in the circumcision frequency rate at about 85% from 1975 to 1978. During the next 6 years, there was a steady, significant decrease of 1.4% to 4% per year, at which time circumcision frequency rate reached its nadir of 70.5%. There was a concomitant increase in the total number of urinary infections among male infants as the circumcision rate declined. This increase resulted from the increase in the overall number of uncircumcised boys, whose infection rate increased by more than 11-fold compared with uncircumcised boys. During the first half of the study there was a predominance of urinary tract infections in female infants from birth onward. As the percentage of circumcised boys decreased, with the resultant increase in the total number of male infants with infection, the male-to-female ratio of urinary tract infections during the first 3 months of life reversed, demonstrating a movement toward a male predominance for infection in early infancy. It would appear that the number of urinary tract infections in male infants, as well as the male-to-female ratio, is affected by the circumcision practices of the population investigated.

▶ By now, just about everybody has either read or heard about the Wiswell article abstracted above and the prior article from this same group (*Pediatrics* 75:901, 1985), which reported an association between circumcision and a decreased frequency of urinary tract infection in infancy. These reports had all the makings of a pediatric cause celebrè and, indeed, the prediction seems to be coming true. The letters to the editor following the first study came in promptly. Among these letters complaining about the way the pendulum may be swinging back toward circumcision were the following comments: ". . . the possibility still exists that the gene coating for *Escherichia coli* receptor in bladder mucosa is linked to the one that induces non-circumcision-directed behavior in a parent . . ." (Cohen, M.L.: *Pediatrics* 78:951, 1986). Another of his comments was ". . . perhaps each hospital should have a consultant *mohel* (a person trained in ritual circumcision)—either to contract to do all the circumcisions or to suggest ways of carrying out the procedure with a minimum of pain and stress and a maximum of care, comfort, and dignity for the child and family."

Since 1975, the American Academy of Pediatrics' position on circumcision has been that there is no absolute medical indication for the procedures. The anticircumcision movement is supported not only by the American Academy of Pediatrics but also by the American College of Obstetricians and Gynecologists. Nonprofessional groups have also gotten into the act. One such group is called INTACT (how appropriate!). The Wiswell article is among the first to show that there is actually a decline in the frequency of circumcision in the United States (or at least among its hospitals). The estimated percentage of boys born in the United States who were circumcised in 1985 ranged between 70% and 90%, as opposed to a 0.4% rate in Great Britain. One way that has been tried to decrease the rate of circumcision is the presentation of video-taped material summarizing factors related to neonatal circumcision (Enzenauer, R.W., et al.: *South Med. J.* 79:717, 1986). In the latter report, a study was designed to see what the effects would be of showing a video tape to parents prior to the decision regarding circumcision. This video tape specifically included the major reports of the Ad Hoc Committee on Circumcision of the American Academy of Pediatrics and specifically mentioned the fact that there was no medical indication for a routine, neonatal circumcision. The presentation also included the NBC documentary aired in 1981 entitled, "Circumcision: The Casual Cut," as well as a blow-by-blow description of circumcision using a Plastibell device. The only thing it didn't do was to show the whole gory scene itself. The results of this study were astounding. The circumcision rate dropped in one Honolulu hospital from 90% to 70% simply with the showing of this video tape.

Before jumping on the circumcision bandwagon to diminish the rate of urinary tract infections in boys, look at another study from the military. This study shows that circumcised boys had a risk of nongonococcal urethritis 1.65 times that in uncircumcised boys (Smith, G.L., et al.: *Am. J. Public Health* 77:452, 1987).

If the data of Wiswell et al. hold up, a lot of us will have had egg on our faces. My gosh, how things have changed! Ten years ago we were making comments about "The rape of the foreskin," and now we're seeing articles reporting to support the ancient practice of circumcision. Circumcision is a procedure that apparently will always be cloaked with controversy. For now, it appears that the circumcision pendulum is swinging back even before it had a chance to swing forth. Obviously, no one can foresee what will happen to the foreskin in ten more years. I, for one, would like to forestall the foreshortening of the object of all this discussion.—J.A. Stockman III, M.D.

Tachycardia and Heart Failure After Ritual Circumcision
A. Mor, G. Eshel, M. Aladjem, and G. Mundel (Assaf Harofe Med. Ctr., The Sackler School of Medicine, Tel-Aviv Univ., Israel)
Arch. Dis. Child. 62:80–81, January 1987   10–3

Circumcision is a common surgical procedure in neonates, but four newborn infants were seen who sustained acute heart failure a few hours after circumcision. Ritual circumcision was performed at 8 days of age in four normal newborn infants. A sponge soaked in 1:1,000 epinephrine solution was applied to the site of circumcision and left in place for several hours. A few hours later, all four infants had pallor, cyanosis, tachycardia, tachypnea, and grunting respirations. Physical and x-ray findings were compatible with acute heart failure. Metabolic acidosis was present in three newborns, lactic acidosis in one, and hyperglycemia in three. Digoxin and diuretics were administered, and signs of heart failure disappeared within 24–72 hours.

The use of topical epinephrine should be prohibited after circumcision. Epinephrine intoxication, as a result of increased absorption through the open wound, can cause acute heart failure in neonates undergoing circumcision.

▶ Ritual circumcision has been practiced by the Jewish people for the last four millenia. The method that should be used, however, is not laid down in the Bible. *Mohels* who perform the circumcision tend to adopt whatever technique was passed on for generations by their forebears. In the article abstracted above, the *mohel* liberally applied a sponge soaked with 1:1,000 epinephrine solution to the freshly circumcised penis. It's fair to say that *mohels* may be more experienced and skilled than physicians in performing this procedure. Unfortunately, an exhaustive study of Milah practices (ritual circumcision) revealed a wide spectrum, ranging from skilled operators and aseptic conditions to unskilled *mohels* using crude, outmoded, and unsanitary procedures (Wallerstein, E.: *Circumcision: An American Health Fallacy*. New York, Springer, 1980). The United States and Israel are the two countries that have the highest rates of circumcision. Perhaps we should emulate the state of Israel, where *mohels* are licensed and lists of approved operators are published by the government.

If the data hold up that support the value of circumcision, perhaps we will pay more attention to how both ritual and nonritual circumcisions are done. If the data hold up, we will also potentially see the demise of the lay group that supports preservation of the foreskin (INTACT; see commentary with Abstract 10–2). I never did like the INTACT group, and never thought they did a lot to help their cause. They seem to be proof positive of the rule that "When the going gets weird, the weird turn pro."—J.A. Stockman III, M.D.

Improvements in Self-Concept After Treatment of Nocturnal Enuresis: Randomized Controlled Trial
Michael Edward Knowler Moffatt, Caroline Kato, and Ivan Barry Pless (McGill Univ. and Montreal Children's Hosp.)
J. Pediatr. 110:647–652, April 1987   10–4

Most children with enuresis are regarded as not substantially different emotionally from other children, but the disorder itself may act as a chronic stressor and, if persistent, have adverse effects on the child's personality. Children aged 8–14 years with primary nocturnal enuresis were entered into a randomized trial of conditioning treatment based on an alarm and "overlearning" procedure. Sixty-six treated children were compared with 55 assigned to a 3-month waiting period. The Piers-Harris Self-Concept Scale, State-Trait Anxiety Scale, and Nowicki-Strickland Locus of Control test were administered, and parents completed the Achenback Child Behavior Checklist. The two groups were comparable demographically.

Forty-two treated children became completely dry at night, for a success rate of 69%. Most of the others improved to some degree. Parental ratings of behavior improved in both groups. Treated children rated themselves as more improved on the Piers-Harris Scale. Changes toward more internal locus of control and less anxiety were evident in the treated group. Controls exhibited similar changes in self-concept when subsequently treated.

Improved self-concept is evident after successful conditioning treatment for nocturnal enuresis. Poor self-concept may be a secondary effect of chronic stress in this setting, rather than a cause of enuresis. The findings can be generalized only to middle-class children in private practice settings. The durability of the change in self-concept remains to be determined.

Factors Related to the Age of Attainment of Nocturnal Bladder Control: An 8-Year Longitudinal Study
D.M. Fergusson, L.J. Horwood, and F.T. Shannon (Christchurch Public Hosp., New Zealand)
Pediatrics 78:884–890, November 1986   10–5

The exact causes of nocturnal enuresis remain unknown, but it is widely believed that the condition is multicausal, involving a combination of organic, genetic, developmental, and psychosocial factors. It has been suggested that the etiology of primary enuresis is predominantly biologic, whereas the causes of secondary or onset enuresis are mostly psychosocial. An 8-year longitudinal study was undertaken of the patterns of the de-

PROPORTIONS OF CHILDREN STILL TO ATTAIN
NOCTURNAL BLADDER CONTROL AND
PROPORTIONS OF CHILDREN WITH NOCTURNAL
ENURESIS BY AGE OF CHILD

Age (yr)	Children Still to Attain Bladder Control (%)	Children With Nocturnal Enuresis (%)
2	92.5	92.5
3	42.8	43.2
4	18.6	20.2
5	11.0	15.7
6	7.6	13.1
7	5.2	10.3
8	3.3	7.4

(Courtesy of Fergusson, D.M., et al.: Pediatrics 78:884–890, November 1986.)

velopment of nocturnal bladder control in 1,265 New Zealand children born in the Christchurch urban region; 1,092 children (86%) still resided in New Zealand after an 8-year follow-up. The children were studied at birth, at age 4 months, and at annual intervals up to the age of 8 years. The age of attainment of nocturnal bladder control was defined as the first age at which the mother reported that the child remained dry throughout the night.

By age 8 years, only 3.3% of the children had not attained nocturnal bladder control (table). However, because some children subsequently relapsed, the overall incidence of those who were bedwetting at age 8 years was 7.4%. Factors predictive of the age of attainment of nocturnal bladder control included a family history of enuresis, the child's developmental level at age 1 year and 3 years, and the child's early sleeping patterns. However, attainment of bladder control was not related to psychosocial factors, e.g., family social and economic background, family life-event measures, changes in parents in the family, or residential changes. Apparently, the etiology of primary enuresis is mainly biologic, with psychosocial factors playing only a small role in this condition.

▶ The two previous articles (Abstracts 10–4 and 10–5) look at the problem of enuresis from differing perspectives. It is heartening to note that when enuresis is successfully dealt with there is improvement in self-concept and self-worth. The conclusion of the Fergusson report may not be all that valid, however. As was noted, these investigators believe that psychosocial issues play only a minimal role in the causality of enuresis. This is probably correct when it comes to primary enuresis. Most do agree that maturational factors, and perhaps genetic factors, underlie this form of enuresis. In secondary enuresis, when the child is continent for a period of time and then begins bedwetting again, psychological factors become more important. We are all taught that secondary enuresis should be more thoroughly investigated. Often there is a need to regress or to receive excessive attention when a significant event threatens to disrupt the child's life, e.g., the birth of a new sibling or the parent's separation or divorce. However, bedwetting may also be a symptom of diabetes mellitus, diabetes insipidus, nocturnal epilepsy, severe mental retardation, or neurologic disorders.

A report from Great Britain demonstrates that intranasal desmopressin may be even better than we had originally thought in the management of nocturnal enuresis. (Dimson, S.B.: *Arch. Dis. Child.* 61:1104, 1986). Children were studied who had failed all other forms of nocturnal enuresis control including failure to respond to imipramine and amitriptyline. When everything else had failed, about 50% of the children were either cured or showed considerable improvement. No side effects were noted. The principles that underlie the management of primary enuresis are basically fivefold: physiologic approaches, psychological approaches, conditioning, pharmacologic measures, and tincture of time. The latter seems to be the most effective. Most of us have come to respect the tenacity of this disorder, if it is even a disorder. The four least credible sentences in the English language are (1) "The check is in the mail"; (2) "Of course I'll respect you in the morning"; (3) "I'm from the government and I'm here to help you"; and (4) "I'm an enuresis device and I work."—J.A. Stockman III, M.D.

Sequential Study of the IgA System in Relapsing IgA Nephropathy
John Feehally, T. James Beattie, Paul E.C. Brenchley, Beatrice M. Coupes, Netar P. Mallick, and Robert J. Postlethwaite (Manchester Royal Infirmary and Royal Manchester Children's Hosp., England)
Kidney Int. 30:924–931, December 1986   10–6

Increased levels of serum polymer IgA and IgA circulating immune complexes have been described in patients with IgA nephropathy. Studies were made in eight children and seven adults with biopsy-proved IgA nephropathy and recurrent macroscopic hematuria, usually precipitated by infection, often of the upper respiratory tract. Nine age-matched children and six adults without clinical abnormalities also were studied. The cellular and immunochemical characteristics of the IgA system were investigated.

No abnormalities of the IgA system were apparent during remissions, but increases in IgA-bearing B lymphocytes occurred during relapse, when gross hematuria was associated with upper respiratory tract infection. In addition, the T helper/suppressor cell ratio and pokeweed mitogen-induced IgA production increased during relapse. Total serum and salivary IgA levels were unchanged. Serum IgA profile studies by high-performance liquid chromatography and enzyme-linked immunosorbent assay showed increases in polymer IgA. No such changes were evident in controls with upper respiratory tract infections.

Gross hematuria in IgA nephropathy is associated with abnormal activation of the IgA system, which is not apparent in periods of remission. Activation may lead to increases in circulating polymer IgA. Because mesangial IgA in IgA nephropathy may be polymeric, deposition of circulating polymer IgA may be an important factor in glomerular damage and hematuria in IgA nephropathy.

▶ This study provides interesting clues into the goings-on in IgA nephropathy. Perhaps it also gives us a diagnostic tool to determine which child is going to relapse based on changes in the amount of circulating polymer IgA.

With the help of the Japanese we are learning a great deal more about what the natural history is of IgA nephropathy. The reason for this is based on the fact that in 1974 the Japanese government initiated yearly school screenings of the urines of all Japanese children between the ages of 6 and 15 years (Yoshikawa, N., et al.: *J. Pediatr.* 110:555, 1987). This unique opportunity led to a series of 818 biopsies performed at the Tokyo Metropolitan Children's Hospital. Of these specimens, 25% showed evidence of IgA nephropathy, the single most common glomerulonephritis in children. The findings in IgA nephropathy include diffuse mesangial deposits of IgA, frequently accompanied by C3 and sometimes by IgG and IgM; various degrees of focal or diffuse mesangial proliferation; and electron-dense mesangial deposits in the absence of systemic disease. It should be noted that similar findings are present in most patients who have Henoch-Schönlein syndrome with renal involvement. The Japanese report made several points: The incidence of subsequent renal failure, hypertension, and persistent heavy proteinuria was much greater in children with older age at onset; the clinical and laboratory findings at onset of disease and the pathologic findings at the time of first biopsy were similar in patients who turned out to have a good prognosis and those who did not; and serum IgA levels were increased above normal in about a third of patients with IgA nephropathy. In addition, spontaneous IgA synthesis was noted in peripheral blood lymphocytes in children with IgA nephropathy. The Japanese initially thought that IgA nephropathy was a benign disorder, but long-term follow-up suggests that progression to renal failure may occur in 20% to 50% of adult patients. Among children in Japan, renal failure developed in 7% of the older children with IgA nephropathy.

What to do about IgA nephropathy is more problematic. There is no evidence that treatment with corticosteroids, cyclophosphamide, or anticoagulants favorably alters the course of the renal disease. At present, there is no specific therapy. This is not to say that some patients should not be treated with steroids. Lai et al. (*Clin. Nephrol.* 26:174, 1986) found that corticosteroids could induce a remission in 80% of children with IgA nephropathy if the only expression of the disorder was the nephrotic syndrome and if the renal biopsy specimen showed only mild abnormalities. Apparently, only time will tell us how bad an actor this disease is. We just haven't had enough experience with it since its description in 1968.—J.A. Stockman III, M.D.

Immune-Complex Glomerulonephritis in Crohn's Disease
Mark Glassman, Matthew Kaplan, and William Spivak (Cornell Univ. and New York Hosp.)
J. Pediatr. Gastroenterol. Nutr. 5:966–969, November–December 1986   10–7

Crohn's disease is often associated with extracolonic manifestations in other organs, including the skin, joints, and liver. A patient with Crohn's disease associated with immune-complex glomerulonephritis was seen.

Girl, 13 years, had a history of fever, arthritis, conjunctivitis, abdominal pain, diarrhea, and weight loss. Colonoscopy and barium enema were consistent with Crohn's disease. Initial urinalysis showed proteinuria, hematuria, and granular casts that persisted despite resolution of other symptoms after methylprednisolone therapy. Renal biopsy revealed diffuse proliferating necrotizing glomerulonephritis. Immunofluorescent studies showed deposition of C3 and immunoglobulins G and M on the basement membrane of the involved glomeruli. Circulating immune complexes, i.e., positive rheumatoid factor and increased titer of serum immune complexes by the Raji cell method, were present in the serum. The patient recovered and was maintained with a lactose-free diet and prednisone. However, hematuria and mild proteinuria persisted.

Immune-complex glomerulonephritis represents a previously unreported extraintestinal manifestation of inflammatory bowel disease. Patients with Crohn's disease should be evaluated for hematuria, proteinuria, and granular casts.

▶ This may well be the very first case description of immune-complex nephritis in association with Crohn's disease. It's a bit surprising, because extraintestinal manifestations are seen in approximately 25% of patients with this disease. Thus, there is no reason to presume that the kidneys should be spared. The upshot of all this is that we really should be paying much more careful attention to the urinary sediment of patients with Crohn's disease. That may become easier soon. Shichiri et al. (*Lancet* 2:781, 1986) have shown the value of an autoanalyzer in examining urinary red blood cell (RBC) morphology as part of the diagnosis of glomerulohematuria. Phase-contrast microscopy of the urine has been used to distinguish glomerular bleeding from other causes of hematuria. Glomerular RBCs have distorted shapes and variations in size, whereas nonglomerular RBCs have smooth surfaces and are uniform in size. What you do here is to get a specimen of urine that is dip-stick and microscopically positive for RBCs and then run it through a Coulter counter that can display a histogram of the RBC size. This is the equivalent of an RBC distribution width when doing routine hematology tests. If the patient has glomerular hematuria, the RBCs will be distorted enough in size and shape to produce a very broad irregular spectrum on the Coulter counter histogram of RBC size. Nonglomerular RBCs in the urine form a very homogeneous size and shape to the histogram.

This is an important observation, especially relative to the article abstracted above. Most patients with Crohn's disease with hematuria have it on a urologic basis, i.e., as a result of urinary calculi or fistulas attached to the urinary tract. Any hematuria related to the latter causes of heme-positive urine should show up as nonglomerular in terms of size distribution on the RBC counting equipment. Patients with the glomerular-size distribution can be spared needless urologic invasions and can be referred directly to a nephrologist for consultation about the necessity for a renal biopsy. Those with nonglomerular distribution are more likely in need of urologic examination.

This is an interesting finding, and I certainly hope it holds up. It sounds better than lemonade on a hot summer day. It is intriguing how the RBC provides so much information about the kidney. Last year we commented on the fact that RBCs in patients with minimal-change nephropathy often lose their negative surface charge. The same is true of albumin. Presumably, it is this loss of surface charge that allows protein to sneak through the glomerulus into the urine rather than being repelled by the similarly charged surface of the capillary wall cell. The story related to variation in charge on RBCs in the different forms of nephritis appears to be holding up (Boulton-Jones, J.M., et al.: *Lancet* 2:186, 1986).—J.A. Stockman III, M.D.

Thromboembolic Complications in Children With Nephrotic Syndrome: Risk and Incidence
P.F. Hoyer, S. Gonda, M. Barthels, H.P. Krohn, and J. Brodehl (Med. School Hannover, West Germany)
Acta Paediatr. Scand. 75:804–810, 1986   10–8

Nephrotic syndrome is associated with a high incidence of thromboembolic complications. In adults, reported rates are 19% to 70%, but pediatric data are largely anecdotal. Laboratory studies have revealed abnormalities in the concentrations of almost every coagulation factor and inhibitor as well as in platelets and the fibrinolytic enzyme system. These findings have been interpreted as being characteristic of a hypercoagulable state, but almost all patients in these studies were adults. Coagulation factors were investigated in children with nephrotic syndrome, and the incidence of thromboembolic episodes was studied scintigraphically.

Sixteen children with corticosteroid-sensitive nephrotic syndrome were studied during the acute phase of a relapse. A renal biopsy in 12 showed minimal-change disease in each. Plasma samples were taken before corticosteroid treatment was started. Fibrinogen and α_2-macroglobulin concentrations were inversely correlated with serum albumin concentrations,and antithrombin III values were correlated positively. The factor VIII:R:AG concentration was elevated. The coagulation disturbances in children were no less severe than those in adults with nephrotic syndrome. In a second study, 26 children with nephrotic syndrome were evaluated retrospectively for the occurrence of thromboembolic events by combined scintigraphic pulmonary ventilation and perfusion studies. A pattern consistent with pulmonary embolism was present in seven patients (27.9%), residual changes were found in ten (38.5%), and findings were normal in nine (34.9%). The incidence of thromboembolic complications in children with severe nephrotic syndrome is as high as that reported in adults. Pulmonary symptoms are probably caused by pulmonary embolism.

▶ This report is enough to scare the dickens out of anybody. I suppose that the next time I see a child with nephrotic syndrome, if that child coughs, displays any respiratory symptoms, or has chest pain, he'll be off for a pulmonary ventilation/perfusion scan to see if a pulmonary embolus has arisen. At one time, the coagulopathy of nephrotic syndrome was thought to be fairly straightforward. Specifically, we thought that it was loss of certain coagulants into the urine that caused the hypercoagulable state. The presumption was that the capillaries leaked antithrombin III, producing a deficiency of this substance and a consequent tendency toward thrombus formation. Obviously, the story is much more complex than that. These authors suggest that there is actual in vivo activation of the coagulation schema within the kidney itself. This is supported by two other recent studies. Alkjaersig et al. (*Kidney Int.* 31;772, 1987) examined blood coagulation function in 84 children with the nephrotic syndrome. Plasma fibrinogen concentration and high-molecular-weight fibrinogen complexes were grossly elevated. These returned to normal during remission states. The antithrombin III concentration was diminished, especially in the group with focal glomerulosclerosis. Mehis et al. (*J. Pediatr.* 110:862, 1987) found that 5% of children with nephrotic syndrome had thromboembolic complications. These were equally divided between arterial thrombi and venous thrombi (the latter mostly in the lung). Antithrombin III concentrations and activities were abnormal in 70% of the children. The protein C level was significantly elevated and thus did not account for the hypercoagulable state. Many children also demonstrated subtle findings consistent with disseminated intravascular coagulation (elevated soluble fibrinogen monomeric complexes and fibrin degradation products). There was also an indication of in vivo platelet activation (elevated β-thromboglobulin). The latter phenomenon led investigators from Japan (Ueda, N., et al.: *Nephron* 44:174, 1986) to use a platelet inhibiting agent, dipyridamole, as a treatment for proteinuria. No toxicity was noted with the use of dipyridamole, and many patients had marked decreases in their proteinuria. Presumably, this effect was based on inhibition of platelet adhesion or activation within the kidney itself.

It is a shame that the story relating a tendency toward clotting and the nephrotic syndrome has become so complex. It's like opening a can of worms when you really aren't ready to go fishing. In essence, we have information overload and not a lot of knowledge of what to do with it.—J.A. Stockman III, M.D.

Prediction of the Progression of Chronic Renal Failure in Children: Are Current Models Accurate?
Michael A. Tabak, Peter C. Christenson, and Richard N. Fine (Univ. of California at Los Angeles)
Pediatrics 78:1007–1012, December 1986   10–9

In the past decade, mathematical models have been developed for the purpose of predicting when children with chronic renal failure will need dialysis and kidney transplantation because of end-stage disease. These mathematical models are based on serial determinations of serum creatinine plotted against time. The prospective use of these models was advocated to measure response to treatment in the hope of delaying end-stage renal disease. However, there is controversy about the accuracy of these mathematical models when used for forecasting purposes.

To test the accuracy of predictive mathematical models, a review was made of the case histories of 37 children whose condition progressed to end-stage renal disease. Five of the 24 boys and 13 girls were aged younger than 1 year. Only patients with a creatinine clearance value of between 5 ml/minute/1.73 sq m and 20 ml/minute/1.73 sq m prior to initiation of dialysis were included. The children were grouped according to their respective primary diseases.

Individual patients within each disease category had wide variation in predictive values and, although any individual patient might follow the course predicted by the mathematical model, it was not possible to identify these children prospectively. The findings indicate that predictive models that use serum levels of creatinine are of limited clinical use.

▶ To know or reasonably predict when children with chronic renal failure will need dialysis and kidney transplantation has been desired by many investigators. The eagerness with which this question has been pursued has been comparable (on the part of some) to the search for the holy grail. As this report in *Pediatrics* shows us, that search will have to continue for a while at least. Each patient seems to do his own thing in his own way and in his own good time.

As disappointing as this *Pediatrics* article was, many good things have happened in the past year or so with respect to our understanding of the management of chronic renal failure. For example, the French have developed a new monoclonal antibody. This antibody is not intended to destroy T lymphocytes; rather, the antibody is directed against interleukin-2 receptors. Interleukin-2 is a growth factor needed for T lymphocyte function and acts as a specific high-affinity receptor for the T lymphocyte. The beauty of this particular monoclonal antibody is that it does not alter lymphocyte counts, only the function of lymphocytes. It therefore differs from the existing monoclonal antibodies that are used for rejection of kidneys. The current monoclonal antibodies are against those T cell subsets that are involved with graft rejection, essentially removing them. With antibody against interleukin-2 receptors, the T cells remain but they do not reject. One study has now shown that the graft-kidney-graft rejection rate fell from 67% to approximately 6% with the use of the interleukin monoclonal antibody (Soulillou, J.P.: *Lancet* 1:1339, 1987). Now if rejection seems imminent despite cyclosporine therapy there are a variety of monoclonal antibodies that can be used to help a patient get through the rejection episode.

Another problem that has responded to a novel approach is in the management of patients with chronic renal failure who have severe anemia. Almost all patients with end-stage renal disease undergoing dialysis are anemic and many are transfusion dependent. This ultimately produces problems because of iron overload from the repetitive transfusions. The anemia of chronic renal failure has been thought of mostly as the anemia of chronic disease. Not necessarily so, say Eschback et al. (*N. Engl. J. Med.* 316:73, 1987). These investigators used human erythropoietin made from recombinant technology. High doses of human erythropoietin administered to patients with end-stage renal disease can effectively turn on the bone marrow to produce sufficient numbers of red blood cells to correct the anemia completely. Recombinant human erythropoietin is effective and can eliminate the need for transfusions with the risk of immunologic sensitization, infection, and iron overload, and can restore the hematocrit to normal in many, if not most, patients with the anemia of end-stage renal disease. Certainly, this product will be studied in other conditions to see how well it works.

A few fast facts about other aspects of renal failure: For one, acute peritoneal dialysis is now possible even for the tiny neonate. Thirteen infants weighing less than 1,500 gm underwent simple peritoneal dialysis procedures because of renal failure. The technique, in fact, appears to work (Steele, B.T., et al.: *J. Pediatr.* 110:126, 1987). Another facet of renal transplantation is our better understanding of what happens to living donors who now have only one kidney. Recently, there has been much concern about these donors because in laboratory models removal of a kidney causes increased blood flow to the other kidney, which can result in proteinuria, hypertension, and progressive azotemia. Not necessarily so, say Williams et al. (*Ann. Intern. Med.* 105:1, 1986). They examined kidney donors for periods of 10–20 years and could find no significant difference between the kidney donors and controls with the exception of a mild increase in urinary protein excretion of unknown clinical significance. It should be noted that adults and children who had nephrectomies for reasons other than renal donation have shown no significant renal functional or structural abnormalities when evaluated up to 46 years after surgery.

Regarding cyclosporine, we are seeing a few new aspects of this important drug that is used to prevent kidney rejection. The drug is now being used in other immune-mediated states. For example, preliminary results of a double-blind randomized trial have shown that cyclosporine is an effective therapy in some patients with myasthenia gravis (Tindall, R.S.A.: *N. Engl. J. Med.* 316:719, 1987). The drug also has been formulated by some investigators into a cream and has shown some early promising results in the management of contact dermatitis and alopecia areata. Finally, with respect to cyclosporine, watch out if you're using it in conjunction with verapamil. The latter drug remarkably inhibits cyclosporine metabolism and can cause marked increases in blood levels of cyclosporine (Lindholm, A., et al.: *Lancet* 1:1262, 1987). As a last comment on end-stage renal disease, there are reports of continuing problems with aluminum intoxication in children with end-stage renal disease. Aluminum intoxication in children with renal insufficiency most commonly occurs as a result of the use of aluminum-containing phosphate-binding compounds. The clinical manifestations of aluminum intoxication include vitamin D-resistant osteomalacia, microcytic anemia, and dementia. Recently, the high aluminum content of an infant milk formula was implicated as a cause of aluminum toxicity in two patients with neonatal anemia (Freundlich, M., et al.: *Lancet* 2:527, 1985). A study from Australia examined the variation in aluminum content among infants fed formulas: The variation is huge. Whereas breast milk contains only 30 μg of aluminum per liter, several formulas contain more than 1,000 μg/L. The unfortunate part about this is that if a child does become aluminum intoxicated the only way of getting the drug out may be by intraperitoneal dialysis with desferrioxamine (*Pediatrics* 78:651, 1986). In the 1986 YEAR BOOK OF PEDIATRICS (p. 274) it was queried: "With all the bad luck associated with aluminum these days, can you guess its atomic number?" In case you have forgotten, it still is 13—what an appropriate atomic number for something that causes so many problems!—J.A. Stockman III, M.D.

Vesicoureteral Reflux in Asymptomatic Siblings of Patients With Known Reflux: Radionuclide Cystography

Annick D. Van den Abbeele, S. Ted Treves, Robert L. Lebowitz, Stuart Bauer, Royal T. Davis, Alan Retik, and Arnold Colodny (The Children's Hosp., Boston, and Harvard Univ.)
Pediatrics 79:147–152, January 1987   10–10

The incidence of familial vesicoureteral reflux, symptomatic or asymptomatic, ranges from 8% to 32%. Its incidence was studied in 60 asymptomatic siblings aged 2 months to 15 years (mean, 4.2 years) of patients with known vesicoureteral reflux using radionuclide voiding cystography. Reflux was classified as occurring in the ureter only or reaching the renal pelvis. Vesicoureteral reflux was detected in 27 (45%) siblings; it was unilateral in 15 and bilateral in 12. The male to female ratio was 2:4. In the group with unilateral reflux, 8 of the 15 patients had reflux reaching the renal pelvis, as did 11 of the 12 with bilateral reflux.

Radionuclide voiding cystography allows prospective identification of the early refluxer prior to the first urinary tract infection. It is highly sensitive in the diagnosis of vesicoureteral reflux, but the radiation dose is low (gonadal dose, 1.0–2.0 mrad). All siblings of a known refluxer who are younger than 10 years of age should be screened with radionuclide cystography. Ultrasonography may be used to screen asymptomatic siblings older than age 10 years. Ultrasonographic evaluation of the kidneys should suffice if screening radionuclide reveals mild reflux and drains promptly from the upper urinary tract, whereas a conventional voiding cystourethrogram may be necessary if the child is a boy or if the reflux is severe.

Urolithiasis in Childhood: Current Management

Hwang Choi, Howard M. Snyder III, and John W. Duckett (Seoul Natl. Univ., Korea, and Children's Hosp. of Philadelphia)
J. Pediatr. Surg. 22:158–164, February 1987   10–11

Urinary stone disease in children is relatively rare in the United States. There are geographic variations in the incidence of urinary stones in childhood, and the high incidence of bladder stones reported in Southeast Asia seems to be related to a high-carbohydrate, low-purine diet.

During the past 12 years, 62 children aged 10 months to 15 years with urinary stones were treated at the Children's Hospital of Philadelphia. A positive family history for stones was noted in 13 patients. All patients

TABLE 1.—PRESENTING SYMPTOMS AND SIGNS

	No. of Patients (%)
Abdominal or flank pain	28 (45)
Pyuria	22 (35)
Gross hematuria	13 (21)
Microscopic hematuria	4 (6)
Nausea and vomiting	4 (6)
Fever	3 (5)
Retention	3 (5)
Failure to thrive	1 (2)

(Courtesy of Choi, H., et al.: J. Pediatr. Surg. 22:158–164, February 1987.)

TABLE 2.—LOCATION OF STONES

	No. of Patients (%)	Neurogenic Bladder	Others
Kidney	29 (47)	1	28
Ureter	14 (23)		14
Bladder	15 (24)	12	3
Urethra	2 (3)		2
Vagina	1 (2)	1	
Kidney and bladder	1 (2)	1	
Total	62 (100)	15	47

(Courtesy of Choi, H., et al.: J. Pediatr. Surg. 22:158–164, February 1987.)

had radiologic studies, and most had stone analysis. The most frequent presenting symptoms were abdominal or flank pain, recurrent or persistent pyuria, and gross hematuria (Table 1). Forty-four children had calculi in the upper urinary tract (Table 2), and 22 had associated congenital urologic anomalies (Table 3). Infection-related struvite stones were most common and were found in 18 children, of whom 15 had anatomical abnormalities. Eighteen of 28 patients evaluated for a metabolic cause had an abnormality, usually hypercalciuria. No predisposing factors could be found in 16 children.

Treatment was directed to correction of anatomical and metabolic predisposing conditions, in addition to removing the stones. Fifteen patients passed stones ranging in size from 2 mm to 6 mm. Forty-six surgical procedures were carried out in 43 patients (Table 4, p. 277). Pyelolithotomy and cystolithotomy were the most frequently performed procedures. There were three residual stones and five recurrences. Five patients were lost to follow-up. Of 29 operations for upper urinary stones, 17 might be considered today as suitable for percutaneous nephrostolithotripsy or extracorporeal shock wave lithotripsy. These less invasive methods of stone removal may be helpful in children and lessen the need for open surgical procedures.

TABLE 3.—PREDISPOSING FACTORS AND ASSOCIATED URINARY INFECTION

	No. of Patients (%)	Urinary Infection	Stone Composition						
			O	P	M	S	U	C	N
Congenital urologic anomalies	22 (35)								
Ectopic ureter	1	1				1			
Horseshoe kidney	2		1		1				
UPJ obstruction	2	1	1			1			
UVJ obstruction	1	1				1			
Vesicoureteral reflux	1	1				1			
Bladder exstrophy	1								1
Prune-belly syndrome	1	1				1			
Dysfunctional voiding	1	1				1			
Meningomyelocele	12	12				8			4
Neurogenic bladder, acquired	3 (5)	3		1	2				
Immobilization	2 (3)	1	1		1				
Metabolic causes	18 (29)								
Renal tubular acidosis	2	2				1	1		
Hypercalciuria	9		2		5				2
Hyperuricosuria	1						1		
Cystinuria	1							1	
Intestinal malabsorption	1						1		
Short bowel	1		1						
Steroid administration	3	1				1	1		1
Infection alone	1 (2)	1				1			
Not found (idiopathic)	16*(26)		3	1	3	3			6
Total	62 (100)	26	9	2	12	18	6	1	14

Abbreviations: O, calcium oxalate; P, calcium phosphate; M, mixed calcium oxalate and phosphate; S, struvite; U, uric acid; C, cystine; N, not known; UPJ, ureteropelvic junction; UVJ, ureterovesical junction.

*Six of these 16 patients had a negative metabolic workup.

(Courtesy of Choi, H., et al.: J. Pediatr. Surg. 22:158–164, February 1987.)

Extracorporeal Shock Wave Lithotripsy and Percutaneous Nephrolithotomy in Children

S-A.M. Boddy, M.J. Kellett, M.S. Fletcher, P.G. Ransley, A.M.I. Paris, H.N. Whitfield, and J.E.A. Wickham (London Stone Clinic and Lithotripter Centre and Inst. of Urology, London)

J. Pediatr. Surg. 22:223–227, March 1987 10–12

Only about 100 new pediatric patients with urinary stones are seen each year in the United Kingdom. Most have renal stones secondary to infection. Seventeen children were treated by percutaneous nephrolithotomy, extracorporeal shock wave lithotripsy (ESWL), or a combination of these methods. Ten children underwent percutaneous stone removal. Ultrasonic disintegration of the stone was necessary in a few of these patients. Six children were treated primarily by ESWL, whereas a combination of the two methods was used electively to treat a child with spina bifida who had a staghorn calculus.

The hospital stay for patients having percutaneous nephrolithotomy

TABLE 4.—MODES OF TREATMENT

	No. of Patients (%)
Passed spontaneously	15 (24)
Removed surgically	43 (69)
Pyelolithotomy	19
Nephrolithotomy	3
Partial nephrectomy	3
Ureterolithotomy	4
Cystolithotomy	11
Litholapaxy	3
Urethrolithotomy	1
Meatotomy	1
Removal of vaginal stone	1
Dissolution of cystine stone	1 (2)
Observation	3 (5)
Total	62 (100)

(Courtesy of Choi, H., et al.: J. Pediatr. Surg. 22:158–164, February 1987.)

alone was 3–8 days, and for those having ESWL alone, 3–5 days. Nine children were cleared of stones by nephrolithotomy. The child having combined treatment required further percutaneous nephrolithotomy for residual fragments. Three children were cleared of stones by ESWL alone. Two others were treated too recently to assess stone clearance fully. Minor complications attended both procedures.

Children more than 5 years of age can safely undergo percutaneous removal of renal stones. Use of the lithotripter also is feasible in many children. The hospital stay is much shorter with these methods than with open surgery, and the convalescent period is greatly reduced. Complication rates are lower when experienced operators perform the procedures. One third of the children can be expected to have underlying urologic abnormalities, and less invasive treatment makes subsequent surgery less dangerous.

▶ The preceding two articles (Abstracts 10–11 and 10–12) tell us a great deal about renal stones in kidneys. The second of the two is a real shocker.

Infection still seems to be the predominant cause of renal stones, even in children. Many of these infections presumably are related to anatomical defects that would also result in poor urinary flow and consequent calculus formation. Among the metabolic causes of stone formation that were uncovered, hypercalciuria, as one might suspect, was the most prevalent.

In the second report, the entire gamut of methodologies for stone removal was discussed. Stones now can be removed in children by a percutaneous nephrolithotomy technique done under general anesthesia. A needle is inserted into the renal pelvis percutaneously through the back. Over the needle, dilators are passed and then, ultimately, a grasping forceps, which is used to pull out a stone or stones.

The most recent development, of course, is ESWL, a fascinating technique. A shock wave is generated by passing an ultrashort high tension electrical discharge underwater to form an arc between two electrodes. The fluid surrounding the arc path vaporizes to form a rapidly expanding gas bubble. As a result of this rapid expansion, a shock wave is created in the surrounding fluid that radiates from its source in a circular manner. These shock waves can be accurately focused to produce a high tensile pressure precisely at a very small area on the body. If you think this hurts, you're absolutely right. It is probably the worst kidney punch anyone could ever get. The procedure, in fact, must be performed under general anesthesia.

In case you're worried that there aren't other reports of the use of lithotripsy in children, fear not. Another study was recently published in which this technique was used in 14 patients under the age of 18 (Cramolowsky, E.V., et al.: J. Urol. 137:939, 1987). I've never had a chance to see lithotripsy in action. As soon as I get up the nerve I'll go and learn how this interesting technology works first hand. I think I'll stand back quite a ways though and bring along a couple of shock absorbers.—J.A. Stockman III, M.D.

Epididymitis in Children and Adolescents: A 20-Year Retrospective Study
Sasithorn Likitnukul, George H. McCracken, Jr., John D. Nelson, and Theodore P. Votteler (Univ. of Texas at Dallas)
Am. J. Dis. Child. 141:41–44, January 1987   10–13

Although epididymitis among adults is common, it is considered rare among prepubertal boys. However, awareness of its occurrence is essential in evaluation of the child with acute scrotal swelling. A review was made of experience with 35 boys aged 8 days to 17 years treated for epididymitis from 1965 through 1984. Twenty-two patients had involvement on the right side, 11 had involvement on the left side, and 2 had bilateral involvement.

Symptoms included swelling, pain, erythema, nausea, vomiting, urinary symptoms, and fever. The duration of symptoms before hospital admission ranged from a few hours to several weeks, but 22 patients (63%) had onset of symptoms within 24 hours of hospital admission. Surgery was performed in 31 patients; in 22 cases cultures were taken from the epididymis at the time of surgery. No patient was treated with antibiotics prior to surgery.

Positive bacterial cultures were obtained from 13 patients; coagulase-negative staphylococci were found in 9. Two patients had multiple bacteria in their cultures. Four had abnormal findings on intravenous pyelography and six had abnormal findings on voiding cystourethrograms. Of 11 patients with abnormal findings at urinalysis, 3 had concurrent urinary tract infections. Although epididymitis is considered to be rare in prepubertal boys, urologic examination should be performed in all children with scrotal swelling who are younger than age 2 years and in all older patients who have recurrent episodes possibly as a result of reflux of urine and associated genitourinary tract abnormalities.

▶ The causes of epididymitis can be classified as follows: (1) bacterial, (2) viral, (3) traumatic, (4) chemical (reflux of urine into the ejaculatory ducts), (5) associated with systemic diseases, e.g., sarcoidosis, Kawasaki syndrome, or Henoch-Schönlein purpura, or (6) idiopathic. The most common causes of epididymitis in older men (more than 35 years of age) are gram-negative bacilli, whereas sexually transmitted organisms (e.g., *Chlamydia* and *Neisseria*) are responsible for a higher portion of episodes in the slightly younger man. In the series reported above, seven patients did have gram-negative organisms as a cause of epididymitis. Half of these were associated with urinary tract infections. Several patients had abnormal urinary tracts on urologic examination. Although it is rare, *Salmonella* has been reported as a cause of testicular infection. *Hemophilus influenzae* type b has also been reported as a cause, but it is usually only one manifestation of systemic illness. The significance of coagulase-negative staphylococci cultured from eight patients in this series is debatable. About half of the patients had no definite or probable predisposing factor; however, viral studies were not done.

The most important aspect of epididymitis is the overlapping clinical picture of this inflammation state with torsion of the testis or its appendix. Although testicular scanning and Doppler ultrasonic tests have been reported to improve diagnostic accuracy, the differential diagnosis has not always been possible between these two entities without surgical exploration. If epididymitis is the clinical diagnosis, urine should be cultured and, in infants, blood as well. Initial empiric treatment with antibiotics appropriate for gram-negative and gram-positive bacteria should be started after culture specimens are obtained if an obvious bacterial cause seems to be present. Otherwise, the results of cultures should be awaited, because the systemic effects of epididymitis are usually minimal. Urologic evaluation consisting of an intravenous pyelography and vesicourethrography is indicated in children younger than 2 years of age and in older patients with recurrent episodes of epididymitis suspected to be caused by reflux of urine. Fortunately, testicular atrophy after epididymitis in boys is rare, and the prognosis in children seems to be much more favorable than in adults.

As noted, the most important aspect of the care of these children is making the differential diagnosis between epididymitis and torsion of the testis. If torsion is suspected, one can go ahead and do the noninvasive studies to diagnose this. However, if there will be any delay because of these studies, it is probably preferable to go right to the operating room. The next issue concerns what should be done with a testis that has had an insult in terms of a cut-off blood supply. Recent evidence (Madarikan, B.A.: *J. Pediatr. Surg.* 22:231, 1987) suggests that if one testis is severely damaged and is left in situ, there may be autoimmune damage to the contralateral testis. This is similar in concept to contralateral autoimmune damage in the eye after injury to the opposite eye. In Madarikan's study, pubescent rats were evaluated. Several ways were found to protect the contralateral testis, one of which was by removal of the damaged testis. Obviously, in human beings we would like to preserve that testis unless it is absolutely "shot" at the time of exploration. Other ways of protecting the contralateral testis were with the use of hydrocortisone, azathioprine, or cyclosporine. The safest among these was a 5-day course of steroids that was completely protective of the normal kidney. I think we shall be hearing a great deal more about this phenomenon of contralateral autoimmune orchitis following torsion of a testis.

We men seem to have great reverence for the objects of these discussions. When you think about it, this reverence may not be well placed. Did you know, for example, that 0.5 cc of human semen is worth only about half as much as 0.5 cc of a Holstein bull's semen ($40.00 vs. $75.00)? Do you know which has a larger testis, man or a Great Dane? It's the Great Dane (45 gm vs. 19 gm).—J.A. Stockman III, M.D.

Undescended Testis: The Effect of Treatment on Subsequent Risk of Subfertility and Malignancy

Clair Chilvers, N.E. Dudley, M.H. Gough, M.B. Jackson, and M.C. Pike (Inst. of Cancer Res., Sutton, John Radcliffe Hosp., Oxford, and Radcliffe Infirmary, Oxford, England)
J. Pediatr. Surg. 21:691–696, August 1986   10–14

At present, 15% of operations for undescended testis are carried out before age 3 years, a further 18% are performed between ages 3 and 5 years, and 50% are carried out before age 7 years. Orchidopexy is performed to reduce the possibility of infertility and the risk of testicular cancer, and for psychological reasons. The literature was reviewed for information on the long-term effects of cryptorchidism on fertility and cancer incidence.

In unilateral cryptorchidism, orchidopexy alone, and human chorionic gonadotropin therapy followed if necessary by orchidopexy, have resulted in similar levels of reduced fertility (15% azoospermia and another 30% oligospermia). Results were closely similar in unilaterally cryptorchid men who had no treatment (and were still cryptorchid at the time of semen examination). Conversely, no untreated bilaterally cryptorchid men had normal fertility, whereas of those treated, one fourth had normal fertility. In some series, as many as half of bilaterally cryptorchid testes descended after hormone treatment, a finding probably resulting from the frequent difficulty in deciding, on clinical examination, whether these testes were truly cryptorchid. Operation early rather than late within the age range of 4 and 14 years does not affect subsequent fertility. Histologic studies indicate that orchidopexy should be carried out before age 2, but there are no follow-up data with which to evaluate the results of early operation. Because there is evidence in a small number of cases that orchidopexy may lead to testicular atrophy, a trial of luteinizing hormone-releasing hormone is recommended.

Little information was found concerning the effect of age at orchidopexy on subsequent risk of testicular cancer. Testes that cannot be brought into the scrotum should be excised.

▶ The preceding article is a classic example of armchair research. What these investigators did was to review 27 papers that considered adult fertility in patients who had an undescended testis. Furthermore, they examined 27 papers that reported the occurrence of cryptorchidism in a series of testicular cancer patients. Put any ten people into a room with 54 papers and you're bound to come up with differing conclusions. Thus, the validity of the interpretation of these papers is open to criticism.

What the authors are suggesting is that the literature gives no indication that orchidopexy does anything to improve fertility in a patient with unilateral undescended testis. About 15% of patients remain azoospermic and 30% will be oligospermic. For those with bilateral undescended testes, there was improvement in fertility with orchidopexy. However, the authors note that many bilateral undescended testes, in fact, are simply retractile testes and thus do not have decreased production of sperm in any event.

With regard to cancer, although it is unequivocal that there is an increased risk of testicular cancer in patients with undescended testes, there is no information at all to suggest that this risk is decreased by orchidopexy done at any age. That is not to say that doing the procedure earlier is not beneficial, just that there are few data to substantiate this. There are at present virtually no follow-up data concerning fertility, malignancy, or testicular atrophy in boys having an orchidopexy when very young. These authors suggest that the current practice of operating at age 4 or 5 years as is done in Great Britain appears to be justifiable, but long-term follow-up of a group of boys treated at around 1 year of age is needed if there is going to be any further understanding of this problem with all of its ramifications. It is also interesting to note that the use of human chorionic gonadotropin (hCG) was recommended, especially in bilaterally affected patients. The merit of hCG or luteinizing hormone-releasing hormone is that these agents may allow the testes to descend without the patient undergoing the risk of orchidopexy, which in fact can damage an otherwise normal testis in a small percentage of cases. A review of 724 patients with testicular cancer seen at the Royal Marsdon Hospital in a 10-year period also has shown that the age at treatment of undescended testes appears to have no effect on the risk of testicular cancer (Pike, M.C., et al.: *Lancet* 1:1246, 1986).

While on the topic of undescended testes, there was an interesting report this past year (Schiffer, K.A., et al.: *Am. J. Dis. Child.* 141:106, 1987) that dealt with the problem of "acquired undescended testes." Now the classic teaching is that boys born with both testes fully descended are not at further risk for the development of cryptorchidism. In each of three cases, the boys under discussion were unequivocally found to have descended testes in the first few months of life. However, as the boys grew, one of the two testes was subsequently found to be high up in the inguinal canal and could not be brought down on physical examination. One of the three responded promptly to hCG and the other two required surgery. This phenomenon indeed must be rare and is called "testicular reascent." The assumption with these testes is that there is a differential body growth with failure of elongation of the spermatic cord. If that is true, then I would prefer to call this the "tethered testis syndrome." These are apparently definitely different from the retractile testes, which I prefer to call the "yo-yo testes" or the "bouncing ball syndrome." (Apologies.)—J.A. Stockman III, M.D.

Hematospermia in Adolescents and Young Adults

Tomas J. Silber and Maria Kastrinakis (Children's Hosp. Natl. Med. Ctr., Washington, D.C., and George Washington Univ.)
Pediatrics 78:708–710, October 1986   10–15

Hematospermia, or blood in the ejaculate, has never been described in the pediatric or adolescent literature. Three such patients aged 14 years, 21 years, and in young adulthood, were the only ones seen during a period of 15 years with this condition. All three were healthy, had no prior genitourinary tract symptoms, and denied a past history of urinary tract infection, venereal disease, prostatitis, renal calculus, or previous instrumentation. Prostatitis was diagnosed in two patients, although infection was not confirmed. All three patients experienced recurrences over periods of weeks to years, ending in spontaneous resolution.

Hematospermia is a condition that can provoke extreme anxiety, but it is usually benign and self-limiting. Clinical assessment is sufficient in evaluation of a patient with uncomplicated hematospermia. Treatment consists of supportive follow-up, with emphasis on the benign nature of the hematospermia.

▶ Actually, despite what the abstract says, blood in the ejaculate, known as hematospermia or hemospermia, was described by both Galen and Ambroise Pare (Parker, G.: *Proc. R. Soc. Med.* 35:659, 1942). In the United States it was first reported by Lydston in 1894, who attributed the condition to "unbridled license." The authors suggest that the adolescent who seeks medical attention for a complaint of blood in his ejaculate should be evaluated with the knowledge that significant disease is exceptional. If he is otherwise asymptomatic; his external genitalia, prostate, and seminal vesicles are normal on examination; and his urinalysis and appropriate cultures for sexually transmitted diseases are negative, no further workup is required because the disease, if it is a disease, appears to be benign and self-limited. I really cannot add anything to the above comments. I know very little about hematospermia except I would speculate that it is extremely anxiety provoking. I would also add the comment that you can reassure these patients that hematospermia is better than no spermia at all.—J.A. Stockman III, M.D.

11 The Respiratory Tract

Treatment of Tracheomalacia: Eight Years' Experience
G.K. Blair, R. Cohen, and R.M. Filler (Hosp. for Sick Children, Toronto)
J. Pediatr. Surg. 21:781–785, September 1986   11–1

Tracheomalacia is often seen in association with esophageal atresia and tracheoesophageal fistula or other thoracic lesions, but is may also occur in isolation. The trachea is soft and collapsible, and severely affected children may have apneic episodes with cyanosis and bradycardia. Recurrent pneumonia is also a problem. Twenty patients were treated for tracheomalacia (group I) and four for tracheobronchomalacia (group II) between 1978 and 1985. The five children with cardiovascular anomalies (table) also had esophageal atresia.

Most group I patients were operated on for life-threatening "dying spells" occurring during or shortly after feeding. Four patients had multiple episodes of pneumonia previously. All group II patients had severe pulmonary parenchymal disease. Aortopexy alone eliminated airway collapse in 15 of 19 group I patients. Another infant with an unrecognized vascular ring had recurrent spells and died unexpectedly after a meal. In two group I patients a tracheal splint was implanted, preventing airway collapse and relieving obstructive symptoms. Splint removal was necessary in one of these. All surviving group I patients were free from significant respiratory symptoms a median of 4 years after operation. Two of three group II patients were not extubated after aortopexy alone and have since died. A patient who also had splint placement could not be extubated and died.

External airway splinting may be used when aortopexy alone is inadequate in patients with tracheomalacia. Treatment of tracheobronchomalacia is more difficult, but aortopexy may relieve tracheal collapse and reduce expiratory airway resistance in this condition, reducing the tendency toward bronchial collapse.

ASSOCIATED ANOMALIES

Associated Anomalies	Group I Tracheomalacia (n = 21)	Group II Tracheobronchomalacia (n = 4)
Esophageal atresia and TEF	18	0
Cardiovascular	5	1
Other	0	1*

*Cervical teratoma.
(Courtesy of Blair, G.K., et al.: J. Pediatr. Surg. 21:781–785, September 1986.)

Respiratory Illnesses in Survivors of Infant Respiratory Distress Syndrome

Martin G. Myers, Gail A. McGuinness, Peter A. Lachenbruch, Franklin P. Koontz, Rachel Hollingshead, and Daniel B. Olson (Univ. of Iowa and Children's Hosp. Res. Found., Cincinnati)

Am. Rev. Respir. Dis. 133:1011–1018, June 1986   11–2

An increasing number of infants now survive respiratory distress syndrome (RDS), but many are thought to be at increased risk of frequent, severe respiratory illnesses. The extent of this risk was examined in a prospective study of respiratory morbidity in preterm infants surviving RDS, preterm infants without RDS, and groups of term infants matched with the study groups for sex, date of birth, and the presence or absence of preadolescent siblings in the home. Twenty-two preterm infants with RDS and 17 without RDS participated.

No significant increase in respiratory illnesses was documented in the preterm infants with RDS within a year of discharge (Table 1). Lower respiratory illnesses were more severe in RDS survivors than in matched term infants. Lower respiratory illnesses also occurred earlier in this group. A survivor of RDS with residual lung disease had more frequent and more severe lower respiratory illnesses than those without persistent roentgenographic abnormalities. Similar agents were recovered from nasal wash cultures in all groups of infants (Table 2).

Any risk of respiratory illness in survivors of RDS appears not to be

TABLE 1.—Frequency and Severity of Respiratory Illnesses Occurring After Discharge From the Hospital of Preterm and Full-Term Infants

	Preterm Infants		Full-term Infants Matched to	
	RDS	No-RDS	RDS	No-RDS
First 6 months				
Infants, n	19	13	18	10
URI, n	3 (0–5)*	3 (0–4)†	3 (0–7)	3 (1–4)
LRI, n	0 (0–3)	0 (0–2)	0 (0–5)	0 (0–1)
RI, n	4 (0–5)	3 (0–4)‡	3 (0–7)	3 (1–4)
First 12 months				
Infants, n	18	7	17	4
URI, n	7 (3–11)	6 (3–11)‡	7 (0–11)	7.5 (4–8)
LRI, n	2 (0–3)	0 (0–2)	0 (0–7)	0 (0–2)
RI, n	7 (3–11)	6 (3–11)‡	7 (0–11)	7.5 (4–8)
Mean severity of URI	2 (1.2–2.8)	1.9 (1.3–2.5)	2.1 (0–2.8)	1.9 (1.5–2.6)
Mean severity of LRI	2.5 (0–3.5)§	0 (0–3.5)	0 (0–3)	0 (0–3)
Mean severity of RI	2 (1.5–2.8)	1.9 (1.3–2.5)	2.1 (0–2.8)‖	1.9 (1.5–2.6)

*Median (range). Differences for RDS and No-RDS case-control pairs were not significant ($P > .20$) by two-tailed, paired t test except where noted. There were 15 and 13 RDS and 9 and 2 No-RDS case-control pairs in the first 6 and 12 months, respectively.
†$P = .11$
‡$P = .07$. When illnesses were adjusted for length of time on study, $P = .01$ for 11 case-control pairs.
§$P = .11$. When illnesses were adjusted for length on study, $P = .03$ for 16 case-control pairs.
‖Two infants who had no illnesses were assigned a severity of 0.
(Courtesy of Myers, M.G., et al.: Am. Rev. Respir. Dis. 133:1011–1018, June 1986.)

TABLE 2.—Illnesses Associated With Agents Recovered From Nasal Wash Culture From Study Infants

	URI Only*		LRI†		Other Febrile Illness‡		Asymptomatic	
	Preterm	Full-term	Preterm	Full-term	Preterm	Full-term	Preterm	Full-term
Respiratory syncytial virus	2	4	4	2				1
Parainfluenza virus	2	4	1	1		1	6	2
Adenovirus	3§	5‖					1	1
Rhinovirus	3	5	2				3	1
Enterovirus¶	1	3				1		1
Influenza A virus	1		1				1	1
Herpes simplex virus	1							
Cytomegalovirus	1§							
Varicella zoster virus**	1				1			
Chlamydia trachomatis		1‖					1	

*Excludes children with simultaneous LRI.
†Includes children with simultaneous URI.
‡One preterm and two full-term infants had occult pneumococcal bacteremia.
§both cytomegalovirus and adenovirus recovered from a child with otitis media.
‖Both *C. trachomatis* and adenovirus recovered.
¶Vaccine-strain poliovirus recovered from 2 additional asymptomatic children.
**One child with varicella and associated otitis media.
(Courtesy of Myers, M.G., et al.: Am. Rev. Respir. Dir. 133:1011–1018, June 1986.)

related to birth at an early gestational age. Earlier and more severe lower respiratory illnesses in RDS survivors are associated with residual lung disease, because similar risks are not found in preterm infants without RDS.

▶ We are obviously seeing an increasing number of infants who survive RDS. For a long time it has been believed that many of these surviving infants, with or without x-ray residua, are at increased risk for the development of more frequent and more severe subsequent respiratory illnesses than are preterm infants without RDS. This study, which was carefully controlled and matched, was unable to demonstrate any increased risk of respiratory illness frequency for preterm infants with or without RDS when compared with term infants matched for sex, date of birth, and the presence of young children within the home. Specifically, both the frequency and the agents associated with respiratory illnesses were similar in both groups. The difference was, however, that RDS survivors experienced their first lower respiratory tract illness sooner and had increased severity of lower respiratory illness than did full-term control infants.

It should be noted that, among the data derived from this study, no differences in respiratory morbidity were found between breast-fed and formula-fed infants. Obviously, critically ill newborns with RDS may not have received breast milk, particularly early in their lives (more on this in a moment). It was also noted that many survivors of RDS have been exposed to multiple transfusions and might have postnatally acquired cytomegalovirus lung infections. But there was no evidence in this study to account for the postdischarge severity of lower respiratory illness. From this study I think it is fairly clear that it is RDS and its sequelae that place premature infants at risk for more severe lower respiratory illness subsequent to discharge. Premature infants who are fortunate enough to make it through the nursery without this complication seem to do perfectly well in this regard.

There are several kinds of infections that one wishes these infants not contract, the most obvious, of course, being respiratory syncytial virus (RSV) infection. Premature infants with residual lung disease are certainly candidates for the use of ribavirin, and it does appear to be effective in helping to control the duration of symptomatology (Conrad, D.A., et al.: *Pediatr. Infect. Dis. J.* 6:152, 1987). The latter study in particular notes the safety of this agent. Similar results were shown by Rodriguez et al. (*Pediatr. Infect. Dis. J.* 6:159, 1987). When you pull out the ribavirin, you would do well to note the words on the package insert so that you don't necessarily overuse this drug. That insert says: "The vast majority of infants and children with RSV infection have no lower respiratory tract disease or have disease that is mild, self-limited, and does not require hospitalization or antiviral treatment." The guidelines for the use of ribavirin, although not entirely clear-cut, do indicate that it is best used for infants who are at high risk for serious infection (those with cardiopulmonary disease, or progressive pulmonary involvement, and perhaps those with underlying immune abnormalities).

Because this drug is aerosolized, a number of hospital personnel, particularly nurses, often express concern over the teratogenic effects of ribavirin described in animals. Indeed, although there are no human data, ribavirin has been found to be teratogenic in nearly all species in which it was examined. This kind of information must be shared with all hospital personnel but with appropriate guidelines as to its significance. It obviously cannot and should not be made "confidential." Anyway, if something is confidential, you can be sure it will be left in the copier machine.

Certainly, any child with significant pulmonary residual disease after RDS who has evidence of RSV is a candidate for ribavirin therapy. In healthy children, RSV can produce residual lung disease. Its effects in RDS survivors can only be worse. We have also recently become aware of the fact that *Chlamydia trachomatis* can also cause residual lung disease after infection, but this may not show up for some years (Weiss, S.G., et al.: *J. Pediatr.* 108:659, 1986). Adenovirus-caused lower respiratory tract disease may very well do the same thing. Fortunately, pertussis does not seem to have any lasting effects on lung function and bronchial reactivity (Johnston, I.D.A., et al.: *Am. Rev. Respir. Dis.* 134:270, 1986).

Although breast-feeding may not protect these infants from subsequent lower respiratory tract illness, there is increasing evidence that it may be protective of subsequent wheezing episodes in infants. McConnochie et al. (*Pediatr. Pulmonol.* 2:260, 1986) noted that among children in whom a family history of allergy is negative, non-breast-feeding does increase the number of wheezing episodes. In this same study, in children in whom the family history was positive for allergy, maternal smoking significantly increased wheezing among infants and children.

The latter part of the preceding paragraph allows this author to make one or two comments about asthma, which is generally dealt with in the allergy and immunology chapter. Exercise-induced asthma has always fascinated me, and recently we have seen some suggestions that acupuncture is able to reduce by almost half the fall in FEV_1 and FVC in asthmatics stressed by exercise (Fung, K.P., et al.: *Lancet* 2:1419, 1986). If you want to give this type of therapy a whirl, insert a needle in the acupoint called *dingechuan,* which is located 0.5 CUN lateral to the midpoint between C7 and T1 spinus processes. This is a specific point for asthma in the practice of traditional Chinese medicine. You also have to put a needle at *kongzui* (7 CUN above the wrist crease on the radial aspect of the forearm) and at *taixi* (located midway between the medial malleolus and the tendocalcaneus). Before you start needling somebody, recognize two factors: First, one CUN is a unit of length with reference to the dimensions of the patient and equals approximately 3 cm; second, realize that acupuncture in the treatment of exercise-induced asthma is about as likely to be successful as a coat check concession in a nudist colony. I rather doubt that anyone can run very far with a needle sticking out of his neck, forearm, or ankle. Just remember where there's a will, there's a won't.—J.A. Stockman III, M.D.

Neonatal Diagnosis of the Immotile Cilia Syndrome

Joseph Ramet, Jeannine Byloos, Marc Delree, Liliane Sacre, and Peter Clement (Vrije Universiteit Brussel, Brussels)
Chest 90:138–140, July 1986   11–3

The immotile cilia syndrome is a congenital, probably recessively inherited disorder characterized by recurrent bronchitis, sinusitis, nasal polyposis, otitis, mastoiditis, and reduced fertility. About half of affected

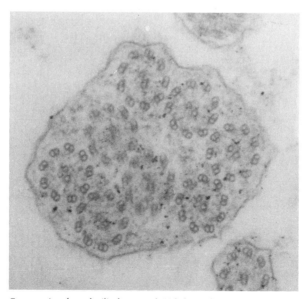

Fig 11–1.—Cross-section through cilia from nasal epithelium of patient. Note compound cilia. (Courtesy of Ramet, J., et al.: Chest 90:138–140, July 1986.)

patients have sinus inversus. A neonate was seen in whom immotile cilia syndrome was documented on the third day of life.

Male, born to a healthy mother after a normal pregnancy, had tachypnea and retractions 2 days after birth. Dextrocardia was observed, but there were no x-ray signs of pulmonary disease. Lung maturation was normal. Bronchoscopy and ultrasonography showed total situs inversus. Nasal biopsy on the third day of life showed absent dynein arms from the outer doublets and an abnormal orientation of cilia (Fig 11–1). Compound and other abnormal cilia were seen. Phase-contrast microscopic study of a second biopsy revealed that only a few ciliated cells were motile and that ciliary beating was uncoordinated. Physiotherapy was performed twice daily. The child had no pulmonary or ear, nose, and throat infections during 37 months of follow-up.

The changes in ciliary ultrastructure in this child must be congenital. Early diagnosis may be important, because appropriate measures may delay or prevent the onset of bronchiectasis. Neonates with respiratory distress should undergo early study of the ciliary ultrastructure if immotile cilia syndrome is suspected.

▶ It has been estimated that the number of scientific and technologic articles published each day worldwide is about 17,000. This is the first that I have ever seen that dealt with the topic of the immotile cilia syndrome in the neonatal period. This is a disorder that is usually missed until later in life. As you may be aware, the immotile cilia syndrome is characterized by an inappropriate motility of the cilia in the airways and any other ciliated organ of the body. Electron microscopy shows architectural abnormalities in the cilia. You don't have to take a biopsy specimen from way down in the respiratory tract. A simple nasal biopsy specimen will do. These investigators also helped us by performing ultrastructural studies on the cilia of a healthy newborn as well, showing that a normal structural pattern is seen in normal infants. They also found that various neonatal pulmonary diseases of the common nursery variety were not associated with structural abnormalities.

The implications of this report, I think, are fairly obvious. We should be doing ciliary biopsies more frequently in infants who have respiratory disease that is not well explained, and certainly in those who have part of the syndrome complex that frequently includes immotile cilia (the situs inversus complex). A note of caution is in order, however. About 5% of the cilia in healthy children and adults can have ultrastructural abnormalities, and Lee and Rossman (*Am. Rev. Respir. Dis.* 129:190, 1984) described an infant with hyaline membrane disease associated with ciliary defects; the lesions disappeared over time, however, so that this was not a true case of the immotile cilia syndrome. Nonspecific structural changes can be seen in patients with asthma and sinusitis and in some smokers. As far as ciliary function is concerned, simple upper respiratory tract disease can cause a wipeout of the cilia and their function.

The point of all this, I hope, is to make us more aware of the fact that when we have babies in our nurseries with complex courses that involve less than straightforward respiratory tract complications, maybe we should be doing more ciliary biopsies. After all, these babies are around for a long time, so perhaps we can expend a little more effort thinking about these rare birds once in awhile.

While speaking of effort and time, recall the Edward's Law of Time/Effort, which reads as follows:

Effort X Time = Constant

    a. Given a large initial time to do something, the initial effort will be small.

    b. As the time goes to zero, the effort goes to infinity.

The obvious corollary to Edward's Law is this: "If it weren't for the last minute, nothing would get done."—J.A. Stockman III, M.D.

A Three-Year Cohort Study of the Role of Environmental Factors in the Respiratory Health of Children in Hamilton, Ontario: Epidemiologic Survey Design, Methods, and Description of Cohort

Anthony T. Kerigan, Charles H. Goldsmith, and L. David Pengelly (McMaster Univ., Hamilton, Ontario)

Am. Rev. Respir. Dis. 133:987–993, June 1987   11–4

A cohort study was carried out to assess the relative roles of certain outdoor environmental factors (e.g., suspended particulates and sulfur dioxide) and indoor factors (e.g., parental smoking and gas cooking) on the respiratory health of children. An interviewer-administered questionnaire was used to obtain data in Hamilton, Ontario, in 1978–1981. The 3,345 children, aged 7–10 years, studied in the first year represented a response rate of 95%. About 76% of the initial group were restudied in both the second and third years. Pulmonary function was assessed from forced expiration and both single-breath and multiple-breath nitrogen washout measurements.

Nearly 5% of the children smoked in the third year of the study. The prevalence of parental smoking and gas cooking was highest in an industrial region with the highest particulate pollution. Repeatability was acceptable apart from variables derived from the single-breath nitrogen washout study.

A comprehensive network of air quality monitors provided accurate estimates of pollution exposure. A nonuniform distribution of such covariables as parental smoking complicates detection of the effects of environmental pollutants, particularly when the effects of current levels of pollutants are likely to be small.

▶ One of the obvious problems in this study is clearly noted by its authors: It is difficult to demonstrate the relative effect of outdoor environmental factors such as suspended particulates and sulfur dioxide, and indoor factors such as gas cooking when these environmental factors tend to be overwhelmed by passive smoking among our children. The passive smoking, of course, is related to smoking on the part of parents or other individuals occupying the child's environment.

One cannot turn around and not find something written about the dirty weed tobacco. There has been a rapid rise in the use of smokeless tobacco among teenagers. Among native American adolescents there has been a veritable explosion in its use. Forty percent of all native American adolescent girls and almost 50% of boys have reported using snuff or chewing tobacco on at least 20 occasions (Schink, S.P.: *JAMA* 257:781, 1987). The role of the pediatrician in regulating tobacco use by children and adolescents was the topic of some discussion recently in *Pediatrics* (79:479, 1987) in a commentary by the Committee on Adolescents of the American Academy of Pediatrics. This should be on everyone's reading list. This is especially true at a time when we are learning more about the consequences of cigarette smoking. Cutting down on cigarettes, say, from an average of 37 cigarettes per day to only 5 cigarettes per day (Benowitz, N.L., et al.: *N. Engl. J. Med.* 315:1310, 1986), doesn't produce as much of an effect as you might think. If you attempt to figure out what the reduction would be in terms of exposure to tar, nicotine, and carbon monoxide, you would come up with the conclusion that you should reduce your intake of tobacco toxins to about 15% or so of what you were originally taking in. Not so, says this study from the *New England Journal of Medicine*. The overall reduction is only about 50%. It is assumed that the intake of tobacco toxins per cigarette actually increased by threefold to account for this discrepancy. Obviously, what these smokers were doing was "dragging" down the butt of the cigarette to a shorter length. Unfortunately, as cigarettes are smoked to shorter lengths, the delivery of tar and carbon monoxide increases logrithmetically while nicotine increases arithmetically. Perhaps we shouldn't be attempting to break habits, but rather to start habits. One such beneficial habit might be to kick the butts of the cigarette companies' chief executive officers once in a while.

This is not to say that attempting to lower one's smoke intake is not good and that people aren't doing it. Indeed, they are. In the last 4 years there has been a decline in the number of smokers here in the United States. The greatest percent decrease is in the District of Columbia (8.1%). For the record, the state of Utah has the best smoking record; only 13% of Utah's adult population smokes, compared with a national average of 26%. Idaho was the next closest at 19.9%. Only four states in the United States have shown a rise in the percent of smokers (Ohio, New York, Indiana, and Montana) (Editorial comment: *JAMA* 257:165, 1987).

If you are attempting to stop smoking, there are two now demonstrated effective ways of doing it. Nicotine gum does appear to be cost effective. It has been shown that the cost per year of lives saved with this intervention ranges from $4,103 to $6,465 for men and from $6,880 to $9,473 for women, depending on age. (Oster, G., et al.: *JAMA* 256:1315, 1986; unfortunately, this study did not enter into the economic data regarding the additional cost of dental care necessitated by replacement of fillings). Also, clonidine may be useful in decreasing the craving for cigarettes in those who are trying to stop (Pearce, K.I.: *Lancet* 1:810, 1986).

Never let it be said that this commentator did not present the opposite side of this picture, i.e., the beneficial effects of smoke as documented in the literature. One such beneficial effect is the fact that when appropriately controlled for, infants born of mothers who smoke have a reduced incidence of the respiratory distress syndrome. Smoking on the part of the mother is equivalent to a 1.5-week acceleration in lung maturity for their infants (White, E.: *Obstet. Gynecol.* 67:365, 1986). This study adds support to the theory that adverse pregnancy conditions may lead to an acceleration in pulmonary maturity and allow earlier extrauterine adaptation. If stress is what is needed, a pregnant woman who smokes might have been better off if she stopped smoking and just shot herself in the foot. One benefit of smoking that cannot be denied is the fact that cigarette smoking has a very potent antiestrogenic effect. (Michnovicz, J.J., et al.: *N. Engl. J. Med.* 315:1305, 1986). This antiestrogenic effect also results in a decreased risk of endometrial cancer (Editorial comment. *Lancet* 2:1433, 1986). One last potential benefit of smoking may be a decreased risk for the development of ulcerative colitis (Boyko, E.J., et al.: *N. Engl. J. Med.* 316:707, 1987). Smokers have 0.6 times the chance of ulcerative colitis developing compared with nonsmokers. However, among former smokers the risk of ulcerative colitis is 2.0 times higher than in nonsmokers. Before running out to buy a pack of cigarettes, realize that these data most likely result from the fact that people who smoke a great deal probably don't have time to go to the bathroom. In any event, smoking doesn't immunize anyone against ulcerative colitis, because if you have smoked and then stopped, your risk of ulcerative colitis actually increases. Unfortunately, I'm sure some smart advertising firm for a cigarette company will read the aforementioned *New England Journal of Medicine* article and incorporate this into some ad copy. We can see it now: "The Marlboro man doesn't have ulcerative colitis, do you?" This isn't as far fetched as it seems. For the period from 1974 through 1984, total expenditures increased by approximately threefold, even after adjustment for the consumer price index, in the area of cigarette advertising. The fastest growing markets in advertising are for discounted cigarettes and for brands containing 25 cigarettes per pack instead of the traditional 20.

In 1984, cigarette manufacturers spent $2.1 billion in advertising. The entire amount that the United States government spent for all of its advertising in the same year was exactly 10% of that and obviously only a fraction went for the campaign against smoking. What did the cigarette manufacturers' $2.1 billion buy? It bought smoking-related diseases annually accounting for $22 billion in health care costs and $43 billion in lost productivity. It bought reports linking sore throats in children to parental smoking (Willat, D.J.: *Clin. Otolaryngol.* 11:317, 1986). It bought a better definition of the relationship between passive smoking and wheezing in children (Burchfield, C.M., et al.: *Am. Rev. Respir. Dis.* 133:966, 1986). It bought a study that clearly shows that infants of breast-feeding mothers have distinctive amounts of cotinine and nicotine in their urine (Woodward, A., et al.: *J. Epidemiol. Community Health* 40:309, 1986). It resulted in a study that has documented that smoking during pregnancy increases the level of fetal thyroid function, perhaps accounting for an increased metabolic rate in oxygen consumption in such infants (Meberg, A., et al.: *Acta. Paediatr. Scand.* 75:762, 1986). It also resulted in another study showing that maternal smoking exerts a pronounced effect on the IgE system in fetal life (*J. Allergy Clin. Immunol.* 78:898, 1986); and lastly, and fortunately, it has resulted in public health laws now having been passed that, in several states, clearly ban the sale of tobacco to individuals under the age of 18 years. Less than fortunate, however, is the fact that these laws don't work, as attested to in a study by DiFranza et al. (JAMA 257:3387, 1987). These investigators sent an 11-year-old girl to 100 different locations to attempt to purchase cigarettes. She was successful 75% of the time!

I apologize for this long-winded commentary. I am quite confident that it is the longest in this year's YEAR BOOK. Let's hope that quantity is not the inverse of quality.—J.A. Stockman III, M.D.

Pulmonary Vascular Lipid Deposition After Administration of Intravenous Fat to Infants

Robert J. Shulman, Claire Langston, and Richard J. Schanler (Baylor College of Medicine and Texas Children's Hosp., Houston)
Pediatrics 79:99–102, January 1987   11–5

The use of intravenous fat emulsions as part of total parenteral nutrition in neonates is cause for concern because of their potentially deleterious effect on pulmonary function. A review was made of the pulmonary histopathology and clinical course of 39 hospitalized infants who died during a 2-year period; an attempt was made to determine whether pulmonary vascular lipid deposits were associated with the use of fat emulsions intravenously that were given to some of these infants as part of total parenteral nutrition. The effect of serum triglyceride levels on the development of pulmonary vascular lipid deposits also was evaluated.

Of the 39 newborns who died during their initial hospitalization after surviving for at least 7 days, 13 had received no lipids and 26 had received lipid infusions. There was no difference between the two groups as to birth weight, gestational age, incidence of small-for-gestational-age infants, number of sepsis episodes, lung disease diagnoses, and number of infants who received nasogastric feedings.

All 39 infants had lipid in pulmonary macrophages, chondrocytes, and interstitial cells. However, the incidence of pulmonary vascular lipid deposition in the group given lipids was significantly greater than in the other group. The grade of pulmonary vascular lipid deposits in infants in the lipid infusion group correlated positively with the percentage of the infants' lives during which lipids were administered and with mean intake, whereas there was no correlation with the peak serum triglyceride level, frequency of elevated triglyceride levels, birth weight, gestational age, or type and severity of lung disease. These findings demonstrate that the pulmonary vascular lipid deposits probably were associated with the use of fat emulsions intravenously and their judicious use in small, premature infants, who require additional energy, is recommended.

▶ Hyperalimentation has saved the life of many an infant. Unfortunately, it continues to produce problems, as noted in this report. For a previous comment on hyperalimentation-induced cholestasis in premature infants, see the 1983 YEAR BOOK OF PEDIATRICS, p. 183.—J.A. Stockman III, M.D.

Systemic Amyloidosis Complicating Cystic Fibrosis: A Retrospective Pathologic Study

Ronald C. McGlennen, Barbara A. Burke, and Louis P. Dehner (Univ. of Minnesota)

Arch. Pathol. Lab. Med. 110:879–884, October 1986   11–6

Reactive systemic amyloidosis results from an imbalance in the production and degradation of acute-phase inflammatory proteins and the subsequent deposition of insoluble fibrils in body organs. The longer survival of children with cystic fibrosis is often complicated by acute infections and chronic low-grade inflammation, as well as stimulation of acute-phase inflammatory reactants, a condition ideal for the development of amyloidosis. A retrospective study was conducted on autopsies performed between 1957 and 1983 on 33 patients with cystic fibrosis at least 15 years of age at the time of death to determine the occurrence of reactive systemic amyloidosis complicating cystic fibrosis.

Amyloid deposits in multiple organs were found in 11 children (33%). The spleen, liver, and kidneys were affected principally, with amyloid deposits localized mainly in blood vessels. The amyloid was assumed to be of the reactive systemic type. All patients had recurrent and persistent respiratory infections from which *Pseudomonas* species and *Staphylococcus aureus* were commonly cultured. Amyloidosis was suspected clinically in only one patient with advanced amyloidosis of the kidneys. Liver and/or spleen enlargement was documented in five patients. None of the 22 patients with cystic fibrosis who were younger than 15 years of age at the time of death had reactive systemic amyloidosis. There were no differences between the groups with and without reactive systemic amyloidosis with respect to age at diagnosis of cystic fibrosis; number, severity, and types of infections; and longevity.

Amyloidosis is a common phenomenon in older patients with cystic fibrosis and may emerge as an overt complication of this disease as the life span of these patients continues to increase. Cystic fibrosis patients older than 15 years are particularly at risk and should be evaluated for amyloidosis should suggestive clinical findings emerge.

▶ Primary amyloid is derived from kappa or lambda light chains, and primary amyloidosis is usually caused by neoplastic B cell disorders. In adult patients, amyloidosis is associated with chronic infections or inflammatory states, e.g., rheumatoid arthritis, tuberculosis, and bronchiectasis. In children, however, amyloidosis is uncommon, but it is a well-documented complication of tuberculosis in underdeveloped areas of the world, and of juvenile rheumatoid arthritis and familial Mediterranean fever in other populations. Prior to the article abstracted above, there were only 16 reports of amyloidosis complicating cystic fibrosis. Chances are that amyloidosis is a common phenomenon in older patients with cystic fibrosis, and that we will be seeing much more of it as these patients live longer.

Interestingly, there have been reports that we still continue to misdiagnose cystic fibrosis either by overdiagnosis or underdiagnosis. In the latter category are children who present with nothing more than simple clubbing of their fingers.

Can you name 18 causes of clubbing? Many intrathoracic conditions are known to be associated with finger clubbing, including bronchial and esophageal carcinoma, mesothelioma, bronchiectasis, lung abscesses, empyema, fibrotic lung diseases, subacute bacterial endocarditis, and cyanotic congenital heart disease. Extrathoracic causes of clubbing include tumors of the upper gastrointestinal tract, ulcerative colitis, Crohn's disease, achalasia of the cardia, polyarteritis nodosa, alpha chain disease, Hodgkin's disease, cirrhosis of the liver, and the Zollinger-Ellison syndrome (Taube, M.: *Br. Med. J.* 293:1346, 1986). While on the topic of quizzes, can you name 17 conditions reported with elevated sweat chlorides? These include cystic fibrosis, malnutrition, celiac disease, untreated adrenal insufficiency, anorexia nervosa, renal diabetes insipidus, ectodermal dysplasia, fucosidosis, familial cholestasis, untreated hypothyroidism, type I glycogen storage disease, hypoparathyroidism, atopic dermatitis, pupillotonia-areflexia and segmental hypohidrosis, mucopolysaccharidosis, Klinefelter's syndrome, and hypogammaglobulinemia (Ruddy, R.M., et al.: *Clin. Pediatr.* 26:83, 1987).

As far as systemic amyloid is concerned, I would refer you to the adult textbooks. There's not very much you can do about it as far as I know.—J.A. Stockman III, M.D.

Pneumatosis Intestinalis in Cystic Fibrosis
Marta Hernanz-Schulman, John Kirkpatrick, Jr., Harry Shwachman, Thomas Herman, Gerald Schulman, and Gordon F. Vawter (Children's Hosp., Harvard Univ., Brigham and Women's Hosp., and Massachusetts Gen. Hosp., Boston)
Radiology 160:497–499, August 1986   11–7

The incidence and time course of pneumatosis intestinalis and its association with extrapulmonary and intrapulmonary ectopic air among patients with cystic fibrosis have not been evaluated. To address these issues, the clinical and radiographic findings in 23 patients with pneumatosis intestinalis among 441 patients who died of cystic fibrosis in a 40-year period were reviewed retrospectively. The findings were compared with those in 41 patients with cystic fibrosis but without pneumatosis intestinalis.

The incidence of pneumatosis intestinalis increased from 1% between 1944 and 1964 to 11% between 1978 and 1984. In addition, the age at onset of the disease increased: 7% of the patients were younger than 20 years when detected at autopsy between 1944 and 1977, whereas 19% were aged at least 20 years when pneumatosis intestinalis was detected between 1978 and 1984. Except in two patients, the disease was confined to the colon. Pneumomediastinum, pneumothorax, or pulmonary interstitial emphysema was found in 95% of patients with pneumatosis intestinalis compared with 62% of patients without it. Moreover, a striking temporal relationship was evident between the appearance of pneumatosis intestinalis and a documented episode of extrapulmonary air in 48% of the patients. The type, distribution, and severity of the disease often changed with time.

Pneumatosis intestinalis in patients with cystic fibrosis is correlated with the development of obstructive pulmonary disease. It is secondary to a "leak" phenomenon, which dissects infradiaphragmatically, probably along vascular sheaths on a path of least resistance to rest in the colonic wall. Dissection of air is often clinically silent and tends to be self-perpetuating.

Circulating Immune Complexes in Cystic Fibrosis and Their Correlation to Clinical Parameters

Mary L. Disis, Thomas L. McDonald, John L. Colombo, Roger H. Kobayashi, Carol R. Angle, and Sandra Murray (Univ. of Nebraska)
Pediatr. Res. 20:385–390, 1986   11–8

The possibility of an immunologic defect in cystic fibrosis has been studied widely. Reportedly, circulating immune complexes (CIC) are elevated in 40% to 86% of patients with cystic fibrosis. The progress of 25 patients with cystic fibrosis was followed for a 10-month period to determine which, if any, clinical parameters correlated with the occurrence or concentration, or both, of CIC (table). Immune complex determinations were done using a coprecipitation method with equine rheumatoid-complement complex.

All of the cystic fibrosis patients had CIC levels elevated above normal; however, CIC levels did not correlate with the severity of a patient's acute exacerbation. Clinical parameters, including pulmonary function tests, vital signs, total serum IgG levels, and other laboratory studies, were obtained for each patient and analyzed in connection with their relationship

---

CLINICAL PARAMETERS THAT CORRELATED WITH
CIC LEVELS IN CYSTIC FIBROSIS PATIENTS

Moderately elevated (CIC, 30–50 μg/ml)	Highly elevated (CIC, 50–80 μg/ml)
Hospitalizations*	NIH score*
NIH score*	Systolic blood pressure†
Wt*	PEFR*
Lung sounds*	FEV1†
White blood cells*	FEF†
FEV1†	P_{CO_2}†
FVC*	pH†
Total serum IgG†	Total serum IgG*
	Age*
$n = 7$	$n = 12$

*$P <.05$.
†$P <.10$.
(Courtesy of Disis, M.L. et al.: Pediatr. Res. 20:385–390, 1986.)

to CIC. Only 4 of 38 parameters investigated reached a significance of $P < .05$. Factors that demonstrated significant correlation with elevated CIC levels included poor National Institutes of Health score, older patient age, low peak expiratory flow rate, and elevated total serum IgG level. These clinical values were associated more with the measurement of chronic disease.

These findings suggest that CIC levels cannot be used as an indication of short-term prognosis or as a monitor to follow the course of acute severe lung infections in the cystic fibrosis patient. An interesting fact is that all patients who died during the course of the investigation had CIC levels higher than 80 µg/ml. The findings and resultant analysis indicate that CIC may have a more important role in cystic fibrosis than just a physiologic reaction to chronic lung infection.

▶ What is that mystical test that will tell us how badly off our patients are with cystic fibrosis? Is it something as simple as measuring CICs? Apparently not. Virtually 100% of patients with cystic fibrosis have elevations of CICs. Presumably, these are somehow related to the pathogenesis of the lung disease or in some way reflect this process. Nonetheless, there were in this study no significant differences in immune complex levels between patients clinically stable enough to be followed on an outpatient basis and patients in exacerbation of their pulmonary disease. Further, levels of CICs determined in an individual over a period of time did not vary widely from the baseline levels despite changes in the patient's overall condition. Finding that there was no significant difference in CIC levels between outpatients and inpatients is important. Previous studies have attempted to link increased levels with microbial lung infections. Apparently, this is not necessarily so.

Not being able to find specific correlations with CICs does not indicate that these are not a primary factor in the development of the serious sequelae associated with cystic fibrosis. Careful analysis of this study does reveal a strong association between increased CICs and the chronicity of the disease process, if you look at the group of patients overall.

I suppose we will have to wait awhile for additional studies to answer the very basic question of whether the immunologic abnormalities seen in cystic fibrosis are a result of the disease, or may be part of the cause of the disease. A clue to that answer will come when newly diagnosed patients are tested for CICs. If these are not related solely to ongoing infection, then perhaps immune suppressive drugs may have the same effect on cystic fibrosis patients as antibiotics did 20 years ago. You may be aware that studies are underway that show some preliminary evidence of the positive benefits of the use of steroids in patients with cystic fibrosis.

Although CICs may not have any prognostic implication in most cases, serum antibodies to *Pseudomonas aeruginosa* may. High titers against this organism were found to be associated with a poor clinical state, whereas low titers were associated with a better clinical outcome in both chronic and intermittently infected patients with cystic fibrosis (Brett, M.M., et al.: *Arch. Dis. Child.* 61:1114, 1986). The latter results suggest that this test may be a specific and sensitive measure for the severity and progress of different stages of pulmonary infection by *P. aeruginosa* in patients with cystic fibrosis.—J.A. Stockman III, M.D.

Cystic Fibrosis Carrier Detection Using a Linked Genetic Probe
Martin Farrall, Peter Scambler, Katherine Wood Klinger, Kevin Davies, Cate Worrall, Robert Williamson, and Brandon Wainwright (St. Mary's Hosp. Med. School, Univ. of London, and Integrated Genetics, Inc., Framingham, Mass.)
J. Med. Genet. 23:295–299, August 1986   11–9

Genetic linkage between the cystic fibrosis locus and cloned DNA markers that recognize restriction fragment length polymorphisms has been reported recently. There are currently two probes, pJ3•11 and met, that are tightly linked to the cystic fibrosis locus that together are sufficiently informative for carrier detection in 80% of families with a living child with cystic fibrosis and unaffected siblings. The application of the linked probe pJ3•11 to carrier detection or exclusion was demonstrated in 16 families.

Carrier detection was possible in five families with unaffected siblings and carrier exclusion in one family. Not all unaffected siblings in a given sibship are necessarily helped by analysis with a single linked marker, but data from additional markers permit haplotype analysis in most families. Estimation of risks for families with unresolved phase may be complex, but identification of the haplotypes will resolve phase in many families and simplify the calculations markedly.

Risk calculations for cystic fibrosis using linked DNA probes can provide useful information for counseling, particularly when carrier status may be excluded. In some extended pedigrees, carrier determination may give phase data helpful for couples seeking prenatal diagnosis who already have an affected child. In addition, DNA carrier determination in unaffected siblings and other relatives will provide additional family material to assess the various carrier detection methods based on enzymes and antigens.

▶ The technology for carrier detection with respect to cystic fibrosis has been generally elusive until recently. Cystic fibrosis is obviously one of the most common genetic diseases in the world. Among those of northern European extraction, the carrier frequency is about 1 in 20. The article abstracted above shows us that one can use genetic linkage involving DNA probes to detect the carrier state in a family in which an individual has already been identified as having cystic fibrosis. Furthermore, subsequent pregnancies can be examined prenatally to make this diagnosis using the same DNA probes. Previously, the antenatal diagnosis for parents with a 1 in 4 risk required microvillar enzyme analysis. (*Prenat. Diagn.* 5:93, 1985) The latter test is usually done by enzyme analysis performed at 17–18 weeks of gestation, which permits the second-trimester diagnosis of cystic fibrosis in a pregnancy at high risk of recurrence. To date, the data suggest that the false negative and false positive rates of this type of test are about 10% and 5%, respectively. With DNA probes, risk calculations show that the expected false negative and false positive rates are

2% and 6%, respectively, for typical families with one affected living child (Farrall, M., et al.: *Lancet* 2:1402, 1986). All of these DNA probes are based on polymorphisms about the presumed genetic defect on chromosome 7.

In a more recent report, researchers from the Cystic Fibrosis Genetic Research Group in London indicate that they have identified, through a variety of genetic and molecular techniques, what appears to be the actual gene for cystic fibrosis (Estivill, X., et al.: *Nature* 326:840, 1987). Initial studies of the isolated DNA sequence suggest that it indeed represents all or at least part of the gene responsible for the development of cystic fibrosis. If these data hold up and are more fully clarified, the gene itself will have been identified. With that information, it may soon be possible to provide cystic fibrosis screening for the general population, unlike polymorphism studies that are done within specific kindreds of families once an identified individual is found.

With the diagnosis of a heterozygote state occurring so frequently in the general population, if there is a specific carrier state detectable among the general population, it would mean roughly that 1 in 400 pregnancies in individuals of northern European background now at risk for cystic fibrosis would have prenatal testing available to them as well. Obviously, all of us are tuning our channel in to chromosome 7 and are awaiting further news and developments.—J.A. Stockman III, M.D.

Prenatal Diagnosis of α_1-Antitrypsin Deficiency by Restriction Fragment Length Polymorphisms, and Comparison With Oligonucleotide Probe Analysis
J.F. Hejtmancik, R.N. Sifers, P.A. Ward, S. Harris, T. Mansfield, and D.W. Cox (Baylor College of Medicine, Houston, Texas; Hosp. for Sick Children and Univ. of Toronto, Toronto, Canada)
Lancet 2:767–770, Oct. 4, 1986   11–10

The technical complexities associated with oligonucleotide analysis have restricted the use of this method for the prenatal diagnosis of α_1-antitrypsin deficiency. The discovery of restriction fragment length polymorphism (RFLP) in the α_1-antitrypsin gene and the strong linkage dysequilibrium of several of these RFLPs with the Z allele provide an alternative means of prenatal diagnosis. The RFLP analysis with the 6.5 kb 3′ genomic probe was used in 16 consecutive pregnancies at risk for α_1-antitrypsin deficiency and the results were compared with those using hybridization of M and Z specific oligonucleotides.

Both oligonucleotide analysis and RFLP analysis provided identical results for all samples and were able to assist decisions about continuation of the pregnancy. However, RFLP analysis was more reliable under routine laboratory conditions and rarely needed to be repeated, giving results reliably within 7–10 days after DNA sampling. Because RFLP analysis does not depend on the type of mutation, it was possible, in the product of an MZ and SZ mating, to predict an MZ rather than an MS phenotype using the RFLP method. In addition, the strong linkage between an *Ava*II RFLP and the Z allele increased its diagnostic value. Oligonucleotide analysis, however, may prove more useful when no affected or normal siblings are available for comparison.

In informative families with an affected sibling available, RFLP analysis with the 6.5 kb 3' genomic probe is as accurate and reliable as oligonucleotide analysis in the prenatal diagnosis of α_1-antitrypsin deficiency. It is technically easier, making it the preferred method of diagnosis.

▶ There is a law of inanimate reproduction that reads as follows: "If you take something apart and put it back together enough times, eventually you will have two of them." Now we have two technologies for the prenatal diagnosis of α_1-antitrypsin deficiency.

α_1-Antitrypsin deficiency, also known as α_1-antiprotease deficiency, can result in severe early-onset emphysema and fatal cirrhosis of the liver. The most common form of this disease results from the PI ZZ phenotype, which has a prevalence of roughly 1 in 7,600 in North American whites and up to 1 in 2,000 in Scandinavians. Severe emphysema develops in 80% to 90% of PI ZZ individuals, although this is markedly influenced by the smoking status of the affected person. About 14% to 17% of PI ZZ infants will have neonatal hepatitis, with a poor prognosis in about one third of them. The risk of severe liver disease in a PI ZZ child is about 40% if the index child has severe liver disease and about 13% if the index child already diagnosed has no or already resolved liver disease. Thus, the prenatal diagnosis of α_1-antitrypsin deficiency may be indicated, especially when the parents have had a child with severe neonatal hepatitis and subsequent cirrhosis.

Prenatal diagnosis was first achieved by PI typing of fetal blood samples. However, even when the new sampling techniques are used for this procedure there is a risk somewhere of up to 3% of fetal losses directly related to the technology that is used. Another technique involves prenatal diagnosis of α_1-antitrypsin deficiency by direct analysis of the mutation with oligonucleotide probes for the M and Z alleles. This technology has also been extended to the S allele and the sensitivity has been improved so that as little as 1 μg of genomic DNA is required. This type of analysis provides a reliable and accurate means for prenatal diagnosis of α_1-antitrypsin deficiency, but it is technically more difficult than the usual RFLP analysis used for traditional DNA probing. What the study abstracted above, shows us is how the last mentioned technique can be applied to the prenatal diagnosis of α_1-antitrypsin deficiency.

If all of this seems a bit complex to you, don't fret; I think it is to everybody except for the molecular biologist and geneticist. That's why these individuals exist, and it takes me no time at all to make a referral to them when questions involving these types of diagnoses arise. It is not that reports involving fairly sophisticated DNA probe analysis are over one's head; it is just that they don't sink into one's head very well. When I walk by the genetics lab at our hospital, I always have a pile of papers in my hand so that if somebody comes out and asks a question in these sophisticated areas, I can always claim I'm in a hurry, on my way to a meeting. It's not a bad trick.

If you want to read a more lucid commentary on α_1-antitrypsin deficiency and prenatal diagnosis, see the excellent editorial comment that appeared last year in the *Lancet* (1:421, 1987). It's really a good one.—J.A. Stockman III, M.D.

12 The Heart and Blood Vessels

Pediatric Cardiology Manpower in the 1980s
James H. Moller and Forrest H. Adams (Univ. of Minnesota and Children's Hosp. and Health Ctr. of San Diego)
Am. Heart J. 112:599–604, September 1986   12–1

In 1980 the Graduate Medical Education National Advisory Committee issued a report on the number of physicians and their geographic distribution required to meet the nation's health care. This report included a projected need for 1,150 pediatric cardiologists by 1990. Because the American Academy of Pediatrics believed that this number was too high, the Sub-Board of Pediatric Cardiology carried out a survey among current pediatric cardiologists to collect up-to-date information about the nature of their professional activities, total amount of time spent on clinical care, and number of residents who enter the field annually.

Of 519 physicians certified by the Sub-Board of Pediatric Cardiology as of 1979, 444 returned their completed questionnaires, 53 did not reply or could not be located, 19 practiced outside the United States, and 3 had died. Of 444 who completed the questionnaires, 367 worked full time in an academic or hospital setting, 64 were in private practice, and 13 were retired. The 444 respondents lived in 44 states: California, Florida, Illinois,

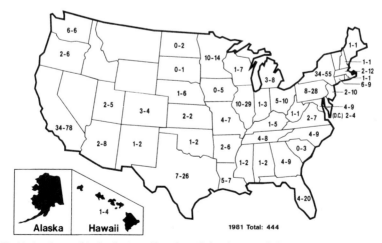

Fig 12–1.—Geographic distribution of board-certified pediatric cardiologists in 1967 and 1981. Left numeral, number of pediatric cardiologists in 1967; right numeral, number of pediatric cardiologists in 1981. (Courtesy of Moller, J.H., and Adams, F.H.: Am. Heart J. 112:599–604, September 1986.)

New York, Pennsylvania, and Texas had more than 20 pediatric cardiologists, whereas Alaska, Idaho, Montana, Nevada, Vermont, and Wyoming had none (Fig 12–1). There was a 10% increase in time spent on clinical activities, with a corresponding decrease in other activities, e.g., research and teaching. Of 444 respondents, 27 spent more than 22% of their time on cardiology research with patients, and 38 spent more than 22% of their time on other cardiology-related research.

An average of 40 physicians enter pediatric cardiology each year, and an average of 14 leave the field each year. On the basis of this survey, the projected number of pediatric cardiologists available for 1990 comes to 901, which is less than the estimated need of 1,150.

▶ Norman S. Talner, M.D., Professor of Pediatrics and Diagnostic Imaging, Yale University School of Medicine, comments.—J.A. Stockman III, M.D.

▶ Of major concern after reviewing this assessment of pediatric cardiology manpower in the 1980s is the decline in time spent on research and teaching in a subspecialty that is for the most part university based. This bodes poorly for academic advancement and for the research training of young individuals now entering the field. This problem has been addressed by the Sub-Board of Pediatric Cardiology and the parent Board, who have extended fellowship training to 3 years with emphasis on a hands-on extended research experience in an environment with a proven track record in basic and/or clinical investigations. Areas of research interest have been targeted and include such items as cardiac morphogenesis, the molecular biology of the heart, developmental cardiovascular physiology, electrophysiology, and the epidemiologic aspects of atherosclerosis and hypertension. Recognized is the need for research training beyond the fellowship years in laboratories of demonstrated excellence using funding approaches such as the clinician scientist program, the young investigator awards, and the newly initiated starter grants from the Society for Pediatric Research, American Society of Pediatrics, and the Medical School Departmental Chairmen. This will require the commitment of a large block of time for research while at the same time reimbursing these individuals at appropriate salary levels. If successful, these programs will infuse into the specialty talented, trained young investigators who will fill the current void and permit research productivity to keep pace with the high performance in the clinical arena.—N.S. Talner, M.D.

The Heart Is Under the Lower Third of the Sternum: Implications for External Cardiac Massage
David A. Finholt, Robert G. Kettrick, Henry R. Wagner, and David B. Swedlow (Univ. of Pennsylvania and Children's Hosp. of Philadelphia)
Am. J. Dis. Child. 140:646–649, July 1986   12–2

It is thought that the infant's heart lies under the sternum at the nipple line, whereas in adolescents it is beneath the lower third of the sternum, and in children it is in an intermediate location. External chest compres-

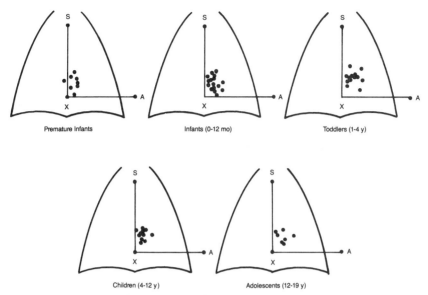

Fig 12–2.—Scattergrams displaying centers of cardiac silhouettes for all 55 patients, divided by age group. *S,* suprasternal notch; *X,* xyphoid; and *A,* abscissa. (Courtesy of Finholt, D.A., et al.: Am. J. Dis. Child. 140:646–649, July 1986.)

sion, when necessary for cardiopulmonary resuscitation (CPR), should be performed at the age-appropriate site. Age-dependent variation in the site of the heart was sought in 25 patients aged 1 day to 19 years who underwent elective cardiac catheterization and right-sided angiography. Chest roentgenograms of 30 patients aged 1 day to 15 years, including 8 premature infants, were also evaluated.

In the angiographic study, the center of the cardiac silhouette corresponded closely with the center of the right ventricle. There was no significant difference between the average site of the cardiac silhouette and the average location of the right ventricle in the total group or in the different age groups (Fig 12–2). The average right ventricle sites were similar in the various age groups. Right ventricle location, however, did differ with the presence of volume overload. No significant age differences in site of the cardiac silhouette were found when data from the two studies were combined. The nipple line bisected the sternum at a mean of 43% of the distance from the xiphoid to the sternum, with no age-related differences.

The heart is uniformly located beneath the lower third of the sternum in all pediatric age groups. Further physiologic studies are needed to determine the most effective means of CPR in children.

▶ This is an important little article. It's amazing how we've come from Galen right up to the present time without being able to state unequivocally where the heart lies. Clearly, the nipple line cannot be taken as an estimation of the heart's intrathoracic location in young children. As important as this study is, the admonishment in the last sentence of the abstract is absolutely critical. It really doesn't matter where the heart lies: It is how effectively compression empties the heart that is important. This requires careful physiologic determinations to be done. We shall all await these before forever saying that the best place to put your hands for external cardiac massage is over the lower third of the sternum.

The only thing I did not like about this article is the imprecise wording of the title. A thousand years from now someone may stumble across this article and think that we all believed that the heart lay directly under the sternum. Even the guys who shot it out in Tombstone, Arizona, knew that the majority of the heart was in the left hemithorax. Thus, the article should more appropriately be titled, "That part of the heart which is under the sternum lies under the lower third of the sternum: Implications for external cardiac massage."

(Quiz: Do you know the number of tombstones in Tombstone, Arizona? The answer is 792.)—J.A. Stockman III, M.D.

Intravenous and Oral Amiodarone for Arrhythmias in Children
Clifford A. Bucknall, Barry R. Keeton, Paul V.L. Curry, Michael J. Tynan, George R. Sutherland, and David W. Holt (Guy's Hosp., London, and Southampton Gen. Hosp., England)
Br. Heart J. 56:278–284, September 1986   12–3

Amiodarone reportedly is effective in children with cardiac arrhythmias, and adverse effects may be less frequent than in adults. Thirty children with a mean age of 7 years received amiodarone therapy in 1979–1984. Nineteen children had supraventricular tachycardia, four had atrial flutter, and seven had ventricular tachycardia. Eight patients had congenital structural heart disorders. Other drugs had been ineffective in 29 children. Five children initially received amiodarone intravenously, but all were treated orally.

Intravenous doses of amiodarone controlled arrhythmia in all five children treated, two of whom had ventricular tachycardia. Oral treatment suppressed arrhythmias in 28 of the 30 children, and it was the only antiarrhythmic agents used in 19 of them. Eight children required digoxin in addition to amiodarone. The mean oral dose of amiodarone associated with initial suppression of arrhythmia was 10 mg/kg daily, and the mean maintenance dose was 6 mg/kg daily. Young infants required higher doses for control of arrhythmia. Adverse effects were frequent, particularly photosensitivity. One child experienced complete heart block. Sleep disorder and corneal deposits also were noted. Treatment was withdrawn from five patients because of side effects.

Amiodarone is an effective antiarrhythmic drug for use in children, but only those with resistant life-threatening arrhythmias should be given it. The oral dose should be calculated by surface area estimation; more data on plasma levels are needed. Particular care is needed in infants, who require a higher weight-related oral dose of amiodarone for suppression of arrhythmia.

▶ Dr. D. Woodrow Benson, Professor of Pediatrics, Northwestern University Medical School, and Chief, Division of Cardiology, Children's Memorial Hospital, comments.—J.A. Stockman III, M.D.

▶ Amiodarone hydrochloride was initially evaluated in Europe about 20 years ago. The drug was first introduced as a coronary artery vasodilator exhibiting weak α- and β-adrenergic antagonist activity. The anti-arrhythmic actions of amiodarone have become known gradually; it is not chemically related to any other antiarrhythmic drug. Much remains to be learned of its pharmacokinetic and pharmacodynamic properties.

Amiodarone was recently approved by the Food and Drug Administration for use as an antiarrhythmic drug in adults; approval has not been granted for children because safety and efficacy have not been established. This is a common scenario for many of the newer medications used in treating cardiovascular disease. The rationale, apparently, is that the market is small (not many children need them) and the risk is high (potentially serious side effects in growing children). Nevertheless, amiodarone is establishing a position of importance in the treatment of a variety of rhythm disturbances in young patients. In recent years, several papers have reported on the amiodarone experience in young patients. The importance of the paper by Bucknall et al. is the more extensive period of follow-up than previously reported. These observations are important for tailoring the method of monitoring children who take amiodarone.—D.W. Benson, M.D.

Maternal Antibodies Against Fetal Cardiac Antigens in Congenital Complete Heart Block
Pamela V. Taylor, James S. Scott, Leon M. Gerlis, Eva Esscher, and Olive Scott (Leeds Maternity Hosp., Univ. of Leeds, and Killingbeck Hosp., Leeds, England, and Univ. Hosp., Uppsala, Sweden)
N. Engl. J. Med. 315:667–672, Sept. 11, 1986   12–4

Previous studies have suggested a strong association between maternal connective tissue disease and congenital complete heart block as a consequence of the transplacental passage of antibodies to soluble tissue ribonucleoprotein antigens. A study was conducted to search for antibodies directed against fetal cardiac conducting tissue by examining serum samples from women who had given birth to an infant with heart block and from normal controls.

The study was done with serum samples obtained from 41 mothers of infants with congenital complete heart block, 44 mothers who had given birth to infants with cardiac anomalies other than complete heart block, and 50 mothers who had given birth to normal infants. In addition, serum samples were collected within 3 months after birth from infants with congenital complete heart block and from 50 normal infants. Fetal heart, liver, kidney, and skin tissue from various sources was also available for examination. Of the 41 mothers of infants with heart block, 17 were found previously to have connective tissue disease.

TABLE 1.—RESULTS OF FLUORESCENCE MICROSCOPY OF FETAL CARDIAC TISSUE WITH
MATERNAL SERUM AT A DILUTION OF 1:10

Serum–Sample Source	Total	No. Positive
Mothers of babies with isolated congenital complete heart block	41	21
Normal controls	50	0
Other groups studied		
Mothers of babies with "miscellaneous" congenital heart block (second degree, intermittent, late diagnosis, or associated with cardiac structural or other malformations)	19	3
Mothers of babies with congenital cardiac malformations not associated with congenital heart block	11	2
Mother of baby with familial type of heart block	1	0
Women with various types of connective tissue disease who had not had babies with isolated congenital heart block	13	4

(Courtesy of Taylor, P.V., et al.: N. Engl. J. Med. 315:667–672, Sept. 11, 1986.)

Of the 41 mothers, 21 (51%) had IgG antibody that was reactive with fetal heart tissue (Table 1), but only 9 (10%) of the 94 control mothers had IgG antibodies. Seventeen of the 21 reactive maternal serum samples were positive for anti-Ro (SS-A). Of the eight samples available from the infants with complete heart block, three were positive for the antibody; all control serum samples were negative. A higher occurrence of antibodies to cytomegalovirus was found in the 41 mothers than in the controls, but Epstein-Barr virus antibodies were not present (Table 2). The data support the concept that maternally derived antibody may often, but not always, be involved in the pathogenesis of congenital complete heart block.

▶ The antibodies described in this article were predominantly IgG and therefore were able to cross the placenta. The antibodies did not, however, react selectively with the conducting tissue of the heart. No antibody specifically related to the pathogenesis of congenital heart block has yet been unequivocably identified, but the findings in this study support the idea that one, or possibly more than one, closely related antibody is involved. Also, maternal antibody that reacted with fetal heart tissue also reacted with other fetal tissues, in keeping with earlier reports that the pathologic process leading to congenital heart block may be diffuse, involving extensive fibrosis of other organs. In most sites, antibody-mediated damage is probably of little clinical relevance, but in cardiac conducting tissue the damage is clinically important and irreversible.

Why all this happens is not known. Some consider that it is most likely caused by viral infection in which autoantibodies are formed directly against antibodies made in reaction to virus infection. One such virus could be cyto-

TABLE 2.—Antibodies to Viruses and Smooth Muscle, and Biologic False Positive Serologic Tests for Syphilis in Maternal Serum

GROUPS	ANTIBODY			FALSE POSITIVE SEROLOGIC TESTS
	CYTOMEGALOVIRUS	EPSTEIN–BARR VIRUS	SMOOTH MUSCLE	
	no. positive/no. tested			
Mothers of babies with isolated congenital complete heart block	17/24	20*/21	2/17	11/24
Normal controls	10/23	21†/23	8/50	1/50
Other groups studied				
Mothers of babies with "miscellaneous" congenital heart block	8/11	7†/7	0/10	Not done
Mothers of babies with congenital cardiac malformations not associated with heart block	6/7	6†/7	Not done	1/7
Women with connective-tissue disease who had not had babies with isolated congenital complete heart block	6/10	Not done	0/7	0/11

*All IgG and one also IgM.
†All IgG.
(Courtesy of Taylor, P.V., et al.: N. Engl. J. Med. 315:667–672, Sept. 11, 1986.)

megalovirus because an increased frequency of antibody to cytomegalovirus has been reported in the mothers of babies with congenital heart block.

Although it was originally thought to be a benign problem, congenital complete heart block is sometimes associated with syncope, sudden death, a need for a pacemaker, or a combination of these. The small subset of patients who are at risk for sudden death has traditionally represented a serious management problem. There have been no reliable markers that permit physicians to predict which asymptomatic patients with congenital complete heart block may need a prophylactic permanent pacemaker. That statement was true until the report of Dewey et al. appeared (*N. Engl. J. Med.* 316:835, 1987). These investigators set about the challenge of identifying high-risk patients. To define the long-term natural history of congenital heart block, they followed 27 patients prospectively by means of frequent ambulatory ECG recordings for a mean of 8 years. During that time, 8 of the 13 patients with a mean daytime heart rate of less than 50 beats per minute had cardiac complications, e.g., sudden death, syncope, presyncope, or excessive fatigue. Six of eight patients had additional ECG findings that suggested instability of the junctional escape mechanism. None of the 14 patients with a mean daytime heart rate of at least 50 beats per minute had an adverse clinical outcome. It was concluded that patients with a mean daytime junctional rate of less than 50 beats per minute and other evidence of an unstable junctional escape mechanism should probably undergo prophylactic pacemaker implantation. Because junctional exit block and tachyarrhythmias sometimes appear first during follow-up, the method of risk identification used in this study depends on the ability to do serial ambulatory ECG recordings.

Thus, we can see from work performed in the last year and a half that we now have a little bit better insight into what may cause congenital heart block and what we have to do about it.—J.A. Stockman III, M.D.

Diagnosis of Fetal Arrhythmias Using Echocardiographic and Doppler Techniques

Leonard Steinfeld, Howard L. Rappaport, Hans C. Rossbach, and Eulogio Martinez (Mount Sinai School of Medicine, New York, and the Paulista School of Medicine, São Paulo, Brazil)

J. Am. Coll. Cardiol. 8:1425–1433, December 1986   12–5

The correct diagnosis of fetal arrhythmias appears to be necessary because certain prenatal tachyarrhythmias respond to pharmacologic intervention. With the aid of two-dimensional echocardiographic imaging, an M-mode cursor can be aligned to record atrial and ventricular motion, either independently or simultaneously. The onset of atrial wall motion serves as a marker for the timing of the ECG P wave, whereas onset of the ventricular wall thickening best approximates the timing of onset of the QRS complex. A time plot of the relationship between derived P waves and QRS complexes provides the basis for reconstruction of the fetal ECG. This diagnostic method was applied in 57 fetuses with irregular heartbeats.

Recurrent atrial (in 12 fetuses) and ventricular (in 21) ectopic beats were the most common prenatal arrhythmias. Atrial flutter, ventricular tachycardia, atrial and ventricular bigeminy, and atrial and ventricular bradyarrhythmias were correctly identified in the remaining fetuses. In one instance, supraventricular tachycardia was satisfactorily controlled with digitalis therapy. Recognition of fetal atrial flutter in the last trimester of three pregnancies forewarned the staff about subsequent management at birth. Low-dosage electrical cardioversion terminated the atrial flutter. Pressure by an echocardiographic transducer on the maternal abdominal wall induced intermittent bradycardia in eight fetuses; lessening the pressure normalized the heart rate and rhythm. Echocardiography and gated pulsed Doppler studies offer the most reliable methods for interpreting fetal arrhythmias, thereby allowing appropriate treatment in some instances.

▶ Samual Gidding, M.D., Assistant Professor of Pediatrics, Northwestern University Medical School, and member, Division of Cardiology, Children's Memorial Hospital, comments.—J.A. Stockman III, M.D.

▶ This article and other recent reports (Strasburger, J.F., et al.: *J. Am. Coll. Cardiol.* 7:1386, 1986; Kleinman, C.S., et al.: *Am. J. Cardiol.* 51:237, 1983; and Allan, L.D., et al.: *Br. Heart J.* 50:240, 1983) review the spectrum of cardiac arrhythmias that can be recognized by the obstetrician as a result of fetal heart rate monitoring. Accurate diagnosis of the arrhythmias can be made by a skilled fetal echocardiographer using 2-dimensional directed M-mode echocardiograms and Doppler ultrasonography. Appropriate therapy may be initiated as a consequence of these studies. Fetal hydrops has been treated successfully in utero as a result of such antiarrhythmic therapy.

Now that a tool is available for the accurate assessment of cardiac rhythm, much remains to be learned about the natural history of arrhythmias in the fetus so that guidelines for therapy can be developed and unnecessary or inappropriate drug therapy can be avoided. Steinfeld et al. make important contributions with respect to abnormal cardiac rhythm. They show that intrauterine supraventricular tachycardia may be nonsustained and does not always lead to hydrops, suggesting that some fetuses with this rhythm disorder may not require therapy. Further, the etiology of tachycardia is multifactorial and can be related to atrial flutter or to a reentrant mechanism. Thus, therapy will have to be guided by an understanding of the etiology of the particular rhythm disturbance. Premature contractions, either atrial, junctional, or ventricular, are common and have a benign prognosis. Fetal bradycardia may be induced by pressure on the abdominal wall; this probably represents a normal finding. Complete heart block may be associated with connective tissue disease in the mother or structural heart disease in the infant.

Fetal echocardiography, now in its embryogenesis, will have a major impact on the management of pediatric heart disease. The diagnosis and treatment of fetal arrhythmias represent one of its earliest successes. Future fetal research will be directed toward understanding the natural history of rhythm disturbances, determining the best pharmacologic agents for the treatment of rhythm disturbances, developing new technology to obtain fetal ECGs, and attempting interventional therapy, e.g., fetal cardiac pacing.—S. Gidding, M.D.

Acute Pediatric Digoxin Ingestion: A Ten-Year Experience
William J. Lewander, Pierre Gaudreault, Arnold Einhorn, Fred M. Henretig, Peter G. Lacouture, and Frederick H. Lovejoy, Jr. (Children's Hosp. and Harvard Univ., Boston, Children's Hosp. Natl. Med. Ctr., Washington, D.C., and Children's Hosp. of Philadelphia)
Am. J. Dis. Child. 140:770–773, August 1986   12–6

An effective antidote, the digoxin-specific Fab antibody fragments, is now available for acute digoxin poisoning. Whether there is a widespread need for this antidote in pediatric emergencies or a need to increase availability for isolated acute pediatric digoxin poisoning remains to be clarified. Findings in 41 children with acute digoxin ingestion admitted from 1972 to 1982 to three major pediatric teaching hospitals were reviewed retrospectively to determine the epidemiology, initial presentation, and clinical course of acute digoxin poisoning. Most of the patients were younger than 5 years of age (mean, 3 years). The majority (90%) were seen within 6 hours of ingestion. All but three episodes involved single drug ingestions and 38 patients underwent gastrointestinal tract decontamination.

SERUM DIGOXIN CONCENTRATIONS IN RELATION TO SIGNS AND SYMPTOMS
AND ECG ABNORMALITIES*

Range of Initial Serum Digoxin Concentration, ng/mL (nmol/L)	No. of Patients	Presence of Signs and Symptoms or ECG Changes, No. (%) of Patients	ECG Changes
0-2 (0-2.6)	15	1 (7)	1° AV block
>2-4 (>2.6-5.1)	11	4 (36)	Bradycardia; ST depression
>4-6 (>5.1-7.7)	5	3 (60)	Increased PR interval; bradycardia
>6-8 (>7.7-10.2)	6	4 (66)	1°, 2° AV block; bradycardia
>8 (>10.2)	4	4 (100)	Increased PR interval; 1°, 2° AV block; bradycardia

*ECG, electrocardiographic; AV, atrioventricular.
(Courtesy of Lewander, W.J., et al.: Am. J. Dis. Child. 140:770–773, August 1986.)

The amount of digoxin ingested ranged from 0.5 mg to 7.5 mg (mean, 2.9 mg). Signs and symptoms (i.e., vomiting, lethargy, bradycardia) or ECG evidence of digoxin poisoning occurred primarily in patients with digoxin concentrations of more than 2 ng/ml (table). However, 44% of the patients remained asymptomatic and had no ECG abnormalities despite serum concentrations of more than 2 ng/ml. Symptoms and ECG abnormalities increased in proportion to increasing digoxin concentration. Eleven (27%) patients had ECG abnormalities, i.e., bradycardia and conduction disturbances; four (35%) had abnormalities documented within 5 hours of ingestion and seven (65%) had delayed-onset ECG abnormalities (Fig 12–3). None of the ECG abnormalities was life threatening. Serum digoxin concentrations ranged from 0.2 ng/ml to 11.6 ng/ml. Peak serum concentrations occurred within 6 hours of ingestion in most patients. Serum half-lives were rapid, approximately 3 hours (primarily distribution), in an initial phase and longer, approximately 20 hours (primarily elimination), in a second phase. Only one patient had transient elevation of the serum potassium concentration.

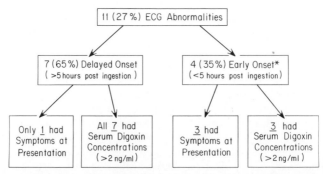

Fig 12–3.—Electrocardiographic (ECG) abnormalities in 11 patients with acute digoxin ingestion. One patient (*) presented with 1–degree atrioventricular block that did not progress or resolve. The serum digoxin concentration was 0.6 ng/ml (0.8 nmole/L) and patient remained asymptomatic. Following evaluation, he was discharged with persistent 1-degree atrioventricular block. (Courtesy of Lewander, W.J., et al.: Am. J. Dis. Child. 140:770–773, August 1986.)

Acute pediatric digoxin ingestions are not common and are usually not severe. Although signs and symptoms on presentation predict a digoxin concentration of more than 2 ng/ml, the absence of signs and symptoms of ECG abnormalities in the presence of a serum digoxin concentration of more than 2 ng/ml does not accurately predict their occurrence later in the course. A correlation between the serum potassium level and digoxin concentration is not apparent. Only nonlife-threatening bradycardia and conduction disturbances are observed. These findings do not support the widespread use of the digoxin antidote in acute pediatric digoxin poisonings, but it should be made available for the isolated severe case.

▶ After reading this article several times, I'm not entirely comfortable with my own feelings of when to be secure in not treating a child who has had a digoxin overdose. It seems reasonably certain that patients who are initially asymptomatic with serum digoxin concentrations of less than 2 ng/ml will remain asymptomatic. However, the absence of symptoms in the presence of a serum digoxin concentration of more than 2 ng/ml cannot be used to predict anything accurately. A major problem with this study is the fact that serum concentrations were measured only once in about half of the patients, so we don't know which way the level might have been going. It seems fair to say that the serum digoxin concentration alone is not as important as the presence of symptoms or ECG abnormalities.

Although hypokalemia is frequently observed with long-term digoxin and diuretic therapy, hyperkalemia is well documented in patients with acute massive digoxin overdose. Elevation of serum potassium concentrations results from inhibition of the sodium-potassium adenosine triphosphate pump by digoxin. Generally, hyperkalemia occurs only with a severe digoxin overdose and therefore may be a clue to the need for additional therapy.

The only absolute conclusion that I personally would want to draw from this study is the fact that patients with a serum digoxin concentration of less than 2 ng/ml within 6 hours after ingestion who remain asymptomatic without ECG abnormalities during a 6-hour period of observation and monitoring may be discharged. It is impressive that in a 10-year period at three major institutions in the United States (Children's Hospital Medical Center at Boston, the Children's Hospital of Philadelphia, and National Children's Hospital Medical Center in Washington) no reports of severe acute digoxin poisoning could be found. In hindsight, then, it would be a rare occasion when these institutions would presumably have used the digoxin-specific Fab antibody fragments were they available during that period of time as an antidote against digoxin toxicity. If you're not entirely familiar with the antigen-binding fragments (Fab) derived from specific antidigoxin antibodies, these were approved in the spring of 1986 for use in the United States by the Food and Drug Administration. They were developed as an orphan product under the trade name of (believe it or not) Digibind by Burroughs Wellcome, Ltd. The antibody, produced in sheep, blocks digoxin in the circulation and the entire complex is then excreted. It works 95% of the time within 30 minutes of administration to reverse life-threatening digitalis toxicity. Even though it is a sheep antibody, hypersensitivity has not yet been reported. Presumably, a patient would not have to be subjected to this more than once in his or her lifetime. It is recognized that the rapid removal of digoxin from the circulation could compromise patients with poor cardiac function who require digoxin. Also, in theory, the antibody could remain in the body long enough to block any therapeutic digoxin that one might want to administer quickly should the patient decompensate. Other forms of therapy presumably could be introduced to correct myocardial dysfunction, however.

The greatest problem with this drug surrounds the issues raised by the article abstracted above, i.e., what criteria should be used for its administration. I personally think that this drug should be available to almost all hospitals. The reason I say this is not because self-administration of digoxin is the major cause of acute life-threatening toxicity. It is not, as the article above notes. Acute life-threatening digoxin toxicity probably occurs more commonly from inadvertent iatrogenic parenteral overdose (i.e., by mistake). One can never tell when that problem will occur, and to have the drug available for this problem means that it must always be available. However, recognize that each 40 mg vial of Digibind costs $150, and it is estimated that 10, 20, or more vials will be needed to treat most life-threatening ingestions, at a cost of as much as $3,000 or more per treatment. That is a lot of inventory to carry on the books for something that will be used extraordinarily infrequently. However, $3,000 seems like a small price to pay to save a life and at the same time avoid a law suit.—J.A. Stockman III, M.D.

Cardiac Involvement in Congenital Acquired Immunodeficiency Syndrome
Laurel J. Steinherz, Joel A. Brochstein, and June Robins (Mem. Sloan-Kettering Cancer Ctr., New York)
Am. J. Dis. Child. 140:1241–1244, December 1986   12–7

Cardiac abnormalities have been reported in 25% to 73% of adults with acquired immunodeficiency syndrome (AIDS). Two recent studies reported a significant incidence of cardiac abnormalities in children with AIDS. A child was seen who had congenital AIDS and findings of cardiac abnormalities.

Male infant, aged 6 weeks, the son of a woman aged 32 years with a 5-year history of intravenous heroin abuse, began to have recurrent episodes of diarrhea, otitis media, and oral moniliasis at age 6 weeks. At age 6 months, he contracted pneumonia and meningitis and was found to have adenopathy and hepatosplenomegaly. At age 11 months, AIDS was diagnosed after an immunologic workup. At age 14 months the child was hospitalized with pneumonia and *Staphylococcus aureus* sepsis. Chest films revealed cardiomegaly. An ECG showed left ventricular hypertrophy and T wave abnormalities. An echocardiogram showed left ventricular dysfunction and dilatation. There were no structural cardiac abnormalities and no increased thickness of the septum or left ventricular free wall.

The patient was treated with low doses of digoxin, and the congestive signs and symptoms resolved. He was maintained with digoxin therapy after discharge and did not require vasodilators for control of his congestive symptoms. The patient died at age 34 months of pulmonary insufficiency.

Children with congential AIDS should be screened periodically to rule out cardiac involvement.

▶ Even though cardiac involvement in children at the time the above article was published appeared to be an uncommon phenomenon, we are seeing it now much more often. In the child described, the heart was uniformly enlarged with dilatation of all four chambers. The ventricles were hypertrophied to such a degree that the heart weighed four times its normal amount. All four valve rings of the heart were dilated. Microscopic examination revealed fibrosis of the spongiosa of the tricuspid and mitral valves. The myocardium was abnormal with marked variation in myocyte nuclear size. There was no inflammation observed. The cause of the cardiac abnormalities seen in patients with AIDS, other than those stemming from involvement with Kaposi's sarcoma, is yet unclear. Direct relationships with ongoing infection, as evidenced by positive concurrent viral or bacterial cultures or viral titers, have been absent in most adult patients.

Even with the increased research funding provided by the National Institutes of Health in the area of human immunovirus infection, perhaps more investment should be made in specifically targeted areas, such as addressing the CNS complications of AIDS or perhaps the cardiac involvement noted here. Most of the investment is now going toward study of the virus itself. If you don't think federal money exists, simply realize that the amount the military spent on recruiting and training the 1,800 homosexuals it discharged in 1985 was $22,138,200.—J.A. Stockman III, M.D.

Development and Progression of Left Ventricular Hypertrophy in Children With Hypertrophic Cardiomyopathy
Barry J. Maron, Paolo Spirito, Yvonne Wesley, and Javier Arce (Natl. Heart, Lung, and Blood Inst., NIH, Bethesda)
N. Engl. J. Med. 315:610–614, Sept. 4, 1986   12–8

Hypertrophic cardiomyopathy, a primary myocardial disease, is characterized by a hypertrophied, nondilated left ventricle. Previously, autopsy of infants with the disease demonstrated that marked left ventricular (LV) hypertrophy developed in utero. An attempt was made to determine whether the morphological expression of this disease can appear later in life.

Thirty-nine patients aged 4–15 years were selected. Criteria for entry included a family history or echocardiograph suggestive of hypertrophic cardiomyopathy, clinical and echocardiographic follow-ups continued for at least 2.5 years, and two-dimensional echocardiographs of sufficient quality to permit accurate measurement of LV wall thickness.

At the outset, 16 patients had normal wall thickness throughout the left ventricle. During the 2.5 to 6.8 years of follow-up, 11 of these 16 did not have ventricular hypertrophy. Six patients with hypertrophy at the outset had no progression of the disease. The remaining 22 patients, 5 who were originally normal and 17 who had ventricular hypertrophy on first evaluation, had marked increases in LV wall thickness. The average increase was 12.1 mm, or a change of 101%, which significantly exceeded the expected change resulting from normal body growth. The most common change was in the anterior ventricular septum. Less commonly, wall thickening occurred in the posterior septum, anterior free wall, and posterior free wall.

The increases in wall thickness were seen most commonly in adolescence and appeared to be spontaneous. Almost 70% of the patients had no basal outflow tract obstruction despite increased wall thickness. Increased LV hypertrophy was not associated with clinical deterioration. Thus, to diagnose hypertrophic cardiopathy, asymptomatic children with a family history of LV hypertrophy should undergo echocardiography every 3 years until they reach adulthood.

▶ Hypertrophic cardiomyopathy is a primary myocardial disease usually transmitted as an autosomal dominant trait. It was not known, at least until now, whether hypertrophic cardiomyopathy is a congenital cardiac malformation in which LV hypertrophy is evident at or shortly after birth, or whether the morphological expression of the disease may first appear in later life. What we see in this study is that many patients who were at risk for hypertrophic cardiomyopathy did not have it at birth but did manifest the problem later in life. Fortunately, none of these patients had associated symptomatic deterioration or related subaortic obstruction.

I think we have a great deal more to learn about the nature of this disorder. Is it possible that individuals who do not manifest the disease until later in childhood will in fact transmit it to their children as an autosomal dominant trait? Even though the children who were picked up well beyond infancy had no significant problems, how will they do late in life? What is the role of cardiac transplantation for infants who have a progressive problem?

For an excellent discussion of cardiac transplantation in children, see the review by Allen (*Am. J. Dis. Child.* 140:1105, 1986).—J.A. Stockman III, M.D.

Phototherapy Effect on the Incidence of Patent Ductus Arteriosus in Premature Infants: Prevention With Chest Shielding
Warren Rosenfeld, Shashi Sadhev, Verlaine Brunot, Ramesh Jhaveri, Ignacio Zabaleta, and Hugh E. Evans (State Univ. of New York/Downstate Med. Ctr., Brooklyn)
Pediatrics 78:10–14, July 1986   12–9

In vitro studies demonstrate that room lights prevent the closure of isolated ductal rings in the lamb. These findings suggest that phototherapy, which is used for the prevention of jaundice and usually begun on the first day of life, may influence the incidence of patent ductus arteriosus in premature infants. To verify this hypothesis, the incidence of patent ductus arteriosus was evaluated among 74 premature infants who received prophylactic phototherapy for hyperbilirubinemia from day 1 of life: 36 had their left chest covered with folded aluminum foil while receiving phototherapy and 38 had no shield. Phototherapy was administered with the Air Shields model PTU 78-1, maintaining irradiance at >4.0 $\mu W/cm^2/nm$. All infants were exposed to radiant warmers and received mechanical ventilation for respiratory distress syndrome.

Birth weights, gestational ages, severity of respiratory distress syndrome, intravenous fluid intake, and duration of phototherapy were similar in both groups. However, the incidence of patent ductus arteriosus was significantly less in the shielded group than in the nonshielded group (23 of 38 infants vs. 11 of 36 infants). Shielding was most effective in infants weighing less than 1,000 gm. In addition, when the patent ductus arteriosus did appear in the shielded group, it tended to be of shorter duration, appeared at a later date, and required less vigorous therapy (i.e., indomethacin). Shielded infants required significantly shorter hospitalization times. Although there was a trend for higher late mortality in the shielded group, the deaths did not appear to be related to use of the shield. All patients who died had had shielding discontinued for a mean of 38 days.

Phototherapy may play a role in the occurrence of patent ductus arteriosus in premature infants. Should this initial observation be confirmed, phototherapy may be a practical method of decreasing the incidence of this common major complication in premature neonates.

The Silent Ductus: Its Precursors and Its Aftermath
Cathy Hammerman, Elene Strates, and Sandra Valaitis (Univ. of Chicago)
Pediatr. Cardiol. 7:121–127, 1986   12–10

Prophylactic closure of the silent patent ductus arteriosus (PDA) in the very-low-birth-weight neonate has been recommended on the assumption that it can improve overall morbidity and mortality in these infants. Thirty-one infants with birth weights of 1,000 gm or less were evaluated on days 2–3 of life to determine potential risk factors in the development of silent ductus, its clinical impact on the subsequent morbidity of the premature neonate, and the potential benefit of prophylactic closure in this presymptomatic stage. Infants with no evidence of ductal shunting received no treatment, whereas those with early evidence of silent left-to-right PDA were randomized to receive indomethacin prophylactically (0.2 mg/kg/dose every 12 hours for three doses) or placebo.

The incidence and extent of elevation of the plasma levels of the dilator prostaglandin metabolite 6-keto-$PGF_1\alpha$ were significantly increased in infants with silent PDA. No other risk factors for PDA were identified. Silent PDA correlated most highly with the later development of symptomatic PDA and overall morbidity and mortality. Prophylactic closure with indomethacin decreased the incidence of subsequent PDA development, but had no effect on overall morbidity and/or mortality.

An elevated plasma level of the dilator prostaglandin metabolite 6-keto-$PGF_1\alpha$ is the only identifiable risk factor associated with PDA development. Silent PDA within the first 2–3 days of life is associated with subsequent symptomatic PDA. Prophylactic closure decreases the subsequent incidence of symptomatic PDA, but not overall morbidity and mortality.

Response of the Patent Ductus Arteriosus to Indomethacin Treatment

James M. Ramsay, Daniel J. Murphy, Jr., G. Wesley Vick, III, James T. Courtney, Joseph A. Garcia-Prats, and James C. Huhta (Baylor College of Medicine, Houston)
Am. J. Dis. Child. 141:294–297, March 1987   12–11

The response of the patent ductus arteriosus (PDA) to indomethacin treatment has been studied previously. However, the findings were based predominantly on physical signs and indirect M-mode echocardiographic measurements. Because these factors have a low sensitivity and specificity in low-birth-weight premature infants on mechanical respirators, the response of PDA to indomethacin treatment was studied with the aid of serial, two-dimensional and pulsed Doppler echocardiography.

The series included 19 preterm infants with confirmed PDA; gestational ages ranged from 26 to 31 weeks and birth weights ranged from 600 gm to 1,680 gm. Patients with congenital heart disease were excluded. All infants underwent two-dimensional and pulsed Doppler echocardiography before and after indomethacin administration until the day after the last dose was given. Blood levels were measured 24 hours after the last dose of indomethacin.

The PDA closed initially in 11 infants (58%), constricted in 7 (37%), and had no effect in 1 (5%). However, it reopened in four infants in the closed duct group and in five in the constricted duct group. The eight patients with reopened ducts and the nonresponding infant subsequently required surgical ductal ligation (table). One patient died after the PDA had constricted originally. One patient whose ductus arteriosus reopened after closing originally responded to a second course of indomethacin treatment.

Serial two-dimensional and Doppler echocardiogaphic study is useful in monitoring PDA patients who are treated with indomethacin, because it can distinguish between ductal closure and ductal constriction. However, the initial response does not predict which ductus arteriosus will reopen, as both groups had occurrences of reopening ducts.

▶ Dr. William F. Friedman, Executive Chairman, Department of Pediatrics, and J.H. Nicholson Professor of Pediatrics (Cardiology), UCLA School of Medicine, comments on the preceding three reports.—J.A. Stockman III, M.D.

RESPONSES TO INDOMETHACIN

Response	No. (%) of Patients
Initial closure	11/19 (57)
Initial constriction	7/19 (37)
Sustained closure	8/19 (42)
Ligation	9/19 (47)

(Courtesy of Ramsay, J.M., et al.: Am. J. Dis. Child. 141:294–297, March 1987.)

▶ Review of these three reports (12–9, 12–10, and 12–11) concerning PDA in the preterm infant reinforces the fact that meaningful conclusions cannot be reached if nonspecific methods are used to evaluate ductal patency when seeking to assess therapeutic interventions, biochemical correlates, or natural or unnatural history. Indeed, that is the most valid point of the Ramsay report and an important failing in the Hammerman and Rosenfeld articles. The low sensitivity and specificity of either clinical examination or M-mode echocardiographic measurements create serious problems with the report of the efficacy of phototherapy, as well as with the patient follow-up component of the Hammerman report on the "silent" ductus. The latter paper used the highly specific and sensitive technique of contrast echocardiography for initial detection of PDA and then, unfortunately, resorted to the unreliable approaches of measuring systolic time intervals or the left atrium/aortic root dimension to analyze findings thereafter (*J. Pediatr.* 92:474, 1978). Conversely, *serial* high-resolution two-dimensional echocardiography and Doppler ultrasound examinations permitted Ramsay and his colleagues to evaluate PDA responses to indomethacin treatment critically.

Studies of the photoactivity spectrum of the ductus arteriosus have not been done. Red light is likely to reach the ductus arteriosus via phototherapy or thoracic transillumination; white light, at the opposite end of the photoactivity spectrum, is the suspected factor in the photodynamic effect of light on the dustus arteriosus. Further, the aluminum foil covering the chest and much of the abdomen of the preterm babies in the Rosenfeld study disallowed blinding of observers to the intervention. This lack of blinding, as well as insensitive detection methods (the LA/AO ratio), limit the value of the report. It is hoped that further evaluation of the effectiveness of shielding the chest from light will use ductus detection methods similar to those employed by Ramsay and co-workers.

Although the Ramsay group used excellent methods to detect the status of the caliber of the ductus arteriosus, their report unfortunately is yet one more paper adding to the confusion concerning the value of indomethacin levels in treatment (*N. Engl. J. Med.* 305:67, 1981, and *Eur. J. Pediatr.* 141:71, 1983). Indomethacin closed or importantly constricted the ductus arteriosus in all but one infant in the Ramsay study. Interestingly, when the ductus reopened in infants in this study, a second course of indomethacin proved successful in the only infant to whom it was offered. Why every other baby whose ductus reopened went to the operating room was unclear, but presumably it was unrelated to the emphasis by the surgeons at the Texas Children's Hospital on the large number of cases they do.

The Hammerman report suggests that plasma levels of a stable metabolite of the vasodilator, prostacyclin, may be an identifiable risk factor for PDA but, unfortunately, these workers assayed the metabolite from unextracted plasma. Moreover, greater production or reduced excretion of prostacyclin does not help to elucidate cause and effect, because the open ductus and high prostacyclin levels may both be reflections of organ immaturity. We know of no studies of prostacyclin kinetics, let alone in an immature animal model. More importantly, the Hammerman report is the latest in a series of papers concerned with prophylactic use of indomethacin. These reports are fairly uniform in telling us that the prophylactic, early administration of indomethacin reduces the incidence of the subsequent development of symptomatic PDA and later reopening of the pharmacologically closed ductus; however, ultimate neonatal morbidity and mortality may not be influenced, although there is some suggestion that intracranial hemorrhage may be a lesser problem in babies given indomethacin prophylactically. Thus, it remains conjectural whether it makes any difference if indomethacin is administered to infants of very low birth weight within the first 2–3 days of life, or until days 6–8 when clear signs of hemodynamic derangement exist. We continue to employ the logic that earlier, rather than later, administration of indomethacin is advisable because the very-low-birth-weight infant is especially vulnerable to any magnitude of left-to-right shunt, because its limited myocardial reserve is easily affected adversely as a result of the immature heart's intrinsic structural and functional characteristics (*Pediatr. Clin. North Am.* 31:1197, 1984).—W.F. Friedman, M.D.

Atrial Septal Defects That Present in Infancy
Larry T. Mahoney, Susie C. Truesdell, Thomas R. Krzmarzick, and Ronald M. Lauer (Univ. of Iowa)
Am. J. Dis. Child. 140:1115–1118, November 1986   12–12

Symptomatic atrial septal defect has been reported in infants, many of whom died or underwent surgical closure; spontaneous closure of an atrial septal defect may also occur in childhood. The course of 26 infants with confirmed isolated atrial septal defect was reviewed. The infants were younger than age 18 months, and the defect was diagnosed by cardiac catheterization between 1969 and 1983. The cases represented 0.7% of all catheterizations done in this period.

One third of the infants were born prematurely. A similar proportion was seen in congestive failure, and about one fourth had frequent respiratory tract infections. Half failed to thrive. The cardiothoracic ratio exceeded 0.6 in half of the patients. The mean age at catheterization was 9 months; in only three infants was the diagnosis made correctly before catheterization. The mean pulmonary-systemic flow ratio was 2.3. Only four patients had definite elevation of left ventricular end-diastolic pressure. The defect closed spontaneously in 39% of the patients, as confirmed at a mean age of 5.1 years. The left-to-right shunt was decreased clinically in all of these patients. Another infant had a decreasing shunt. Twelve patients had surgical closure at a mean age of 4 years. A patient who was not operated on died of respiratory failure at age 1 month, with pulmonary edema and an isolated atrial septal defect observed at autopsy. Clinical features did not differ substantially between patients having spontaneous closure of the defect and those undergoing surgical closure.

Spontaneous closure of an atrial septal defect is frequent and this, with the success of medical treatment, allows most infants with symptomatic defects to be followed medically to see whether spontaneous closure occurs. The mechanism of spontaneous closure is unknown. It seems appropriate to defer elective operation until age 5 years unless intractable symptoms persist.

► Isolated atrial septal defects of the secundum type are diagnosed in less than 1% of all infants with congenital heart disease. Because atrial septal defect is one of the most common forms of congenital heart disease in older children and adults, its rare recognition in infancy suggests that there are mechanisms that increase flow across the defect with age, that defects increase in anatomical size with age, or that the clinical features in infants are not easily recognized. The patients described in the abstracted article are atypical for the presentation of atrial septal defect. Most had very high pulmonary to systemic blood flow ratios when catheterized in infancy. This suggests that they had a sort of precocious mechanism that resulted in an early left-to-right shunt across the atrial septal defect. The five findings that usually make us think of this defect (a widely split and fixed second heart sound, a systolic pulmonic ejection murmur, a diastolic tricuspid flow murmur, cardiomegaly, and right ventricular hypertrophy observed on ECG) may not be present in infants with serious atrial septal defects.

So what do we learn from this article? Whereas an atrial septal defect typically is asymptomatic in childhood, infants who present with such conditions are often symptomatic. More than half have heart failure, and a body weight of less than the tenth percentile was common. Spontaneous closure of isolated atrial septal defects has been reported to occur in up to half of these infants. Closure appears to be unrelated to symptoms, physical findings, and data obtained at cardiac catheterization. In this study, the closure of the defect was demonstrated at 2–8 years of age. The authors are probably correct in suggesting that, whenever possible, surgery should be avoided during infancy. Certainly, surgical mortality is greater than that reported in older children. The high rate of spontaneous closure in infants suggests that vigorous medical management, as opposed to surgical closure, should be tried whenever possible to allow sufficient time for spontaneous closure to occur. That leaves surgical intervention reserved for infants with severe symptoms or older children in whom there is evidence of a large left-to-right shunt and the possibility of pulmonary hypertension. So, the next time one of our colleagues suggests that an atrial septal defect be closed, say no, then negotiate.—J.A. Stockman III, M.D.

Prosthetic Heart Valve Replacement in Children: Results and Follow-Up of 273 Patients
A. El Makhlouf, B. Friedli, I. Oberhänsli, J.-C. Rouge, and B. Faidutti (Univ. of Geneva, Switzerland)
J. Thorac. Cardiovasc. Surg. 93:80–85, January 1987   12–13

Rheumatic fever is uncommon in Western countries, but it remains a serious problem in Third World nations. Conservative surgery of valvular lesions is the treatment of choice, but prosthetic valve replacement is often unavoidable when scarring and calcification have made valve reconstruction impossible. A review was made of the surgical results and long-term follow-up data concerning a large group of children with valvular disease, mostly from North Africa and the Middle East, who underwent prosthetic heart valve replacement.

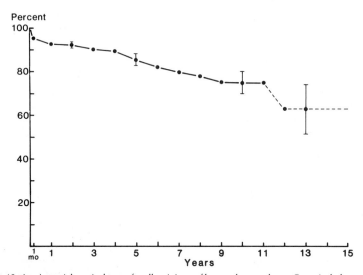

Fig 12–4.—Actuarial survival curve for all recipients of heart valve prostheses. Curve includes operative mortality. Five-year survival was 86% and 10-year survival, 75%. Total number followed up at 5 years was 120, at 10 years, 22; only seven have been followed longer than 11 years, thus the drop at 12 years is of questionable significance (large standard error). (Courtesy of Makhlouf, A.E., et al.: J. Thorac. Cardiovasc. Surg. 93:80–85, January 1987.)

The 273 children (126 boys, 147 girls) were aged from 2 years to 15 years; 253 had rheumatic valvular disease, 19 had congenital valve anomalies, and 1 had endomyocardial fibrosis. A single valve was replaced in 211 children, two valves were replaced in 60, and three valves were replaced in 1 child. A Starr-Edwards prosthesis was implanted in 266 patients, a Björk-Shiley valve in 58, a St. Jude Medical valve in 7, and a Hancock valve in 6 patients.

Four patients died during the operation and nine died within 1 month after operation, for an early mortality of 4.7%. Of 260 survivors, 48 (18%) were lost to follow-up. Causes of 23 late postoperative deaths occurring 2 months to 12 years after operation (Fig 12–4) included thrombosis and embolism (eight patients), heart failure (five), bacterial endocarditis (two), and prosthetic valve detachment (one). The main complication encountered was thromboembolism. None of the patients has yet needed valve replacement because of somatic growth.

Valve replacement in children can be done with a low operative mortality and satisfactory late survival. Although children with advanced rheumatic heart disease benefit enormously from valve replacement operations, eradication of rheumatic fever would be the ultimate solution to this serious problem in Third World countries.

▶ Philip J. Spevak, Assistant in Cardiology, The Children's Hospital, Boston, comments.—J.A. Stockman III, M.D.

▶ Recent advances in the management of congenital heart disease have resulted in a larger pediatric population with prosthetic cardiac valves.

The above series represents one of two larger reviews of children who have required valve replacement. The Boston study (Abstract 12–14) was limited to patients less than 5 years of age who for the most part had congenital heart disease. The series reported by El Makhlouf included older children (mean age, 12 years) primarily with rheumatic disease. The differences in patients influenced surgical technique. El Makhlouf reported good results using the Starr-Edwards Ball and cage device, but we have implanted mostly low-profile tilting disk valves. We encountered early problems with subaortic obstruction when the higher profile devices such as the Starr-Edwards were used. This complication is more likely to occur in small children, especially those with atrioventricular (AV) canal defects when the AV annulus is displaced apically so that the left ventricular outflow dimensions are decreased.

All patients in the El Makhlouf series were anticoagulated (roughly a third received Coumadin and the remainder a combination of aspirin and Dipyridamole). No difference in the incidence of thromboembolic or hemorrhagic complications was noted. This is in contrast to the report of Bradley et al. who found that patients treated with aspirin/Dipyridamole were at increased risk of serious thrombotic events (the group treated with Coumadin did have more frequent, but minor hemorrhagic events) *Am. J. Cardiol.* 56:533–535, 1985. Our policy is to anticoagulate all children who have prosthetic valves with Coumadin (sometimes adding Dipyridamole).

In addition to thromboembolic and hemorrhagic events, other complications of valve replacement include heart block (which occurs around the time of surgery), endocarditis, and intravascular hemolysis. Valves can fail acutely when they are obstructed by thrombus or are prevented from closing by pannus. More commonly in our experience, valve failure is related to patient growth, when relative prosthetic valve stenosis develops gradually over time. Often the signs and symptoms of valve dysfunction are accentuated by an unrelated infectious illness. This is especially true with mitral prostheses when fever increases cardiac output but the associated tachycardia shortens the diastolic time when blood can flow across the valve. Consequently, the gradient across the prosthesis will increase.

Children with prosthetic valves may require urgent attention and often referral to a center experienced in the surgical management of congenital heart disease if they experience respiratory distress, hemodynamic instability, focal neurologic signs, or unexplained anemia or fever.—P.J. Spevak, M.D.

Valve Replacement in Children Less Than 5 Years of Age
Philip J. Spevak, Michael D. Freed, Aldo R. Castaneda, William I. Norwood, and Phyllis Pollack (Children's Hosp., Boston; and Harvard Univ.)
J. Am. Coll. Cardiol. 8:901–908, October 1986   12–14

Valve replacement in small children younger than age 5 years is becoming increasingly common, but little has been reported on the risks and benefits of this type of surgery in young children. A review was made of the records of 63 patients younger than age 5 years when they underwent a total of 70 valve replacements, which included 6 aortic, 49 mitral (5

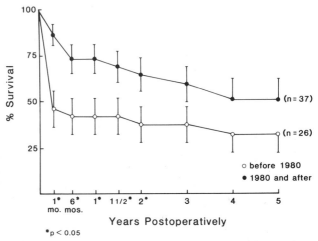

Fig 12–5.—Actuarial survival curves for 26 patients operated on before 1980 and 37 operated on in 1980 or afterward. (Courtesy of Spevak, P.J., et al.: J. Am. Coll. Cardiol. 8:901–908, October 1986.)

repeat), 11 tricuspid (systemic ventricle, 2 repeat), 2 tricuspid (pulmonary ventricle), and 1 multiple (mitral-aortic). One patient was lost to follow-up. Follow-up of the 46 surviving patients ranged from 1 month to 12 years 8 months.

Half of the valves inserted before 1980 were tissue valves, either porcine or dura mater; the other half were either high-profile (31%) or low-profile (69%) mechanical valves. Since 1980 mechanical low-profile valves, either Björk-Shiley or St. Jude, have been used exclusively.

The 1-year survival rate for the 26 patients operated on before 1980 was 42%, compared with 73% for the 37 patients operated on in 1980 and thereafter. The 4-year survival rates were 32% and 51%, respectively (Fig 12–5). Ages of the patients from the two time periods did not differ significantly. More than two thirds of all fatalities were operative deaths, usually occurring within 3 days of surgery. Nine patients required a pacemaker when complete heart block developed after replacement of an aortic valve. Although valve replacement in young children generally results in significant postoperative hemodynamics, mortality, although declining over time, remains higher than that observed in adults.

▶ Valve replacement has been performed in children for quite some time. The above report is important in that it provides a great deal of information about how things are going. It is only during this decade that we have seen major improvements in operative mortality and an improvement in long-term survivorship after valve replacement in children. There are late deaths, though, and these authors note that some of these result from valve failure. Fortunately, there was a very low thromboembolic complication rate in this series—only 1.6 episodes per 100 patient-years. Presumably, this represents an increased use of the Björk-Shiley and St. Jude prosthetic valves. These investigators protect prosthetic valves with warfarin, but many other centers simply use aspirin and

Dipyridamole. Other investigators using the St. Jude cardiac valve replacement achieved similar results using anticoagulation with warfarin (Schaffer, N.S.: *J. Am. Coll. Cardiol.* 9:235, 1987). McGrath et al. (*Ann. Thorac. Surg.* 43:285, 1987) examined in detail the effectiveness of aspirin and Dipyridamole. They found significant problems with adequate anticoagulation and recommended that all patients who receive valve replacement of the type noted above should be completely anticoagulated with full-dose warfarin sodium therapy. On the other hand, Verrier et al. (*J. Thorac. Cardiovasc. Surg.* 92:1013, 1986) unequivocally state that children with mechanical aortic valves in normal sinus rhythm can be treated safely with aspirin (with or without Dipyridamole) with little risk of thromboembolic events, valve thrombosis, or valve failure. This seems a little like the battle of the universities trying to decide what is right. Maybe I'll wait for a powerhouse like the University of Alabama to settle the issue. Then again, they spend eight times as much on their athletic department than they do on their physics department.

Data from Canada suggest that perhaps they have the right answer. Callaghan et al. report on a 6-year clinical study of the use of the "Omniscience" valve prosthesis. (*J. Am. Coll. Cardiol.* 9:240, 1987). They describe a superb clinical performance with this valve. With a name like "Omniscience," what can you expect? We should be learning more about the experience in the United States with the "Omniscience" valve because it was given full approval for use here by the Food and Drug Administration in May 1985. Stay tuned.— J.A. Stockman III, M.D.

The Arterial Switch Operation: An Eight-Year Experience
Jan M. Quaegebeur, John Rohmer, Jaap Ottenkamp, Tjik Buis, John W. Kirklin, Eugene H. Blackstone, and A.G. Brom (Univ. Hosp., Leiden, The Netherlands)
J. Thorac. Cardiovasc. Surg. 92:361–384, September 1986   12–15

An arterial switch repair has been performed in 66 patients since 1977. Twenty-three neonates had transposition with an intact ventricular septum; 33 infants and children had transposition and a large ventricular septal defect (VSD); and 10 patients had a double-outlet right ventricle with a subpulmonary VSD. Forty-eight of these patients had associated cardiac anomalies (table).

The actuarial survival at 11 months, including hospital and later deaths, was 81%. Lower birth weight and a patent ductus arteriosus of any size increased the risk of death, as did an earlier date of operation. Systolic left ventricular function was normal late after operation in all but 1 of 36 patients having two-dimensional echocardiography. Three survivors had evidence of mild semilunar valve incompetence. Sinus rhythm was present at last follow-up in 96% of the patients. Most children gained weight relative to normal for age after surgery. All but 2 of 55 patients were in New York Heart Association class I at last follow-up, the exceptions being in class II. Two patients had reoperations for complications related to the

ASSOCIATED CARDIAC LESIONS PRESENT AT THE TIME OF THE
ARTERIAL SWITCH OPERATION

Associated cardiac anomaly	No.	% of 66
None	18	27%
Patent ductus arteriosus	29	44%
Small	10	15
Moderate	11	17
Large	7	11
Coarctation of aorta	2	3%
Left superior vena cava	3	5%
Left juxtaposition of atrial appendage	4	6%
Left ventricular outflow tract obstruction (dynamic)	4	6%
Pulmonary artery bifurcation stenosis (iatrogenic)	5	8%
Small distal pulmonary artery	1	1.5%
Bicuspid aortic valve	1	1.5%
Bicuspid pulmonary valve	1	1.5%
Small tricuspid valve	1	1.5%
Straddling tricuspid valve	2	3%
Nonfacing intercoronary commissures	1	1.5%
Eccentric coronary orifice	1	1.5%
Dextrocardia	1	1.5%
Interrupted aortic arch	1	1.5%

In patients with patent ductus arteriosus, coarctation of the aorta, pulmonary artery bifurcation stenosis, straddling tricuspid valve, or interrupted aortic arch, repair was performed at the time of the arterial switch operation. Some patients had more than one associated cardiac anomaly.

In nine additional patients (14%) a patent ductus arteriosus was repaired at a previous operation; in six (9%) a coarctation was previously repaired.

(Courtesy of Quaegebeur, J.M., et al.: J. Thorac. Cardiovasc. Surg. 92:361–384, September 1986.)

arterial switch procedure, and three patients underwent repair of a residual VSD.

The arterial switch operations is anatomically applicable to nearly all patients having transposition with a VSD, an intact septum, or a double-outlet right ventricle with subpulmonary VSD. Hospital mortality is low. The results are superior to those of the atrial switch operation. Surgery is indicated in the first 2 weeks of life in patients with transposition and an intact ventricular septum, with or without patent ductus arteriosus. Patients with transposition and a large VSD should have closure of the defect and an arterial switch repair at about age 3 months, or earlier if congestive failure or rapidly progressive pulmonary vascular disease develops. Pulmonary artery banding is not indicated, but it does not contraindicate an arterial switch operation.

▶ Dr. Farouk Idriss, Professor of Surgery, Northwestern University Medical School, and Chief, Division of Cardiovascular Surgery, Children's Memorial Hospital, Chicago, comments.—J.A. Stockman III, M.D.

▶ Surgical repair of transposition of the great arteries has oscillated over the years between atrial venous rerouting and anatomical repair, the two basic approaches that could be used to effect correction. In atrial venous rerouting (Senning, Mustard), the great arteries remain in their transposed position (aorta to right ventricle and pulmonary artery to left ventricle); however, the venous return to the heart is rerouted so that the pulmonary venous blood returns to the right ventricle, which remains the sytemic ventricle. This approach was the most commonly used until the past 10 years, when anatomical repair was revived. Anatomical repair in the early 1960s by switching the great arteries and coronary arteries did not initially result in survival, and the technique was abandoned in favor of the more successful atrial venous rerouting. Long-term results of this atrial approach, however, proved unsatisfactory because of the occurrence of troublesome arrhythmias, systemic venous return obstruction, and, most importantly, significant right ventricular dysfunction, because the right ventricle remains the systemic ventricle with these techniques. Because of these problems, and after the success reported by Jatene 10 years ago, many centers returned to the arterial switch for complete repair of this defect. At present, there is definite evidence that with this anatomical approach, when the left ventricle is returned to its systemic pumping function, there is preservation of ventricular function and lack of the significant complications encountered in the atrial rerouting. Thus, at present we recommend the arterial switch as the procedure of choice.

In infants with an intact ventricular septum, the repair should be performed in the neonatal period—definitely before the third week of life and preferably in the first few days after birth—for the left ventricle not to adapt to the lowered pulmonary resistance after birth and thus not be capable of suddenly assuming the systemic load after the arterial switch. In those infants with a large VSD, the left ventricle remains exposed to right ventricular pressure and may be repaired at a later stage after pulmonary artery banding to limit the left-to-right shunt and keep the left ventricular pressure at a high level. We tend at present to repair the VSD and perform an arterial switch early in infancy.

Other less common complex forms of transposition of the great arteries may not be amenable to this approach, and other procedures using conduits may have to be used, e.g., the Rastelli procedure when the flow from the left ventricle is directed to the aorta through the VSD and the right ventricle connected to the pulmonary artery by a valved conduit, thus accomplishing an anatomical repair without switching the great arteries.

Although the results of anatomical repair are excellent at present and very encouraging with decreasing mortality and morbidity, there is need for very long-term follow-up to determine if late complications develop.—F. Idriss, M.D.

Aortic Dilation, Dissection, and Rupture in Patients With Turner Syndrome

Angela E. Lin, Barbara M. Lippe, Mitchell E. Geffner, Antoinette Gomes, Juan F. Lois, Catherine W. Barton, Amnon Rosenthal, and William F. Friedman (Univ. of California at Los Angeles, and Univ. of Michigan)
J. Pediatr. 109:820–826, November 1986   12–16

The incidence of cardiac defects in patients with Turner's syndrome is 20% to 44%. Although a bicuspid aortic valve may be the most common, and aortic coarctation the most recognized, anomaly, aortic dissection and aneurysmal rupture are the most devastating. Of 57 patients with Turner's syndrome examined with M-mode, two-dimensional, and Doppler echocardiography, either at first presentation (33 patients) or at follow-up visits (24), 5 (8.8%) had significant aortic root and vessel abnormalities that were distinct from coarctation. Three patients had a bicuspid aortic valve, one had stenosis and regurgitation, and one had regurgitation alone. Magnetic resonance imaging was performed in four of these five patients. Of four patients with a dilated aortic root, two had a dilated aortic segment of the sinus of Valsalva; one of these two patients had a bicuspid valve (Fig 12–6).

On the basis of these findings, aortic abnormalities represent a source of potential morbidity and mortality in patients with Turner's syndrome that is often overlooked. Cardiologic evaluation should begin in childhood in all patients with Turner's syndrome.

▶ The factors that predispose patients with Turner's syndrome to cardiac and vascular problems are not known. It is probable that, before aortic dissection occurs, there is cystic medial necrosis of the aorta such as what is seen in Marfan's syndrome. That patients with Turner's syndrome may have a similar primary mesenchymal defect is suggested by abnormalities in other mesenchy-

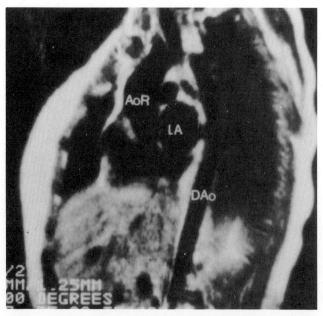

Fig 12–6.—Sagittal magnetic resonance imaging scan of thoracic aorta. Aortic root (AoR) is dilated significantly compared with descending thoracic aorta (DAo), which is of normal caliber. LA = left atrium. (Courtesy of Lin, A.E., et al.: J. Pediatr. 109: 820–826, November 1986.)

mal tissues (e.g., bone matrix and lymphatic vessels) in these patients. The presence of coarctation of the aorta is also a risk factor for dilatation, dissection, and rupture of the aorta. For what it's worth, aortic dilatation correlated fairly well with having the webbed-neck phenotype of Turner's syndrome. This is relatively important, because the occurrence of aortic dissection has been reported with Noonan's syndrome, another condition in which neck webbing may be a consequence of fetal lymphatic obstruction.

These authors suggest that every patient with Turner's syndrome have a full cardiologic examination including chest x-ray studies and Doppler echocardiograms. If no abnormalities are found, a similar repeat examination would be done every 3–5 years. If abnormalities are found, particularly those of the aortic root or arch dilatation, magnetic resonance imaging (MRI) should be used to delineate further the extent of the abnormality, and MRI should be the procedure for following these patients at regular intervals. If a patient has significant dilatation, every measure must be instituted to prevent complications. If hypertension is present, it must be rigorously controlled. The patient will have to receive prophylaxis against infectious endocarditis and probably should be advised to avoid contact sports and sustained isometric exercise. Some also advocate the use of propranolol to slow the progression of aortic dilatation. This recommendation is commonplace in children and adults with Marfan's syndrome. Needless to say, all patients with Turner's syndrome should be educated about the life-threatening significance of unexplained chest pain, dyspnea, or hypotension that can signal aortic rupture.—J.A. Stockman III, M.D.

Minoxidil for Control of Acute Blood Pressure Elevation in Chronically Hypertensive Children
C. Frederic Strife, Monica Quinlan, F. Bryson Waldo, Cheryl J. Fryer, Elizabeth C. Jackson, Thomas R. Welch, Paul T. McEnery, and Clark D. West (Univ. of Cincinnati)
Pediatrics 78:861–865, November 1986   12–17

Minoxidil is a potent vasodilator that acts directly to relax arteriolar smooth muscle. It has generally been reserved for treatment of refractory hypertension. Minoxidil has rarely been used for long-term treatment of hypertensive children, because of the side effects of hypertrichosis, tachycardia, and sodium retention. Recently, minoxidil given orally in combination with propranolol and furosemide was reported to lower blood pressure to acceptable levels within 8–12 hours in severely hypertensive adults. It was hypothesizesd that the slow decrease in blood pressure with oral minoxidil treatment, in contrast with the rapid decrease obtained by intravenous diazoxide or sodium nitroprusside administration, was advantageous. The oral use of minoxidil in hypertensive emergencies in pediatric patients was explored.

Twenty-three episodes of acute blood pressure elevation related to renal disease in 13 chronically hypertensive children aged 2–18 years were treated with one oral dose of minoxidil. All patients except for one were receiving a β blocker at the time minoxidil was administered. The goal of lowering blood pressure to or below the 95th percentile for age within 4 hours of minoxidil administration was achieved in 14 of the 23 treatment episodes. When the dose of minoxidil was at least 0.2 mg/kg, the goal was achieved in 9 (82%) of 11 patients; when the dose was less than 0.2 mg/kg, the goal was achieved in 5 (42%) of 12. Patients who were treated with at least 0.2 mg/kg had a substantial decrease in mean systolic and diastolic blood pressures within 1 hour. However, patients who received less than 0.2 mg/kg never experienced a significant change in mean systolic blood pressure and had no marked change in mean diastolic blood pressure for 2 hours. The adverse effects of the drug were minimal. Minoxidil in one dose of 0.2 mg/kg in combination with a diuretic and a β blocker appears to lower blood pressure to safe levels within 4 hours in most patients who have severe hypertension related to renal disease; side effects are minimal.

▶ One of the beautiful aspects of minoxidil is that it is rapidly absorbed after oral administration and produces peak blood levels in just 60 minutes. Its half-life is approximately 4 hours. Internists frequently use the oral form of minoxidil in contrast to intravenous forms of diazoxide or sodium nitroprusside, particularly in patients with incipient hypertensive encephalopathy with malignant hypertension, or with hypertension complicated by renal insufficiency, cerebral infarction, cerebral ischemia, or ischemic heart disease. The reason for using minoxidil as opposed to these other two agents is that it lowers the blood pressure gradually but has a relatively rapid onset of action. The gradual reduction of blood pressure in the conditions just mentioned is far more safe than sudden drops in blood pressure. The investigators in the study abstracted above also used minoxidil successfully in acute hypertensive emergencies. This is what encouraged them to use it on a chronic basis in children. What we see in chronically hypertensive children is that minoxidil, when used with a diuretic and a β-blocking agent, is extremely helpful in controlling hypertension. If you don't care how quickly you lower the initial blood pressure, the calcium channel blocker nifedipine can be used; it can be given sublingually and lowers the blood pressure extremely rapidly.

The implications of this report are pretty straightforward. The use of single-dose minoxidil therapy for control of severe hypertension not only obviates parenteral therapy but avoids the rapid, precipitous blood pressure changes that can occur after treatment with diazoxide or sodium nitroprusside. In addition, minoxidil can be used advantageously when patients are being transported or in the home, assuming adequate blood pressure monitoring is available.

It's curious that such an excellent antihypertensive as minoxidil receives more attention as the drug that is the final hope for the "bald." The manufacturer of minoxidil, Upjohn, has marketed a topical preparation containing 2% minoxidil ("Regaine") for the treatment of male baldness (androgenic alopecia) in Belgium, Canada, and France, and is about to do so in many other countries. Before running out to buy some minoxidil for yourself or your loved one, read the excellent review of this drug by deGroot (*Lancet* 1:1019, 1987). It is noted that topical application of minoxidil can, in some men with androgenic alopecia, induce the growth of terminal hair. A cosmetically satisfactory result is achieved in only a small proportion of users, probably less than 10%. The costs are considerable, especially because the treatment apparently cannot be stopped without loss of the hair gained. Despite the unimpressive results of treatment with minoxidil, licensing of the drug for this indication will create a great demand for it. The British view of the results of a cost-benefit analysis of treatment of male baldness with topical minoxidil raises doubts about the wisdom of permitting its use for this purpose, but the argument is that it is, in effect, a cosmetic and not a drug.

To quote an editorial in the *New York Times,* the low chance of success with minoxidil should be stated clearly on the packaging and Upjohn should define better who is likely to benefit and by how much. Heed ye these words, or a lot of us Americans are going to be "scalped."

(Incidentally, be wary of minoxidil as an antihypertensive for use in pregnant patients. Hypertrichosis and congenital anomalies have been associated with its use during pregnancy. *Pediatrics* 79:434, 1987.)—J.A. Stockman III, M.D.

Lipoproteins in the Progeny of Young Men With Coronary Artery Disease: Children With Increased Risk
Julia Lee, Ronald M. Lauer, and William R. Clarke (Univ. of Iowa)
Pediatrics 78:330–337, August 1986   12–18

Genetic and environmental interactions play important roles in the age of onset and severity of ischemic heart disease. A study was undertaken to determine whether examination of progeny with a parental history of premature onset of coronary heart disease will identify a group of children and young adults at high risk for future ischemic heart disease. In all, 173 progeny from 63 families in which the father had angiographically diagnosed coronary artery disease by age 50 were studied. Age-specific and sex-specific data from the Lipid Research Clinic Prevalence Study were used as references for total lipids, lipoproteins, Quetelet Index, and systolic and diastolic blood pressures.

FATHERS AND PROGENY WITH ABNORMAL LIPIDS AND LIPOPROTEINS*

Category	Fathers (N = 52)			Progeny (N = 173)		
	n	% Total	% Abnormal	n	% Total	% Abnormal
LDL-C	13	25	39	20	12	23
HDL-C	6	12	18	29	17	33
LDL-C, HDL-C	1	2	3	7	4	8
Triglyceride	5	0	15	13	8	15
Triglyceride, LDL-C	2	4	6	7	4	8
Triglyceride, HDL-C	5	10	15	5	3	6
Triglyceride, LDL-C, HDL-C	1	2	3	6	3	7
Total abnormal	33	65%	100%	87	51%	100%

*Categories are mutually exclusive. Abnormality defined as a level >90th percentile of the Lipid Research Clinic age-specific and sex-specific data for low-density lipoprotein cholesterol (LDL-C) or triglyceride or < tenth percentile for high-density lipoprotein cholesterol (HDL-C). % Total = percent of the total group (fathers, n = 52; progeny, n = 173) with abnormal levels of lipids or lipoproteins as defined above. % Abnormal = percent among those with abnormal levels of lipids or lipoproteins (fathers, n = 33; progeny, n = 87).

(Courtesy of Lee, J., et al.: Pediatrics 78:330–337, August 1986.)

Overall, 65% of the affected fathers and 51% of the progeny had elevated levels of triglycerides and low-density lipoprotein cholesterol (LDL-C), diminished high-density lipoprotein cholesterol (HDL-C) or a combination thereof (table). Distribution of the total lipids and lipoproteins in the progeny bore a striking resemblance to those in their affected fathers. In both, the distribution of total cholesterol, total triglyceride, and LDL-C was shifted upward with excessive numbers of patients in the upper decile of these variables; the distribution of HDL-C was shifted downward with a significantly increased number of patients with low HDL-C. A significant number of mothers had diminished HDL-C, which appeared to be related to their obesity.

Children with a parental history of premature coronary heart disease or hyperlipidemia are at unusually high risk for the development of lipid and lipoprotein abnormalities and future coronary artery disease. Early identification of these children offers an opportunity for early initiation of preventive measures.

▶ Familial hypercholesterolemia is a genetic disorder of lipoprotein metabolism characterized by elevated plasma levels of LDL and premature atherosclerosis. These elevations appear to result from a defective gene that either produces no LDL receptors or abnormal receptors that cannot bind LDL, causing a consequent rise in the plasma cholesterol concentration that accelerates the formation of atherosclerosis. Heterozygotes with one defective gene have plasma cholesterol levels usually in the range of 300–500 mg/dl and clinically apparent atherosclerosis begins to occur in the fourth decade of life. Homozygotes with two defective genes have a more severe clinical picture, with plasma cholesterol levels of 700–1,000 mg/dl and onset of atherosclerotic disease in the first or second decade of life. Almost all of the latter patients are dead before the age of 20.

What are some of the things that contribute to the risk of atherosclerosis? Some have suggested that "fast foods" are one contributor. The average American man, woman, and child now spend about $200 a year on fast foods. It has been estimated that one person of every seven visits a McDonald's each day. With regard to fast foods, topping the chart for burgers with respect to calories is Wendy's triple cheeseburger at 1,040 calories; it contains just under 2 gm of sodium and 15 teaspoons of fat. In contrast, a plain McDonald's hamburger has 263 calories, 3 teaspoons of fat, and 500 mg of sodium. With respect to fish sandwiches, if you believe in omega-3, watch out! By the time mayonnaise, other dressings, cheese, and so forth are piled on, a Burger King Whaler sandwich winds up with twice the calories of Arthur Treacher's broiled fish. If you want to get your maximum daily allowance of cholesterol (as recommended by the American Heart Association), simply have an Arby's sausage and egg croissant. In fact, you'll get 2 days worth of maximum daily cholesterol. If you think you'll save your heart by having a breakfast at Jack in the Box, think again—their egg breakfast contains 10 teaspoons of fat. How can you ward off all these complications of fast foods? The answer is simple: Either stop eating them or learn to skip the mayonnaise, tartar sauce, cream dressings, and hold the cheese. Having a Whopper without mayo reduces calories by 150. While on a holding pattern, hold the barbeque sauce. That little ounce of McDonald's barbeque sauce for your Chicken McNuggets contains almost triple the amount of salt as a regular order or French fries. If you're wondering where all this information is contained, see a book entitled, *The Fast Food Guide* by M. Jacobson.

What to do about adult heart disease prevention during childhood has been extremely controversial. I'm sure that the readers of the YEAR BOOK are well versed in all aspects of the issues related to these controversies. If you wish to refresh yourself, see the following three references: McNamara, D.G.: *Am. J. Dis. Child.* 140:985, 1986; Committee on Nutrition: *Pediatrics* 78:521, 1986; Nader, P.R., et al.: *Pediatrics* 79:843, 1987. Much of the controversy centers around who should be screened. Griffin, T., Christoffel, K., and the Pediatric Practice Research Group of Children's Memorial Hospital in Chicago have shown that screening for hyperlipidemia based solely on a family history of early coronary artery disease is inadequate to detect coronary disease in most children with hyperlipidemia (*Proceedings* of the Midwest Society for Pediatric Research, November 1987). These investigators recommend universal screening of all children if the goal is early detection of hyperlipidemia. Indeed, we have seen recommendations appearing during the past year for universal neonatal screening for hypercholesterolemia (Asami, T., et al.: *Lancet* 1:1038, 1987).

We now have many options available to us to help manage children who have hyperlipidemia. For example, hypercholesterolemia can be treated with a soybean protein diet. This can achieve a reduction of more than 20% in total cholesterol (Gaddi, A., et al.: *Arch. Dis. Child.* 62:274, 1987). Activated charcoal is capable of reducing LDL-C by 25% to 40% (Kuusisto, P., et al.: *Lancet* 2:366, 1986). If necessary, we can use cholesterol-binding resins. We've all heard about trying to eat more fish with omega-3 fatty acids, which tend to lower total lipid levels and also reduce platelet aggregation (Weiner, M.A.: *N. Engl. J. Med.* 315:833, 1986).

Many of the above measures will no longer be necessary (except the recommendation for a prudent diet) with the introduction of Lovastatin (mevinolin). This is the drug that everybody waited for last year. It is able to stimulate LDL receptor activity and consequently lower the LDL-C concentration. This appears to be an extremely effective agent. For example, there was reported a 6-year-old child who, because of homozygous familial hypercholesterolemia and severe coronary artery disease, underwent cardiac and liver transplantation. The cardiac transplantation was necessitated because of the severity of this child's coronary artery disease and the liver transplantation was intended to provide enough LDL receptors to lower the patient's LDL-C level. Even though the child did well with the surgery and the LDL-C level fell by 80% after the transplantation, it remained significantly elevated for the child's age and sex. At this point, treatment with Lovastatin was initiated. The LDL-C level moved into the normal range (East, C., et al.: *JAMA* 256:2843, 1986). If this is typical of what can happen with homozygous familial hypercholesterolemia, gone will be the days of recommending portacaval shunts, plasmapheresis, and all the other relatively ineffective methodologies that had been used heretofore.

In closing, everyone wishes there were a more simple way to tell who's at risk for early heart attacks. It's a shame that simple obesity isn't a good enough screen: Being a "blimp" isn't enough. The only reason I mention the latter is because the word "blimp" has always been a fascinating one, at least to me. I thought that corpulent individuals were called "blimps" because they had a shape similar to the lighter-than-air airships. Not so, says John Ciardi (*A Second Browser's Dictionary,* New York, Harper and Row, 1983, p. 25). An obese person is called a "blimp" after a certain Colonel Blimp, a complacently dogmatic, fat, and fat-headed, elderly British clubman who retired from service in India during this past century. His pompous attitudes and ponderous size introduced the word "blimp" into the English language very quickly. Believe it or not, the lighter-than-air airship called a blimp isn't named after Colonel Blimp at all. It stands for type *B, limp* airship, as distinguished from the rigid dirigible. How odd the English language works! Some have claimed that we are damaged angels, others that we are improved apes. If we began as angels, the damage is obvious. If we began as apes (or cousins to the ape), the improvement is not as readily visible, at least when it comes to language.

With this rather lengthy commentary, so closes the chapter on the heart and blood vessels.—J.A. Stockman III, M.D.

13 The Blood

Neonatal Polycythemia: Frequency of Clinical Manifestations and Other Associated Findings
Thomas E. Wiswell, J. Devn Cornish, and Ralph S. Northam (Brooke Army Med. Ctr., Ft. Sam Houston, Tex.)
Pediatrics 78:26–30, July 1986   13–1

Neonatal polycythemia remains a diagnostic and management problem. The frequency of clinical features and associated findings of neonatal polycythemia was evaluated in two large groups of newborns. All infants born from 1981 through 1984 at the Brooke Army Medical Center were screened for polycythemia in the first part of the study, and all infants born in United States Army hospitals during a 5-year period were evaluated in the second part of the study.

Of the 3,768 infants born at Brooke Army Medical Center, 55 (1.46%) had neonatal polycythemia. Most of these infants were full term and appropriate for age, but the incidence of polycythemia was significantly higher in small-for-gestational-age infants and large-for-gestational-age infants. Overall, 85% of these infants had features associated with the disorder. The most common signs and symptoms were "feeding problems" (21.8%), plethora (20%), lethargy (14.5%), cyanosis (14.5%), respiratory distress (9.1%), jitteriness (7.3%), hypotonia (7.3%), and heart murmur (5.5%). Laboratory findings included hypoglycemia (40%), hyperbilirubinemia (21.8%) and thrombocytopenia (5.5%). Only 14.5% of these polycythemic infants had no clinical or laboratory abnormalities. Of the 220,050 infants born in all army hospitals, 932 (0.42%) had neonatal polycythemia. The disorder was also frequent among preterm infants (6.3%) and those who were small (12.3%) and large (13.6%) for gestational age (table). Frequent findings were hyperbilirubinemia (33.5%),

PATIENT PROFILE OF 932 POLYCYTHEMIC INFANTS

	No. (%) of Infants
Gestational age	
Preterm (<38 wk)	59 (6.3)
Term (38–42 wk)	841 (90.2)
Postterm (>42 wk)	32 (3.4)
Growth status	
Small for gestational age	115 (12.3)
Appropriate for gestational age	690 (74.0)
Large for gestational age	127 (13.6)

(Courtesy of Wisell, T.E., et al.: Pediatrics 78:26–30, July 1986.)

hypoglycemia (13%), and respiratory distress (6.6%). Only 1.4% of infants had necrotizing enterocolitis, 1.0% were thrombocytopenic, and 0.5% had seizures. Several findings were unexpected: intracranial hemorrhages in 0.6% of infants, gonadal dysgenesis in 0.3%, and cystic fibrosis in 0.3%. Although most of the associated findings were evident in infants who were full term and appropriate for gestational age, several findings, i.e., hyperbilirubinemia and hypoglycemia, were common in premature infants and those large or small for gestational age.

Most infants with polycythemia have clinical signs and symptoms, and more than 20% of polycythemic infants have laboratory abnormalities without overt symptoms. Polycythemia is not rare among premature infants, but its overall frequency appears to be lower than previously reported. Because of the frequency of significant morbid complications, routine screening for polycythemia is warranted as part of normal neonatal care.

▶ I don't think anyone will disagree with the fact that neonatal polycythemia can be associated sometimes with life-threatening insults to the brain, heart, kidneys, lungs, and intestines. Despite the "plethora" (pardon the pun) of literature describing this, that, or another manifestation of polycythemia/hyperviscosity, we still see reports such as the one abstracted that go a little bit further to aid our understanding but never really quite hit the mark. What are the issues? They are to screen or not to screen? If to screen, by what technique, and at what age? Should the polycythemic baby be treated prophylactically, or treated only if symptoms develop?

Some would challenge the value of the capillary hematocrit as being an adequate screening tool, such as what was done in this study. Another series, which examined cord hematocrits and capillary hematocrits (Ramamurthy, R.S., et al.: *J. Pediatr.* 110:929, 1987) found that the mean ± 2 SD capillary hematocrit was 64% ± 12% in infants without polycythemia and 71% ± 8% in infants with polycythemia. If the latter authors had used the criteria reported in the abstract above, i.e., capillary hematocrit of 65%, they would have done a lot of venous samplings. Thus, it is difficult even to gauge what one would mean by a "normal" capillary hematocrit, much less what would be considered a hematocrit associated with polycythemia. If a capillary sample is obtained after elevating the skin temperature of the foot to 40 C, a better correlation with a venous hematocrit is seen. Capillary hematocrits are also significantly influenced by pH and systolic blood pressure.

The military study above reports what may be the highest association between symptoms and the presence of polycythemia (using their criteria). Only 20% of polycythemic infants did not have any symptomatology. In the *Journal of Pediatrics* article by Ramamurthy et al., only 1 infant of 16 with polycythemia became symptomatic.

What can be made of all this? I don't have the slightest idea. What I think is needed is the complete "full service" study. This would be one in which the data from the *Journal of Pediatrics* article are duplicated showing that cord hematocrits are as useful as capillary hematocrits in screening for polycythemia. I personally believe that it should be relatively easy to obtain cord heparinized blood with a relatively low clot rate. That seems like a better initial screening test. It is true that the highest hematocrits will be seen at 2 hours, but they should be predictable from the cord sample in most instances. If one wants to do a comparative study, let him go ahead and reproduce the *Journal of Pediatrics* data. Because most nurseries do not have the ability to determine viscosities, all of the numbers generated should be correlated with clinical signs and symptoms in their infant population. Those signs and symptoms then should be used to decide what are appropriate cutoffs at what age to define polycythemia. The last part of the study is the most difficult. That would involve taking a control group of infants in whom no exchange transfusions were performed to lower the hematocrit and compare them with a group of infants in whom prophylactic exchange was performed. The overall outcome of both groups would then be examined. The probability of all this actually happening is almost nonexistent. And, thus we will be stuck with seeing more reports, albeit very well intended, that do not necessarily add a great deal more information to our present knowledge base. What that knowledge base tells us right now is that maybe we should be screening all infants, and those who are unequivocally polycythemic should be watched like a hawk.—J.A. Stockman III, M.D.

Oral Vitamin E Supplementation for the Prevention of Anemia in Premature Infants: A Controlled Trial
A. Zipursky, E.J. Brown, J. Watts, R. Milner, C. Rand, V.S. Blanchette, E.F. Bell, B. Paes, and E. Ling (Hosp. for Sick Children, Toronto, Univ. of Toronto, and McMaster Univ., Hamilton)
Pediatrics 79:61–68, January 1987   13–2

Newborn infants have reduced serum vitamin E concentrations. It has been asserted that vitamin E deficiency is partly responsible for the development of anemia in premature infants during the first 6 weeks of life. Earlier workers reported that vitamin E administration prevents anemia in premature infants, but the validity of these findings has been questioned. A randomized, controlled, double-blind trial was conducted to assess the effectiveness of vitamin E therapy in the prevention of anemia in premature infants.

The 178 premature infants, all weighing less than 1,500 gm at birth, were assigned to either a treatment group or a control group. The treatment group included 46 sick and 44 well infants, and the control group included 48 sick and 40 well infants. The infants were treated daily during the first 6 weeks with 25 international units of *dl*-α-tocopherol (study group) or a placebo solution (control group).

Starting on day 3 of treatment, vitamin E concentrations in the treated group were significantly higher throughout the 6-week study than in the control group. However, 6 weeks, there was no significant difference between the treated and untreated groups with regard to hemoglobin concentration, reticulocyte count, platelet count, or erythrocyte form. Both sick and well infants in the vitamin-E supplemented group had increased

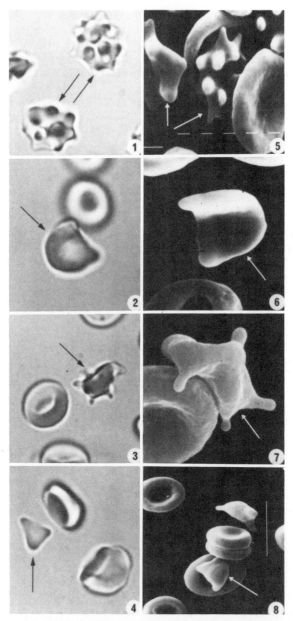

Fig 13–1.—Appearance of abnormally shaped erythrocytes in peripheral blood of premature infants. All preparations were glutaraldehyde fixed. 1 to 4, Light microscopy; 5 to 8, scanning electron microscopy; 1 and 5, echinocytes; 2 and 6, keratocytes; 3 and 7, acanthocytes; and 4 and 8, schizocytes. (Courtesy of Zipursky, A., et al.: Pediatrics 79:61–68, January 1987.)

numbers of echinocytes during the first week (Fig 13–1). The significance of this finding is unknown, but it may have been a toxic effect associated with vitamin E therapy. Because of a lack of hematologic response and a finding of possible vitamin E toxicity, administration of vitamin E to premature infants cannot be recommended.

▶ Lewis A. Barness, M.D., Professor and Chairman, Department of Pediatrics, College of Medicine, University of South Florida, is this country's resident expert on vitamin E. He comments.—J.A. Stockman III, M.D.

▶ This carefully controlled study indicates that with presently available infant formulas in the United States, prematurely born infants have little likelihood of vitamin E responsive hemolytic anemia developing, and that further supplements of vitamin E are unnecessary to modify this effect of vitamin E.

Lest this result in relaxation of infant formula standards, caution is needed. Present formulas have lesser amounts of polyunsaturated fats than those used in 1966 and have supplemental vitamin E, so that the E/PUFA ratio is significantly different. The iron content is similar at both times (iron is a pro-oxidant). The red blood cell membrane mimics ingested fats; it is likely that the present combination of low PUFA and some tocopherol is sufficient to protect the red blood cells of the 1987 babies from hemolysis caused by peroxidation. Support for this is the finding that peroxide hemolysis gives falsely negative results in those vitamin E-deficient infants who are given vitamin E within 3 days of performing the hemolysis test.

The study of Zipursky et al. confirms the desirability of the present E/PUFA ratio, but does not negate the previously documented vitamin E-responsive hemolytic anemia of prematurity. Let vitamin E remain a vitamin!—L.A. Barness, M.D.

Evaluation of the Capillary Microhematocrit as a Screening Test for Anemia in Pediatric Office Practice

Paul C. Young, Barbara Hamill, Richard C. Wasserman, and Joseph D. Dickerman (Univ. of Vermont and Med. Ctr. Hosp. of Vermont, Burlington)
Pediatrics 78:206–208, August 1986   13–3

The microhematocrit measurement of a capillary blood sample is frequently used to screen children for anemia. This technique requires no special skill or expensive equipment, and results are rapidly available. However, recent reports have suggested that the capillary microhematocrit gives values markedly higher than simultaneous venous hematocrits obtained with an electronic counter. The capillary microhematocrit has been used for many years to screen for anemia in children, and experience has indicated that the venous Coulter hematocrit value is usually higher than the capillary value. A study was designed to evaluate the capillary microhematocrit as a screening test for anemia in a pediatric office practice.

The study population consisted of 66 children, aged 9 months to 14 years, whose capillary hematocrits were less than, equal to, or one or two points higher than the lower limit of normal for age. Simultaneous with the capillary sample, venous samples were obtained, and the hemoglobin concentration, hematocrit, and mean corpuscular volume were determined with a Coulter electronic counter. Published standards of venous hemoglobin concentration were used, and the sensitivity, specificity, and predictive values of the capillary microhematocrit were assessed in this patient population.

Of the 66 patients, 20 had venous hemoglobin values less than the lower limit of normal. The sensitivity of the microhematocrit was 90.0% and the specificity was 43.5%. The predictive value for a normal (negative) hematocrit was 90.1%, and the predictive value for a low (positive) hematocrit was 40.9%. The microhematocrit method using capillary blood misses few patients with significantly low venous hemoglobin values and is therefore an acceptable screening test for anemia.

▶ A capillary microhematocrit test as usually performed in an office setting is quick, inexpensive, and does not require special skill. The results are immediately available. To understand the study abstracted above, please realize that "sensitivity" refers to the percentage of patients with a low venous hemoglobin value whose capillary hematocrit value also was low. "Specificity" refers to the percentage of patients with a normal venous hemoglobin value whose capillary microhematocrit also was normal. The predictive value of a positive test, i.e., a low hematocrit, refers to the percentage of patients with a low hematocrit value whose venous hemoglobin was also low and the predictive value of a negative test designates the percentage of patients with a normal hematocrit whose venous sample also was normal. Thus, "sensitivity" here at 90% refers to the percentage of patients with a low venous hemoglobin and a low capillary hematocrit. The capillary technique, therefore, picked up 90% of those with an abnormal venous specimen. More important are the predictive values of the test. If the data in this study hold up, they are reasonably acceptable. Their data do suggest that the microhematocrit as routinely performed is an acceptable test for anemia. It is a sensitive test, but on the other hand it has a high false positive rate, which makes evaluation of a child with a low hematocrit value very important. This might consist of then drawing a venous specimen for full Coulter counts, including red blood cell indices. Obviously, if one is working in a setting in which iron deficiency has a reasonably high prevalence, a therapeutic trial of iron would be an alternative that is acceptable as well as cost effective. What I would like to see done is a modern study that compares the ability to detect iron deficiency using all the powers that exist with the Coulter counter vs. a simple office microhematocrit test.

Continuing information evolves showing that iron-deficiency anemia does affect infant developmental test performance (Lozoff, B., et al.: *Pediatrics* 79:981, 1987). Studies earlier than the latter one also suggest that iron deficiency in the absence of anemia can do the same thing. It is the latter category that would be missed with screening techniques that involve a simple microhematocrit. The Coulter is able to give us a mean corpuscular volume, a mean corpuscular hemoglobin, and, depending on the instrumentation, a red cell distribution width (RDW) all of which can give us clues to the presence of iron deficiency, even in the absence of anemia. What is the additional advantage of a complete set of red blood cell indices over the hemoglobin or hematocrit alone in the detection of iron deficiency in 1988? Are we missing a small and insignificant percentage of iron-deficit patients, or is the number large enough to warrant shifting our thinking about the way we screen for anemia (and ergo iron deficiency)?

As with the study on neonatal polycythemia, let's go back and really do it right, making all these comparisons in 1988. The reason for mentioning the year has to do with the fact that iron deficiency is clearly on the wane, and we have to decide just how we're going to go to wipe out the last case in our practices. If the data are correct that depleted iron stores may be associated with certain functional abnormalities of cognitive performance, and if the only way we can detect depleted iron stores might be by early and subtle changes in the RDW, then maybe it is worthwhile going that last step, even though we are seeing fewer patients with iron deficiency. Notice the "if" in the prior sentence. I am a believer in the concept that iron deficiency does produce cognitive defects. The data, in addition to that already mentioned, continue to accumulate. Groner et al. (*J. Adolesc. Health. Care* 7:44, 1986) found that the use of iron in a randomized trial of oral iron on tests of short-term memory and attention span in young pregnant women was associated with significant improvement in these parameters in nonanemic individuals. A study in Texas has confirmed prior studies by Oski and by Lozoff et al. that preschool children with iron deficiency, with or without anemia, are less likely to pay attention to relevant clues in problem solving and that this situation can be corrected with iron treatment. (Pollitt, E., et al.: *Am. J. Clin. Nutr.* 43:555, 1986). One could go on and on with these comments. It is again stressed that the microhematocrit alone is a relatively crude way of detecting iron deficiency, if that is the goal. Maybe a full set of blood counts isn't good enough either, but it's got to be better than the microhematocrit.

The least one can do as part of these examinations is to get a careful look at the sclerae. Among 169 hospital inpatients studied to assess the association between blue sclerae and iron-deficiency anemia, blue sclerae were seen more often in patients with iron deficiency (87%) than in those with other anemias (7%) or without anemia (5.3%) (*Lancet* 2:1267, 1986). The specificity of blue sclerae in iron-deficiency anemia was 0.94, with a sensitivity of 0.87. By comparison, mucosal pallor was noted in only 30% of patients with iron-deficiency anemia, with a specificity of 0.96 and a sensitivity of only 0.20. Maybe a look at the sclerae (again after a study done in children) will turn out to be as good as anything else. Note that blue sclerae are associated with osteogenesis imperfecta, inherited disorders of connective tissue, collagen disorders, corticosteroid therapy, and myasthenia gravis. All of these disorders are uniformly less common than iron deficiency in the pediatric population. Let's see that study done in children. In the meantime, the presence of a bluish tinge to the sclerae should alert the clinician to possible underlying iron deficiency. It was Osler in 1908 who first described blue sclerae in iron-deficient undernourished teenage girls. Almost 90 years later, Kalra et al. (*Lancet* 2:1267, 1986) reconfirmed this finding.—J.A. Stockman III, M.D.

Intravenous Treatment of Autoimmune Hemolytic Anemia With Very High Dose Gammaglobulin

J.B. Bussel, C. Cunningham-Rundles, and C. Abraham (New York Hosp.-Cornell Med. Ctr.; and Mem. Sloan-Kettering Cancer Ctr.)
Vox Sang. 51:264–269, December 1986   13–4

Intravenous γ-globulin (IVGG), in doses (2 gm/kg) that are effective in immune thrombocytopenic purpura and autoimmune neutropenia, has not been effective in patients with autoimmune hemolytic anemia. Therefore, a higher dose of IVGG was used in four patients with severe autoimmune hemolytic anemia.

Four patients, three children and one adult, had severe autoimmune hemolytic anemia unresponsive to conventional doses of IVGG, corticosteroids, azathioprine (two patients), and red blood cell transfusions (three). A total dose of IVGG of 5 gm/kg was given over 5 days. Two patients had sustained remission; they received 435 gm and 305 gm of IVGG, respectively. They were able to discontinue corticosteroid therapy and did not require red blood cell transfusions. The third patient had a transient response. Treatment failed in the fourth. Both of the latter patients continued to receive transfusions even with high-dose prednisone. Neither responded to splenectomy. Toxicity was minimal. In one patient transient worsening of preexisting hepatitis developed, but transaminase activity did not change in the other three.

Higher doses of IVGG may be effective for some patients with severe autoimmune hemolytic anemia, particularly those refractory to conventional treatment or those who require prolonged immunosuppressive therapy. A high dose of IVGG is required, possibly because of the enlarged reticuloendothelial system in these patients.

▶ Intravenous gammaglobulin has been widely used to treat idiopathic thrombocytopenic purpura refractory to steroids or when a rapid response was desired. In selected cases, IVGG may also be useful in the treatment of immune neutropenias (Ventura, A., et al.: *Helv. Paediatr. Acta.* 41:495, 1986). There have been scattered case reports of its use in autoimmune hemolytic anemia, with varying results. As the abstract indicates, perhaps some of that variability may have occurred because of the dose of IVGG used. The report from Cornell shows that if massive doses of IVGG are administered, a response may be obtained. The amount used was 2.5 times the highest doses generally given in management of idiopathic thrombocytopenic purpura. It would also be expected to be quite a bit more expensive as well. Pocecco et al. (*J. Pediatr.* 109:725, 1986) also found that high-dose IVGG could be effective in refractory autoimmune hemolytic anemia. Refractory generally means disease that has not responded to steroids. This mode of therapy can also be used for patients who are immunocompromised, in whom one may not wish to use steroids.

Just in case you think everything is all right in Gotham City, read the report of Richmond et al. (*J. Pediatr.* 110:917, 1987). They describe an 8-month-old black infant with severe autoimmune hemolytic anemia. This child initially responded to IVGG with a rise in hemoglobin. However, the more IVGG that was used, the more problems developed. Apparently, the IVGG enhanced hemolysis over time in this patient, who then had a gradually progressive decline in hemoglobin despite continuation of therapy. It was suggested that the immunoglobulin therapy potentiated a warm antibody that was present, which was causing the hemolysis. It should be noted that immunoglobulin-enhanced hemolysis has been reported in two patients with immune thrombocytopenia. Subclinical hemolysis has also been observed in patients with uncomplicated immune thrombocytopenia given IVGG.

From all this one can deduce a few things: Autoimmune hemolytic anemia that is unresponsive to steroids is not a particularly good disease. It is probably worth a shot at using immunoglobulin intravenously as part of the subsequent management. It may work. It may not work. It might make the situation worse, but it may well be worth the attempt.—J.A. Stockman III, M.D.

Transient Erythroblastopenia of Adolescence
Theodore Zwerdling, Jonathan Finlay, and Bertil E. Glader (Stanford Univ., Children's Hosp. at Stanford, and Univ. of Wisconsin at Madison)
Clin. Pediatr. (Phila.) 25:563–565, November 1986   13–5

Transient erythroblastopenia of childhood, an acquired red blood cell (RBC) aplasia, is seen most commonly in children aged 2–6 years. When a 16-year-old girl with pure RBC aplasia of 7 months' duration was seen, it was feared initially that she had the chronic disorder most commonly seen in adults.

Girl, 16 years, presented with malaise and pallor. Her past medical history was unremarkable. Hematologic evaluation disclosed decreased hemoglobin levels, reticulocytopenia, and normal leukocyte and platelet counts. The peripheral blood smear showed no abnormalities, and the bone marrow aspirate was normal except for marked depletion of erythroblasts with no erythroid precursors. Other pertinent laboratory findings were unremarkable. In vitro culture of peripheral blood revealed adequate but slightly reduced BFU-E growth. The patient's hypoproliferative anemia was caused by intrinsic RBC failure. Idiopathic acquired RBC hypoplasia was diagnosed and therapy was instituted with RBC transfusions and prednisone. The patient was discharged but required RBC transfusions every 3–4 weeks. A brief hemolytic episode was noted 2.5 months after diagnosis; however, no cause of hemolysis could be discerned. After 5 months of transfusion-dependent RBC hypoplasia, epigastric pain, fever, and jaundice developed as well as non-A, non-B hepatitis, which later resolved. About 7 months after diagnosis, the patient's transfusion requirements abated and hemoglobin levels stabilized. No RBC abnormalities were noted in the 3 years subsequent to bone marrow recovery.

These findings may well represent the adolescent equivalent of transient erythroblastopenia of childhood. The erythrocyte characteristics and in vitro culture of erythroid progenitors are similar to that found in transient erythroblastopenia; however, the clinical course is relatively longer, though shorter than that of the adult types of RBC aplasia. Pure RBC aplasia in adolescents should be managed like transient erythroblastopenia of childhood.

▶ Transient erythroblastopenia of childhood is a relatively common cause of acquired RBC aplasia. It is self-limited and of unknown etiology. In adults, however, acquired pure RBC aplasia is a much more complex disease that may or may not be associated with thymoma. It often results in a life-long need for RBC transfusions. Death may ultimately result from transfusion-related hemosiderosis. The problem is, what do you do when RBC aplasia develops in a 16-year-old? This is an unusual age for onset of transient erythroblastopenia of childhood but younger than that of pure RBC aplasia of adults. The authors suggest that watchful waiting and supportive transfusions will allow the appropriate diagnosis to be made.

Red blood cell aplasia generally falls into one of four categories. One is that associated with congenital hypoplastic anemia (or the Diamond-Blackfan syndrome), usually diagnosed in the first 6 months of life (sometimes much later) and often associated with congenital abnormalities. If you have the ability to do so, you can demonstrate that these children have abnormal RBC characteristics such as high mean corpuscular volumes, increased levels of fetal hemoglobin, the presence of "i" antigen, and elevated activity of adenosine deaminase. In many cases life-long steroid therapy or RBC transfusions are required. A second form of RBC aplasia is a variety acquired in association with chronic hemolysis, commonly seen in both adults and children. The degree of anemia in these patients is often severe, because hemolysis continues unabated while RBC production is impaired. This kind of RBC aplasia is transient and is the one associated most commonly with infections with parvovirus. Transient erythroblastopenia of childhood is a third form of RBC aplasia and generally affects children under the age of 6 years. The anemia commonly follows ill-defined viral illnesses. No other hematologic problems should be present. The disorder is self-limited and rarely requires more than a single transfusion. Adult-acquired pure RBC aplasia is the rare fourth entity, seen in adults usually over the age of 50. It is in the latter group that thymoma may occur in 50% of patients, although pure RBC aplasia develops in only 5% of those with thymoma. Pure RBC aplasia in adults can also be seen in association with a variety of immunologic disorders (rheumatoid arthritis, systemic lupus erythematosus), drugs (Dilantin, chloramphenicol), infections (hepatitis), and malignancies.

The reason for including the case abstracted above is the unusual age of the patient, her negative medical history, and ultimately the transient nature of her illness. One case does not a series make, but there is a lot to be learned here. Bide your time. While waiting and supporting with transfusions, it is usually worthwhile to use corticosteroids to see if a "remission" can be induced. Androgens have also been used, although the response to androgens is unpredictable. Immunosuppressives other than steroids have been used in individual cases but response to these is also unpredictable. There are a few patients who have also received intravenous doses of immunoglobulin, with sporadic responses.

Before closing out the story on RBC aplasia, a commentary such as this would be incomplete without some update on parvovirus infection. We have learned that human parvovirus infection during pregnancy can result in serious risk to the fetus with hydrops fetalis (Anand, A., et al.: *N. Engl. J. Med.* 316:183, 1987). This peculiar virus, the causative agent of erythema infectiosum or fifth disease, can wreak havoc with a pregnant woman and her fetus. Carrington et al. (*Lancet* 1:433, 1987) reported two patients with hydrops fetalis and intrauterine death associated with human parvovirus B19 infection that produced very few symptoms during the second trimester of pregnancy before the hydrops was ultimately diagnosed by ultrasound. Coincidentally, maternal α-fetoprotein levels were raised long before any other abnormalities were found. Thus, there is increasing evidence that human parvovirus (B19) harms the fetus, resulting in spontaneous abortion in the first trimester, hydrops fetalis in the second trimester, or stillbirth at term. However, there is no certainty that maternal parvovirus infection will have an adverse effect on the fetus and, for this reason, markers such as α-fetoprotein levels may serve as a useful tool in indicating which pregnancies are going to go awry. You can bet a great deal that we're going to hear more about parvovirus in the fetus.—J.A. Stockman III, M.D.

Marrow Transplantation in Patients With Advanced Thalassemia

Guido Lucarelli, Mariella Galimberti, Paola Polchi, Claudio Giardini, Patricia Politi, Donatella Baronciani, Emanuele Angelucci, Flavia Manenti, Constante Delfini, Giovanni Aureli, and Pietro Muretto (Ospedali Riceniti di Pesaro, Pesaro, Italy)
N. Engl. J. Med. 316:1050–1055, Apr. 23, 1987   13–6

Allogeneic marrow transplantation was carried out in 40 patients aged 8–15 years with advanced homozygous β-thalassemia. Twenty-two of the sibling donors were heterozygous for β-thalassemia. The median dose of marrow cells administered was 4.1×10^8/kg. Patients were prepared with

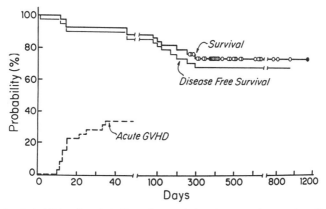

Fig 13–2.—Probabilities of survival, disease-free survival, and acute graft-versus-host disease. *Open circles* represent patients surviving without thalassemia; *closed circles*, patients surviving with thalassemia. (Courtesy of Lucarelli, G., et al.: N. Engl. J. Med. 316:1050–1055, Apr. 23, 1987.)

busulfan and cyclophosphamide, and cyclosporine and methotrexate were given perioperatively.

The disease-free survival rate was 69% (Fig 13–2). All patients but one had normal performance status at the time of evaluation. Two patients were alive with thalassemia at follow-up. Five deaths were caused by infectious complications related to graft-vs.-host disease. Two patients with transient rejection died with marrow aplasia. Of 37 evaluable patients, 14% were not engrafted or rejected their grafts within 4 months. Risk factors for graft failure could not be identified. Liver failure was not an important contributing cause of death in this series.

Long-term disease-free survival is possible after allogeneic marrow transplantation in patients with advanced homozygous β-thalassemia. There are risks of morbidity and early death, but the improving outcome of marrow transplantation warrants its consideration if a suitable donor is available, particularly in younger patients. The merits of early vs. late transplantation remain to be determined.

▶ Few reports have created more interest in hematology communities than this one. This is the first large series in the world reporting the value of bone marrow transplantation in patients with transfusion-dependent thalassemia. It is not the first report, however. The first patient to undergo transplantation for thalassemia major is now hematologically normal and growing more than 5 years after bone marrow transplantation (Thomas, E.D., et al.: *Lancet* 2:227, 1982).

As impressive as these data are and as compelling a case as they make, anyone caring for a child with thalassemia is left with a major quandary. More efficient iron chelation programs with deferoxamine have been used in the United States and elsewhere for more than 10 or 15 years. Although improvement has been noted in many children who are vigorously chelated, the truly long-term benefits of this rigorous form of therapy are still not available. The drug is expensive, and compliance with its subcutaneous administration has proven a major impediment to its effectiveness. So what is the dilemma? The dilemma is the fact that you have two options: You can go the bone marrow transplantation route with an up to 25% chance of doing in a child as a consequence of the procedure and/or its subsequent problems, or go the transfusion and chelation route with all of its uncertainties. This is less of a dilemma in other parts of the world. Regular transfusion and chelation therapy are not options for many children on this earth. Their only chance of survival would be referral to some center in another part of the world that is willing to perform a bone marrow transplant. But what to do here in the United States? Thus far, most individuals have stuck with the concept that transfusion therapy along with chelation treatment will buy time for the patient, during which, it is hoped, some innovative, less risky treatment will come along, e.g., gene therapy. The dilemma mentioned is one that we gladly accept, in the sense that at least more and more options are open to children with this genetic disorder. It's a shame that the options are not a little more appealing.

While on the topic of thalassemia major and iron overload, let's mention a few other things that are going on. One is that 1,2-dimethyl-3-hydroxypyridone may be an effective oral chelator for the treatment of iron overload. Its use in a small number of children has shown some significant promise (*Lancet* 1:1294, 1987). It is not yet known whether it has nearly the capability of deferoxamine, however. We also are learning that deferoxamine may be significantly toxic to both the eye and the ear. Current data suggest that chelation of copper by this drug may be the cause of this problem (Pall, H., et al.: *Lancet* 2:1279, 1986). We need more studies on that topic. Also, some patients with thalassemia who are not well transfused will experience complications as a result of spinal cord pressure by heterotopic bone marrow. This can also produce problems in the airway. Fortunately, one study has now defined the role of radiation therapy in this. Small doses of radiation (10–26 Gy) will relieve symptoms (Papavasiliou, C., et al.: *Lancet* 1:13, 1987).

While we're on a roll here, talking about thalassemia, let's note that partial splenic embolization as part of the management of hypersplenism can produce responses that last at least 5 or more years (Politis, C., et al.: *Br. Med. J.* 294:665, 1987). Maybe we can put away those knives and leave the spleen in and just make it a little bit smaller. As a last comment on iron chelation, patients who have received long-term treatment with iron chelation may indeed have a good outlook when it comes to preservation of the integrity of the ACTH-cortisol axis. (Sklar, C.A., et al.: *Am. J. Dis. Child.* 141:3327, 1987).

And last, and possibly least, although this has nothing to do with thalassemia, note that bone marrow transplantation in the youngest patient was recently reported. This was a 17-week-fetus born of a pregnancy complicated by severe Rh immunization. The fetus was transfused in utero with maternal bone marrow cells in the hope that the mother's bone marrow would allow the infant to produce Rh-negative red blood cells. The bone marrow graft did not take, but fortunately the baby was able to be supported in the usual traditional fashion with intrauterine transfusions and was discharged from a neonatal unit in good health (Linch, D.C., et al.: *Lancet 2:1453, 1986*). I'm not sure if the latter investigators are to be congratulated or criticized for this form of human experimentation. The idea was a novel one, but the procedure indeed was investigative.—J.A. Stockman III, M.D.

Rapid Prenatal Diagnosis of Sickle Cell Anemia by a New Method of DNA Analysis
Stephen H. Embury, Stephen J. Scharf, Randall K. Saiki, Mary Ann Gholson, Mitchell Golbus, Norman Arnheim, and Henry A. Erlich (San Francisco Gen. Hosp., Univ. of California at San Francisco, and Northern Calif. Comprehensive Sickle Cell Ctr., San Francisco, Cetus Corp., Emeryville, Calif., and Univ. of Southern California)
N. Engl. J. Med. 316:656–661, March 12, 1987   13–7

A new method for increasing the sensitivity of restriction DNA analysis is based on in vitro enzymatic amplification of the genomic β-globin gene sequences to be analyzed. The method increases sensitivity by more than two orders of magnitude while reducing the laboratory time for DNA analysis to less than 1 day. Only a small amount of DNA is required when the modified method is used to distinguish the genotypes of SS or AS patients from normal AA individuals.

A 200,000-fold enzymatic amplification of the specific β-globin DNA sequences that may carry the sickle mutation first is carried out. A short radiolabeled synthetic DNA sequence homologous to the normal β^A-globin gene sequence then is hybridized to the amplified target sequences and the hybrid "duplexes" are digested with two restriction endonucleases. The presence of β^A-globin or β^S-globin gene sequences in the amplified target DNA from the patient determines whether the β^A-hybridization probe anneals perfectly or with a single nucleotide mismatch. This affects digestion of the DNA and the size of the labeled digestion products, which are distinguished by electrophoresis and autoradiography.

Prenatal diagnosis of sickle cell anemia now can be made on the day that fetal DNA is available. Successful prenatal diagnosis was carried out in two couples at risk of an SS child. The method also can be applied to diagnosing hemoglobin C disease.

▶ The difference between this and prior prenatal methods for diagnosis of sickle cell anemia (or other hemoglobinopathies) is the method of DNA analysis. Read the article in more detail if you are a true aficionado of this type of topic. The essence of it, however, is the fact that you can have a diagnosis the same day that you are obtaining a specimen for diagnostic purposes. This allows for a more speedy turnaround in terms of utilization of the information and doesn't leave two parents sitting and wondering for any significant length of time what the results will be. Old et al. (*Lancet* 2:763, 1986) have also reported on first-trimester fetal diagnosis of hemoglobinopathies by analysis of chorionic villus DNA. They reported on their experience with more than 200 patients. They found an "acceptably" low fetal loss rate (6.7%, debatable whether or not low). There were no deleterious serious long-term effects on fetal development. Other centers have reported loss rates in the 2% range with chorionic villus biopsy.

Obviously, the reason for wanting to gain this knowledge is to allow parents to make an informed decision regarding abortion. For whatever reason, prenatal diagnosis has not been seized upon in large numbers by parents who are at risk for having a child with sickle cell anemia. That is a decision that only the parents can entertain. What is important beyond that pregnancy is the ability to detect sickle cell anemia as soon as possible. As of this past year, only ten states offered newborn screening for sickle cell disease. A National Institutes of Health (NIH) panel in March 1987 recommended that such screening be made available for all babies. The purpose of early detection is to be able to counsel parents as to the risk of an infection resulting from functional hyposplenia. Newly diagnosed patients should be given prophylactic penicillin orally because this has been shown to decrease by approximately 85% the number of episodes of septicemia and other serious infections that patients with sickle cell anemia experience. If your state does not have a newborn screening program for sickle cell disease, read the NIH panel report (*Science* 236:259, 1987). Also, keep your eyes open for any new information that's coming down the pike regarding gene therapy. There was an excellent review of this by Ledley this past year (*J. Pediatr.* 110:1, 1987). See also the excellent commentary on penicillin prophylaxis for babies with sickle cell disease (Editorial comment: *Lancet* 2:1432, 1986).—J.A. Stockman III, M.D.

Pitted Red Cell Counts in Sickle Cell Disease: Relationship to Age, Hemoglobin Genotype, and Splenic Size
Oluyemisi J. Fatunde and Roland B. Scott (Howard Univ.)
Am. J. Pediatr. Hematol. Oncol. 8:329–333, 1986   13–8

Earlier studies showed that a palpable spleen in children with homozygous sickle cell anemia (HbSS) marks the onset of its diminishing function. Decreased splenic reticuloendothelial function is associated with increased susceptibility to severe, overwhelming infection. Thus, early recognition of splenic hypofunction may help to identify patients with sickle cell anemia who are in potential danger of contracting severe infections. The pitted red blood cell (RBC) count correlates well with results from splenic scans. Therefore, the relationship between splenic function and pitted RBC counts was studied in 114 children aged 1–18 years with sickle cell disease. Also studied were 100 black controls with hemoglobin genotype AA aged 2 months to 60 years. In all, 500 RBCs were counted in each specimen. A pitted cell was defined as an erythrocyte having at least one crater-like indentation on its surface, regardless of the size or number of indentations (Fig 13–3).

Controls had a mean pit count of 0.08%. Patients with HbSS had a

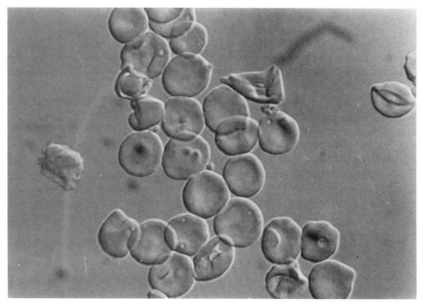

Fig 13–3.—Pitted erythrocytes in sickle cell disease. (Courtesy of Fatunde, O.J., and Scott, R.B.: Am. J. Pediatr. Hematol. Oncol. 8:329–333, 1986.)

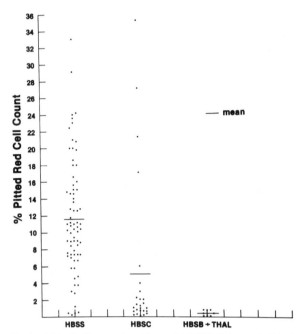

Fig 13–4.—Pitted red blood cell counts in patients with HBSS, HbSC, and HbS-β⁺-thalassemia hemoglobinopathies. (Courtesy of Fatunde, O.J., and Scott, R.B.: Am. J. Pediatr. Hematol. Oncol. 8:329–333, 1986.)

mean pit count of 11.8%; the count increased with age. Patients with sickle cell hemoglobin C disease (HbSC) had a mean pit count of 4.9%; the count was not affected by age. Patients with HbS-β⁺-thalassemia had a mean pit count of 0.4% (Fig 13–4). One patient with HbS-β⁺-thalassemia, one with HbSS-α-thalassemia, one with HbS-O Arab, and one with HbS-Lepore had pit counts of 12%, 4.9%, 31.4%, and 0.4%, respectively. Patients with HbSS and HbSC who had palpable spleens had significantly lower pit counts than those who did not have enlarged spleens. The pitted RBC count may be used to predict disease severity in patients with sickle cell disorders.

▶ Richard H. Sills, M.D., Associate Professor of Pediatrics, Children's Hospital of Buffalo, State University of New York at Buffalo, comments.—J.A. Stockman III, M.D.

▶ This study reconfirms the importance of recognizing hyposplenia in patients with sickling disorders. The incidence and mortality of hyposplenia-related septicemia in these patients can clearly be decreased with prophylactic penicillin, immunization against pneumococcus and *Hemophilus influenzae,* and aggressive treatment of significant febrile episodes with antibiotics intravenously.

The study also emphasizes the importance of the erythrocyte pit test as a means to evaluate splenic function. Although radionuclide scans have been the traditional test to measure splenic function, these studies are more expensive, more invasive, and probably no more (if not less) accurate than the pit test. The pit test simply requires a drop of peripheral blood, which can be studied even months later if it is appropriately fixed. The percentage of RBCs containing pits is determined by examining the blood as a wet preparation using a special light microscopic system (direct interference contrast microscopy). When more than 3% of the RBCs contain pits, the sulfur-colloid radionuclide scan will generally demonstrate diminished uptake consistent with hyposplenia.

The pit test does what radionuclide scanning cannot: It allows for the study of individual hyposplenic patients on a longitudinal basis and for screening large populations for individuals with hyposplenia. This latter function becomes more important when one considers the increasing variety and number of conditions associated with hyposplenia other than surgical splenectomy and the sickle hemoglobinopathies. Hyposplenia has now been associated with inflammatory bowel disease, collagen-vascular disorders, glomerulonephritis, celiac disease, graft-vs.-host disease, and many others. Although the risk of septicemia associated with hyposplenia in these disorders remains unclear, several case reports of sepsis are very concerning. Many instances of septicemia in the past may have gone unreported because the association with hyposplenia was unrecognized, or because the septicemia was blamed on the underlying disorder and not on the resulting hyposplenia.

The pit test provides an ideal means of screening patients with the aforementioned disorders to determine who has hyposplenia and what is the consequent risk of septicemia. Its use will become increasingly important in making decisions concerning the need for prevention and treatment of overwhelming septicemia, not only in sickle hemoglobinopathies, but in many other disorders as well.—R.H. Sills, M.D.

Bacteremia in Sickle Hemoglobinopathies
Harold S. Zarkowsky, Dianne Gallagher, Frances M. Gill, Winfred C. Wang, John M. Falletta, William M. Lande, Paul S. Levy, Joel I. Verter, Doris Wethers, and the Cooperative Study of Sickle Cell Disease (Washington Univ. and other major institutions in the United States)
J. Pediatr. 109:579–585, October 1986   13–9

Young patients with sickle cell anemia (SS) or sickle cell-hemoglobin C disease (SC) often contract bacterial infections, of which the pneumococcal infections are considered particularly serious. The occurrence and outcome of bacteremia in SS and SC have been studied previously, but only in small numbers of patients. A review was made of the results of a prospective study of age-specific incidence rates and clinical features of bacteremia in a large population of patients with sickle hemoglobinopathies.

The series included 3,451 patients, all participants in the Cooperative Study of Sickle Cell Disease (CSSCD). During 13,771 patient-years of follow-up, 178 episodes of bacteremia were reported to the CSSCD. There were 134 patients who experienced a single episode of bacteremia and 20

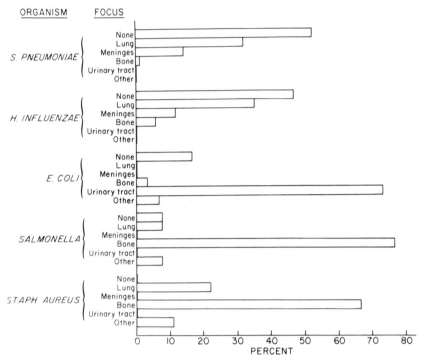

ORGANISM   FOCUS

Fig 13–5.—Frequency with which focus of infection was associated with specific bacteremia. (Courtesy of Zarkowsky, H.S., et al.: J. Pediatr. 109:579–585, October 1986.)

who had more than one episode. The incidence rate of bacteremia was highest among children with SS and SC who were younger than age 2 years. *Streptococcus pneumoniae* accounted for 67% of the bacteremic episodes in children younger than age 6 years, but for only 19% of such episodes in patients older than age 6 years. Gram-negative organisms were responsible for 50% of the bacteremic episodes in patients aged 6 years and older (Fig 13–5). Infection was the cause of death in 18 patients with SS, of which 15 were sepsis related deaths caused by pneumococcal infection. The prophylactic use of penicillin appears to reduce the risk of pneumococcal bacteremia in children younger than age 3 years.

Acute Chest Syndrome in Children With Sickle Cell Disease: A Retrospective Analysis of 100 Hospitalized Cases
Robert H. Sprinkle, Thomas Cole, Susan Smith, and George R. Buchanan (Univ. of Texas at Dallas)
Am. J. Pediatr. Hematol. Oncol. 82:105–110, 1986   13–10

Little is known about the clinical, radiographic, and microbiologic features of acute chest syndrome in younger patients with sickle cell disease. A retrospective review was conducted of 100 hospitalizations of 57 pe-

---

KNOWN AND PROPOSED CAUSES OF THE SICKLE CELL CHEST SYNDROME

I. Pulmonary vascular occlusion
  A. Thrombosis in situ
  B. Pulmonary arterial embolism
    1. Thromboembolism
    2. Bone marrow embolism
II. Pulmonary infection
  A. Pneumonia
    1. *Streptococcus pneumoniae*
    2. *Hemophilus influenzae*
    3. *Mycoplasma pneumoniae*
    4. Other infectious agents
  B. Other pulmonary infections

III. Hypoventilation
  A. Secondary to painful chest cage lesions
    1. Bone infarction
    2. Osteomyelitis
    3. Trauma
  B. Secondary to subdiaphragmatic pain
    1. Hepatobiliary disease
    2. Abdominal wall incisions
  C. Secondary to narcotic administration
IV. Intravascular volume overload
  A. High-output congestive heart failure
  B. Iatrogenic volume overload

(Courtesy of Sprinkle, R.H., et al.: Am. J. Pediatr. Hematol. Oncol. 82:105–110, 1986.)

---

diatric patients with symptoms and clinical signs of acute chest disease associated with radiographic evidence of pulmonary infiltration, pleural effusion, or pulmonary edema. The mean age was about 8.5 years.

Symptoms on admission included fever (77%); pain (67%), most commonly in bony areas; chest distress (pain or dyspnea (70%); and cough (57%). Radiographic findings consisted of pulmonary infiltration more commonly in the lower lobes (86%), pleural effusion in 38%, and pulmonary edema in 5%. The chest syndrome was recognized on presentation in 79% of the patients, but it was recognized only later in 21% admitted for other indications. Patients in whom chest syndrome was recognized initially were more often febrile on admission (68%) than those who were recognized subsequently (33%). The median number of days of fever and hospitalization were fewer for those whose disease was diagnosed initially. The median hospital stay was significantly longer (7 days) for 58 patients who received narcotics than for 42 patients not treated with narcotics (4 days). Polyvalent pneumococcal vaccine was administered to 44 patients at some time before hospitalization, and 18 patients had received penicillin prophylaxis orally. Only 2 of 93 blood cultures grew *Streptococcus pneumoniae*. Serologic evidence of *Mycoplasma pneumoniae* infection was found in eight patients and of *Hemophilus influenzae* infection in two others. There were two deaths and one major neurologic complication.

Sickle cell chest syndrome in children is an acute febrile pulmonary disease frequently associated with pain and/or narcotic analgesia, but infrequently associated with bacterial infection. Known and proposed causes of this syndrome include pulmonary vascular occlusion, pulmonary infection, hypoventilation, and intravascular volume overload (table).

▶ The child with sickle cell disease who presents to the clinic, office, or emergency room with respiratory symnptoms, with or without a fever, poses a dilemma. The patient may have a simple cold, or may progress to a full-blown sickle cell chest syndrome. This is one of the most common clinical problems in patients with sickle cell anemia. The typical features are those of cough, dyspnea, chest pain, fever, pulmonary infiltration, and a poor response to antibiotics. Its etiology is not known. It was once thought that these findings represented pulmonary vascular occlusive phenomena, but this is no longer entirely clear. Infectious etiologies (e.g., Mycoplasma pneumoniae) could account for similar changes. I tend to favor the former, but it makes little difference in individual patients.

These patients are usually quite febrile and should be admitted to the hospital promptly where intravenous antibiotics and fluids can be started. We like to follow these patients' blood gases closely. When it becomes obvious that arterial oxygenation is compromised, we move to exchange transfusion promptly. These children can get sick in a hurry and can die extremely quickly. Exchange transfusion may or may not make a great deal of difference in terms of the course of the pulmonary problem, but when the arterial Po_2 is in the range associated with spontaneous sickling, you have little choice except to use that procedure. In essence, it really doesn't make a great deal of difference whether the known or proposed causes of sickle cell chest syndrome are present in any particular patient: You may well wind up managing the patient in exactly the same way.

I agree with these authors when they say that a prospective study of all aspects of the sickle cell chest syndrome, including a critical investigation of the etiologic role of narcotic analgesics, is badly needed. We use a lot of narcotics in the management of sickle cell disease, and this may lead to hypoventilation and sickling, which only further complicate the course. If you would like to read more about pain relief in sickle cell crisis, see the editorial comment in *Lancet* 2:320, 1986.—J.A. Stockman III M.D.

Incidence of Ocular Abnormalities in Patients With Sickle Hemoglobinopathies

Thomas R. Friberg, Craig M. Young, and Paul F. Milner (Univ. of Pittsburgh and Med. College of Georgia, Augusta)
Ann. Ophthalmol. 18:150–153, April 1986   •   13–11

Patients with sickle hemoglobinopathies may have a spectrum of ocular abnormalities that can be categorized as proliferative or nonproliferative. Proliferative lesions include peripheral vascular occlusions; arteriovenous anastomoses; peripheral neovascularization, including "sea fans"; associated vitreous hemorrhage; and retinal detachment. Nonproliferative lesions include sunbursts, salmon patches, schisis cavities, vascular tortuosity, and iridescent spots. It is generally thought that black sunbursts, schisis cavities, and iridescent spots are the residua of previous intraretinal hemorrhages (salmon patches), secondary to the sickling of blood within the retinal vessels. The incidence of various ocular lesions associated with sickle hemoglobinopathies was investigated.

Of 110 consecutive unselected patients in a sickle cell clinic, 92 had SS, 8 SC, and 10 Sthal hemoglobin. The most prevalent retinal abnormality was the conjunctival comma sign, followed by black sunbrusts in the retina, which occurred in 46% of SS, 63% of SC, and 37% of Sthal patients. The data suggested that retinal lesions become more prevalent up to the fifth decade of life. Included in this series was a patient, aged 8 years, with SS hemoglobin, who had a dense vitreous hemorrhage secondary to a large salmon patch that had bled into the vitreous and that reduced her vision to 20/200.

Unless one is accustomed to the subtleties of the comma sign, it is easily overlooked. Therefore, a more valuable diagnostic sign is the presence of a black sunburst within the fundus. The diagnosis of sickle hemoglobinopathy should be suspected in any black patient with an unexplained, flat, pigmented lesion with ragged borders in the midperiphery. If SS, SC, or Sthal hemoglobin is diagnosed, the fundi should be examined at least annually to detect the early development of proliferative retinopathy. Laser photocoagulation, cryoablation, and vitrectomy should be considered whenever appropriate.

Recurrent Mutations in Hemophilia A Give Evidence for CpG Mutation Hotspots

Hagop Youssoufian, Haig H. Kazazian, Jr., Deborah G. Phillips, Sophia Aronis, George Tsiftis, Valerie A. Brown, and Stylianos E. Antonarakis (Johns Hopkins Univ., Athens (Greece) Univ., and Collaborative Research Inc., Lexington, Mass.)
Nature 324:380–382, Nov. 27, 1986   13–12

Many different molecular lesions probably result in hemophilia A; all nine mutations described to date appear to be unique changes. A study of 83 patients with hemophilia A yielded two different point mutations, in exons 18 and 22, that recurred independently in unrelated families. Each of the mutations produces a nonsense codon by a change of CG to TG, and each occurred de novo on the X chromosome from the maternal grandfather. Nine of the ten point mutations were detected with *Taq*I, which has the dinucleotide CpG in its recognition sequence. The findings support the view that CpG dinucleotides are mutation hotspots.

Reports of a given mutation in different ethnic groups and in different β-globin gene frameworks indicate that recurrent mutations occur in various β-globin gene alleles. There is strong circumstantial evidence that CpG dinucleotides are hotspots for mutation in man. It was estimated that more than 1,000 persons are alive today with different recurrent origins of the C-T mutation at codon 1,960, or of the C-T mutation at codon 2,135 of the factor VIII gene. The estimated total number of recurrences of each type of mutation in man is about 10,000.

▶ Hemophilia A is a common disorder of blood coagulation caused by a deficiency of factor VIII. It is inherited as an X-linked recessive trait, and one third of all cases are thought to result from de novo mutations. The clinical severity of hemophilia A varies markedly among different families, and a subset of these patients with severe disease has antibodies against factor VIII, called inhibitors. Because of this heterogeneity, it is likely that many different molecular lesions result in hemophilia A. Indeed, of the nine mutations described to date, all appear to be unique changes. The study abstracted above was performed in 83 patients with hemophilia. The investigators were able to identify two different point mutations that have occurred independently in unrelated families. Each mutation produces a nonsense code by a change in base sequences in the X chromosome. For most patients with hemophilia A, the diagnosis can be made prior to birth using a variety of non-DNA techniques measuring the amounts of factor VIII that are present. Soon we should be able to learn from studies such as the one abstracted above how prenatal diagnosis on a DNA basis can be accomplished. Similar progress is being made in hemophilia B (Nisen, P., et al.: *N. Engl. J. Med.* 315:1139, 1986).

One of the "hottest" things to come along has been the ability to sex the human pre-embryo by DNA-DNA in situ hybridization (West, J.D., et al.: *Lancet* 1345, 1987). If individual blastomeres of a preimplantation human pre-embryo could be obtained by biopsy without compromising the pre-embryo's developmental potential, genetic tests could be carried out on these cells for prenatal diagnosis. The term "pre-embryo" refers to the definition proposed by McLaren (Ciba Foundation: *Human Embryo Research. Yes or No?* London, Tavistock Publications, 1986, pp. 5–23). (At this point we won't enter into the ethical debate about what is or is not an embryo.) By the McLaren definition, pre-embryos could be obtained during the course of an in vitro fertilization program, or normally fertilized pre-embryos could be collected by uterine lavage. Diagnosis of genetic disorders at this early stage would allow selection of unaffected pre-embryos for transfer back to the uterus, thus avoiding the need for abortion of affected fetuses recognized at later stages of development. The *Lancet* report has used this technique to show that you can determine male sex without damaging the pre-embryo. Nothing more has been done with this information as yet. It has obvious implications for any disorder that is X linked, however. The distinction between abortion and the discarding of a "pre-embryo" is one that I have great personal difficulties with. This, however, does not negate the importance of the *Lancet* report.—J.A. Stockman III, M.D.

Intracranial Hemorrhage in Patients With Hemophilia

Uri Martinowitz, Michael Heim, Rina Tadmor, Amiram Eldor, Irit Rider, Gideon Findler, Abraham Sahar, and Bracha Ramot (Chaim Sheba Med. Ctr., Tel Hashomer, Ichilov Hosp., Tel-Aviv Med. Ctr., Tel-Aviv, and Hadassah Univ Hosp., Jerusalem)

Neurosurgery 18:538–541, May 1986   13–13

Intracranial hemorrhage is a significant cause of death in hemophiliacs. The diagnosis, clinical course, and management of eight such episodes that occurred in 7 of 288 (0.27%) registered hemophiliacs in Israel from 1972 to 1982 were reviewed.

All intracranial hemorrhages occurred in patients with hemophilia A. Three of the episodes occurred in patients with factor VIII inhibitor, for an incidence of 0.86%, compared with 0.1% in hemophiliacs without inhibitor. A history of trauma was present in four episodes, with a symptom-free interval ranging from 6 hours to 10 days. The presenting symptoms included changes in level of consciousness in five episodes, headaches in four, and personality changes in two. Neurologic findings were abnormal in five patients. The diagnosis was confirmed by CT scan in all but one patient. All seven patients received immediate replacement therapy. The plasma level of factor VIII ranged from 30% to 75%. Two patients improved within a few hours and recovered, although one of them experienced seizures. Rebleeding, in the absence of trauma, occurred in another patient 5 weeks after the first episode of intracranial hemorrhage, who recovered after early craniotomy. Four patients died despite adequate factor replacement and supportive therapy, probably because of a conservative and hesitant neurosurgical approach. All three patients in whom operation was delayed for 1–4 days died.

Correction of factor VIII to hemostatic levels alone is inadequate in most episodes of intracranial hemorrhage in hemophiliacs. Operation is strongly recommended when no improvement is noted within a few hours.

▶ Hemophilia was reported by Rabbi Simon Ben Gamiel in the Talmud in the second century A.D., long before its first description in the medical literature by Otto in 1803. Hemophilia A is among the most common of the hereditary bleeding disorders, with an incidence of about 1/10,000. Intracranial hemorrhage is experienced by 2% to 8% of all hemophiliacs during their life-time. It is certainly the leading cause of death, accounting for one third of all deaths among hemophiliacs. The risk of a hemophiliac experiencing intracranial hemorrhage after even minor head trauma ranges up to 13% in various series. Prior to the use of factor concentrates and cryoprecipitate, the mortality rate after intracranial hemorrhage was more than 70%. This is now decreased to approximately 25% in most centers. Actually, if you look at truly current data, the percentage is even much smaller than this with the availability of CT scanning.

In our center, a patient with any symptomatologies that might be consistent with intracranial hemorrhage or with a history of any degree of head trauma is corrected immediately with factor VIII concentrate to raise the level of factor VIII coagulant activity to 100%. A CT scan is performed to see if there is evidence of intracranial bleeding. This is pretty much what most centers are now doing. The CT scan is done after the treatment, not before. When the CT scan does not demonstrate intracranial hemorrhage but symptoms or signs are present, repeated doses of replacement therapy are given to maintain appropriately high factor VIII levels and a repeat CT scan is usually done later. If intracranial hemorrhage is diagnosed, therapeutic amounts of factor VIII concentrates should be given for at least 10 days. Many centers will treat patients prophylactically for much longer than that, although there is no controlled study to indicate clearly how long such treatment should be given. The role of surgery and antifibrinolytic agents is left to the discretion of the individual center. The rule here is pretty straightforward: When in doubt, treat and then make a diagnosis.

With respect to hemophilia care these days, the most prominent issue, of course, is transfusion-associated acquired immunodeficiency syndrome (AIDS). As of this past year, hemophiliacs made up approximately 1% of all patients with AIDS. On the other hand, most hemophiliacs who were treated with factor VIII concentrates prior to the introduction of the heat-treated variety a few years back are likely to be human immunodeficiency virus (HIV) antibody positive. We do not yet know what percentage of that group of patients will ultimately turn out to have AIDS. Hilgartner (*Am. J. Dis. Child.* 141:194, 1987) recently reviewed AIDS in the transfusion patient. This is well worth reading.

The whole issue of what to do with HIV antibody-positive asymptomatic hemophiliac patients should be revolutionized once we have availability of antigen testing. Currently, hemophiliacs who are antibody positive are usually counselled about the risk of transmission of AIDS during intercourse, and so on. This has produced a major problem for most patients, especially since we do not even know if they are contagious. Again, a little time should sort all this out, with better techniques to tell who is and who is not infectious.—J.A. Stockman III, M.D.

Transmissibility of Human Immunodeficiency Virus in Haemophilic and Non-Haemophilic Children Living in a Private School in France
A. Berthier, R. Fauchet, N. Genetet, M. Pommereuil, S. Chamaret, J. Fonlupt, M. Gueguen, A. Ruffault, and L. Montagnier (Internat. d'hemophiles Rey-Leroux, La Bouexière, Centre Hospitalier Régional and Centre Régional de Transfusion Sanguine, Rennes, and Institut Pasteur, Paris)
Lancet 2:598–601, Sept. 13, 1986   13–14

Hemophiliacs are at high risk for acquiring infection with the human immunodeficiency virus (HIV) through exposure to contaminated blood products. Although transmission of the virus from infected hemophiliacs to their sexual partners has been reported, transmission by casual contact has not been established. The transmissibility of HIV was studied in children with and without hemophilia living together in a private school in France that accommodates children with various disorders, including epilepsy, diabetes, and hemophilia. The children are either full-time boarders or they live at home and attend the school during the day. Serologic testing was done in three groups of children with hemophilia that varied in degree of severity and in two groups of nonhemophiliac children who had never received any blood products.

At the end of the 3-year study, half of the patients with severe hemophilia living in the school and half of those treated at home had seroconverted. However, no seroconversion was noted in any of the nonhemophiliac children living with the hemophiliacs in the school. Transmission of HIV among casual contacts appears to be low, and there is no reason to exclude children who are HIV-antibody carriers from any community.

▶ Dr. James Bussel, Assistant Professor of Pediatrics, Division of Pediatric Hematology/Oncology, Cornell University Medical School, New York, comments.—J.A. Stockman III, M.D.

▶ Transmission of HIV by those infected with it to other people is a critical problem in view of the continued spread of the acquired immunodeficiency syndrome (AIDS) epidemic. This article helps to define which restrictions of infected persons are appropriate and which are not.

Initially, it was thought that the population infected with the virus would be restricted to known high-risk groups, i.e., homosexuals, intravenous drug abusers, and recipients of infected blood, especially hemophiliacs. Subsequent investigation demonstrated that sexual contacts of infected persons also could become infected, and that bisexual men and intravenous drug abusers were avenues by which the virus could enter the general population. A key question remained: How much contact with an infected individual would result in virus transmission if persons were not sexual partners and did not share an infected needle? Virologic investigation showed that the HIV virus could be isolated from stool and saliva, but studies have been unanimous in indicating that the HIV virus is not transmissible via casual contact. The first reports studied hospital workers in contact with infected patients and found that other than by inoculation of infected blood or needles directly into the worker, there was no risk of HIV transmission. Subsequent studies confirmed these reports by looking at the families of hemophiliacs at home, including those members who assisted with factor concentrate administration; there was no transmission in this setting. Even wives of infected husbands were not always themselves infected.

The current study bears on another important area of possible transmission: school contact. Parents of normal children have become hysterical with the fear that their children would contract AIDS if they came into contact with infected children. This is the first study to emphasize the lack of risk of school transmission of HIV, even in a boarding school setting. This finding is not surprising in view of the lack of transmission of HIV in the other, more intimate settings mentioned earlier. Although clinical disease can take a long time to develop after HIV infection, seroconversion occurs within 6 months and therefore the study is reliable for demonstrating the lack of infection in children in intimate contact with hemophiliacs. Another interesting point about the study is that hepatitis B, known to be transmitted via stool, was apparently transmitted at a low rate even though HIV was not, indicating that stool and saliva are not routes of HIV transmission. The conclusion of this study is that children infected with HIV do not need to be secluded from other children to keep the normal children safe; therefore, these children should be allowed to continue in school.—J. Bussel, M.D.

Spontaneous Deep Vein Thrombosis in Childhood and Adolescence
L.T. Nguyen, J.-M. Laberge, F.M. Guttman, and D. Albert (McGill Univ.)
J. Pediatr. Surg. 21:640–643, July 1986   13–15

Thrombosis of the deep veins of the lower extremities is common and well described in adults, and the morbidity and mortality remain significant, particularly when it is complicated by thrombosis of the inferior vena cava or by pulmonary embolism. In children, superficial thrombophlebitis and, less frequently, deep vein thrombophlebitis (DVT) may result from prolonged use of intravenous catheters. In addition, spontaneous DVT in children has been described in the presence of various indirect factors, e.g., trauma, sepsis, surgery, tumor, heart disease, systemic lupus erythematosus, effort, obesity, pregnancy, and oral contraceptive use. A review was made of experience with DVT in children and adolescents to evaluate the changes in associated factors since the 1970s and to assess the incidence of pulmonary embolism and postphlebitic changes.

Between 1970 and 1984, spontaneous DVT was diagnosed in 15 patients seen at the Montreal Children's Hospital; the female to male ratio was 2:1, and ages ranged from 10 years to 17 years. Venography was positive in all 14 patients tested. In 12 patients there were significant factors related to DVT, including use of oral contraceptives (7 patients), pelvic fracture (1), nephrotic syndrome (1), and ulcerative colitis (2 patients, in 1 of whom DVT developed 3 months prior to onset of gastrointestinal tract symptoms). The sites of thrombophlebitis were the left iliofemoral vein (11 patients), right iliofemoral vein (2), right tibial vein (1), and left subclavian vein (1). In three patients pulmonary emboli developed that were recurrent in two children and required iliac vein ligation or inferior vena cava clipping. Treatment usually included intravenous doses of heparin followed by anticoagulants orally for 3–6 months; two patients were given streptokinase, with good results. All of the patients recovered. In a limited follow-up (6 months to 5 years), there were no postphlebitic sequelae.

▶ We are seeing an increase in the number of DVTs in children and adolescents. Actually, the emphasis should be on adolescents. The reason I say this is because the greatest increase is seen among those who are using oral contraceptives. This is not to say that oral contraceptives should not be used. On the whole, the risk of DVT is small versus the risks of early pregnancy. In younger children, DVT is usually related to the problems noted in the abstract: trauma, sepsis, surgery, tumor, polycythemia, vasculitis, or indwelling catheters. The management of these problems is similar in both adults and children. It involves heparinization followed by a period of warfarin anticoagulation. The role of systemic thrombolytic or local thrombolytic therapy is much more vague. Extensive experience with the use of thrombolytic (fibrinolytic) agents such as streptokinase and urokinase in adults has provided a basis for their use in neonates and older children. These agents are usually administered in treatment of aortic thrombi consequent to catheter placement. Results with the use of fibrinolytic agents in the pediatric age group have been variable (Miemami, A., et al.: *Pediatrics* 79:773, 1987). The best thing that can be done for any thrombus is to try to prevent it. In this case, an ounce of prevention is well worth a cure that's not even proven to work.—J.A. Stockman III, M.D.

Autoimmune Neutropenia of Infancy

Parviz Lalezari, Manoochehr Khorshidi, and Margarita Petrosova (Montefiore Med. Ctr., Bronx, N.Y., and Albert Einstein College of Medicine)
J. Pediatr. 109:764–769, November 1986   13–16

When chronic benign neutropenia of infancy and childhood was first described in 1941, it was suggested that the abnormality was a chronic state of mature neutrophil depletion with a compensatory increase in the immature granulocytes in the bone marrow, analogous to erythroid hyperplasia in hemolytic anemia. However, an attempt to demonstrate leukocyte antibodies was unsuccessful. More recently, various immunologically induced neutropenias among infants and young children have been described.

Neutrophil antibodies were demonstrated in 119 of 121 infants and young children with chronic neutropenia, thereby establishing the diagnosis of autoimmune neutropenia of infancy. The median age at diagnosis was 8 months (range, 3–30 months). Autoimmune neutropenia of infancy was expressed by recurrent fever and infection. All patients had selective neutropenia (absolute neutrophil count 0–500), and many had monocytosis. Fifteen of 16 patients tested did not respond to epinephrine and hydrocortisone stimulation. The bone marrow had myeloid hyperplasia and reduced numbers of mature neutrophils. All 81 patients who passed age of 5 years recovered, except for 1 who is recovering at age 6.5 years. The estimated median duration of the disease was 20 months. Neutrophil antibodies were detected early in the neutropenic phase by using a combination of immunofluorescence and agglutination tests; 10% of these antibodies had specificity for NA1 or NA2. Twelve serum samples reacted strongly in the flow cytometer; ten of these reacted only with neutrophils. Two also reacted with an unidentified subpopulation (30%) of lymphocytes. Lymphocyte subsets were normal in ten patients. However, abnormal amounts of circulating immune complexes were detected in serum from 11 (44%) of 25 patients tested. All eight patients who received intravenous IgG therapy experienced temporary remission .

Autoimmune neutropenia of infancy is probably the most common chronic neutropenia in infancy and early childhood and can be diagnosed by immunologic techniques. The disease requires only conservative treatment, because spontaneous cure seems to be the rule.

▶ Dr. Pedro A. deAlarcon, Assistant Professor of Pediatrics, The University of Iowa, comments.—J.A. Stockman III, M.D.

▶ Chronic benign neutropenia of childhood is a rare disorder. However, unlike other severe neutropenias, it is not associated with an increased incidence of severe and lethal infections despite an absolute neutrophil count of less than 0.5/cu mm in most patients. In one of the early reports of this condition, Stahlie concluded: "Be this as it may, the only thing that can be done to throw more light on this peculiar condition is to collect more data." (*J. Pediatr.* 48:710–720, 1956). This article has done just that.

In the first review of the literature concerning chronic benign neutropenia of childhood, five clinical diagnostic criteria were suggested (Salomonsen, L.: *Acta Pediatr.* 35:189–201, 1948). Of these, four are still applicable: (1) chronic, marked, selective granulocytopenia with a correspondent leukopenia; (2) normal bone marrow; (3) lower resistance to infection, but otherwise little constitutional involvement; and (4) spontaneous cure. After reading this article we can add to these criteria two more: (5) presenting during the first 2 years of life, and (6) presence of antineutrophil antibodies.

Benign chronic neutropenia has been compared with autoimmune hemolytic anemia of childhood and idiopathic thrombocytopenic purpura. It has been suggested that the mechanism of neutropenia in chronic benign neutropenia is an increased destruction of neutrophils. (Zuelzer, W.W., Bajoghli, M.: *Blood* 23:359–374, 1964). The increased myeloid activity in the bone marrow with the absence of the most mature forms, the segmented neutrophils, has been a uniform finding that supports this theory. The presence of an intact process of proliferation, differentiation, and maturation in these patients has also been used to explain their ability to produce and mobilize cells when special demands (e.g., infection) arise. Although autoimmune neutropenia has been reported previously, attempts to document destruction of neutrophils in chronic benign neutropenia were unsuccessful until now. Evidence for the autoimmune nature of chronic benign neutropenia was long overdue.

In this article, 15 of 16 patients tested did not respond to a steroid stimulation test, but previously reported patients with a similar clinical picture, including the one reported by Stahlie, responded to a steroid stimulation test.

The clinical spectrum of patients reported to have chronic benign neutropenia varies from asymptomatic to recurrent infections. The patients in this article, like the previously reported patients, had recurrent infections, but life-threatening invasive infections were unusual and most patients recovered. Antibiotic therapy for the infections was effective. Although those patients who were treated with intravenous gammaglobulin responded, the course of the disease is such that this expensive therapy should be limited to patients with more severe infections who may experience serious sequelae. Steroid therapy is another alternative, because it has also given neutrophilic responses in some patients with this disorder. (Nepo, A.G., et al.: *J. Pediatr.* 87:251–254, 1975).

Virally induced transient neutropenia is a common finding in pediatrics. The neutropenia usually is mild, but severe neutropenia can occur. The mechanism for the neutropenia is not yet clear, and one can speculate that autoimmune neutropenia of childhood when it is "chronic" may represent only the tip of the iceberg of postinfectious autoimmune neutropenias. If Dr. Lalezari chooses to study these more common transient neutropenias, given the more frequent use of white blood cell counts and differential cell counts in febrile infants, it should keep him busy for the next 12 years.—P.A. deAlarcon, M.D.

Severe Hemorrhage in a Patient With Gray Platelet Syndrome
Joseph E. Gootenberg, George R. Buchanan, Christine A. Holtkamp, and Catherine S. Casey (Georgetown Univ., Univ. of Texas at Dallas, and Southwestern Med. School, Dallas)
J. Pediatr. 109:1017–1019, December 1986   13–17

Gray platelet syndrome is characterized by large, almost agranular platelets that have a peculiar gray color on stained blood smears. These platelets contain normal numbers of mitochondria, dense bodies, and lysosomes, but they are selectively deficient in other constituents. Only 30 patients with gray platelet syndrome have been reported in the literature, and data on clinical parameters are scanty. A new patient with gray platelet syndrome was seen at Georgetown University Hospital.

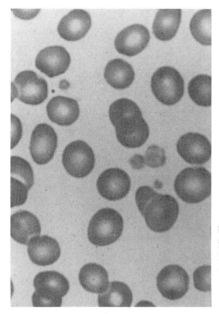

Fig 13–6.—Photomicrograph of peripheral blood smear demonstrates large size, gray color, and hypogranular character of platelets. Romanovsky stain: original magnification, × 1,000. (Courtesy of Gootenberg, J.E.: J. Pediatr. 109:1017–1019, December 1986.)

Girl, 3 years with a lifelong history of easy bruising, had large, gray, barely discernible platelets that lacked distinctive granules in the peripheral blood smear (Fig 13–6). Results of in vitro platelet function studies and additional testing confirmed a diagnosis of gray platelet syndrome. The patient was hospitalized at age 4 years after striking her head on a concrete surface. Examination revealed a massive subgaleal hemorrhage with left periorbital ecchymosis but no other physical or neurologic abnormalities. The platelet count was 94,000/cu mm; hemoglobin, 6.1 gm/dl; and hematocrit, 18.5%. Transfusion of platelets and red blood cells was carried out. On the third hospital day the child experienced a marked increase in head pain as well as scalp and facial swelling. Examination showed no increase in the intracranial hematoma. She was treated with ε-aminocaproic acid and an additional transfusion of platelets. The subgaleal hemorrhage slowly resolved during the next 2 weeks. Follow-up studies at 1 month revealed complete resolution of both the subgaleal and intracranial components.

The gray platelet syndrome may be more common than previously thought because its clinical features can mimic idiopathic thrombocytopenic purpura.

14 Oncology

Unsuspected Non-Hodgkin's Lymphoma of the Tonsils and Adenoids in Children
Derry Ridgway, Lawrence J. Wolff, Robert C. Neerhout, and David L. Tilford
(Oregon Health Sciences Univ. and Bess Kaiser Hosp., Portland)
Pediatrics 79:399–402, March 1987   14–1

Non-Hodgkin's lymphoma accounts for about 10% of pediatric cancers. Fifty-eight children were seen in a 13-year period with newly diagnosed non-Hodgkin's lymphoma, including five with disease arising in the tonsils and/or adenoids. Another child had undergone tonsillectomy 2 months before acute lymphoblastic leukemia was diagnosed and the tonsils were found to contain a lymphoblastic infiltrate. In no case was cancer suspected before surgery, and in two instances a long delay resulted. Three patients had lymphoblastic lymphoma, two had Burkitt's lymphoma, and one had mixed large cell and small cell lymphoma. All of the tumors had a diffuse histologic pattern.

Large cell types predominate in adults with lymphoma of the tonsils and adenoids. Diffuse mixed cell lymphoma is diagnosed infrequently in pediatric patients. Asymmetric involvement and progressive painless enlargement of the tonsils or adenoids without direct evidence of infection might suggest malignant disease. Careful review of the microscopic findings may be necessary to make a diagnosis of non-Hodgkin's lymphoma. Awareness of the possibility of tonsillar lymphoma by surgical pathologists will promote early diagnosis.

▶ This is a very scary article. Most of us have seen children with enlargement of the tonsils without a particularly significant history of recurrent infections. Less frequently, we see asymmetric enlargement of the tonsils. Nevertheless, these were the only two clinical hallmarks associated with a lymphoma in these removed tonsils. I suppose every time now that asymmetric, painless enlargement is seen a little red flag should go up in our minds to forewarn of the possible discovery of malignancy.

Tonsillectomy, with or without adenoidectomy, remains a common surgical procedure despite a decline in its incidence in all regions of the United States. The number of such operations reported annually in this country exceeds 100,000. The usual indications for surgery are persistent enlargement of the tonsils and recurrent tonsillitis and pharyngitis, or both. None of the patients reported in this series were even suspected of having a lymphoma. When that red flag goes up, it is important to have a prior consultation with the pathologist. Normally, tonsils, when removed, are either reviewed grossly without cut sections, or only a few cut sections are made for histology. If there is even a chance that a lymphoma will be discovered, then a great deal more should be done with the tissue at the time it is removed. Marker studies to define the cell origin of the lymphoma would normally be obtained if there was significant suspicion that a lymphoma were present in a tonsil. Thus, it is up to us and the otolaryngologist to bear responsibilities for these patients.

So what else is new in the world of non-Hodgkin's lymphoma? Probably the most remarkable are the data that are being derived from adult lymphoma studies. It is generally agreed that patients with intermediate and high-grade non-Hodgkin's lymphoma who have a relapse after initial therapy have a grave prognosis. Despite attempts at secondary therapy with irradiation or chemotherapy, or both, the likelihood of cure is nowhere nearly as great as the first time around with therapy. We've seen a great deal written in the past year about the use of autologous bone marrow transplantation in non-Hodgkin's lymphoma in adults. The use of this procedure has obvious advantages and certain disadvantages. The principal advantage, of course, is the avoidance of serious problems of graft vs. host disease when using another individual's marrow as the donor. The obvious disadvantage is the possibility that the patient's own bone marrow may contain lymphoma cells that will reseed the patient.

Two papers in *The New England Journal of Medicine* this past year (Takvorian, T., et al.: *N. Engl. J. Med.* 316:1499, 1987; Philip, T., et al.: *N. Engl. J. Med.* 316:1493, 1987) show the value of autologous bone marrow transplantation. The two series are very different in terms of the way their patients were selected and the way the treatments, other than autologous transplants, were given. The article by Philip et al. can be viewed as a paper reflecting the art of autologous transplantation after first replacement for non-Hodgkin's lymphoma, again, largely in adults. The results of this study were that 21% of patients died of toxicity induced by the treatment, 13% had severe nonfatal morbidity, and 19% were judged to be free of the disease 3 years after transplantation. An additional cohort of patients were still within 3 years of diagnosis. These results, although seemingly poor, do represent the state of the art, at least in adults. The article by Takvorian et al. reflects a different experience. The overall numbers of patients studied were smaller and all were followed in a single institution. The patients were extremely highly selected and a uniform management technique was applied. The procedure was a bit more innovative in that autologous bone marrow was treated in vitro with monoclonal antibodies and complement in an effort to eliminate any known or occult lymphoma cells. The results of this latter study were surprisingly good, with 34 of 49 patients remaining in remission and only 2 dying of treatment-related complications. This study also suffers from certain flaws, but its contribution to our overall knowledge is important in the sense that it shows that bone marrow can be treated significantly in vitro and reinfused without decreasing its ability to reconstitute the patient who presumably may be free of lymphoma after systemic intensive therapy.

Autologous bone marrow transplantation is being done in children with "purging" using monoclonal antibodies. But we will have to wait awhile to accumulate the large numbers seen in adult series, however. My bet is that the data will be not only as good, but probably better.—J.A. Stockman III, M.D.

Bone Marrow Transplantation for Children With Acute Leukemia and Down Syndrome

Charles M. Rubin, Maura O'Leary, Penelope A. Koch, and Mark E. Nesbit, Jr. (Univ. of Minnesota, Roswell Park Mem. Inst., Buffalo, and Montreal Children's Hosp.)
Pediatrics 78:688–691, October 1986   14–2

In 1957 it was first reported that Down's syndrome and leukemia occur in combination at a frequency greater than that expected by chance alone. Among children the risk that leukemia will develop appears to be up to 30 times greater for those with Down's syndrome. Among a large number of children treated for acute lymphoblastic leukemia and acute nonlymphoblastic leukemia, 2.1% had Down's syndrome, the incidence of which is about 1/660 births. Bone marrow transplantation is a promising approach to the management of patients with poor-risk leukemia and, occasionally, patients with Down's syndrome are also considered to be candidates for this procedure. A review was made of experience with four children who had acute leukemia and Down's syndrome and who underwent bone marrow transplantation

All four patients received high-dosage cyclophosphamide therapy and total body irradiation in preparation for marrow transplantation. They experienced significant skin and mucous membrane toxicity. Three children died during the immediate posttransplantation period of infectious and hemorrhagic pulmonary complications. One patient had hematologic recovery and is surviving disease free 1 year after transplantation.

These preliminary observations agree with previous data suggesting that children with Down's syndrome are at higher risk of toxicity, pneumonitis, and possibly death after administration of intensive therapy for leukemia than are children who do not have Down's syndrome. Future improvement in management of these children will depend on better understanding of the biologic and pathophysiologic aspects of Down's syndrome and further clinical experience.

▶ Dr. F. Leonard Johnson, Professor and Chief of the Division of Pediatric Hematology-Oncology, the University of Chicago Medical Center and Wyler Children's Hospital, comments on the topic of transplantation and Down's syndrome.—J.A. Stockman III, M.D.

▶ Time is finally beginning to tell how effective allogeneic bone marrow transplantation is in the treatment of children with life-threatening hematologic and immunologic diseases. The best results are in infants given transplants because of immunodeficiency disorders and children with severe aplastic anemia given transplants before they have been multiply transfused. Between 70% and 80% of these transplants are successful when the donor is "completely" matched (i.e., matched at the A, B, and D loci of the major histocompatibility complex). The need to eradicate malignant cells, in addition to obtaining engraftment, complicates the procedure in the treatment of acute leukemia and other pediatric malignant diseases. Nonetheless, in the past decade, with transplantation done earlier in the course of the disease, approximately 30% of children who receive transplants in the treatment of acute lymphoblastic leukemia in second remission and 50% of children given transplants for acute nonlymphoblastic leukemia during a first remission have remained leukemia free for more than 5 years and are potentially cured.

Three major problems need to be solved, however, before marrow transplantation will have a greater impact as a therapy for childhood cancer. The first is graft-vs.-host disease, which generally limits the availability of marrow transplantation to only the one patient in four who has a "completely" matched donor. Even in this "perfectly matched" setting, 20% of children treated with marrow transplantation will contract a fatal infection or sustain other severe organ damage because of graft-vs.-host disease.

Transplantation between less well-matched donors and recipients remains experimental. Two promising research directions for mismatched transplantation in leukemia include removing T lymphocytes, known to be involved in the pathogenesis of graft-vs.-host disease, from the donor marrow before it is infused into the patient, and use of the patient's own marrow (autologous marrow transplantation). Currently, the T cell depletion approach is associated with a high risk of failure of the graft to take, and autologous marrow transplantation is hampered by a lack of efficient methods for complete removal of malignant cells contaminating the marrow.

Relapse is the second stumbling block in transplantation for leukemia, occurring in up to 50% of patients given transplants because of acute lymphoblastic leukemia and 20% of those given transplants in treatment of acute nonlymphoblastic leukemia when the "standard" antileukemic preparative regimen of cyclophosphamide and total body irradiation is used.

The third problem, toxicity resulting from the preparative regimen, usually accounts for less than 10% of the mortality after marrow transplantation. The paper by Dr. Rubin and his colleagues suggests that such toxicity, however, may be the major cause of mortality after the procedure in children with Down's syndrome. The complications of severe skin and gastrointestinal tract toxicity, rapidly fatal bacterial or fungal sepsis, and severe hemorrhagic cystitis occurring in the patients with Down's syndrome given transplants in management of acute leukemia, after cyclophosphamide and total body irradiation, are very reminiscent of the complications observed when children with Fanconi's aplastic anemia are treated by marrow transplantation after high-dose cyclophosphamide therapy.

Skin fibroblasts and lymphocytes from patients with Fanconi's anemia or Down's syndrome have increased chromosomal sensitivity to mutagenic agents and abnormal DNA repair. It is not too surprising, then, that these patients are predisposed to more severe toxicity after transplantation when the preparative regimen involves irradiation or alkylating agents, e.g., cyclophosphamide. In addition, patients with Down's syndrome appear to be particularly sensitive to methotrexate, which is used as an immunosuppressive agent in these patients to prevent graft-vs.-host disease (Peeters, M.A., et al.: *Lancet* 2:1279, 1986).

Thus, the therapeutic difficulty of treating leukemia in children with Down's syndrome by marrow transplantation appears to mirror that observed with conventional therapy. The challenge in children with certain constitutional chromosomal abnormalities is the design of specific antileukemic and immunosuppressive therapy before transplantation and graft-vs.-host disease preventive measures afterward that are less toxic, but as effective, as the best "standard" approaches.—F.L. Johnson, M.D.

Detection of Residual Acute Lymphoblastic Leukemia Cells in Cultures of Bone Marrow Obtained During Remission

Zeev Estrov, Tom Grunberger, Ian D. Dubé, Yao-Ping Wang, and Melvin H. Freedman (Hospital for Sick Children, and Univ. of Toronto)
N. Engl. J. Med. 315:538–542, Aug. 28, 1986   14–3

Approximately half of all patients with childhood acute lymphoblastic leukemia (ALL) can be cured with chemotherapy. The others have recurrent disease that is ultimately fatal unless bone marrow transplantation is successful. Currently, most centers predict which patients will have an early relapse by means of hematologic, clinical, and cytogenetic prognostic factors. However, there are a number of instances when predicted and clinical outcomes differ. To determine why ALL recurs in some patients and not in others, a colony-culture assay was developed for quantitation of blast cells in the marrow of patients with ALL.

The semisolid culture assay was used to quantitate leukemia cells in the bone marrow of 40 patients with childhood ALL. In all of the bone marrow cultures, the colonies that developed in vitro consisted of lymphoblasts with the same surface markers and abnormal karyotype as the original diagnostic marrow specimens. When marrow cultures of specimens obtained from 13 patients in chemotherapy-induced remission were studied, it was found that six of these, including one obtained from a patient during successful engraftment after marrow transplantation, also yielded lymphoblast colonies in culture with the same immunologic phenotype or abnormal karyotype as the original leukemic marrow. Four of these patients, including one who underwent marrow transplantation, relapsed within 2–30 months of the abnormal cultures; the other two remain in remission. Bone marrow cultures from eight normal controls and from the other seven patients in remission did not yield lymphoblast colonies.

This assay appears to detect small numbers of residual leukemic cells. This technique will probably be useful in monitoring the efficacy of chemotherapy and allogeneic bone marrow transplantation in ALL, as well as in evaluating the quality of purged marrow for autologous marrow transplantation.

▶ Slightly more than 50% of patients with ALL are cured with routine chemotherapy. Currently, most centers use a number of hematologic, clinical, and cytogenetic prognostic factors determined at the time of diagnosis to predict which patients will have early relapse. To date, these prognostic factors, while useful, have not been entirely satisfactory. What has been sought for quite some time is a marker of disease activity during the remission phase. The authors of this article have attempted to learn why ALL recurs in some patients and not in others by using a newly developed colony-culture assay for quantitation of blast cells in the marrow of patients with ALL. Their data indicate that clinical and hematologic remission in childhood ALL does not always mean that the patient is free of leukemic cells. This would have been predictable, because relapse occurs at a steady frequency in this disease. What they note is that such cells are present in the bone marrow but are not in a proliferative phase. If these data hold up, it would indicate that bone marrow from every patient who is in remission or who has undergone bone marrow transplantation should be assayed and cell cultured in an attempt to detect small numbers of residual leukemic blasts. It would then be possible for specific follow-up of these patients to provide a basis for selection of subgroups who would benefit from more intensive or alternate forms of therapy prior to the onset of clinical relapse. Thus, this assay would become an essential tool as part of the overall management of patients. It would then also be used in patients who were undergoing autologous bone marrow transplantation to make sure that no contaminating leukemic cells were returned to the patient or, if they were present, that they be destroyed by some of the newer technologies noted in the preceding commentary.

If we do find leukemic cells during remission, we will probably have a difficult time determining the best way to manage this. We still aren't entirely sure about the best way to manage overt relapse in terms of trying to achieve a "total cure." Although between 50% and 70% of patients remain in continuous first remission for 5 years or more, the prognosis for children who have relapse in the bone marrow is poor. Although 70% to 90% experience a second complete remission, long-term disease-free survival is only between 10% and 20%. The treatment of children in second or later remission with high-dose chemotherapy and radiation followed by HLA-identical bone marrow transplantation bumps these numbers up to about 30% to 50% with disease-free survival, but it has not proved easy to compare the results of conventional therapy with those of bone marrow transplantation, specifically adjusting for all variables to make certain that there are appropriately matched patients in each group.

A recent analysis of data on 871 children treated by bone marrow transplantation or chemotherapy for a relapse state now in second remission showed that outcome was correlated with risk factors at diagnosis and with length at first remission. Bone marrow transplant seemed superior in patients who relapsed within 18 months of first remission while taking maintenance chemotherapy. Bone marrow transplant was not demonstrably superior in patients who relapsed more than 18 months after first remission. The choice of treatment in childhood ALL in second remission must therefore be based on prognostic variables at diagnosis and on the circumstances of the relapse (Butturini, A., et al.: *Lancet* 1:429, 1987). To show what bone marrow transplantation in high-risk ALL can do in first and second remissions, see the report of Herzig, R.H., et al. (*Lancet* 1:786, 1987). Data from 444 ALL patients with one or more high-risk features at diagnosis were analyzed to evaluate the outcome after HLA-identical bone marrow transplantation during the first or second remission. The 4-year probability of leukemia-free survival was 45% for patients in first remission and 22% for those in second remission. Overall, for high-risk ALL, transplantation in first remission had clearly superior results to transplantation in second remission.

Obviously, further studies are needed to determine whether patients with high-risk ALL should receive transplants as the procedure of choice during first remission as opposed to chemotherapy. Would that we all could be clairvoyant and titer our therapies upfront accordingly. No one has such a snapshot of the future. (Speaking of snapshots, do you know what percentage of all snapshots taken in the United States are taken at Disneyland, Disney World, or Epcot Center? The answer is approximately 4%. I really don't know why I needed to provide you with that information, but it struck me as curious when I ran across it. Thank goodness that so many photos are taken at theme parks. When the camera goes off in the professional baseball park, it is usually isolated on a male athlete. As one might expect from Murphy's laws, when a camera focuses on a male athlete, he will spit, pick, or scratch.)—J.A. Stockman III, M.D.

Intensive Retreatment of Childhood Acute Lymphoblastic Leukemia in First Bone Marrow Relapse: A Pediatric Oncology Group Study
Gaston K. Rivera, George Buchanan, James M. Boyett, Bruce Camitta, Judith Ochs, David Kalwinsky, Michael Amylon, Teresa J. Vietti, and William M. Crist (St. Jude Children's Res. Hosp., Memphis, Univ. of Texas at Dallas, Univ. of Florida, Midwest Children's Cancer Ctr., Milwaukee, Stanford Univ., Washington Univ., and Univ. of Alabama at Birmingham)
N. Engl. J. Med. 315:273–278, July 31, 1986   14–4

Children with acute lymphoblastic leukemia (ALL) who have a relapse in bone marrow during initial therapy or shortly thereafter typically have had a poor prognosis. Conversely, children in whom relapse occurs more than 6 months after elective cessation of therapy have better prospects for inducing and maintaining a remission. It was hypothesized that the length of the first hematologic remission directly reflects the degree of drug sensitivity, or perhaps the intrinsic growth potential of leukemic cells. A plan of intensive chemotherapy was devised to correct the problem of inadequate results of treatment in children with ALL in first bone marrow relapse.

This plan of chemotherapy was tested in 43 children with ALL who were in first bone marrow relapse and had no prior leukemic involvement of the CNS. Immediately after remission was induced using four conventional drugs, a 2-week intensification course of teniposide and cytarabine was administered to eradicate subclinical leukemia. Patients in remission then were treated for 2 years with rapid rotation of pairs of drugs that were not cross resistant, and periodic courses of the same agents were used to induce remission. A second complete remission was induced in 31 of the 39 patients in whom response to chemotherapy could be assessed. The mean probability of maintaining bone marrow remission in these patients for 1 year was 0.38, and the 2-year probability was 0.29. The treatment program was completed by seven patients, five of whom have been in continuous cessation of therapy. The children whose initial bone marrow remission lasted for less than 18 months had markedly poorer responses to retreatment than did those whose first remission lasted for a longer period of time. Intensive chemotherapy may save half of the children with ALL in whom bone marrow relapse occurs after a relatively long initial remission.

▶ Bruce M. Camitta, M.D., Professor of Pediatrics, The Medical College of Wisconsin, comments.—J.A. Stockman III, M.D.

▶ Optimal treatment regimens produce permanent complete remission (cure) in 60% to 75% of children with ALL. However, if relapse occurs during (or shortly after completing) therapy, second remissions are achieved less frequently and are usually shorter than with the initial treatment regimen. Reasons for the ineffectiveness of secondary treatment include selection of patients with high initial tumor burdens, leukemia cell types (B, preB, T) responding poorly to chemotherapy, leukemia cell chromosome arrangements (translocations) favoring genetic instability, and drug resistance (caused by gene amplification, altered drug transport, and so on).

The paper by Rivera et al. confirms the dismal prognosis for children whose initial complete remission was shorter than 18 months. In contrast, 50% of children with longer initial remissions remained disease free and may be cured. However, several caveats must be considered: The study size was relatively small; preceding therapy was modern but not uniform; 20% of the patients did not experience a second remission; the efficacy of each component of the regimen is unknown; and the method for detecting initial bone marrow relapse was not specified. It is possible that leukemia relapse detected only by regularly scheduled marrow examination may have a better prognosis (lower tumor burden) than relapse that is suggested by the presence of leukemic cells in the blood.

An alternative treatment for children in second remission of ALL is bone marrow transplantation. Reports from single institutions show long-term disease-free survivals of 30% to 60%. Two comparative studies suggest that bone marrow transplantation results in superior long-term disease-free survival when compared with chemotherapy (35% to 60% vs. 0%, respectively) for children with ALL in second remission (*N. Engl. J. Med.* 310:263, 1984; *Proc. Am. Soc. Clin. Oncol.* 6:163, 1987). However, once again, certain caveats must be considered: Patients given marrow transplants are selected for survival in remission until transplantation and for referral biases; bone marrow transplantation is associated with long-term toxicities; only one third of the patients have a matched sibling donor; unrelated and partially matched marrow transplantation is still experimental; and as chemotherapy and bone marrow transplantation regimens rapidly evolve, their realtive efficacy will change.

Love may be wonderful the second time around, but treatment of recurrent ALL is not. This should not lead to therapeutic nihilism. Cure is possible. More effective, less toxic treatments are required. Biologic response modifiers (e.g., interferons) are being investigated. In the future, molecular biologists may give us the tools to turn off aberrant oncogene activation.—B.M. Camitta, M.D.

Acute Lymphoblastic Leukaemia Under 2 Years
A.D. Leiper and J. Chessells (Hosp. for Sick Children, London)
Arch. Dis. Child. 61:1007–1012, 1986   14–5

Infants first seen with acute lymphoblastic leukemia (ALL) at younger than age 2 years tend to have a worse prognosis than older children. It is thought that infants with ALL who are younger than age 1 year fare especially poorly.

Between 1972 and 1980, ALL was diagnosed in 396 children. Of these, 48 were younger than age 2 years at diagnosis; 16 were younger than age 1 year (group 1), and 32 were between 1 and 2 years (group 2). Results in these 48 were compared with those in 348 aged 2–14 years (group 3).

Children in group 1 had a higher prevalence of null cell ALL, leukocyte counts of more than $100 \times 109/L$, and hepatosplenomegaly, and had a higher CNS relapse rate and shorter duration of remission than those in the other two groups. Disease-survival and overall survival in group 2 paralleled that in group 3, although group 2 patients had a markedly higher CNS relapse rate. Neurologic toxicity resulting from methotrexate and irradiation was common in patients younger than age 2 years as a whole.

Children younger than age 1 year have a particularly poor prognosis; those between ages 1 year and 2 years have a prognosis similar to that of older patients. Alternative approaches to CNS prophylaxis are needed to reduce the high prevalence of CNS disease and toxicity.

▶ There are a variety of reasons why young infants don't do well with treatment for ALL. Even though they have a higher prevalence at presentation of null cell leukemia (a favorable form under other conditions), their white blood cell counts tend to run very high and splenomegaly and hepatomegaly is much more common than in older children. They also have a much higher prevalence of CNS disease. Because of the concurrence of all of these unfavorable points, it is sometimes difficult to tell whether it is age alone or the massive number of other unfavorable features that makes the prognosis so poor in young children. Why CNS involvement is so high is not known. Some believe that it results from the fact that CNS radiation therapy is not usually given for young infants because of the sequelae of this form of CNS prophylaxis. It is precisely the high risk of long-term sequelae that ties the hands of treatment providers even in this high-risk condition state.

A report from The Netherlands profiles a unique aspect of children with ALL: There were more first-born children among patients [relative risk (RR), 1.8 times], more children from one child families (RR, 1.4), more children of parents with higher education (RR, 1.2), and more rooms in the patients' houses (RR, 1.4). Curiously, common colds, periods of fever, and primary childhood infections led to a much lower RR during the first year of life in children in whom leukemia subsequently developed. This study (van Steensel, H.A., et al.: *Am. J. Epidemiol.* 124:590, 1986) suggests that lack of early exposure to infectious agents may increase one's risk of subsequent malignancy—a novel thought at best.

An increased incidence of leukemia was reported recently in the vicinity of two nuclear instillations in the United Kingdom. The reason for mentioning this is that ongoing studies are attempting to see if there is any relationship between childhood leukemia and radiation doses near these power plants. One such study to date (Darby, S.C., et al.: *Br. Med. J.* 294:603, 1987) raises all of the usual concerns, but was unable to conclude that radiation exposure was the cause of the increased incidence of ALL, at least thus far.—J.A. Stockman III, M.D.

Malignant Tumours in the Neonate
A.N. Campbell, H.S.L. Chan, A. O'Brien, C.R. Smith, and L.E. Becker (Hosp. for Sick Children, Toronto, and Univ. of Toronto)
Arch. Dis. Child. 62:19–23, January 1987   14–6

Cancer in the neonate is rare and its management poses unique problems. A review was made of the prognosis and management of 102 patients with neonatal cancers seen during a 60-year period at The Hospital for Sick Children, Toronto. These cancers represented 2% of all pediatric malignancies seen at this institution. The male to female ratio was 1.7:1.

Neuroblastoma was the most common neonatal tumor (47%), followed by retinoblastoma (17%), soft tissue sarcoma (12%), CNS tumor (9%), leukemia (8%), and in a few children, Wilms' tumor, liver tumors, and miscellaneous tumors. The overall mortality was 41%. Children with retinoblastoma, Wilms' tumor, and neuroblastoma had the best prognosis, whereas those with leukemia, CNS malignancies, and soft tissue sarcomas had the worst. All 43 survivors underwent operation, radiochemotherapy, or both. None had severe mental or physical disabilities as a result of treatment. In only one child did thyroid carcinoma develop in an irradiated field.

A large percentage of neonates with malignant tumors can be cured successfully with minimal long-term handicaps as a result of treatment. Physicians should discuss with parents the possible risks of treatment before it is implemented.

▶ Tumor masses are fairly common findings in the neonatal period, but they are rarely malignant. In this series from one institution, malignant tumors in the newborn period comprised only 2% of all childhood malignancies. Most of these tumors are evident on the first day of life. Nonetheless, about one tumor in five will be found as an incidental notation at autopsy. Why boys have an almost 2:1 predominance over girls with respect to neonatal tumors is not known. Even though you might suspect that there would be an association with neonatal tumors and various syndromes known to predispose to malignancy, this was not observed in the series from Toronto. In fact, in this series, there was nothing that clearly distinguished why these infants were more likely to have early malignancies.

It should be noted that the long-term survivors in this series did well. Specifically, only 1 of 43 had a second malignancy. This is different from experience with older children in whom it is suspected that there is approximately a 10% to 12% cumulative probability of a second cancer developing in an irradiated field in patients of all ages who survived for 5 years or more after their first cancer.

There is another way of looking at neonatal malignancy, and that is to use data derived from collaborative or cooperative group studies. One such study is the National Wilms' Tumor Study. Twenty-seven patients were registered who presented with renal masses at less than 30 days of age. Of this overall number, 18 had mesoblastic nephroma, 1 had a malignant rhabdoid tumor of the kidney, 4 had non-neoplastic lesions, and the remaining 4 had Wilms' tumors of favorable histology. All patients did well except for the patient with stage 1 rhabdoid tumor, who died at 8 weeks of age.

Obviously, childhood cancer is a puzzle with respect to why it occurs and what to do about it. One thing to do about it is to advise mothers to stop smoking during pregnancy. The data on that topic emerge in a very clear-cut manner. Stjernfeldt, M., et al. (*Lancet* 1:1350, 1986) examined a large number of children with cancer in Sweden. A dose-response relationship was found between the number of cigarettes smoked per day by the mother during pregnancy and risk of cancer in the offspring. When all tumor sites were considered, the cancer risk was 50% higher for the most exposed group than for controls. The risk was double for non-Hodgkin's lymphoma, acute lymphoblastic leukemia, and Wilms' tumor. In this day and age when everybody is suing everybody else, it might not be unheard of to see a child suing his or her parents for smoking. Maybe that's what it takes to get the point across.—J.A. Stockman III, M.D.

Survival of Children with Brain Tumors: SEER Program, 1973–1980
Patricia K. Duffner, Michael E. Cohen, Max H. Myers, and Herman W. Heise (Children's Hosp., Buffalo, and Natl. Cancer Inst., Bethesda)
Neurology 36:597–601, May 1986   14–7

Reports of prolonged survival of children with brain tumors have appeared, but experience with these tumors often is discouraging. Data were reviewed on 887 children with brain tumors in Surveillance, Epidemiology, and End Results (SEER) registries in 1973–1980. The registries cover about 10% of the population in the United States. The children, aged 14 years or less, were followed through 1983. The most frequent tumor types were low-grade supratentorial astrocytoma, medulloblastoma, cerebellar astrocytoma, and high-grade supratentorial astrocytoma. There were 112 patients younger than 2 years of age at the time of diagnosis.

FIVE-YEAR SURVIVAL BY TUMOR TYPE

Tumor type	Current series	Literature
Medullo-blastoma	39%	67-77%
Ependymoma	28%	12.5-21% (inc) 44-47% (ex)
Cerebellar astrocytoma	91%	90-100%
Brainstem glioma	18%	17-30%
Low-grade astrocytoma	71%	70%* 40-50%†
High-grade astrocytoma	35%	16-30% grade III 0-3% grade IV

(Courtesy of Duffner, P.K., et al.: Neurology 36:597–601, May 1986.)

Surgery plus irradiation was the most frequent treatment. Nearly one fourth of patients had chemotherapy combined with surgery and/or radiotherapy. No specific treatment was given to 5% of the children. Children with cerebellar astrocytoma had the best survival, and those with brain stem glioma had the worst (table). Children younger than 2 years of age had a 5-year survival of 36%, compared with 57% for those aged 10–14 years at diagnosis.

Lack of central pathologic review is a limitation of the SEER data. The data do, however, provide a chance to follow outcome trends in large numbers of children in whom brain tumor has been diagnosed since the mid-1970s. The poor overall results emphasize the need for continued research into the treatment of children with CNS neoplasms.

Cerebellar Astrocytomas: Therapeutic Management

E.B. Ilgren and C.A. Stiller (Univ. of Oxford)
Acta Neurochir. (Wien) 81:11–26, 1986   14–8

Cerebellar astrocytomas are one of the most common childhood brain tumors. Although some patients with cerebellar astrocytoma have survived for long periods without operation, treatment is almost exclusively surgical, because most patients die if operation is not performed. A review was made of the records of patients with cerebellar astrocytoma treated at their institution between 1938 and 1984. The literature was also reviewed.

Of the 112 patients treated for cerebellar astrocytoma during the study period, 3 underwent biopsy; 45 had subtotal removal, 50 had total removal, and 10 had cyst aspiration or decompression without incision. There was no surgical record for the other four patients. Of the three patients who had only tumor biopsy, two died within 2 years of operation and one patient lived for 10 years without recurrence. Of 43 patients who survived subtotal tumor removal, 11 (26%) received radiotherapy and the other 32 had no further treatment. There was no significant difference in survival or recurrence-free survival rates between these two groups, which was only 35.2% at 5-year follow-up. Of the 50 patients who underwent total tumor removal, 95% were recurrence free for at least 25 years. All ten patients treated by decompression or cyst aspiration had recurrence within 6 years. Radiotherapy did not influence survival, either to first recurrence or to death. Survival rates for patients who undergo total removal of a cerebellar astrocytoma are significantly higher than for those who undergo subtotal removal or any other procedure.

▶ Dr. Henry S. Friedman, Associate Professor of Pediatrics, Duke University Medical Center, comments.—J.A. Stockman III, M.D.

▶ The preceding two articles (14–7 and 14–8) demonstrate the heterogeneous clinical course and outcome for children with brain tumors. The paper by Ilgren and Stiller focuses attention on the therapeutic management of children with cerebellar astrocytomas. Their observations highlight the importance of complete tumor removal (including the mural nodule) and note the excellent prognosis for prolonged survival and cure in patients with these lesions. Unfortunately, as noted in the article by Duffner et al., cerebeller astrocytomas represent only 12% of pediatric brain tumors. The 5-year survival of children with more malignant lesions (e.g., high-grade supratentorial astrocytomas, medulloblastomas, ependymomas, and brain stem gliomas) is far less impressive, with most children ultimately dying of progressive disease.

The advances seen in the treatment of pediatric malignancies such as leukemia, lymphoma, Hodgkin's disease, and Wilms' tumor have not been paralleled with similar success in the treatment of pediatric brain tumors. Although improvements in neurosurgical techniques (e.g., the use of the operating microscope) have enabled safer, more effective tumor resections, surgical intervention alone is not curative for any child with a malignant brain tumor. The addition of radiotherapy may cure a fraction of patients with certain tumors (e.g., ependymoma and medulloblastoma), but it plays a far less effective role in the treatment of tumors such as high-grade gliomas or brain stem gliomas. Nevertheless, recent advances in understanding of the biology and treatment of pediatric brain tumors suggests that a considerable, if not dramatic, increase in survival of children with these tumors will be forthcoming in the next decade.

Three areas of therapeutic research that may play a significant role in the treatment of children with brain tumors are (1) chemotherapeutic intervention, (2) hyperfractionated radiotherapy, and (3) monoclonal antibody delivery of radioisotopes. The role of chemotherapy is perhaps most optimistic in the treatment of children with medulloblastomas because there now appear to be several agents with clear-cut activity (demonstrated in the treatment of children with recurrent disease). These agents, specifically cyclophosphamide, cisplatin, and vincristine, are now being used in adjuvant therapy protocols conducted by the Pediatric Oncology Group (POG) and the Children's Cancer Study

Group (CCSG). These studies may well demonstrate a dramatic increase in survival with the use of current chemotherapeutic regimens. Unfortunately, similar success does not appear to be as imminent in the treatment of glial tumors or ependymomas. With the exception of cisplatin in the treatment of children with ependymoma, no chemotherapeutic agent appears to have any significant degree of activity in the treatment of any of these neoplasms. A recent CCSG report documenting the activity of CCNU, vincristine, and prednisone in the treatment of children with high-grade gliomas is provocative, but will need collaboration in a larger controlled study (currently being conducted by the CCSG).

The role of hyperfractionated radiotherapy designed to increase the total tumor dose without increasing long-term radiotherapeutic toxicity is currently a frontline approach for children with brain stem gliomas treated on CCSG and POG protocols. These studies attempt to duplicate the still early success of the San Francisco Brain Tumor Research Center employing doses between 720 and 7,200 cGy delivered in split daily fractions. The early data from the Brain Tumor Research Center suggests that this intervention may result in an increase in disease-free progression at 1 year, but documentation that this is not merely a right shift of the survival curve (with ultimate failure) remains forthcoming. Nevertheless, this modality offers an exciting new treatment approach for children whose 5-year survival ranges between 15% and 20% in most large series. No chemotherapeutic approach in patients with recurrent disease or at diagnosis appears to have any role in the treatment of children with these tumors. Future studies may well address the role of chemotherapy in conjunction with hyperfractionated radiotherapy.

The role of monoclonal antibodies in the treatment of children with brain tumors represents the most exciting frontier in the treatment of these lesions. The extensive preclinical studies of Bigner's team at Duke Medical Center illustrate the operational specificity of a panel of monoclonal antibodies to human gliomas and medulloblastoma, the localization of these antibodies to subcutaneous and intracranial human CNS xenografts growing in athymic mice and rats, and the therapeutic activity of these monoclonal antibodies when conjugated to radioisotopes (e.g., I131). The early studies by Coakham and Kemshead in London in the treatment of children and adults with leptomeningeal tumor dissemination treated by intrathecal instillation of radiolabeled monoclonal antibodies suggest the potential therapeutic benefit of this approach.

The next decade may well bring a new understanding of the biology and treatment of pediatric brain tumors and, we hope, result in advances similar to those seen in other pediatric malignancies.—H.S. Friedman, M.D.

Thyroid Carcinoma in Children and Adolescents
Eva Tallroth, Martin Bäckdahl, Jerzy Einhorn, Göran Lundell, Torsten Löwhagen, and Claes Silfverswärd (Karolinska Hosp. and Inst., Stockholm)
Cancer 58:2329–2332, Nov. 15, 1986   14–9

Age at diagnosis is an important prognostic factor in patients with thyroid carcinoma, and children in particular are considered to have an excellent prognosis. However, a previous study found that patients who had thyroid carcinoma in childhood may relapse and die of thyroid carcinoma after as many as 20–30 years. Long-term follow-up is thus indicated in these patients. Follow-up was made of 40 children and adolescents with thyroid carcinoma up to 35 years after diagnosis. They were no more than 20 years of age at diagnosis. The mean length of follow-up was 22 years.

All patients had undergone total thyroidectomy (12) or resection (28). There were 34 papillary, 3 medullary, and 3 follicular carcinomas. One patient died during thyroid resection. Lymph nodes with tumor growth were found at operation in 29 patients and removed in 27 of them. All except one patient received thyroid hormone suppressive therapy. Additional primary postoperative radiotherapy was given to 16 patients.

During follow-up, eight patients had recurrence, including two who died of metastatic tumor growth 5 and 14 years after the primary diagnosis, respectively. Of these eight patients, seven had only the tumor and part of the thyroid gland removed during primary surgery. The remaining six patients were treated and survived. At the end of the study, 37 of the 40 patients were alive, with no signs of recurrence.

▶ This study confirms that age at the time of diagnosis is of prognostic importance in thyroid carcinoma. Although several patients in this report had advanced disease at diagnosis, there were few recurrences and only 2 of 40 patients died because of tumor growth. All 34 patients with papillary carcinoma are alive regardless of treatment. The importance of thyroid hormone suppressive therapy seems obvious from this study. Thyroid therapy was given to all patients except one who died of metastatic tumor growth. As importantly, of the other ten patients who were not given thyroid medication immediately after operation, three had recurrences.

What many fear is that there will be a rise in the number of thyroid malignancies consequent to the nuclear accident at Chernobyl. Despite all of the epidemiologic radiation dose data available, it is stated that it probably will not be possible to detect the increased number of malignancies that are consequent to this disaster. They will occur; it's just that they will be spread around so widely that the numbers of affected patients will blend into the background of other malignancies.

It is curious how much emphasis has been placed on Chernobyl as opposed to other radiation exposures. It has been estimated that the number of pounds of plutonium and highly enriched uranium that are missing from inventories in the United States is 9,600 (only 15 lb of plutonium are needed to make an atomic bomb). Of course, it is suspected that most, if not all of this, represents logistical error and not plutonium that is off somewhere. Although we worry about Chernobyl, it should be recognized that the average American consumes 9 lb of chemical additives each year in his or her diet. About the only thing that we don't keep parity with in terms of the Soviet Union is the number of movie theaters. We only have about 10% the number of movie houses here in the United States (18,000 vs. 151,280).—J.A. Stockman III, M.D.

Prognostic Factors in Neuroblastomas Treated in Denmark From 1943 to 1980: A Statistical Estimate of Prognosis Based on 253 Cases
Niels L.T. Carlsen, Ib Jarle Christensen, Henrik Schroeder, Poul V. Bro, Gunna Erichsen, Bente Hamborg-Pedersen, Kaj Bjoern Jensen, and Ole H. Nielsen (Rigshosp., Copenhagen, Finsen Lab., Copenhagen, Univ. Hosp., Aarhus, Univ. Hosp., Odense, and Aalborg Hosp., Denmark)
Cancer 58:2726–2735, Dec. 15, 1986   14–10

Neuroblastoma is the most common malignant tumor in infancy, representing about 7% of all childhood cancers. It does not respond dramatically to modern antitumor therapy, but survival has improved significantly with the general use of chemotherapy. The prognostic significance of age, stage, sex, primary tumor site, calendar year of diagnosis, and treatment was studied in an unselected patient population in Denmark.

The study included 253 children treated for neuroblastomas between 1943 and 1980; 236 of the tumors were histologically proved. In the other 17 tumors, results of histologic examination were inconclusive (12) or absent (5), but the clinical data indicated neuroblastoma. Treatments included palliative irradiation of metastases and biopsy in 64 patients, irradiation of the primary tumor only in 48, tumor excision with or without irradiation in 42, and tumor excision and chemotherapy with or without irradiation in 57.

Prognosis for survival improved significantly from decade to decade. The prognosis became progressively worse with age up to 3 years, but improved again with age for children older than 3 years. Survival also became progressively worse from stage to stage. Survival was significantly affected by the primary tumor site. Multimodal treatment with operation, irradiation, and chemotherapy, especially in stage II patients older than age 1 year, significantly affected survival. That age at diagnosis and chemotherapy have independent prognostic significance is explained by the hypothesis that all neuroblastomas are congenital, and that the difference in age at diagnosis reflects the difference in tumor growth rates.

▶ A number of factors are used to determine prognosis at the time of diagnosis in a child with a neuroblastoma. Age has long been considered an important prognostic factor. Stage of disease is likewise prognostic except for perhaps the curious stage IV-S. You will recall that this is the unique form of disseminated neuroblastoma characterized by remote disease in the skin, liver, or bone marrow. Patients with stage IV-S tumors have a high spontaneous remission rate and a survival rate of 60% to 90%. It should be noted that not all young patients with stage IV-S neuroblastoma do well; five newborn infants were recently seen at Walter Reed Army Medical Center with this age and stage of neuroblastoma and four of them died of mechanical complications associated with massive hepatomegaly (Stephenson, S.R., et al.: *Cancer* 58:372, 1986). Other aspects of this tumor that relate to prognosis include the abnormal expression of the N-myc oncogene. Increased amplification of N-myc is associated with a poor outcome in most studies. This is not an all or none phenomenon, and one recent report of N-myc amplification in a child with stage IV-S tumor was reported. There are also other biologic markers associated with prognosis in neuroblastoma. These include the presence of neuron-specific enolase, the serum ferritin level, neuroblastoma histology, tumor-associated gangliosides, cytogenetic analyses, and cellular DNA content. These are markers of the disease in a general sense but are difficult to apply to single patients in terms of extent of disease or specific prognosis.

If you are interested in reading more about gene amplification in malignancy, see the excellent editorial comment in *The Lancet* (1:839, 1987). The main implications of gene amplification fall into two areas: prognosis and therapy. There are three human tumors in which proto-oncogene amplification correlates with a poor prognosis. One is neuroblastoma with the caveats noted above. Another is small cell cancer, and the third is breast cancer (*JAMA* 258:19, 1987). Another aid to help the physician is a newly developed radiopharmaceutical, I-131-labeled metaiodobenzylguanidine. This radiopharmaceutical has been used to determine scintigraphically the location of adrenal medullary hyperplasia, pheochromocytoma, neuroblastoma, and other neurocrest tumors (Ikekubo, K.: *Clin. Nucl. Med.* 11:780, 1986); Edeling, C.J., et al.: *J. Nucl. Med.* 25:172, 1986).

The most newsworthy item relative to neuroblastoma during the past year has been the strong impetus toward screening all infants in North America for this tumor with spot urine testing for catecholamine. Woods and Tuchman (*Pediatrics* 79:869, 1987) present a potent argument for this. For some time now, many pediatric oncologists in the United States have criticized the Japanese for their routine screening for neuroblastoma. In Japan this is done at 6 months of age with spot urine checks. What Woods and Tuchman have done is to present some preliminary data and then review the Japanese experience in the context of what we can expect here in the United States. As noted, the argument is indeed compelling. Urinary spot tests can be done for $3.50. This works out to about $25,000 per tumor diagnosed. This tumor occurs in about 1 in 7,000 children in the United States. If you don't find the article just mentioned strong enough, then read the accompanying article on page 1048 of the same issue of *Pediatrics*. I, for one, have clearly been on the fence about the issue of universal screening for neuroblastoma. Even I am swayed by the arguments put forth. Sure, there are a lot of unknowns (what is the false positivity rate; the false negativity rate; the best age at screening, and so on). None of those unknowns, however, would remain unknown if carefully designed studies were done as part of mass screening. I think what will happen is that the Woods and Tuchman article will just tip the balance so that those who have been on the fence will fall off. A long time ago, Dr. J. Ryle in his book entitled *The Natural History of Disease*, ed. 2, (Oxford, Oxford University Press, 1948) noted that "the three main tasks of the clinician . . . are diagnosis, prognosis and treatment. Of these, diagnosis is by far the most important, for upon it the success of the other two depends." How apt this is with regard to neuroblastoma.—J.A. Stockman III, M.D.

Outcome of Pregnancy in Survivors of Wilms' Tumor

Frederick P. Li, Kathreen Gimbrere, Richard D. Gelber, Stephen E. Sallan, Francoise Flamant, Daniel M. Green, Ruth M. Heyn, and Anna T. Meadows (Natl. Cancer Inst., NIH, Bethesda, Dana-Farber Cancer Inst., Boston, Harvard Univ., Inst. Gustave Roussy, Villejuif, France, Roswell Park Mem. Inst., Buffalo, C.S. Mott Children's Hosp., Ann Arbor, and Children's Hosp. of Philadelphia)

JAMA 257:216–219, Jan. 9, 1987   14–11

Advances in treatment have resulted in improved survival of children and young adults with cancer. Although antineoplastic agents and radiotherapy can induce gonadal failure and fetal malformations and death when exposure occurs during pregnancy, data on the course of pregnancies occurring years after successful treatment of childhood cancer are scarce. Because data are needed to provide genetic counseling and appropriate antepartum care to these patients, the outcome of pregnancy was studied in patients who survived childhood Wilms' tumor.

A total of 191 singleton pregnancies of at least 20 weeks' duration occurred among 99 patients, including 65 female patients and 34 wives of male patients who had survived Wilms' tumor. Their ages ranged from less than 1 to 18 years at diagnosis of Wilms' tumor. All patients underwent unilateral nephrectomy, and 60 female and 34 male patients received abdominal radiotherapy.

Of 114 pregnancies in the 60 women who underwent abdominal radiotherapy, 34 (30%) had an adverse outcome, including 17 perinatal

OUTCOME OF 191 SINGLETON PREGNANCIES, BY ABDOMINAL RADIOTHERAPY TO THE PARENT WHO HAD WILMS' TUMOR

	No. (%) of Pregnancies			
	Mother With Wilms' Tumor		Father With Wilms' Tumor	
Outcome of Pregnancy*	Radiation	No Radiation	and Radiation	Entire Series
Adverse outcome†	34 (30)	0 (0)	2 (3)	36
Fetal death	11	0	0	11
Low birth weight (2500 g or less)	22‡	0	2	24
Neonatal death; normal birth weight	1	0	0	1
Normal outcome	80 (70)	13 (100)	62 (97)	155
Total	114 (100)	13 (100)	64 (100)	191

*Adverse outcome was defined as fetal death at 20 weeks or more of gestation, neonatal death, or liveborn infant weighing 2,500 gm or less.

†Rates of adverse outcome among first pregnancies of patients with 99 Wilms' tumors: 37% (22/60) for irradiated mothers, 0% (0/5) for nonirradiated mothers, and 3% (1/34) for fathers.

‡Neonatal deaths occurred in 5 of the 22 low-birth-weight infants: in 4 of 7 who were 1,500 gm or less, 1 of 9 between 1,501 and 2,000 gm, and none of 6 between 2,001 and 2,500 gm.

(Courtesy of Li, F.P., et al.: JAMA 257:216–219, Jan. 9, 1987.)

deaths and 17 with low-birth-weight infants, whereas all 13 pregnancies in the 5 women who did not have radiotherapy had a normal outcome. Of 64 pregnancies in the 34 wives of men who underwent abdominal radiotherapy, 2 (3%) had an adverse outcome (table). The perinatal mortality and percentage of low-birth-weight infants among the 114 singleton pregnancies in irradiated female patients significantly exceeded the corresponding figures for singleton pregnancies in white women in the United States. The high risk of adverse pregnancy outcome should be a consideration in the counseling and antepartum care of women who have received abdominal irradiation for Wilms' tumor in childhood.

▶ Read this report in its original form. Look at the data yourself. Some will read this and say the glass is half empty; others will say the glass is half full. Actually, I think it's a tribute to modern medicine that 70% of women who previously had abdominal radiation therapy for Wilms' tumor will have a successful outcome of their pregnancy. Yes, there is a high risk of adverse pregnancy outcome, but I would think of it the other way around and look at this as being a problem of the glass being half full. There are well over 50,000 individuals in the United States who have survived a childhood cancer. I think we need much more time to learn what the pluses and minuses are of these cures.—J.A. Stockman III, M.D.

Hepatoblastoma and Hepatocarcinoma in Children: Analysis of a Series of 29 Cases
Frédéric Gauthier, Jacques Valayer, Bao Le Thai, Martine Sinico, and Chantal Kalifa (Bicêtre Hosp. and Gustave Roussy Inst., Villejuif, France)
J. Pediatr. Surg. 21:424–429, May 1986   14–12

   Hepatoblastoma is the most frequent malignant primitive tumor of the liver in children and is associated with a high mortality. The sole possibly successful treatment is surgical, but only one tumor of every two is usually operable, and cure is obtained in only one of three patients with operable tumors. Experience with hepatoblastoma and hepatocarcinoma was reviewed.

   During a 13-year period the same surgical team operated on 29 children with liver malignancies (26 hepatoblastomas and 3 hepatocarcinomas). Four were found at operation to have nonresectable tumors, even after chemotherapy. The 25 operations consisted of right lobectomy in 14 patients, left lobectomy in 9, and tumorectomy in 2. In five patients a second operation had to be performed because of histologic doubt on the cut section about the presumed normal parenchyma or for local recurrence. Preoperative chemotherapy appeared to facilitate operation on otherwise inoperable tumors, but the benefits of preoperative embolization, performed in three children, were minimal. Ten patients died, one in the immediate postoperative period, eight others of the disease, and one of a complication of chemotherapy. Follow-ups among the 18 survivors, all recurrence and metastasis free and with normal α-fetoprotein values, were less than 2 years for 4 patients and from 2 to 11 years for 14. Although six of seven children operated on without adjunctive treatment are cured, a systematic course of preoperative chemotherapy has been prescribed in more recent patients.

▶ The experience reported by Gauthier et al. is in keeping with that of most oncology centers in the Western world. Malignant hepatocellular tumors in children are associated with a poor prognosis; currently, the best chance of cure lies in opportune and complete surgical excision, with a good margin of safety around the neoplasm. That 10 of 26 patients in this series died (4 with unresectable tumors at diagnosis) is a sobering reminder of the aggressiveness of this disease, even when surgery appears practicable. Recurrence or metastases, signaled by rising titers of the α-fetoprotein level between 4 and 14 months after surgery, virtually always precludes therapeutic success.

The management of unresectable, metastatic, or recurrent malignant hepatocytic tumors is a major preoccupation of interinstitutional collaborative studies in North America at the present time. There is little experience with the new combined therapies proposed by these study groups, as some of the protocols have been in trial officially for a very short time. European oncologists have often resorted to preoperative chemotherapy of malignant pediatric tumors on the plausible contention that it reduces the size of the tumor and prevents early metastases. This apparently was the concept that guided chemotherapy in the patients reported by Gauthier et al., because the more recently treated patients all received preoperative and postoperative chemotherapy regardless of size and location of the tumor.

The wisdom of this approach is now a matter of debate, as avowed by Gauthier and collaborators, considering that (1) surgery alone has been curative in localized neoplasms, and that (2) very few of the unresectable tumors become amenable to surgery. Nevertheless, the patient series described by this French group adequately stresses the difficult quandaries posed by these aggressive tumors.—F. Gonzalez–Crussi, M.D.

Cancer of the Large Bowel in Children
Suk-Jung Gerald Koh and Warren W. Johnson (Univ. of Tennessee, and Le Bonheur Children's Med. Ctr., Memphis, and Univ. of Mississippi)
South. Med. J. 79:931–935, August 1986   14–13

Although carcinoma of the colon and rectum has a high incidence in adults older than age 40, it is rare in children. Large bowel cancer in children is curable, provided that it is diagnosed early enough. However, the diagnosis is often delayed, because this type of tumor has a tendency to produce vague signs and symptoms that mimic those of inflammatory bowel disorders. A review was made of the case histories of 22 children treated for large bowel cancer at St. Jude Children's Research Hospital in Memphis between 1962 and 1979.

The 12 girls and 10 boys (12 blacks, 10 whites) were aged 9–19 years

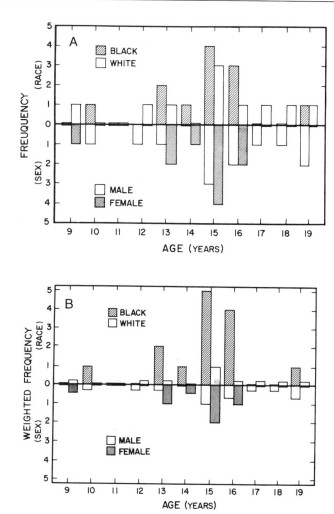

Fig 14–1.—**A**, age-matched racial and sexual frequency of large bowel cancer. **B**, age-matched racial and sexual differences in relative incidence (weighted frequency-frequency/denominator populations) of large bowel cancer. (Courtesy of Koh, S.-J.G., and Johnson, W.W.: South. Med. J. 79:931–935, August 1986.)

(median, 15 years), and had confirmed carcinoma of the large intestine (Fig 14–1). The tumors were fairly evenly distributed throughout the colon and rectum (Fig 14–2). Of 22 carcinomas, 18 were classified as mucinous adenocarcinomas, 3 as well-differentiated adenocarcinomas, and 1 as a poorly differentiated adenocarcinoma. At diagnosis, 18 patients had Dukes' stage C disease, with involvement of regional lymph nodes, peritoneum, omentum, and other abdominal organs; 7 of these patients had evidence of metastasis to the liver, lungs, bone marrow, supraclavicular lymph nodes, and skin. Of these 18 patients, only 1 was alive 12 months

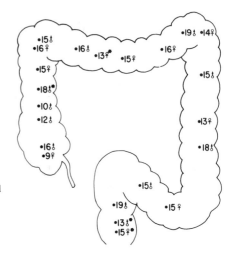

Fig 14–2.—Anatomical sites of large bowel cancer. Numerals represent ages of patients; asterisks denote cases of nonmucinous adenocarcinoma. (Courtesy of Koh, S.-J.G., and Johnson, W.W.: South. Med. J. 79:931–935, August 1986.)

after diagnosis. Of three patients with Dukes' stage B disease, two were alive 16 months and one was alive 7 months after diagnosis. The one patient with Dukes' stage A disease was alive 121 months after diagnosis. In this group of patients, the tumor had no predilection for sex, but it was significantly more frequent in blacks than in whites. Large bowel cancer does occur in children, and awareness of this may lead to early discovery and possible cure.

▶ You might be asking why so many of these colonic carcinomas were missed. It's fairly simple: Of the 22 patients with large bowel carcinoma, only 1 had a history of colonic polyposis and possible familial cancer syndrome (about 20% of his family members had a history of various types of cancer). No other patient in this series had inflammatory bowel disease or other cancer precursors. Thus, when symptoms began there was reason to suspect that the patient had a carcinoma. We, as pediatricians, are not particularly prone to think of this diagnosis. An internist treating a 70-year-old with abdominal complaints will immediately do a stool guaiac examination with the thought that the patient may have a malignancy. The purpose of including such a rare diagnosis in the YEAR BOOK OF PEDIATRICS is simply to remind us all that this disease can occur and that 22 such patients were seen in just one institution, albeit a referral center. We obviously should be very concerned about the likelihood of cancer whenever we care for a child who has had long-standing inflammatory bowel disease or a very strong family history of bowel cancer, particularly in inherited familial polyposis and Gardner's syndrome.

The Peutz-Jeghers syndrome is among the disorders that we rank highest on our list of associations with large bowel carcinoma. This last year has seen a more careful elucidation of the risk of cancer in patients with this disorder. Recall that the Peutz-Jeghers syndrome is an autosomal dominant disease characterized by polyps in the gastrointestinal tract and by mucocutaneous melanin pigmentation. The polyps were thought initially to have little potential for malignancy, but reports in the medical literature have associated the syndrome with cancer of the gastrointestinal tract and malignant tumors of the breast. Giardiello et al. (*N. Engl. J. Med.* 316:1511, 1987) followed 31 patients with the Peutz-Jeghers syndrome. Cancer developed in 15. Four had gastrointestinal tract carcinomas and ten had cancers elsewhere. In one, multiple myeloma developed. Most of the cancers were diagnosed when the patients were relatively young. Thus, whenever you see the typical melanin pigmentation on the lips of a patient that suggests they have the Peutz-Jeghers syndrome, look at the parents, confirm the diagnosis, and sharpen up your diagnostic surveillance tools.—J.A. Stockman III, M.D.

Compliance of Pediatric and Adolescent Cancer Patients

Cameron K. Tebbi, K. Michael Cummings, Michael A. Zevon, Leasel Smith, Mary Richards, and Janis Mallon (Roswell Park Mem. Inst., Buffalo)
Cancer 58:1179–1184, Sept. 1, 1986   14–14

Previous studies on patient compliance for diseases other than cancer have shown that patients tend to be noncompliant in following a prescribed regimen. Undetected noncompliance affects therapy and the therapeutic outcome, often resulting in altered regimens or unnecessary laboratory studies. The level of medication-taking compliance was studied in adolescent and pediatric cancer patients for whom chemotherapeutic agents were prescribed and factors relating to noncompliance were identified.

The series included 40 parents and 46 pediatric and adolescent cancer patients, 26 males and 20 females aged 2.5–23 years; all were being self-treated orally at home with chemotherapy. Diagnoses included acute lymphatic leukemia (in 25), Hodgkin's disease (8), non-Hodgkin's lymphoma (4), and other cancers (8). Chemotherapeutic agents included prednisone, 6-mercaptopurine, methotrexate, procarbazine, and tamoxifen. Patients and parents were interviewed in depth at 2 weeks, 20 weeks, and 50 weeks post diagnosis. The results of self-reported compliance were verified by serum bioassay of the prescribed medications.

Compliance was better in pediatric cancer patients than in adolescent cancer patients. Although compliance appeared to decline during the course of therapy, the decline was statistically not significant. There was no significant difference in noncompliance with regard to the drugs taken. Inpatient-outpatient status and disease phase did not correlate significantly with compliance. There was no significant relationship between compliance and side effects, number of medications, or amount of time a particular medication had been prescribed. However, understanding instructions on how to take medications was significantly related to compliance. The main reasons given for noncompliance included forgetfulness, busy schedules, and nonavailability of medication.

Compliance is a complex issue that interrelates with a large number of medical and social factors. Noncompliance in cancer therapy requires proper patient-parent education and increased awareness of the problem by health care providers.

Psychosocial Consequences of Childhood and Adolescent Cancer Survival

M. Jane Teta, Marianne C. Del Po, Stanislav V. Kasl, J. Wister Meigs, Max H. Myers, and John J. Mulvihill (Union Carbide Corp., Danbury, Conn., Boston Univ., Yale Univ., and Natl. Cancer Inst., NIH, Bethesda)

J. Chron. Dis. 39:751–759, 1986   14–15

As a result of advances in the treatment of childhood cancer, many children survive the disease and live to adulthood. Previous studies of psychological outcome in survivors of childhood cancer have found that most made an excellent adjustment and matured to live essentially normal, fully active lives. However, one extensive study indicated that certain survivors and their family members experienced psychosocial maladjustment. A study was conducted to assess the incidence of depression and realization of selected socioeconomic objectives.

The study included 450 survivors of childhood or adolescent cancer and 587 of their siblings. All were interviewed in person. The participants were selected with similar age-sex frequency distributions for survivors and controls. The findings were compared with incidence rates of depression in the general population by sex.

Male survivors were significantly more likely to experience short-term depression than their brothers were, but the percentages for female survivors and their sisters were nearly identical. However, the frequency of lifetime major depression in male and female survivors did not appear to differ from that in their siblings and was similar to that reported for the general population. Male long-term survivors did experience significantly more rejection from the armed forces, college, and employment than their brothers did (table). Female long-term survivors were significantly more likely than their sisters to be rejected by the armed forces, but no differences were found between females and their sisters with regard to college admission or employment. Survivors of both sexes also had more difficulty in obtaining health and life insurance than their siblings did. Although

PERCENTAGES OF SURVIVOR AND SIBLING APPLICANTS DENIED
MILITARY, EDUCATIONAL, AND OCCUPATIONAL
OPPORTUNITIES BY SEX

	Male		Female	
	Survivors	Siblings	Survivors	Siblings
Military	80 (92)*	18 (130)	75 (8)	13 (8)
$p <$	0.0001		0.05	
College	13 (128)	3 (163)	6 (124)	7 (161)
$p <$	0.01		NS†	
Graduate school	6 (47)	11 (38)	0 (30)	4 (46)
$p <$	NS		NS	
Job	32 (210)	21 (267)	19 (224)	19 (299)
$p <$	0.05		NS	

*Number of applicants in parentheses.
†NS: not significant.
(Courtesy of Teta, M.J., et al.: J. Chron. Dis. 39:751–759, 1986.)

survivors of childhood or adolescent cancer do not appear to be at a higher risk of major depression than their siblings or the general population, they seem to have more problems than their siblings in attaining certain major socioeconomic goals.

▶ Dr. Cameron K. Tebbi, Director, the Adolescent Unit, Roswell Park Memorial Institute, Buffalo, comments.—J.A. Stockman III, M.D.

▶ With an increased number of pediatric and adolescent patients surviving their disease, and their long life expectancy, visible and invisible scars of cancer have found increasing importance. Among major issues for survivors are second malignancies, long-term psychological effects, education, employment, and insurability (Li, F.P., et al.: *J. Natl. Cancer Inst.* 71:1205–1209, 1983; Boyle, M., et al.: *Med. Pediatr. Oncol.* 10:301–312, 1982).

Depression as a consequence of the cancer and its therapy is of major concern in these patients. Adults undergoing active therapy for cancer are found to have approximately a 20% to 40% rate of severe depression, as compared with 10% in those with benign diseases (Plumb, M., Holland, J.: *Psychosom. Med.* 43:243–254, 1981). The prevalence of depression in children with cancer is less clear. In one study, 15.4% of adolescent cancer patients were depressed (Tebbi, C.K., et al.: *J. Clin. Oncol.* 6:259, 1987). Females had significantly more depressive symptoms than males had. The article by Teta et al. indicates that the rate of depression in long-term survivors of cancer declines to a level approximating that of the population at large.

Another major issue for cancer survivors is employability. A study commissioned by the California Division of the American Cancer Society reported that 54% of former cancer patients in white collar occupations and 84% of those in blue collar occupations experienced discrimination (Mellette, S.J.: *CA* 35:360–373, 1985). This problem appears to be a universal finding in reports addressing the vocational status of cancer patients. Such discrimination often stems from the community's fear of the disease, recurrence, and even contagion. The article by Teta et al. confirms the existence of such difficulties among survivors of childhood and adolescent malignant disorders. Although the rate of physical disability in these patients is not stated, the article confirms that a bias against employment of cancer survivors exists.

The prejudice against former cancer patients is clearly evident when these individuals apply for health or life insurance. It appears that many companies consider the prior diagnosis of cancer to be an indication for absolute rejection of the applicant. Some studies have shown that 24% of patients have difficulty in obtaining health insurance, and nearly half are rejected for life insurance (Holmes, G.E., et al.: *Cancer* 57:190–193, 1986). Obviously, the availability of insurance has a direct impact on the financial security of former cancer patients.

The data described by Teta et al. are retrospective and derived from a heterogeneous sample of patients. With the help of aggressive therapy, a much larger number of those with leukemia and solid tumors survive, thus the mix of patients in the 1980s will probably be different. Still, this study is germane with regard to identifying important issues concerning the quality of life of long-term cancer survivors that deserve prospective investigation. The development of methods for preventing stigmatization and employment bias against cancer survivors is warranted.—C.K. Tebbi, M.D.

15 Ophthalmology

Acute Bacterial Conjunctivitis: Bacteriology and Clinical Implications
Pakit Vichyanond, Quinzetta Brown, and Doug Jackson (Labette County Med.
Ctr., Parsons, Kan.)
Clin. Pediatr. (Phila.) 25:506–509, October 1986   15–1

Acute bacterial conjunctivitis is a common eye affliction, especially among children. Studies were made of the incidence rates and sensitivity to antibiotics of various types of bacteria that were cultured from the eyes of children with conjunctivitis.

The microbiologic records of eye culture specimens obtained from pediatric patients were analyzed retrospectively. The patients ranged in age from 1 day to 20 years (mean, 31 months). Most of the patients (26) fell into the age range of 2–12 months, followed by those aged 1–2 years (19). Of 80 specimens examined, 72 were positive for one or more species of bacteria, and 42 were cultured for sensitivity. Serotyping was not performed.

Hemophilus influenzae was the most commonly isolated bacteria (34 strains, 42%), followed by *Staphylococcus epidermidis* (11 strains, 13.75%), and *Streptococcus pneumoniae* (9 strains, 11.25%). *Hemophilus influenzae* was present in 47.2% of all submitted specimens (Fig 15–1). The mean age of the patients with *H. influenzae* was 15 months. Of ten positive cultures from newborns, five grew *S. epidermidis,* four were common surface contaminants, and one was *H. influenzae.* Sensitivity studies showed that chloramphenicol and tetracycline had excellent in vitro activity in all age groups. Ampicillin had acceptable activity only in the younger age group. Erythromycin had poor activity in all age groups. Tetracycline appears to be the preferred drug for the treatment of acute bacterial conjunctivitis.

▶ Have you ever wondered which commentary among the several hundred or

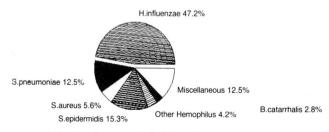

H.influenzae 47.2%

S.pneumoniae 12.5%

Miscellaneous 12.5%

S.aureus 5.6%

S.epidermidis 15.3%

Other Hemophilus 4.2%

B.catarrhalis 2.8%

% = Percentages over all submitted specimens

Fig 15–1.—Distribution and percentages of all bacteria isolated. [Courtesy of Vichyanond, P., et al.: Clin. Pediatr. (Phila) 25:506–509, October 1986.]

so that appear in this book was written first? Well, as far as this editor's half of the YEAR BOOK goes, you would have guessed right if you said this one. The first one always seems to be the hardest to do. Being the first at anything violates one of the basic three rules of nature: never be first, never be last, and never volunteer for anything. However, because something had to be first, here goes:

It's amazing how the controversy still rages over what to do about neonatal eye prophylaxis. It has been 108 years since Credé showed that the ocular instillation of silver nitrate was highly effective in the prevention of gonococcal ophthalmia. Nothing since that time has shown that silver nitrate fails to work. The only problem is that silver nitrate can cause red eyes and, if used in inadvertently high concentrations, corneal damage. Current recommendations of the American Academy of Pediatrics include the topical use of 1% silver nitrate, 0.5% erythromycin ointment, or 1% tetracycline ointment. The Academy considers these equally acceptable for the prevention of gonococcal ophthalmia neonatorum. Obviously, erythromycin or tetracycline may be quite appropriate for prophylaxis of Chlamydia infection (Dillon, H.C.: N. Engl. J. Med. 315:414, 1986). But, as we all know by now, the problem with any form of topical prophylaxis is that it does not eradicate organisms elsewhere.

For example, it has been confirmed that infants with gonococcal conjunctivitis may also have gonococcal infection of the pharynx (Fransen, L., et al.: J. Infect. Dis. 153:862, 1986). This could be a source of reinfection after local prophylaxis of gonococcal ophthalmia and may be also the portal of entry for disseminated gonococcal infection or for lower respiratory tract infection with this organism. Perhaps the use of single-dose ceftriaxone, which is effective in the prevention of gonococcal ophthalmia neonatorum (Laga, M., et al.: N. Engl. J. Med. 315:1382, 1986), will be effective in eradicating the gonococcus no matter where it is in the body of a neonate. Unfortunately, this antibiotic does not do very much for Chlamydia infection. The usual problem here is that if we use erythromycin or tetracycline as eye prophylaxis, the Chlamydia-caused pneumonia will still show up a few weeks later and then require prolonged antibiotic therapy.

Because of problems with chemical conjunctivitis, distribution issues, and cost constraints, the use of silver nitrate or antibiotics is not always practical in developing countries. Bishai and Bishai (N. Engl. J. Med. 316:1549, 1986) noted that for centuries in India, colostrum has been applied topically to the eyes of neonates to prevent ophthalmia neonatorum. Colostrum contains many antibodies, including IgA as well as leukocytes and lysozymes. These authors note that colostrum is free, nontoxic, and readily available. Not quite so: Nothing in life is truly free, and nothing is totally nontoxic. Human immunodeficiency virus (HIV) has been detected in human breast milk, and in certain developing areas, especially in Africa, the high prevalence of HIV infection would compromise that approach because the colostrum used in eye prophylaxis is usually obtained from a woman other than the mother of a newborn infant. Nonetheless, the whole idea of the use of colostrum is intriguing. I have a veterinary friend who claims he never sees conjunctivitis in newborn calves. I wonder if this is because their eyes are bathed in milk as they are attempting to feed?

Much of the above commentary deals with sexually transmitted disease. Obviously, an ounce of prevention is worth a pound of cure. Unfortunately, our legislators are not putting enough money into prevention. Perhaps we can entice the private sector to do so. As a mode of comparison, the annual municipal budget for the Miami vice squad is $1.2 million. In contrast, the budget per single episode of the TV program "Miami Vice" is $1.5 million. There must be a meaning in all this or at least some ad(VICE) for our legislators.

I asked Dr. Arnold Smith, Professor of Pediatrics, University of Washington, and Chief, Division of Infectious Disease, Children's Hospital and Medical Center, Seattle, to discuss further the issue of conjunctivitis in older infants and children.—J.A. Stockman III, M.D.

▶ What do you do if you see a child between 2 and 24 months of age with conjunctival inflammation and exudate for 20 hours? The mother doesn't recall an episode of trauma or foreign body inoculation, and the infant is afebrile and lacks other identifiable foci of infection. Vichyanond and colleagues (1) conclude: "Tetracycline may prove to be the drug of choice for the treatment of acute conjunctivitis if comparative clinical data support its *in vitro* superiority." Is it appropriate to treat acute conjunctivitis without obtaining microbiologic evidence of infection? Don't we obtain cultures in other instances when there is only epithelial infection, i.e., urethritis?

Browning (2) in 1912 also wondered about the value of a Gram stain in cases of acute conjunctivitis. He found that in only 30% of the infections was the smear useful: The correlation with eventual culture results was erroneous or misleading. In 1921 Lindner (3) suggested that certain bacteria can adhere to and invade conjunctival epithelial cells; removing the epithelial cells by scraping and subsequent staining might be a more accurate way of identifying the pathogen. Doing this, Lindner obtained excellent correlation (my calculation of $r = .88$) between smear and culture.

What are the organisms causing conjunctivitis in this age group? Giglotti et al. (4) recovered *H. influenzae* from 42%, adenovirus from 22%, and *S. pneumoniae* from 12% of children with eye redness, with or without exudate. Cultures of the conjunctiva of controls revealed no *H. influenzae* or adenovirus, but 3% harbored pneumococci. The children in Giglotti's study, however, were slightly older than those reported by Vichyanond et al.: The mean patient age was 4.4 years. Sandstrom and colleagues (5) scraped the conjunctiva of 36 infants with palpebral edema, purulent discharge, and conjunctival hyperemia, all of whom were less than 1 month of age. After Gram staining, each oil field contained more than 5 leukocytes in 77% of the smears, whereas 14% of the controls had more than 1 but less than 5 leukocytes per field. Using purulence (i.e., at least 5 leukocytes per field) as an indicator of infection, the etiology was *Hemophilus* in 17%, *S. aureus* in 17%, *Chlamydia trachomatis* in 14%, and *S. pneumoniae* in 11%. Viruses were not sought. So how does one distinguish an infant with bacterial conjunctivitis from one with adenoviral disease? Children with adenoviral disease tend to have concomitant pharyngitis (55% in Giglotti's study), whereas others (6) emphasize the presence of preauricular lymphadenopathy. Our colleagues in ophthalmology (7) believe that adenoviral disease is more often accompanied by hyperplasia of the lymphoid follicles beneath the conjunctiva, hyperemia of the palpebral conjunctiva, and subconjunctival hemorrhages on the globe. Thus, we can sort out adenoviral conjunctivitis from bacterial conjunctivitis on physical examination in more than half of the patients.

So what do we do with the remaining patients? I would treat topically with an ophthalmic ointment. Giglotti and co-workers (8) administered an ointment formulation containing 10,000 units of polymyxin per gm and 500 units of bacitracin per gm four times a day for 7 days. This effected a clinical cure in 31 of 34 patients and a bacteriologic cure in 27 of 34 within 8–10 days. Placebo ointment produced a clinical cure in 23 of 32, but pathogens persisted in 22 of the 32. Thus, after a week of topical therapy, if the eye is not better, the conjunctiva should be scraped and the material processed for *C. trachomatis* antigen and Gram stained and cultured for bacteria. Subsequent antibiotic therapy will probably be by the oral or parenteral route, depending on the pathogen identified (9).—A. Smith, M.D.

References

1. Vichyanond, P., Brown, Q., Jackson, D.: Acute bacterial conjunctivitis. *Clin. Pediatr.* 25:506, 1986.
2. Browning, S.H.: The value of direct smear in the bacteriology of conjunctivitis, with analysis of a thousand cases. *Ophthal. Rev.* 31:97, 1912.
3. Lindner, K.: Uber die Topographie der parasitaren Bindhautkeime. *Grafes Arch. Ophthalmol.* 105:726, 1921.
4. Gigliotti, F., Williams, W.T., Hayden, F.O., et al.: Etiology of acute conjunctivitis in children. *J. Pediatr.* 98:531, 1981.
5. Sandstrom, K.I., Bell, T., Chandler, J.W., et al.: Microbial causes of neonatal conjunctivitis. *J. Pediatr.* 105:706, 1984.
6. Rowe, W.P., Huebner, R.J., Hartley, J.W., et al.: Studies of the adenoidal-pharyngeal-conjunctival group of viruses. *Am. J. Hyg.* 61:197, 1955.
7. Dawson, C., Hanna, L., Wood, T.R., et al.: Adenovirus keratoconjunctivitis in the United States III. Epidemiologic, clinical and microbiologic features. *Am. J. Ophthalmol.* 69:473, 1970.
8. Gigliotti, F., Hendley, J.W., Morgan, J., et al.: Efficacy of topical antibiotic therapy in acute conjunctivitis in children. *J. Pediatr.* 104:623, 1984.
9. Siegel, J.: Eye infections encountered by the pediatrician. *Pediatr. Infect. Dis.* 5:741, 1986.

Metastatic Bacterial Endophthalmitis: A Contemporary Reappraisal
Mark J. Greenwald, Lisa G. Wohl, and Clive H. Sell (Northwestern Univ., Children's Mem. Hosp., Chicago, and Pacific Med. Ctr., San Francisco)
Surv. Ophthalmol. 31:81–101, September–October 1986   15–2

Findings in 67 previously reported patients with metastatic bacterial endophthalmitis and those in five new patients seen from 1981 to 1985 were reviewed. In focal endophthalmitis, inflammation is concentrated in one or a few discrete foci. Anterior diffuse and posterior diffuse forms of metastatic endophthalmitis also are seen, as is a panophthalmitis. A wide range of bacteria have been implicated in metastatic endophthalmitis.

One third of the patients reviewed were younger than 20 years of age, and ten of them were infants. Intravenous injections are associated with *Bacillus cereus* endophthalmitis. Nonocular foci of infection are present in most patients in whom metastatic endophthalmitis develops. Both eyes are involved in one fourth of the patients. The only certain means of determining the cause in a given patient is to aspirate intraocular fluids for culture. Delayed treatment may contribute to poor results. Intravenous administration of antibiotics has been the chief factor in the current success achieved in treating metastatic bacterial endophthalmitis.

Ocular fluids need not be obtained if the patient is septic with a previously identified organism, or if initial smear study or immunologic testing of a nonocular specimen is positive. Initial antibiotic therapy should be as for meningitis and other serious infections, with subsequent adjustment based on serum levels when aminoglycosides are used and according to the sensitivity findings. The value of topical antibiotics is unproved. The role of vitrectomy in these cases is uncertain.

▶ For more than a century it has been recognized that bacteria may infect the eye by way of the bloodstream. Until about 40 years ago, eyes so afflicted nearly always were blinded, and most of the victims died of overwhelming sepsis. That all changed with the introduction of antibiotics. Nevertheless, metastatic bacterial endophthalmitis remains a potentially devastating condition. As recently as 12 years ago, one review noted that about 40% of eyes treated with antibiotics failed to recover useful vision. Controversy currently surrounds the management of this condition because of uncertainty about the value of and indications for surgery of the vitreous. With metastases and ophthalmitis, the infection is actually inside the eye. We now recognize that the meningococcus is no longer the predominant cause of this problem. It has been replaced by a curious bug known as *B. cereus*. The authors of this article have done us a service by telling us what is perhaps the best approach to this problem. They note that systemically administered antibiotics seem to be quite valuable in metastatic endophthalmitis as opposed to that occurring postoperatively or as a result of trauma. They also show that the intraocular injection of antibiotics and vitrectomy make only a limited contribution to a successful outcome with this type of infection.

Fortunately, once a diagnosis of metastatic bacterial endophthalmitis is suspected, it can usually be confirmed or ruled out with confidence on the basis of microbiologic studies performed on ocular or nonocular fluids. For this reason, and because the outcome of treatment in bacterial endophthalmitis may definitely be worsened by delay in diagnosis, the possibility of this condition must be kept in mind by the clinician faced with any patient with inflammation that seems to be arising from inside the eye. More often than not, the etiologic agent in eye infections can be identified with confidence on the basis of positive cultures from nonocular sources, particularly blood. When ocular fluids must be cultured, the anterior chamber of the eye and its aqueous fluid can usually be relied on to yield the organism. The selection of antibiotics prior to definite identification of the causative organism depends on the characteristics of the patient and the likely source of bacteremia. Plain penicillin or ampicillin is generally indicated in previously healthy infants, children, and adolescents, unless there is evidence of meningitis. When infection is believed to have originated in a cutaneous wound or penetrating lesion, a penicillinase-resistant penicillin or a cephalosporin would be more appropriate. The authors also suggest that if the urinary or gastrointestinal tract is the likely source, an aminoglycoside should be included. An easy "cop out" is to recognize that newer "generations" of cephalosporins (e.g., cefuroxime, ceftriaxone, and ceftazidime) are effective against most of the bacteria known to be associated with metastatic endophthalmitis. So, when in doubt, give something beginning with a "C" or a "K." When it comes to antibiotics, the retrospectoscope also helps. Churchill stated, "In any given set of circumstances, the proper course of action is best determined by subsequent events."—J.A. Stockman III, M.D.

Bacterial Infections of the Orbital and Periorbital Soft-Tissues in Children

James R. Spires and Richard J.H. Smith (Baylor College of Medicine, Houston)
Laryngoscope 96:763–767, July 1986   15–3

Bacterial infections of periorbital soft tissues are not unusual in childhood and resolve quickly with antimicrobial therapy. However, orbital soft tissue infection is uncommon and often causes serious morbidity. A retrospective study of children with periorbital and orbital soft tissue infections was conducted to determine the incidence of serious sequelae.

The records of 241 children hospitalized for orbital and periorbital soft tissue infections were reviewed to determine epidemiology, predisposing factors, pathogenesis, microbiology, treatment, and outcome. The infec-

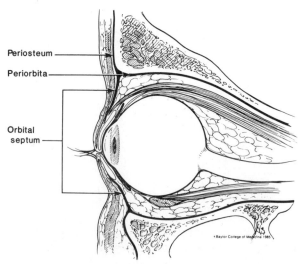

Fig 15–2.—The orbital septum. (Courtesy of Spires, J.R., and Smith, R.J.H.: Laryngoscope 96:763–767, July 1986.)

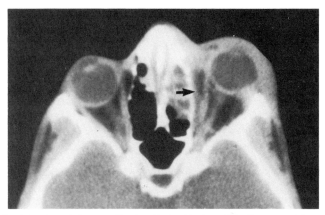

Fig 15–3.—Subperiosteal abscess with ethmoid sinusitis. Lateral displacement of the medial rectus and proptosis are present. (Courtesy of Spires, J.R., and Smith, R.J.H.: Laryngoscope 96:763–767, July 1986.)

tions were classified into five groups as preseptal cellulitis when the orbital septum was involved (Fig 15–2), orbital cellulitis, subperiosteal abscess (Fig 15–3), orbital abscess, or cavernous sinus thrombosis.

Of the 241 children, 226 had periorbital soft tissue infections. All but two responded quickly to antimicrobial therapy. Of the 15 children with true orbital infections, 11 had orbital cellulitis, 3 had subperiosteal abscesses, and 1 had cavernous sinus thrombosis. Sinusitis had occurred previously in 12 of these patients. In 7, treatment included surgical drainage and intensive antimicrobial therapy. Three children experienced complications of blindness and brain abscess, septic shock, or a "psychotic reaction."

Bacterial infections of periorbital and orbital soft tissues range from minor preseptal cellulitis to possibly fatal cavernous sinus thrombosis. Periorbital infections usually occur in children younger than age 2 years and are preceded by trauma or upper respiratory illness in half of the patients. Antibiotics are effective in preventing complications. Older children are more prone to acquire true orbital soft tissue infections. Sinusitis is present in most of these patients. Despite surgical and antimicrobial therapy, significant complications often occur. Computed tomographic scanning is needed to diagnose the extent of the infection. If administration of broad-spectrum antimicrobials is inadequate, surgery should be performed early.

▶ Bacterial infections of the orbital and periorbital soft tissues in children are among the most common problems we pediatricians are involved with. Generally, periorbital soft tissue infections respond promptly to antimicrobial therapy. The possibility of a serious infection carrying severe morbidity or even mortality, however, makes it imperative to assess accurately the extent of the infectious process to allow to modification of treatment if indicated. In the series abstracted above, 94% of the children had periorbital infection that was easy to label "preseptal" cellulitis. This responds quickly. True orbital infections were seen in only 4% of the patients, and in only 1% was there subperiosteal abscesses. In comparison with those children with preseptal cellulitis, children with orbital soft tissue infections tend to be much older. They are rarely less than 6 years of age. The history helps to identify the organism. Trauma and bites around the eye are usually associated with infections by *Staphylococcus aureus* and group A streptococcus. On the other hand, upper respiratory ill-nesses commonly result in preseptal cellulitis caused by *Hemophilus influenzae* or pneumococcus. Although the role of sinusitis was minimized in the report by Spires and Smith, other series report an incidence of sinusitis of at least 85% in children with true orbital cellulitis. Sinusitis is rarely missed these days, because CT scanning is an indispensable diagnostic aid in assessing the full extent of the infectious process.

Before closing out the story on infections in the eye, recognize that as the number of contact lens users increases, we are seeing a great deal in the way of eye infections. There has been an increase of more than 50% in the use of contact lenses in the past 8 years. The major culprit with regard to infection is the wearing of soft contact lenses, especially extended wear varieties. It appears that the number of infections associated with contact lens wear began climbing dramatically around 1981 when extended-wear soft contact lenses were approved by the Food and Drug Administration for persons with myopia. There appear to be two reasons why soft contact lenses, particularly extended wear, may be associated with infections and corneal ulcerations. The first is that, because soft contact lenses are hydrophilic (some extended-wear lenses are almost 75% water), they are extremely likely to pick up debris, including bacteria and fungi. The most implicated organism, bacteria-wise, is *Pseudomonas aeruginosa.* The staphylococci are next in order of identified prevalence. A second reason for infections is the lens care systems that are used. In most systems, there are too many steps involved in the cleaning process. One recent report showed that among 210 randomly selected patients using soft contact lenses, 82% failed to maintain their lenses according to instructions (*JAMA* 258:17, 1987). This is approximately the same frequency with which most people choose the wrong line while waiting for the teller at the bank.

If all this isn't horrific enough, a new actor has come on the scene known as *Acanthamoeba.* Individuals wearing contact lenses may be at unusually high risk for infection with this particular organism. *Acanthamoeba* keratitis is ex-traordinarily difficult to treat. Infection with it often leaves a severely damaged cornea. The first patient was reported with this infection in 1973 and now dozens of patients since the introduction of soft contact lenses have been reported.

As a final warning, beware of "Orville Redenbacher's Gourmet Brand" mi-crowave-popped popcorn. A 10-year-old boy was recently reported who sus-tained burns of his eye when he opened a container of freshly popped popcorn. A rush of released steam got into his eyes. Obviously, Orv is not to be blamed here. Parents should pay more attention to what the microwaves in their homes are doing. In fact, the gourmet brand of popcorn clearly carries the label "Handle the bag carefully—it's hot!" Well, when you're hot, you're hot, but not every child who is capable of using a microwave is additionally capable of reading (Routhier, P., et al.: *N. Engl. J. Med.* 315:1359, 1986).—J.A. Stockman III, M.D.

Incidence and Prognosis of Childhood Glaucoma: A Study of 63 Cases
Magda Barsoum-Homsy and Line Chevrette (Univ. of Montreal)
Ophthalmology 93:1323–1327, October 1986   15–4

Glaucoma in infants and children is classified into three groups: primary congenital or infantile glaucoma (group I), glaucoma associated with congenital anomalies (group II), and glaucoma secondary to other ocular pathology (group III). The relative incidence of glaucoma within each group was examined in 63 children with glaucoma in 95 eyes treated during an 8-year period. Follow-up ranged from 2 months to 10 years (average, 4.4 years).

Fourteen patients (22.2%) had group I glaucoma (24 eyes), 29 (46%) had group II glaucoma (47 eyes), and 20 (31.8%) had group III glaucoma (24 eyes). The presenting signs and symptoms associated with group I childhood glaucoma were mostly a cloudy cornea and tearing. The ocular and systemic anomalies associated with group II childhood glaucoma included iridocorneal dysgenesis and aniridia (Table 1). The primary diagnoses in group III secondary glaucoma included uveitis, aphakia, and congenital rubella (Table 2).

Surgery was performed in 95.8% of the eyes in group I, in 53.2% of the eyes in group II, and in 54.2% of the eyes in group III. Patients in group I had the best visual prognosis, and 77.3% of the affected eyes achieved a visual acuity equal to or better than 20/50. Good pressure control was obtained in all patients. In group II vision equal to or better

TABLE 1.—OCULAR AND SYSTEMIC
ANOMALIES ASSOCIATED WITH GROUP II
CHILDHOOD GLAUCOMA

Pathology	Cases (49 eyes)
Iridocorneal dysgenesis	
Goniodysgenesis	3
Rieger's syndrome	5
Rieger's anomaly	2
Axenfeld syndrome	2
Aniridia	8
Sturge-Weber syndrome	6
Uveal coloboma	1
Neurofibromatosis	1
Larsen syndrome	1
Total	29

(Courtesy of Barsoum-Homsy, M, and Chevrette, L.: Ophthalmology 93:1323–1327, October 1986.)

TABLE 2.—Etiologic Diagnosis in Group III
Secondary Glaucoma

Pathology	Cases (24 eyes)
Uveitis	6
Aphakia	5
Traumatic hyphema	2
Congenital rubella	1
Congenital rubella and aphakia	2
Coats	1
Retrolental fibroplasia	1
Persistant hyperplastic primary vitreous	1
Microphthalmus with congenital retinal fold	1
Total no. of cases	20

(Courtesy of Barsoum-Homsy, M., and Chevrette, L.: Ophthalmology 93:1323–1327, October 1986.)

than 20/50 was achieved in 41.5% of affected eyes, whereas 41.4% had vision of 20/200 or less. The intraocular pressure remained uncontrolled in 19.1%. Group III patients had the poorest prognosis and most morbidity; 30.5% of the affected eyes achieved a visual acuity of 20/50 or better and 47.8% of affected eyes 20/200 vision or less. In 33.3% of group III patients the intraocular pressure remained uncontrolled.

Occurrence of Strabismus in Infants Born to Drug-Dependent Women
Leonard B. Nelson, Saundra Ehrlich, Joseph H. Calhoun, Theresa Matteucci, and Loretta P. Finnegan (Wills Eye Hosp., and Thomas Jefferson Univ., Philadelphia)
Am. J. Dis. Child. 141:175–178, February 1987   15–5

Maternal drug abuse during pregnancy exposes the fetus to the possibility of toxic or addicting effects. When routine ophthalmologic examinations of infants of drug-dependent women in a methadone hydrochloride maintenance program revealed an inordinate incidence of strabismus, a study was undertaken to determine the relationship of prenatal drug addiction and the subsequent development of strabismus.

During a 36-month period, 29 infants exposed prenatally to psychoactive drugs were seen at birth and at a 6-month follow-up examination. Strabismus was diagnosed in seven (24%); four had esotropia and three had exotropia. This incidence was significantly greater than the 2.8% to 5.3% incidence reported in the general population. Mean methadone hydrochloride dosage at the time of delivery was significantly greater for mothers of infants with strabismus than for those of nonstrabismic infants. In addition, in utero exposure to diazepam and "other drugs" (e.g., antidepressants) was a more frequent occurrence in infants with strabismus. Lower mean birth weight and neonatal and obstetric complications appeared to be more common in strabismic infants.

Maternal drug abuse and increased methadone dosage during pregnancy may predispose infants to the development of strabismus.

▶ Dr. Ira J. Chasnoff, Associate Professor of Pediatrics, and Director, Perinatal Center for Chemical Dependence, Northwestern University Medical School, comments on the issue of substance abuse in pregnancy.—J.A. Stockman III, M.D.

▶ Although problems of substance abuse in pregnancy have received increasing attention in the medical literature since the early 1970s, there has recently been a very rapid increase in the number of articles and books published related to this field. The reasons for this new interest are easily understood when current statistics from the National Institute on Drug Abuse are reviewed. Although patterns of abuse of alcohol, marijuana, heroin, and other substances by women of childbearing age have changed very little in the past 10 years, the incidence of cocaine use in this special population has been rising rapidly, a reflection of cocaine's increasing popularity among the general population of the United States.

Use of "hard" drugs (e.g., heroin, methadone, and phencyclidine) during pregnancy is known to be associated with a high rate of spontaneous abortion, intrauterine growth retardation, perinatal morbidity and mortality, and neurobehavioral deficits in the newborn. Cocaine use by the pregnant woman places the pregnancy, fetus, and infant at an even higher level of risk for these complications, and case reports of intrauterine cerebral infarctions, congenital malformations, and sudden infant death among these infants have been appearing in the pediatric literature. No true withdrawal syndrome has been described for cocaine-exposed neonates. Rather, the symptoms mimic those of an adult intoxicated with cocaine: irritability, hyperreflexia, and tremulousness.

Public education and early prenatal detection appear to be the keys to prevention of the perinatal morbidity and mortality associated with drug use in pregnancy, but current efforts are far from adequate and are hampered by the reluctance of physicians to delve into the life-styles of their patients even though these life-styles may place a child at high risk for long-term developmental deficiencies and abnormalities. Until early intervention programs are more successful, pediatricians will continue to see increasing numbers of infants affected by their mothers' drug use. Unfortunately, the fetus is not given the chance to "say no."—I.J. Chasnoff, M.D.

Ocular Findings in Childhood Lactic Acidosis
Seiji Hayasaka, Keiko Yamaguchi, Katsuyoshi Mizuno, Shigeaki Miyabayashi, Kuniaki Narisawa, and Keiya Tada (Tohoku Univ., Sendai, Japan)
Arch. Ophthalmol. 104:1656–1658, November 1986   15–6

There are few reports on ocular findings in childhood lactic acidosis. Nine children aged 5 months to 9 years at onset of lactic acidosis were examined ophthalmologically. Blood lactate concentrations ranged from

18.9 to 117.6 mg/dl (2.1–13.0 mmole/L), and blood or serum pyruvate and alanine concentrations were also increased.

All children had abnormal ocular findings. Optic atrophy or temporal pallor of the optic nerve was present in six and was associated with mitochondrial myopathy, pyruvate decarboxylase deficiency, cytochrome c oxidase deficiency, and an idiopathic form of the disease. Other ocular findings included nystagmus in three patients, blepharoptosis in one, cataract in one, and limitation in abduction in another.

Optic atrophy is the most common ocular finding in childhood lactic acidosis and is possibly secondary to the generalized alteration in carbohydrate metabolism caused by an enzyme defect. Nystagmus and ophthalmoplegia also are common.

▶ Lactic acidosis is defined as a blood lactic concentration of more than 2 mEq/L. Lactic acidosis in childhood is associated with several disorders, some of which are chronic, e.g., Leigh's subacute necrotizing encephalomyelopathy, mitochondrial myopathy, pyruvate decarboxylase deficiency, and cytochrome oxidase deficiency. Congenital lactic acidosis of an idiopathic or unknown nature has also been described. What we see with this report is the fact that children with lactic acidosis can have serious eye problems. The optic atrophy noted is permanent and can lead to significant visual loss.

Lactic acidosis can also occur with jogging and similar perverse forms of exercise. I wonder if anyone has looked at the eye grounds of people afflicted with this form of addiction. It certainly would explain why one sees so many of these individuals bumping into cars, falling over pedestrians, and making a general nuisance of themselves. I know it is not fashionable to criticize those who like to exercise, especially when exercise is "in." I, however, will remain, as you may have noted from prior YEAR BOOKS, with the philosophy of staying in with the outs. Most joggers are probably *deaf* from their Walkman headsets. Now we can theorize that they may be *blind*. Whether jogging itself qualifies as *dumb* is up to you.—J.A. Stockman III, M.D.

Removal of Corneal Crystals by Topical Cysteamine in Nephropathic Cystinosis

Muriel I. Kaiser-Kupfer, Leslie Fujikawa, Toichiro Kuwabara, Sandeep Jain, and William A. Gahl (Natl. Eye Inst. and Natl. Inst. of Child Health and Human Development, NIH, Bethesda)
N. Engl. J. Med. 316:775–779, March 26, 1987   15–7

Nephropathic cystinosis is a rare lysosomal storage disease in which cystine accumulates within cells because of recessively inherited impairment of carrier-mediated cystine transport across lysosomal membranes. The intracellular cystine apparently interferes with the function of various organs, including the cornea, resulting in recurrent erosions and secondary blepharospasm. Cysteamine effectively reduces the cystine content of cystinotic corneal cells in culture. A double-blind, placebo-controlled trial of topical cysteamine drops was carried out in two young children with nephropathic cystinosis.

The patients, both younger than 2 years, were treated with 10 mM cysteamine eyedrops in one eye. A striking reduction in corneal crystals occurred in the cysteamine-treated eye within 4–5 months of onset of treatment. The findings were confirmed by independent ophthalmologists. No clinical toxicity resulted from topical cysteamine therapy.

Topically administered cysteamine is the treatment of choice for young children with cystinosis and corneal crystals, because of its effectiveness in depleting the cornea of crystals and its safety. Further studies are needed to determine whether hourly treatment is necessary and whether older children will benefit.

▶ We've been hearing a lot about cystinosis and cysteamine therapy. This therapy was first used in 1978 as a cystine-depleting agent in cystinosis. Cysteamine can be given orally and passes through plasma and lysosomal membranes. Because it is a weak base it concentrates within acidic lysosomes. There it reacts with cystine to form cysteine and a cysteine-cysteamine mixed disulfide, both of which transverse the cystinotic lysosomal membrane in a normal fashion. Follow that?! This drug is so active that it readily depletes peripheral blood leukocytes of 90% of their endogenous cystine content and it was recently shown to be effective in maintaining renal function and normalizing growth in children with cystinosis (Gahl, W.A., et al.: *N. Engl. J. Med.* 316:971, 1987).

As good as the oral form of cysteamine is, it has several problems. One of them is that it does not prevent corneal crystal accumulation. Thus, enter stage left, topical cysteamine. This drug does seem to work very well to deplete the cornea of cystine crystals. Unfortunately, as noted in the abstract, the drug was administered on an hourly basis, which is not all that acceptable. Whether less frequent intervals can be used, whether a lower concentration will work, and whether patients who are older with this problem will respond are all questions requiring years of study. The above report, however, provides a strong impetus to pursue the answers to these questions. Before cysteamine came along, we really had very little to offer patients with cystinosis. Now perhaps we can abort the onset of the associated renal Fanconi syndrome, severe growth retardation, photophobia, hepatosplenomegaly, hypohidrosis, hypothyroidism, retinal depigmentation, and secondary carnitine deficiency, which are part of the multisystem manifestations of this disease. Whether all of these things will respond remains to be seen. Stay tuned.—J.A. Stockman III, M.D.

Pupillary Responses and Airway Reactivity in Asthma
Pamela B. Davis (VA Med. Ctr., Cleveland)
J. Allergy Clin. Immunol. 77:667–673, May 1986   15–8

Although β-adrenergic responses have long been studied in asthma, only recently has attention been focused on the other branches of the autonomic nervous system. The three major mechanisms of reversible airway obstruction are regulated in part by cholinergic and α-adrenergic systems. Studies of autonomic function in asthma are most easily interpreted if tests are carried out at uninvolved sites in patients who are not taking medication and who have near normal pulmonary function. In one such study increased pupillary cholinergic sensitivity and increased pupillary and peripheral vascular α-adrenergic sensitivity were reported in patients with asthma. To confirm the results of this study the pupillary responses to phenylephrine and carbachol, as well as airway reactivity, were measured in 19 drug-free persons with mild allergic asthma, in 21 nonatopic controls, and in 6 asymptomatic atopic controls. The concentration of phenylephrine necessary to dilate the pupil 1 mm was used as a measure of α-adrenergic sensitivity.

The mean concentration was markedly lower for those with asthma than for atopic or nonatopic controls (1.11%, 1.86%, and 1.52%, respectively). The concentration of carbachol necessary for pupillary constriction of 1 mm was used as a measure of cholinergic sensitivity. The mean value was substantially lower for patients with asthma than for atopic or nonatopic controls (0.23%, 0.41%, and 0.35%, respectively). Pupillary α-adrenergic sensitivity and cholinergic sensitivity were significantly correlated. Both α-adrenergic sensitivity and cholinergic sensitivity of the pupils correlated with airway reactivity when it was expressed as the concentration of methacholine that caused a 20% fall in FEV_1. The autonomic aberrations observed in this study could not be attributed to the use of drugs or to significantly abnormal pulmonary mechanics. Autonomic abnormalities are associated with allergic asthma and may contribute to the airway reactivity characteristic of the disease.

▶ This is a very intriguing study. It is proof positive that if you look a man in the eye you can tell a lot about what's going on with him. Patients with asthma required a lesser concentration of phenylephrine to dilate their pupils than did nonasthmatic individuals. This is taken as a measure of α-adrenergic sensitivity. The same was true of cholinergic sensitivity with carbachol. If the authors are correct, one can speculate that the autonomic abnormalities seen in asthma patients are inborn and contribute to the development of airway reactivity. Another example of the peculiar pupillary responses seen in asthmatics is the fact that the pupil size change in an asthmatic is no way nearly as dramatic when going from light to dark as in nonasthmatics.

Before you run off to purchase these ophthalmic solutions to see what kind of pupillary responses you will find in whatever you are attempting to examine (e.g., siblings of asthmatics to see if they will be prone to the subsequent development of asthma), realize how safe or not safe these ocular drugs are. Read the Palmer's article (*Ophthalmology* 93:1038, 1986), who reviews in detail all of the commonly used eye drops and shows us some of their major side effects. In general, you add the same amount of eye drops to an infant's eyes as you do to an adult's eyes. The adult, however, is able to dilute any absorbed drug to at least twentyfold more than a neonate can because of the differences in blood volume between them. As noted in prior YEAR BOOKS, hypertension and other problems have resulted from the use of eye drops.

Some people have a hard time remembering whether the pupil is supposed to dilate or constrict in response to adrenergic drugs. I always remember which is which because of a cat named Mickey who used to hang around our house when I was a child. Prior to pouncing upon his prey, the cat would assume a typical pointing posture, give a little wiggle to his rump, and then fully dilate his pupils before pouncing. Now that's an adrenergic response. Mickey, by the way, lived to be 23 and God knows how much cat scratch disease and *Toxocara cati* he passed around during that almost quarter of a century. Sorry about this tail from Lake Wobegon.—J.A. Stockman III, M.D.

16 Dentistry and Otolaryngology

Baby Fruit Juices and Tooth Erosion
A.J. Smith and L. Shaw (The Dental School, Birmingham, England)
Br. Dent. J. 162:65–67, Jan. 24, 1987   16–1

Excessive ingestion of fruit drinks and other acidic beverages has erosive effects on dental enamel, and concentrated fruit juices containing vitamin C are now becoming available for use diluted or undiluted. The pH of these juices was determined and an in vitro study of possible erosive effects on human enamel carried out.

Several samples of apple, pear, and orange juices had pH values of 3.22–3.65 undiluted and 3.64–4.12 diluted (table). Overnight immersion of extracted primary teeth in the juices produced "white spot" lesions representing appreciable destruction of enamel and complete loss of the surface enamel. In a girl aged 3 years referred with upper anterior tooth pain, prolonged use of baby fruit juice as a comforter was acknowledged. Extensive erosion was noted, especially palatally (Fig 16–1), and some pulp exposure and associated periapical abscess were observed. Conservative management, including gradual withdrawal of the fruit juice, was effective.

Extensive ingestion by infants of fruit juice may lead to enamel erosion. The juice should not be used for prolonged periods as a comforter, and its daily intake should be restricted.

▶ This report is proof positive that "nature abhors people." We've all heard about baby bottle caries, but now we're seeing reports such as this suggesting that frequent or prolonged exposure to acidic baby fruit juices may be just as harmful. Actually, this should come as no surprise because, as noted in earlier YEAR BOOKS, ingestion of acidic substances (e.g., aspirin) on a frequent basis as part of the management of juvenile rheumatoid arthritis can also produce similar problems with enamel erosion of the teeth.

So what are we supposed to learn from this? I suppose it means that we

MEAN pH VALUES OF BABY FRUIT JUICES

Fruit juice	Undiluted pH (mean + SD, n = 5)	Diluted (1 in 10) pH (mean $\pm$ SD, n = 5)
Apple and pear	3·56 $\pm$ 0·05	3·98 $\pm$ 0·08
Apple and orange	3·33 $\pm$ 0·08	3·73 $\pm$ 0·08

(Courtesy of Smith, A.J., and Shaw, L.: Br. Dent. J. 162:65–67, Jan. 24, 1987.)

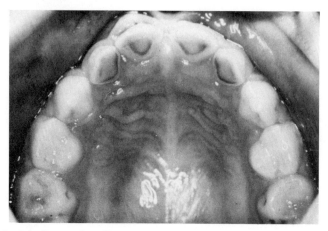

Fig 16–1.—Palatal aspect of maxillary primary teeth showing extensive erosion of enamel of *BA/AB*. Pulp tissue is seen through the thin residual dentine. (Courtesy of Smith, A.J., and Shaw, L.: Br. Dent. J. 162:65–67, Jan. 24, 1987.)

have to add to the list of cariogenic substances baby fruit juices. I would not embrace the results of this study so closely to my own heart as to eliminate fruit juices completely from an infant's diet. For many infants, such juices might be the most consistent way in which they receive vitamin C. As an aside, can you name the occupational disease that has accounted for more deaths than any other? The answer to this is a little unfair because it goes back a bit. Nonetheless, "the explorer's sickness" or scurvy has accounted for more than 2 million deaths documented throughout history, most of it among British sailors. For the medical aficionados in the reading audience, it was William Shakespeare's son-in-law, Dr. John Hall, who was the first to use scurvy grass successfully in treatment of this disease in 1630. It was the single richest source by weight of ascorbic acid found in nature. Individuals wanting to learn more of the history of scurvy and vitamin C should see the book with the same title by Kenneth Carpenter, Cambridge University Press, 1986. In the introduction, the book says it is written for the "intelligent lay-person." Perhaps we qualify.—J.A. Stockman III, M.D.

Fluoride Supplements: Changes in Physicians' Attitudes and Practices Following an Intensive, Multifaceted Educational Program

Frederick J. Margolis, Barbara K. Chesney, and M. Anthony Schork (Wayne State Univ. and Univ. of Michigan)
Am. J. Dis. Child. 141:72–76, January 1987   16–2

In 1978 a survey was conducted among primary care physicians with pediatric patients to assess their knowledge, attitudes, and prescribing practices with regard to fluoride supplements for infants and children. After the results of this survey were analyzed, an intensive, multifaceted

SPECIFIC PRESCRIBING PRACTICES AMONG RESPONDENTS WHO PRESCRIBED
FLUORIDE SUPPLEMENTS*

	Pediatricians		Family Practioners		All Physicians	
	1978 (n=781), %	1981, %†	1978 (n=203), %	1981, %‡	1978 (n=984), %	1981, %§
Homes With Fluoridated Water						
Breast-fed infants						
0 to 6 mo of age	44	56	33	41	42	52
6 to 12 mo of age	54	62	40	58	51	61
Bottle-fed infants						
0 to 6 mo of age	11	11	17	18	12	13
6 to 12 mo of age	12	14	19	22	13	16
Homes Without Fluoridated Water						
Breast-fed infants						
0 to 6 mo of age	79	88	78	84	79	87
6 to 12 mo of age	88	94	80	98	86	95
Bottle-fed infants						
0 to 6 mo of age	79	85	82	84	80	85
6 to 12 mo of age	90	94	84	97	89	95

Increased prescription of fluoride supplements in 1981 for bottle-fed infants living in homes with fluoridated water may reflect increased use of ready-to-feed infant formulas, none of which, to authors' knowledge, contain fluoridated water.
*Percentages are based on total number of respondents who answered each question.
†For eight survey questions represented in table, *n* for pediatricians ranged from 589 to 635.
‡For eight survey questions represented in table, *n* for family practitioners ranged from 191 to 216.
§For eight survey questions represented in table, *n* for all physicians ranged from 780 to 851.
(Courtesy of Margolis, F.J., et al.: Am. J. Dis. Child. 141:72–76, January 1987.)

education program was conducted at Wayne State University. A resurvey of the targeted population was then conducted in 1981. These results were compared with those of the original survey to assess the impact of the educational program.

There were 2,840 questionnaires mailed to 2,428 physicians with MD degrees and 412 physicians with DO degrees; overall, 1,269 (45%) responded and 1,122 responses qualified for analysis. The awareness of fluoride increased between the initial survey in 1978 and the resurvey in 1981 by 3% among pediatricians and by 14% among family physicians. Overall, 45% of the resurvey respondents reported a positive change in attitude about the effects of fluoride on dental caries in children in comparison with results in the original survey; 51% reported no change in attitude, 1% reported a negative change in attitude, and 3% did not reply to the question. The percentage of physicians who reported that they prescribed fluoride supplements for pediatric patients was 86% in 1981 and 76% in the original survey (table). The intense, multifaceted educational program concerning fluoride and childhood dental caries that was carried out may have contributed to the positive changes noted.

Caries Levels and Patterns in Head Start Children in Fluoridated and Non-Fluoridated, Urban and Non-Urban Sites in Ohio, USA

D.C. Johnsen, M. Bhat, M.T. Kim, F.T. Hagman, L.M. Allee, R.L. Creedon, and M.W. Easley (Case Western Reserve Univ., Rainbow Babies and Children's Hosp., Cleveland, Ohio State Univ., Cincinnati Children's Hosp., and Ohio Dept. of Health, Columbus)
Community Dent. Oral Epidemiol. 14:206–210, August 1986   16–3

Earlier comparative studies reported levels of caries of the primary dentition in children from a wide range of socioeconomic backgrounds who resided in urban and nonurban areas. Caries patterns were determined in 1,310 children from low-income families living in urban and nonurban areas that had varying levels of water fluoridation. All were enrolled in Project Head Start in Ohio. Dental examinations to determine the level and prevalence of dental caries patterns were conducted in 505 children from urban fluoridated areas, 395 from urban nonfluoridated areas, 183 from nonurban fluoridated areas, and 227 from nonurban, nonfluoridated areas. The World Health Organization caries diagnostic system was used as a basis for scoring.

Analysis of the data showed that caries scores for the urban and nonurban fluoridated sites were almost identical. Percentages of caries-free children were higher in the urban and nonurban fluoridated sites than in the urban and nonurban nonfluoridated sites. Percentages were similar for urban and nonurban nonfluoridated sites. Percentages of children with smooth surface lesions were higher in nonfluoridated sites, but percentages of children with defect-associated lesions were similar for all four sites. The percentages of caries-free children in all four sites ranged from 36% in the urban nonfluoridated area to 50% in the nonurban fluoridated area.

Amounts of Fluoride in Self-Administered Dental Products: Safety Considerations for Children

Stanley B. Heifetz and Herschel S. Horowitz (Natl. Inst. of Dental Res., NIH, Bethesda)
Pediatrics 77:876–882, June 1986   16–4

Various fluoride preparations are currently available for the prevention of caries. An understanding of the body's mechanism of metabolizing fluoride provides a rational basis for assessing the possible risks of excessive fluoride ingestion. Plasma concentrations of fluoride usually peak within 30–60 minutes after ingestion. In growing children, more than half of the ingested fluoride is incorporated in the bones and the rest is excreted in the urine. A dose of 5–10 gm of sodium fluoride is considered certainly lethal in a 70-kg adult. One quarter of this can be ingested without producing serious acute toxicity and is known as the safely tolerated dose. Less than 1 gm of fluoride is fatal in children aged 12 years or younger and is not safely tolerated by children younger than 18 years of age (Table 1).

The signs and symptoms of toxicity are predominantly gastrointestinal

TABLE 1.—CERTAINLY LETHAL DOSES (CLD)
AND SAFELY TOLERATED DOSES (STD) OF
FLUORIDE FOR SELECTED AGES

Age (yr)	Wt (kg [lb])*	CLD (mg)	STD (mg)
2	10.0 (22)	320	80
4	13.2 (29)	422	106
6	16.8 (37)	538	135
8	20.5 (45)	655	164
10	24.1 (53)	771	193
12	29.1 (64)	931	233
14	37.7 (83)	1,206	301
16	41.8 (92)	1,338	334
18	43.2 (95)	1,382	346

*Third percentile of the normal age-specific weight distribution.
(Courtesy of Heifetz, S., et al.: Pediatrics 77:876–882, June 1986.)

TABLE 2.—COMMON SIGNS AND SYMPTOMS
OF ACUTE FLUORIDE TOXICITY

Low Dosages	High Dosages
Nausea	Convulsions
Vomiting	Cardiac arrhythmias
Hypersalivation	Comatose
Abdominal pain	
Diarrhea	

(Courtesy of Heifetz, S., et al.: Pediatrics 77:876–882, June 1986.)

TABLE 3.—TOXIC EFFECTS OF CHRONIC EXCESSIVE
FLUORIDE INGESTION

Effect	Dosage	Duration
Dental fluorosis	>2 times optimal	Until 5 yr of age (excluding third molars)
Skeletal fluorosis	10–25 mg/d	10–20 yr
Kidney damage*	5–10 mg/kg	6–12 mo

*In animals.
(Courtesy of Heifetz, S., et al.: Pediatrics 77:876–882, June 1986.)

with low dosages; they begin within 30 minutes of ingestion and may persist for 24 hours (Table 2). High dosages are associated with convulsions, cardiac arrhythmias, and coma. If not spontaneous, vomiting should be induced using fluoride-binding liquids, e.g., milk and liquid or gel antacids. The patient should be taken to the nearest emergency care center where the stomach should be washed thoroughly with lime water. Frequent exposure to low but excessive quantities of fluoride can result in dental fluorosis, skeletal fluorosis, and kidney damage (Table 3).

The use of 0.05% sodium fluoride, acidulated phosphate fluoride, or

TABLE 4.—SUPPLEMENTAL FLUORIDE
DOSAGE SCHEDULE*

Age (yr)†	Concentration of Fluoride in Water (ppm)		
	<0.3	0.3–0.7	>0.7
Birth–2	0.25	0	0
2–3	0.50	0.25	0
3–13	1.00	0.50	0

*Schedule approved by the Council on Dental Therapeutics of the American Dental Association. Dosages are in milligrams of fluoride per day.
†Schedule of the American Academy of Pediatrics initiates fluoride supplements at 2 weeks of age and continues them until 16 years.
(Courtesy of Heifetz, S., et al.: Pediatrics 77:876–882, June 1986.)

0.1% stannous fluoride daily at home is safe. Weekly rinsing with a 0.02% sodium fluoride solution is the preferred procedure for school-based programs. Parents should make sure that only a pea-sized portion of fluoride paste is used by preschool children and is followed by rinsing and expectorating thoroughly after brushing. Dentists and physicians should know the fluoride concentration of a patient's water supply before dispensing fluoride supplements (Table 4). Fluoride preparations should be dispensed in appropriate quantities, labeled with cautionary statements, and packaged, when appropriate, with child-proof closures or in tear-proof materials; they should be stored in safe locations. The risk of adverse effects is small when fluorides are used judiciously.

▶ The preceding three abstracts (16–2, 16–3 and 16–4), all dealing with fluorides, represent extreme edges of the spectrum of fluoride status here in the United States. The "Head Start" report shows us clearly that fluoridation of water supplies has had a remarkable effect on the incidence of childhood caries. Even we physicians, as noted by Margolis et al., have begun to accept this principle. What is scary, however, is the report of Heifetz and Horowitz, which shows us how dangerous fluorides can be if we aren't paying some reasonable attention to what our children are doing with the new ubiquitously available fluoride-containing substances in our environment. The risk for the latter begins at around the age of 2 years when children usually develop sufficient motor coordination to open bottles and tubes kept around the house.

Dilute fluoride rinses for use at home or in school-based programs are currently popular as a simple way to expose teeth to fluoride frequently. All products for daily use at home contain sodium fluoride concentrations of about 0.02%. To reach a safely tolerated dose maximum, defined as the amount that can be ingested without producing symptoms of serious acute systemic toxicity, a hypothetical 2-year-old child would have to swallow at one time 360 ml (12 oz) of fluoride rinse. To reach a certainly lethal dose, that same hypothetical child would have to swallow about 1.5 qt of rinse. The largest commercially available bottle of fluoride rinse contains about 118 mg of fluoride, an amount greater than the safely tolerated dose but well below the certainly lethal dose for a 2-year-old child. It is unlikely, however, that a child could consume the contents of an entire bottle (509 ml) without vomiting. Many school-based programs use weekly rinsing with a 0.2% sodium fluoride solution as the preferred procedure for such programs. Obviously, this is a more toxic solution, but the safety of school-based programs is excellent.

Most households do not keep these fluoride mouth rinses around, but most do have fluoride toothpaste. About 90% of all the dentifrices sold in the United States are fluoride-containing toothpastes. The intent is that a single brushing with a full ribbon of paste on a toothbrush provides about 1 gm of toothpaste and 1 mg of fluoride. Note, though, that the largest container of toothpaste manufactured (9 oz), the so-called family size tube, contains about 255 mg of fluoride. This is well above the safely tolerated dose for a 2-year-old child if that child were to ingest the contents of the entire tube. Since 1955 when a fluoride dentifrice was first introduced for sale over the counter, no untoward consequences have been reported with the use of fluoride toothpastes. The reason for this is fairly obvious: Toothpaste contains detergent and flavoring oils that would irritate the stomach if taken in any significant quantity. I would suspect that the frequency with which children ingest excessive amounts of toothpaste is increasing nonetheless. For example, the relatively recently introduced solid upright cylinders of toothpaste made of hard plastic with little pump handles seem to be selling like hot cakes, at least in our neighborhood. They sit on our bathroom counter and look like tiny Atlas rockets. Some way to begin the day!

One aspect of fluoride supplementation that has been subject to much discussion for many years is the value of prescribing fluoride supplements for pregnant women to protect the teeth of their offspring. The rationale and supporting evidence for the use of prenatal fluorides were reviewed at an American Dental Association symposium 8 years ago (see *J. Dent. Child.* 101:1, 1981). It was concluded that, despite encouraging results, particularly in the primary dentition, adequate evidence to support the prenatal use of fluorides is still lacking. More than 20 years ago the Food and Drug Administration put a ban on claims of efficacy for the prenatal administration of fluoride supplements. It would seem that this ban is as justifiable today as it was 20 years ago.

Just how large the problem is with oral fluoride overadministration is not yet defined. Certainly, caries prevention is a large problem in the United States, but as the saying goes, "Inside every large problem is a small problem struggling to get out." Perhaps the safety issue is one of those small problems, struggling to get attention.—J.A. Stockman III, M.D.

A Survey of Biopsied Oral Lesions in Pediatric Dental Patients
Robert L. Skinner, W.D. Davenport, Jr., J.C. Weir, and R. F. Carr (Louisiana State Univ., New Orleans)
Pediatr. Dent. 8:163–167, June 1986   16–5

An attempt was made to determine the most common biopsied oral lesions in children and the age, sex, rate, and site tendency for each lesion.

The retrospective study consisted of 1,525 biopsy specimens of oral lesions obtained from patients aged 1–19 years. The lesions were classified as: inflammatory and reactive, cystic, benign neoplastic, oral developmental anomalies, or normal tissue.

Inflammatory and reactive lesions occurred in 61.3% of all patients. The mucocele, the most common of this group, appeared most often on the lower lip of white females. Cystic lesions, usually dentigerous and radicular cysts, accounted for 17.6% of the total number. Most were found in white males and occurred throughout the oral cavity. The benign neoplastic lesions represented 17.5% of the cases. Squamous papillomas were the most common, usually occurring on the lips of white males.

Mucocele was found most often in children aged 12 years or younger, whereas nonspecific inflammation and radicular cysts occurred in the teen-aged group. Oral developmental anomalies were found in an insignificant proportion of the children. Two malignancies were found among the 1,525 biopsied lesions. One was secondary to leukemia in a child aged 6 years, and the second was found in a boy aged 19 years who had adenoid cystic carcinoma.

▶ I like this study dealing with lumps and bumps in the mouth. As practitioners, we see children who have things that we can't explain or that are puzzlesome, at least in terms of what to do about them. This study tells us a little more about the frequency with which X, Y, or Z causes these lumps and bumps. Far and away, the front leader is the common "mucocele." About a third of all mucoceles are found in the pediatric age group. They occur more frequently in girls than boys, with the lower lip being the most frequent site. Mucoceles occur ten times more frequently in white children than in black children. They are removed if they are unsightly or otherwise cause problems.

Before moving out of the dental area of this chapter, we would be remiss not to comment on the infections that dentists can acquire or spread. It has been estimated that 3,000 dental professionals in the United States are asymptomatic hepatitis B carriers. Such dentists are capable of spreading hepatitis to their patients. One report from the Centers for Disease Control described hepatitis B occurring in nine patients of a dentist practicing in a rural area. Although this particular dentist never had any hepatitis symptoms, his serum was positive for hepatitis B surface antigen and hepatitis B e antigen and negative for hepatitis B core IgM antibody, indicating that he was probably a hepatitis B carrier. Two of the nine patients died of fulminant hepatitis. An additional 15 asymptomatic patients also were found. This particular dentist did not routinely wear gloves when treating patients. He admitted to vigorous hand scrubbing with a surgical brush before and after each patient, and it is assumed that this vigorous scrubbing led to pinpoint bleeding in the dentist's hands, which then became the source of the transfer of hepatitis B to the patients (Shaw, F.E., et al.: JAMA 255:3260, 1986). About 3 years ago only 24% of dentists wore gloves. That number is much higher now because of the risk of acquired immunodeficiency syndrome that has been documented. Needless to say, all dental students and dental technicians should receive hepatitis B vaccine before they have patient contact. They should also wear gloves.

Two years ago my own dentist was not using any preventative measures. Last year I noted that he was wearing gloves. On my most recent visit, not only was he wearing gloves, he was wearing a mask and goggles. As it turns out, it wasn't until after the visit, as I was paying my bill, that I realized that it wasn't even the same dentist. He was that unrecognizable. I suppose the next time I go, unless the human immunodeficiency virus story has settled down, I may be greeting a dentist in a space suit.

While on the subject of gloves, a recent survey of automobile owners was taken to see how many people who own cars have gloves in their glove box. Do you know what the answer was? It was 0%. About 60% kept maps in the glove box. Maybe it's time for a change of names.—J.A. Stockman III, M.D.

The Combined Use of Pit and Fissure Sealants and Fluoride Mouthrinsing in Second and Third Grade Children: One-Year Clinical Results
Louis W. Ripa, Gary S. Leske, and Francine Forte (State Univ. of New York at Stony Brook)
Pediatr. Dent. 8:158–162, June 1986   16–6

Fluoride mouth rinsing affects mostly smooth tooth surfaces, whereas application of sealants protects pits and fissures, suggesting significant additive benefit from the combined use of these procedures. The additive benefits of sealants applied to caries-free first permanent molars were examined in second-grade and third-grade children participating since kindergarten in a school-based fluoride mouth-rinsing program. The first-year findings in the 2-year study were reviewed. The children rinsed with 0.2% sodium fluoride; the 95 study subjects also had sealant placed on first permanent molars 4 months after the baseline examination. Delton autopolymerized Pit and Fissure Sealant was used.

Overall, 97% of the study group and 85% of those who only rinsed were caries free at the first annual examination. Ten of 16 surfaces were occlusal. Two occlusal surfaces had all sealant missing, whereas seven had partial sealant loss. Eight occlusal surfaces had to be resealed. One occlusal surface and two lingual surfaces in the study group required restorations. Among controls, 13 surfaces, 9 occlusal, required restoration.

When sealant therapy was combined with fluoride mouth rinsing in young schoolchildren in this study, there were almost no decayed or filled permanent tooth surfaces at the first annual evaluation. This management is highly recommended for patients in office practices. When sealant is used in children already in a mouth-rinsing program, teeth should be selected for sealing on an individual basis.

▶ Robert D. Cooley, D.D.S., M.S., Head, Division of Dentistry, Children's Memorial Hospital, Chicago, comments.—J.A. Stockman III, M.D.

▶ There are several design weaknesses that may have predetermined the test results in this study. Generally, a 1-year clinical trial is insufficient to determine incremental dental caries incidence variations between two heterogeneous populations. The same examiner performed all oral evaluations in both groups.

Multiple standardized examiners would have eliminated bias tendencies and may have changed the reported results. Further, the figures used to calculate cost-comparative estimates do not reflect professional fees. No cost was included for replacement and repair of missing or deficient sealants (10% in 8 months). Some studies indicate that 50% of sealants are lost or defective after 5 years. No cost projections relevant to length of service are included in the discussion.

Although a combination of fluoride mouth rinse used with pit and fissure sealant may be the most effective method for preventing dental caries, other factors must be considered. When measuring the cost effectiveness of sealants, it is difficult to determine all factors relative to cost. If measured by value of professional services, the cost of sealant placement is approximately one half to two thirds that of a dental restoration. However, it is doubtful that a sealant will have similar longevity to that of a silver amalgam restoration. The cost of placing and maintaining sealants in nonsusceptible teeth would affect the overall cost. It is highly unlikely that the beneficial effects of sealants in children who have received fluoridated water during the critical developmental period would be as great as that portrayed in this study. It is well known that a significant number of teeth in these children will be caries free without sealant use. Children who have frequent preventive services in a well-managed pediatric dental environment would also have less sealant benefit than children without this care.

For children in areas with fluoridated water supplies and good professional preventive services, sealants should be used according to criteria-based evaluations rather than through universal application. The criteria for use of sealants might include prior dental caries in the primary dentition, very deep grooves in premolars and permanent molars, lack of regular preventive dentistry professional services, lack of community water fluoridation or dietary fluoride supplements, and lack of good oral hygiene practices. If none of the above factors are present, I would emphasize frequent preventative professional services, supervised oral hygiene practice including appropriate use of fluoride application and dietary counseling as a more cost-effective practice.

It should be pointed out that occlusal pit and fissure sealants are not completely fail safe. They require preventive maintenance measures, occasional repair or replacement, and periodic restoration with a longer lasting material. If one could accurately predict on which surfaces dental caries would actually develop, placement of sealants exclusively on those teeth would be a most cost-effective measure.—R.D. Cooley, D.D.S., M.S.

Correction of Congenital Auricular Deformities by Splinting in the Neonatal Period
Forst E. Brown, Lawrence B. Colen, Rocco R. Addante, and John M. Graham, Jr. (Dartmouth-Hitchcock Med. Ctr., Hanover, N.H.)
Pediatrics 78:406–411, September 1986   16–7

Congenital deformities of the nonhypoplastic ear include lop ear (Fig 16–2), cup ear (Fig 16–3), Stahl's ear (Fig 16–4), and protruding ear (Fig

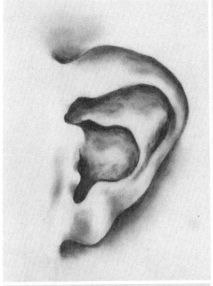

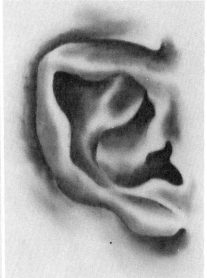

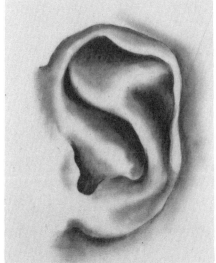

Fig 16–2*(upper left).*—Lop ear.
Fig 16–3*(upper right).*—Cup ear.
Fig 16–4*(lower left).*—Stahl's ear.
(Courtesy of Brown, F.E., et al.: Pediatrics 78:406–411, September 1986.)

16–5). Such deformities can result from abnormalities of morphogenesis or from external pressure or positioning in utero. To correct these problems without operation, neonatal splinting, as recommended by some Japanese clinicians, was used in a number of infants within a few days of birth. Aluwax, a dental compound, was used to correct all of the abnormal folding problems observed. Strips of surgical tape were used with Aluwax to correct a protruding ear (Fig 16–6). Splinting was maintained for a minimum of 2 weeks; if the deformity recurred, the splint was reapplied for another week.

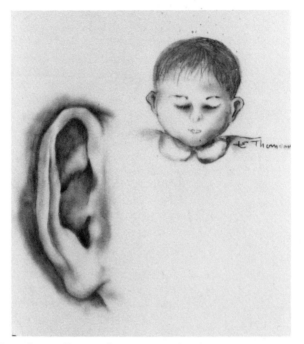

Fig 16–5.—Protruding ear. (Courtesy of Brown, F.E., et al.: Pediatrics 78:406–411, September 1986.)

One patient was a full-term infant born with bilateral lop ears and a left-sided preauricular cyst. Splinting was begun 2 days after birth and continued for 1 month, with excellent results.

The neonatal ear is soft and malleable because of the transiently high concentration of estrogen. Within 3 days of birth, the estrogen concentration falls, and the ear becomes more elastic and firm. Thus, it is crucial to begin correction in the first few days. Aluwax splinting is an effective, noninvasive method to accomplish lasting correction.

▶ Attempts at nonsurgical correction of congenital auricular deformities, especially prominent ears, have been described in "old wives' tales" for years, although most have been little more than good stories. Until recently, professional attempts at correction without surgery have been little better. Hirose et al. in 1980 and later Matsuo et al. applied current understanding of auricular cartilage development and its elastics properties in attempts to achieve a lasting nonsurgical treatment of prominent ears and milder forms of constricted ears (commonly referred to as cup-ear and lop-ear). The critical factor in molding of a deformed ear was clearly the early application of splinting. The auricle was extremely malleable when splinting was started within the first 3 days after birth and became increasingly less so after that time.

The techniques described by the above authors were applied to a small series of patients by Brown et al. and the benefits of this nonsurgical approach

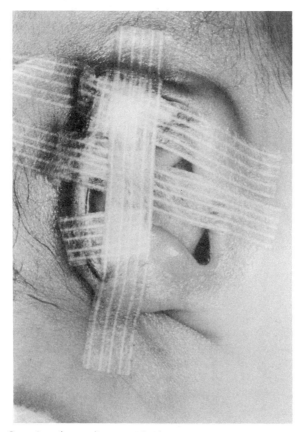

Fig 16–6.—Correction of protruding ear with Aluwax. Ear held in position with surgical tapes. (Courtesy of Brown, F.E., et al.: Pediatrics 78:406–411, September 1986.)

were clearly demonstrated. They have also emphasized the importance of beginning alteration of the abnormal cartilage architecture within the first 72 hours. Delay of treatment beyond the first week or so is likely to lead to incomplete correction. The hypothesis that this change in elasticity is secondary to the dropping estrogen content within the tissues is of interest but still somewhat circumstantial.

Several points remain to be clarified and will likely be so as later long-term follow-up reports are presented. Whereas this paper suggests that splinting be maintained for 2 weeks, with an additional week if needed, 75% of the ears described were splinted for 1 month minimum (as suggested by Matsuo et al.). The longest postsplinting follow-up was 1 month, and the authors have stated neither the number of infants treated nor the longest follow-up period. Previous reports were also hampered by a follow-up of no longer than 6 months. Presumably, the correction is stable once the cartilage is no longer soft, but this also remains to be demonstrated.

The described techniques are relatively simple, but a note of caution is war-

418 / Pediatrics

ranted: The use of a hard material (e.g., a dental impression compound), when taped to the tender skin of a neonate, presents a real risk of ulceration and cartilage exposure. Great caution and care must be exercised in creating a smooth splint and maintaining vigilant observation of the skin adjacent to the mold.

The authors are to be commended for bringing this approach from the plastic surgery literature to the pediatricians who most commonly see these deformities early. It is hoped that this awareness, plus careful long-term follow-up, will widen the application of these techniques to more of the mild ear deformities and avoid the trauma of both the deformity and later surgical correction.—B.S. Bauer, M.D.

Laryngotracheal Foreign Bodies in Children: A Comparison With Bronchial Foreign Bodies
Ramon M. Esclamado and Mark A. Richardson (Univ. of Washington)
Am. J. Dis. Child. 141:259–262, March 1987   16–8

Because of their relatively infrequent occurrence, laryngotracheal foreign bodies are rarely considered separately from bronchial foreign bodies. Findings in 20 children with laryngotracheal foreign bodies seen during an 11-year period were reviewed to determine the clinical features that differentiate them from bronchial foreign bodies.

The patients were aged 6 months to 17 years, with 80% younger than 3 years. A history of choking or aspiration was present in 90%, and the most common presenting symptoms were stridor, wheezing, sternal retractions, and cough. Chest roentgenographic findings were normal in 58%

TABLE 1.—ROENTGENOGRAPHIC FINDINGS IN
LARYNGOTRACHEAL FOREIGN BODIES

Finding	Chest (n=19)	Lateral Neck (n=13)
Normal	11	1
Pneumonia	3	...
Subglottic density/ swelling	...	11
Tracheal soft tissue density	3	...
Metallic foreign body	2	1

(Courtesy of Esclamado, R.M., and Richardson, M.A.: Am. J. Dis. Child. 141:259–262, March 1987.)

TABLE 2.—Diagnostic Accuracy

	No.
Initial diagnosis	
Foreign body aspiration	11
Croup	5
Pneumonia/bronchiolitis	3
Asthma	1
Time to correct diagnosis	
< 24 hours	11
24–48 hours	4
3–7 days	3
8–21 days	1
5-1/2 months	1

(Courtesy of Esclamado, R.M., and Richardson, M.A.: Am. J. Dis. Child. 141:259–262, March 1987.)

of the patients, but the anteroposterior and lateral neck x-ray films suggested the diagnosis in 92% (Table 1). Although the diagnosis was made correctly within 24 hours of presentation in 55% of the children, most diagnoses (90%) were reached within 1 week (Table 2). The overall complication rate was 45%, and the incidence of complications was greater among patients with a delay in diagnosis of more than 24 hours (67%) than in patients whose problem was diagnosed early (27%).

The diagnosis of laryngotracheal foreign body aspiration should be strongly considered in children seen with apparent croup or reactive airway disease. Bronchoscopic evaluation should be considered early in these patients if medical management does not result in early resolution of symptoms.

▶ Lauren D. Holinger, M.D., Acting Head, Division of Bronchoesophagology-Otolaryngology and Department of Communicative Disorders, Children's Memorial Hospital, Chicago, comments.—J.A. Stockman III, M.D.

▶ Esclamado and Richardson have published an important and timely review of laryngotracheal foreign bodies in 20 children. Although the incidence of foreign body aspiration continues to decline in industrialized nations (better parent awareness?), this review is a timely reminder of the potential serious consequences if the problem is left untreated. In patients with a delay in diagnosis of more than 24 hours, the complication rate was 67% (6 of 9). Of two patients with apnea, one sustained cardiorespiratory arrest and died, for a mortality rate of 5%.

In evaluation of children with symptoms of airway obstruction, the importance of a thorough history cannot be overemphasized. A history of choking or aspiration was obtained in 90% (18 of 20). The absence of a positive history, however, should not deter the clinician from recommending endoscopic evaluation. An episode of aspiration may not be observed by an adult, and the child may be unable or unwilling to report such an episode. When a specific history of foreign body aspiration is absent, the clinician should inquire into the possibility of peanut ingestion. Of the laryngotracheal foreign bodies in this series, 7 (35%) were peanuts or peanut shells, a high incidence, but nevertheless lower than that observed with bronchial foreign bodies.

Stridor, wheezing, sternal retractions, and cough were the most common symptoms. Interestingly, there was no mention of the "palpable thud" or "audible slap" that, in addition to the "asthmatic wheeze," were described by Jackson as being pathognomonic for tracheal foreign bodies. The chest roentgenogram was normal in 11 children (58%) (Table 1). As does the possibility of a negative history, this high figure reflects the likelihood of negative findings in airway foreign bodies. Posteroanterior and lateral neck roentgenograms suggested the diagnosis in 92% (12 of 13), emphasizing the importance of these films in arriving at correct diagnosis.

The authors report a 45% incidence of complications in laryngotracheal foreign bodies, a figure at least four to five times greater than that reported for all aspirated foreign bodies, again emphasizing the extremely hazardous potential of this problem. They also conclude that in children with a diagnosis of croup or reactive airway disease who responded poorly or whose condition deteriorates despite appropriate medical management, early endoscopy should be carried out. The authors also correctly point out the advantages of open-tube (rigid) endoscopy over flexible fiberoptic bronchoscopy for management of this hazardous problem. They offer several helpful comments regarding technique, which will be of particular interest to the endoscopist.—L.D. Holinger, M.D.

Post-Tonsillectomy Hemorrhage: Incidence, Prevention and Management
Steven D. Handler, Linda Miller, Kenneth H. Richmond, and Christine Corso Baranak (Children's Hosp. of Philadelphia and Univ. of Pennsylvania)
Laryngoscope 96:1243–1247, November 1986   16–9

Tonsillectomy with or without adenoidectomy is a common operation in children. The reported incidence of posttonsillectomy hemorrhage has varied greatly because definitions of postoperative bleeding have varied. A review was made of the records of 1,445 children who underwent tonsillectomy during a 2-year period to determine the exact incidence and type of postoperative hemorrhage.

INCIDENCE AND DISTRIBUTION OF
POSTOPERATIVE HEMORRHAGE

Category	n	%	
A. Nonbleed	1407	97.38	
B. Immediate major	0	0.00	
C. Immediate minor	2	0.14	38/1445=2.62%
D. Delayed major	15	1.03	
E. Delayed minor	11	0.76	
F. Delayed minor home	10	0.69	
Total	1445	100.00%	

(Courtesy of Handler, S.D., et al.: Laryngoscope 96:1243–1247, November 1986.)

The patients were divided into six groups on the basis of the incidence and type of postoperative hemorrhage (table). Thirty-eight children (2.62%) had postoperative bleeding. The group that had delayed major bleeding was composed of 15 patients who required 18 intraoral explorations of the tonsillar fossae for bleeding. Thirteen required a procedure to stop postoperative hemorrhage. One patient had to be returned twice to the operating room to stop bleeding, and one with factor VIII deficiency hemophilia required three procedures to stop bleeding. No deaths occurred.

The low rate of posttonsillectomy hemorrhage in this series was achieved by performing complete preoperative coagulation screening, paying meticulous attention to surgical technique, and using suction-cautery to obtain hemostasis. Although antibiotics were used routinely in all postoperative tonsillectomy patients to prevent infection, their role in reducing the incidence of postoperative bleeding has not been determined.

▶ The exact incidence of postoperative tonsillar bleeding is difficult to determine. Indeed, every surgeon has his or her own personal criteria for reporting such bleeding. Increased attention to hemostatic control has been most responsible for lowering the rate of postoperative hemorrhage. The routine use of suction-electrocautery to obtain hemostasis is associated with a lower postoperative bleeding frequency. The use of adjunctive hemostatic agents (e.g., topical thrombin) has been advocated by several authors in the literature. In the above study, however, the use of such agents did not seem to make any difference.

Several other issues have arisen recently regarding tonsillectomy and adenoidectomy. One of these is whether or not it is safe to have a same-day discharge for children undergoing these procedures. Crysdale et al. (*Can. Med. Assoc. J.* 135:1139, 1986) studied a total of 9,409 children who were admitted to the Hospital for Sick Children in Toronto between the years 1980 and 1984 for tonsil or adenoid surgery, or both. They found that same-day discharge was possible for children undergoing adenoidectomy alone with only a minimum of 6 hours of observation being required. However, because a substantial number of children bled from their tonsillar fossae, overnight observation with discharge the next day seemed safer. These findings are in agreement with those of Herdman et al. (*J. Laryngol. Otol.* 100:1053, 1986). Another area of controversy has been the routine use of antibiotics during the recovery period from tonsillectomy. A team of dentists from the Children's Hospital of Philadelphia found recently that the intravenous administration of ampicillin at the time of surgery, followed by 7 days of amoxicillin orally, was not only well tolerated and safe but was effective in minimizing fever and other troublesome postoperative symptoms, e.g., pain, lassitude, mouth odor, and poor oral intake after tonsillectomy (Telian, S.A.: *Arch. Otolaryngol. Head Neck Surg.* 112:610, 1986).

One can logically ask the question: "What is the best way to prevent postoperative bleeding with tonsillectomies?" There seem to be three basic methods. One is the use of preoperative coagulation profiles consisting of prothrombin time, partial thromboplastin time, and bleeding times. The second is to use electrocautery during the surgery; this increases the postoperative complication rates of fever and pain, but these effects can possibly be ameliorated by the routine use of antibiotics. A third solution to the problem of postoperative bleeding after tonsillectomy is not to do the tonsillectomy at all. It's difficult to imagine why more than 9,000 children were admitted to the hospital referred to in the above abstract in just a 4-year period solely for tonsillectomies and adenoidectomies. In fact, the latter concept is embraced in the "Star Gazers Guide to Modern Science." This guide has four basic dictums: (1) If it's green or wiggles, it's biology. (2) If it stinks, it's chemistry. (3) If it doesn't work, it's physics. (4) If it may not be necessary, it's a T & A.

My apologies to all of my friends in otolaryngology. Certainly, there are clearcut indications for tonsillectomy and adenoidectomy. (We pediatricians just like to take a few pot shots at these indications once in awhile.)—J.A. Stockman III, M.D.

Deafness: Ever Heard of It? Delayed Recognition of Permanent Hearing Loss
James Coplan (State Univ. of New York at Syracuse)
Pediatrics 79:206–213, February 1987   16–10

Prompt detection of permanent hearing loss remains an unattained goal. Records of about 1,000 children seen for evaluation of developmental delay from July 1979 to December 1985 were reviewed to the determine factors that contributed to prompt or delayed recognition of hearing loss. The diagnosis of hearing loss was based on the results of formal testing by certified audiologists, which included behavioral response audiometry in a sound field, speech awareness, speech reception, pure-tone testing under headphones, and acoustic reflex testing.

Forty-six children (4.6%) had permanent hearing loss. Causes of hearing loss included single-gene defects, chromosomal aberrations, sporadic syndromes, teratogens, and perinatal or postnatal factors, e.g., infection and

---

TABLE 1.—Hearing Loss in a Child Development Clinic Population

Category of Loss	No. (%) of Children	Etiology
Single-gene defect	10 (22)	Waardenberg syndrome [2], autosomal recessive progressive [2], neurofibromatosis [1], Treacher Collins syndrome [1], hypomelanosis of Ito [1], possibly genetic [3]
Chromosomal	2 (4)	45XO (Turner syndrome) [1], ring chromosome-18 [1]
Sporadic syndrome	5 (11)	Hemifacial microsomia [4], McCune-Albright syndrome [1]
Teratogenic	12 (26)	Cytomegalovirus infection: proven [1], suspected [7]; rubella infection [1]; other [3]
Perinatally acquired	5 (11)	Intraventricular hemorrhage: proven [3], suspected [2]
Postnatally acquired	3 (7)	H influenzae meningitis [1], cranial irradiation [1], basilar skull fracture [1]
Multiple factors (2 or more/ child)	6 (13)	Intrauterine growth retardation, recognizable malformation syndrome, parental consanguinity, intraventricular hemorrhage, meconium aspiration and seizures, bacterial meningitis
Unknown	3 (7)	

*Numbers in brackets are numbers of children.
(Courtesy of Coplan, J.: Pediatrics 79:206–213, February 1987.)

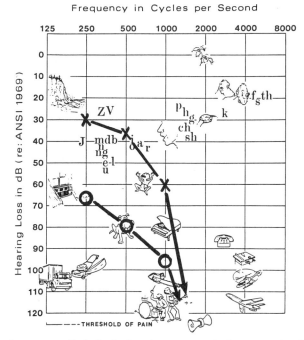

Fig 16–7.—Frequency amplitude distribution of common sounds. Severe to profound midfrequency and high-frequency sensorineural hearing loss of perinatal onset. *Open circles* denote right ear; *crosses* indicate left ear. Partial sparing of low-frequency hearing created false impression of normal hearing on physical examination. Age at audiologic diagnosis: 43 months. (Courtesy of Coplan, J.: Pediatrics 79:206–213, February 1987.)

intraventricular hemorrhage (Table 1). Profound congenital deafness was not diagnosed until a mean age of 24 months, whereas mild to moderate or unilateral hearing impairment was not diagnosed until a mean age of 48 months (Fig 16–7). Nearly half of the children with congenital loss had associated physical anomalies that should have triggered a prompt search for deafness, including neural crest abnormalities, first or second branchial arch abnormalities, or findings diagnostic of specific syndromes known to be associated with hearing loss. Hearing loss was suspected or diagnosed initially by the author in 40% of children; the rest appeared to hear normally during physical examination but were referred for audiologic evaluation because of the medical history or the finding of speech or language delay on developmental testing (Fig 16–8).

Physicians should not place undue confidence in their ability to detect even major hearing impairment during routine physical examination of children, particularly those who are developmentally disabled. Several risk criteria have been formulated to permit timely diagnosis of hearing impairment in all children: high-risk medical or family histories, branchial arch or ectodermal-neural crest defects on physical examination, or delayed speech or other developmental abnormalities (Table 2).

▶ The author of this report does us all a great service. About 1 child in 1,000

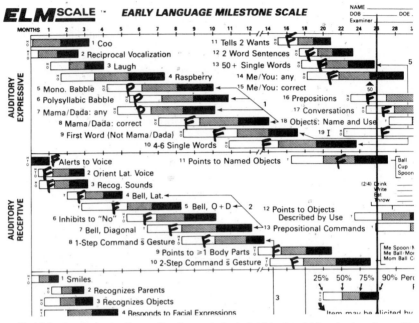

Fig 16–8.—Language-screening profile of congenitally deaf child referred for evaluation of "possible mental retardation." Vocalizations were arrested at 9-month level. Intelligence was normal on psychometric testing. Age at audiologic diagnosis: 25 months. Greater attention to language development would have substantially shortened delay in diagnosis of child's hearing loss. (From Modern Education Corp., Tulsa, Okla; used with permission. Courtesy of Coplan, J.: Pediatrics 79:206–213, February 1987.)

TABLE 2.—INDICATIONS FOR AUDIOLOGIC EVALUATION

Neonatal intensive care
  Birth wt <2,500 g: All cases
  Birth wt >2,500 g: If medical complications (asphyxia, seizures, persistent fetal circulation, intracranial hemorrhage, assisted ventilation, hyperbilirubinemia, ototoxic drugs)
Proven or suspected intrauterine infection
Bacterial meningitis
Anomalies of 1st or 2nd brachial arch (microtia, auricular dysplasia, micrognathia)
Anomalies of neural crest/ectoderm (widely spaced eyes; pigmentary defects)
Family history of hereditary or unexplained deafness
Parental concern regarding hearing loss
Delayed speech or language development
Other developmental disabilities (mental retardation, cerebral palsy, autism, blindness)

(Courtesy of Coplan, J.: Pediatrics 79:206–213, February 1987.)

is born deaf and an additional 2 children per 1,000 are deafened during childhood. The developmental and psychosocial impact of hearing loss can be devastating, particularly if hearing loss is accompanied by other developmental disabilities, or if the diagnosis of hearing impairment is delayed for any significant length of time. The first 36 months of life are a critical period for language learning. Failure to identify hearing loss and provide intervention before this period lapses will needlessly prejudice language development beyond the effect of the hearing loss itself. Unfortunately, on the average there is a delay of about 12 months between the parents' first suspicion of hearing loss and physician referral to an audiologist.

It should be recognized that nearly half of the children with deafness may have other physical anomalies that would have provided an early clue to the associated presence of deafness. Any child with dysplastic external ears, micrognathia, or other cranial or facial anomalies should be evaluated in very early life. The same would be said of children with widely spaced eyes. Infants who are born prematurely may have a sensorineural hearing loss as high as 12%. Whether that's because of all the noise they are exposed to in the nursery or is a consequence of their developmental immaturity at the time of birth is a subject for another commentary.

In addition to ambient noise levels in our nurseries, bouts of acidosis, hypoxia, the use of aminoglycosides, loop diuretics, and hyperbilirubinemia can be problems. Nield et al. (see Abstract 16–12) demonstrated that "graduates" of level III neonatal intensive care units have at least a 3% risk of confirmed hearing loss even in the absence of any other known risk factors. It may be possible to perform hearing screening relatively easy even in the newborn period with the use of the Crib-O-Gram. This is a hearing device designed to be used exclusively in the newborn nursery. The basic element of the Crib-O-Gram is a motion-sensing transducer that lies beneath the mattress of an infant's incubator or bassinet. The output of the transducer is converted to a digital signal and tabulates automatically as an infant's activity is monitored (Webb, K.C., et al.: *Arch. Otolaryngol. Head Neck Surg.* 112:420, 1986). It should be noted that the presence of preauricular tags may also be associated with a high prevalence of hearing loss (Kankkunen, A., et al.: *Acta Paediatr. Scand.* 76:143, 1987). If you are interested in reading more about screening for hearing impairment in the newborn, see the excellent editorial in the *Lancet* (2:1429, 1986). It should be noted that at least one study has indicated that the Denver Developmental Screening Test is not particularly sensitive in picking up speech and language disorders, many of which are caused by hearing deficits (Borowitz, K.C., et al.: *Pediatrics* 78:1075, 1986).

Recently under fire was the concept that children with repeated episodes of otitis media with effusions have a higher frequency of later verbal and academic performance problems. Not so, say Roberts et al. (*Pediatrics* 78:423, 1986). The latter investigators found no evidence of an association between measures of early childhood otitis media with effusion and later measures of verbal or academic functional disorders. This study flies in the face of many prior studies suggesting the opposite. It also flies in the face of a recent National Institutes of Health consensus conference (*Public Health Rep.* 101:189, 1986). The conferees all agreed that the effects of even a "mild" hearing loss of 15–25 dB in early childhood, if persistent and if neglected, may not only disturb the acquisition of language but also adversely affect the social and emotional development of a child with the full implications of these consequences yet to be determined.

The whole issue of the relationship between otitis media with effusion and hearing loss is indeed difficult to understand, but that makes it a modern topic. Once I understand something, it's already become obsolete.—J.A. Stockman III, M.D.

Unexpected Hearing Loss in High-Risk Infants

Toni A. Nield, Shirley Schrier, Angela D. Ramos, Arnold C.G. Platzker, and David Warburton (Univ. of Southern California)
Pediatrics 78:417–422, September 1986   16–11

The incidence of hearing impairment among graduates of the neonatal intensive care unit (NICU) has been reported to be between 2% and 10%. The auditory brain stem response (ABR) is the recommended screening test at discharge from the NICU; however, 7% to 30% of infants with an abnormal ABR on initial screening hear normally on subsequent testing at ages 1–4 months. Infants who pass the initial ABR screening test are not usually retested. Eleven high-risk infants who passed an initial ABR screening test were found on follow-up testing to have significant sensorineural hearing loss.

All 11 infants were products of high-risk pregnancies and deliveries. Birth weights were 890–3,700 gm, and gestational ages were 28–42 weeks. Durations of hospitalization ranged from 45 days to 167 days, and all the infants had respiratory distress, requiring prolonged mechanical ventilation, with resultant chronic lung disease. Each infant was given pancuronium, morphine, ampicillin, and gentamicin, and ten also received furosemide and chlorothiazide. Other clinical complications included abnormal CNS findings during the NICU stay (ten patients), acidosis (pH < 7.25) on the initial blood gas test (eight), and persistent fetal circulation in seven infants whose birth weights were more than 1,500 gm. Developmentally, eight of nine children tested between ages 12 months and 36 months were normal in all respects other than the hearing loss and the related language impairment.

Infants who have been seriously ill in the newborn period, including term infants, may be at risk for the development of substantial sensorineural hearing loss, even though they have passed an initial ABR screening test in the neonatal period.

▶ James Coplan, M.D., Associate Professor of Pediatrics, State University of New York Health Science Center at Syracuse, comments.—J.A. Stockman III, M.D.
▶ This is a very disturbing paper. Were the initial ABRs false negatives, or did these children have progressive hearing loss? Should we be administering something other than ABR for audiologic screening at discharge from the NICU? I asked my audiologic colleague, Charles T. Grimes, Ph.D., for help with these questions. First, the data presented are probably indicative of progressive loss, at least for the two children whose ABRs were shown. Second, in the newborn period, ABRs are still the best screening technique around.

The "gold standard" for audiologic evaluation is pure-tone testing under headphones, which usually cannot be performed until 30–36 months of age because of the degree of voluntary cooperation required. While we do not suggest that all NICU grads undergo pure-tone testing at 36 months, it is evident that some infants should be retested despite perfectly normal ABRs at discharge. Which children? First, any child with delayed speech or language development. Such children often have "normal" Bayley or other test results because of the paucity of language items on these instruments. The Early Language Milestone Scale (Modern Education Corporation, Tulsa) is one useful adjunct to the Bayley for NICU developmental follow-up. Second, certain medical factors probably increase the risk for progressive hearing loss. Intrauterine growth retardation suggests congenital viral infection, which can certainly produce progressive deafness. Perinatal events (e.g., intraventricular hemorrhage) have always been assumed to produce deafness at the time of the bleed, not later. Perhaps this assumption needs to be reexamined. All 11 infants in this series had chronic renal disease and/or chronic lung disease. Perhaps chronic hypoxia is capable of producing progressive hearing loss, or perhaps it can potentiate other factors (do I see a study here?).

It is disturbing to note that most children referred back had bilateral severe to profound deafness. How many more NICU graduates are out there with moderate (and still disabling) hearing loss? Nobody knows. Children at high risk for hearing loss should undergo periodic rescreening of language development and periodic retesting of hearing despite "normal" ABRs at discharge from the NICU.—J. Coplan, M.D.

Sensorineural Hearing Loss in Cordless Telephone Injury
Daniel J. Orchik, Daniel R. Schmaier, John J. Shea, Jr., John R. Emmett, William H. Moretz, Jr., and John J. Shea, III (Shea Clinic and Found. Memphis, and Johnson City, Tenn.)
Otolaryngol. Head Neck Surg. 96:30–33, January 1987   16–12

The results of excessive noise exposure on hearing have been well documented. There are two distinct types of noise-induced hearing loss: One occurs gradually over many years and is related to repeated exposure, and the second can be attributed to a single brief exposure of very high intensity, which is referred to as acoustic trauma. The potential hazard of acoustic trauma produced by cordless telephones has been reported and confirmed in subsequent studies. In the present investigation, 24 children with reported cordless telephone injuries were examined. Three had preinjury audiograms available.

All 24 patients had sensorineural hearing loss as determined by puretone audiometry in the affected ear. Immittance audiometry indicated normal middle ear function. Five patients had histories of severe hearing loss in the ear opposite that injured by the cordless telephone. In two patients with preinjury and postinjury audiograms, the time lapse between these audiograms was about 18 months. In the third patient, the time lapse was 13 years. However, a comparison of the two audiograms revealed no change in hearing in the uninjured ear. The frequency spectrum of the ring of the three cordless telephones was characterized by a peak energy level of about 750 Hz, with subsequent peaks of decreasing sound-pressure levels at frequencies about the second through sixth harmonics of 750 Hz. In all probability, the energy peak in the region of 750 Hz explains why the most frequent audiometric pattern in cordless phone injury is of midfrequency, sensorineural loss.

Of particular importance is the typical audiometric pattern seen in these patients. That a single insult can affect hearing in a frequency region within the speech spectrum is especially alarming. It is believed that the hazard is real, and measures should be taken to recall or modify the potentially dangerous units.

▶ The assault on the ears continues. If it isn't a Huey Lewis concert, it may well be a cordless telephone. Before throwing away your cordless telephone, please realize that not all of these instruments are culpable. Sensorineural hearing loss has been reported only with those instruments in which the ear receiver doubles as the ringing or bell device. In each instance, the patient held the telephone against the ear just at the time the ringing occurred. The loudness of the ring was sufficient to cause permanent and irreversible hearing loss. To make matters worse, in most instances it was a single insult that occurred and the effect was a hearing loss in the frequency region within which the speech spectrum occurs. Obviously, the effects were devastating.

While on the subject of telephones, Dr. Jack W. Finney has come up with an interesting recommendation (*Am. J. Dis. Child.* 140:975, 1986). Because car telephones are becoming so ubiquitous, one way to ensure that adolescents wear their seat belts would be to use interlocking devices between the car telephone and the seat belt. If the seat belt isn't fastened, the car telephone will not work. What a creative idea! Even more creative would be the destruction of all car telephones. Being a creature who of necessity must travel a very busy highway each morning, I enjoy the opportunity of seeing how many "deals" and so forth are being made at 6:30 AM with the use of car telephones. There seems to be an inverse relationship between the presence of a car telephone and how well somebody drives.

When it comes to teenagers, I really don't think that they are all that interested in making calls on telephones in their cars as much as they like the appearance of being observed to be using the car telephone. A neighbor of ours has a creative teenage son who places a cheap antenna on the trunk of his car and pretends he is talking into a nonfunctional hand phone from an old discarded telephone unit. If that sounds a bit perverse, that's probably correct, but some of us who were around in the '50s and '60s can remember when many a teenager would drive around town in the family car with all the windows rolled up on a hot summer day just to make others think that the family was well off enough to afford air conditioning. I think I liked it better when kids eagerly looked forward to braces as a status symbol. Car telephones are a bit too much. I would also like to see the end of some of these ridiculous commercials produced by telephone companies. You know the ones I mean—the one where you can hear a pin drop from outer space via telephone lines, or the one in which a singer seems to get great enjoyment of breaking a glass of fine crystal from 2,000 miles away. If you're not familiar with these ads, you yourself must be from somewhere in outer space.—J.A. Stockman III, M.D.

Adequate Illumination for Otoscopy: Variations Due to Power Source, Bulb, and Head and Speculum Design

Francisco Barriga, Richard H. Schwartz, and Gregory F. Hayden (Georgetown Univ., Children's Hosp. Natl. Med. Ctr., Washington, D.C.; and Univ. of Virginia)
Am. J. Dis. Child. 140:1237–1240, December 1986   16–13

Otitis media is common among sick children and an accurate diagnosis is essential to the primary care physician. The capability and actual performance of office otoscopes were assessed by measuring their light output before and after replacement of the battery and bulb in the instrument. The study group included 91 physicians, 57 pediatricians, 23 family physicians, and 11 allergists, all staff members of 2 suburban hospitals, who owned a total of 221 otoscopes. All were visited by an investigator after

TABLE 1.—LIGHT OUTPUT OF 221 OTOSCOPIES ACCORDING TO OTOSCOPE SITE

Light Output, Foot-candles	Site, No. of Otoscopes		
	Office	Hospital	Total
0–19	5	1	6
20–49	12	1	13
50–99	26	3	29
≥100	119	54	173
Total	162	59	221

(Courtesy of Barriga, F., et al.: Am. J. Dis. Child. 140:1237–1240, December 1986.)

TABLE 2.—EFFECT OF BULB AND BATTERY REPLACEMENT ON ADEQUACY OF LIGHT OUTPUT*

Type of Battery or Bulb Unit	No. Tested	No. Inadequate	No. (%) Adequate After Replacement
Battery Replacement			
Rechargeable	105	27	4 (15)
Nonrechargeable	15	8	5 (63)
Total	120	35	9 (26)
Bulb Replacement			
Halogen/battery	102	28	22 (79)
Halogen/transformer	94	10	9 (90)
Nonhalogen	14	8	6 (75)
Total	210	46	37 (80)

*Adequacy of light output was defined as 100 foot-candles or more.
(Courtesy of Barriga, F., et al.: Am. J. Dis. Child. 140:1237–1240, December 1986.)

TABLE 3.—Light Output of 3.5-V Otoscopes According to Type of Head and Mounting

Type of Mounting	Type of Head		
	Plastic	Metal	Total
Wall			
Light output, foot-candles	372.2	80.8	331.9
No. of otoscopes	81	13	94
Portable			
Light output, ft–c	321.2	127.9	217.0
No. of otoscopes	41	48	89
Total			
Light output, ft–c	355.1	117.9	276.0
No. of otoscopes	122	61	183

(Courtesy of Barriga, F., et al.: Am. J. Dis. Child. 140:1237–1240, December 1986.)

their participation in the study had been requested by mail and confirmed by telephone. However, the physicians did not know the nature of the study beforehand.

After a brief interview to determine the date of purchase of the otoscope, frequency of bulb change, and availability of extra bulbs in the office, otoscopes were measured for light output with a research photometer in an "as is" condition, and again after a new bulb and new battery had been placed in the unit. A light output of at least 100 foot-candles was considered optimal for clinical otoscopy. Of the 221 otoscopes examined, 173 had a light output of at least 100 foot-candles before bulb and battery replacement (Table 1). Replacement of the bulb restored adequate light output in 80% of the 48 otoscopes that initially had given a poor performance, as did replacement of the battery in 26% (Table 2). In 3.5-V instruments with halogen lamps, differences between metal and plastic heads showed that the light output of otoscopes with plastic heads was significantly greater than that of instruments with metal heads (Table 3; Fig 16–9).

▶ The fact that light bulbs burn out and batteries wear out should come as a surprise to no one. Most of us have a subtle hostility about replacing these things before they're on their last legs. Indeed, this study shows that most physicians change an otoscope light bulb only when the light becomes too dim to see the eardrum clearly. As an aside, despite the scientific advantages of pneumatic otoscopy, one third of the physicians were not using this technique routinely. The frequency of replacement for disposable batteries with hand-held otoscopes varies according to the frequency and intensity of otoscopic use, but a busy practitioner will need to change batteries often to ensure good output. In contrast, most rechargeable batteries last for many years. The expiration date printed on the rechargeable battery is usually 2 years. Most batteries appear to perform perfectly well long after that amount of time, so physicians may elect to continue to use a rechargeable battery until it fails to retain a

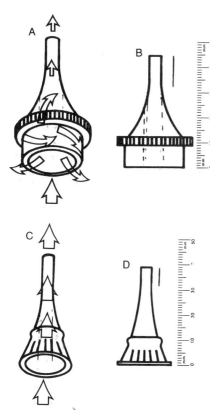

Fig 16–9.—A, in green nylon aural speculum, light does not travel in straight line; some is lost by diffusion outward and backward. B, green nylon aural speculum has 8-mm straight portion from tip to beginning of flared section, permitting sufficient penetration of straight portion into ear canal. Base is cylindrical. C, in black plastic aural speculum light travels in straight path from base to tip. D, although conical base of black plastic speculum concentrates light beam with less loss of foot-candles than with green nylon speculum, straight portion of black speculum measures only 3 mm. This precludes optimal insertion into ear canals of young children and largely counterbalances advantages in light transmission. (Courtesy of Barriga, F., et al.: Am. J. Dis. Child. 140:1237–1240, December 1986.)

charge for a full work day. The duration of light bulb performance depends on the frequency and intensity of use. For the most commonly used light bulb lamps (the 3.5-V halogen lamp), light output starts to diminish after only about 10 hours' use. After about 20 hours most individuals find that the bulb is relatively useless except as a Christmas tree ornament. In a busy practice, this translates into replacement of bulbs as frequently as every 2–4 months.

I think most will agree that the major problem with the ability to examine an ear appropriately has little to do with light bulbs or batteries. It has more to do with getting around the wax that is in the external canal and really understanding what that particular tympanic membrane is trying to tell you. The best otoscopes in the world are no substitute for experience and understanding. Among the cardiologists that I have the greatest fondness for was one whom I first met in my residency. This gentleman had used the same stethoscope for more than 20 years without ever changing the diaphragm. In fact, he used a stethoscope with just a diaphragm and no bell. He could hear things that no one else could hear, even those who had the most sophisticated of stethoscopes. One can say confidently that a little more or a little less brightness coming out of a speculum must be mated with a little more or less brightness on the part of the user. Certainly, never ask a manufacturer's rep if you think you might need a new otoscope. That's like asking a barber if you need a haircut. Trust your own senses.—J.A. Stockman III, M.D.

Efficacy of Amoxicillin With and Without Decongestant-Antihistamine for Otitis Media With Effusion in Children: Results of a Double-Blind, Randomized Trial

Ellen M. Mandel, Howard E. Rockette, Charles D. Bluestone, Jack L. Paradise, and Robert J. Nozza (Children's Hosp. of Pittsburgh and Univ. of Pittsburgh)
N. Engl. J. Med. 316:432–437, Feb. 19, 1987   16–14

The lack of efficacy of an oral decongestant-antihistamine combination in the treatment of otitis media with effusion has been reported. Because middle ear effusion commonly occurs after a middle ear infection and pathogenic bacteria are often recovered from chronic effusions, the efficacy of a 2-week course of amoxicillin (40 mg/kg/day) with and without a 4-week course of an oral decongestant-antihistamine combination was evaluated in a randomized, double-blind, placebo-controlled trial involving 518 infants and children with otitis media with effusion.

Among the 474 children evaluated at 4 weeks after entry, the rate of resolution of middle ear effusion was significantly twice as high in those treated with amoxicillin, with or without the decongestant-antihistamine combination, than in the placebo-treated controls (table). However, about 70% of the patients treated with amoxicillin still had effusion in at least one ear. Moreover, among those without effusion at the 4-week end point, about half of both the amoxicillin-treated and placebo-treated patients had a recurrence of effusion within 16 weeks after treatment. Overall, resolution was more likely in children with initially unilateral effusion, in those who had effusion for 8 weeks or less, and in those without an upper

STATUS OF MIDDLE-EAR EFFUSION IN **460** SUBJECTS AT TWO WEEKS AND FOUR WEEKS AFTER STUDY ENTRY

STATUS OF EFFUSION AT TWO WEEKS	STATUS OF EFFUSION AT FOUR WEEKS		
	ABSENT	PRESENT	TOTAL
	no. (%) of subjects		
Present			
Amoxicillin and decongestant–antihistamine	22 (19.8)	89 (80.2)	111 (100)
Amoxicillin and placebo	18 (16.4)	92 (83.6)	110 (100)
Placebo and placebo	8 (6.2)	121 (93.8)	129 (100)
Absent			
Amoxicillin and decongestant–antihistamine	27 (61.4)	17 (38.6)	44 (100)
Amoxicillin and placebo	28 (62.2)	17 (37.8)	45 (100)
Placebo and placebo	13 (61.9)	8 (38.1)	21 (100)

(Courtesy of Mandel, E.M., et al.: N. Engl. J. Med., 316:432–437, Feb. 19, 1987.)

respiratory tract infection at the 4-week end point. Side effects were more common in patients who received the decongestant-antihistamine combination. Amoxicillin therapy appears to increase to some extent the likelihood of resolution of otitis media with effusion in infants and children.

▶ The Pittsburgh group previously reported the lack of efficacy of an orally administered decongestant-antihistamine combination as a treatment for otitis media with effusion ("secretory" or "serous" otitis media) in children. Because middle ear effusion commonly occurs as an aftermath of frank middle ear infection, and pathogenic bacteria are often acquired from effusions of long duration, these investigators studied the efficacy of an antimicrobial drug in relieving middle ear effusion not apparently associated with the clinical evidence of acute middle ear infection. As the authors suspected, amoxicillin, with or without a decongestant/antihistamine, was effective in helping to resolve middle ear effusions. At the end of 4 weeks, the use of amoxicillin was associated with twice as high a resolution rate as the nonuse of this antibiotic. Although not as well controlled, another study also found that medical treatment of otitis media with antibiotics decreases the duration of secretory otitis media (Gates, G.A., et al.: *Otolaryngol. Head Neck Surg.* 94:350, 1986). Please recognize that although amoxicillin is better than placebo and its use therefore may sound encouraging, it worked in only 30% of the patients. Whether the remainder represent antibiotic failures in the presence of other kinds of bacteria not susceptible to amoxicillin or failures as a consequence of drainage problems of the middle ear, as most have suspected, cannot be answered by this study from Pittsburgh.

Although the findings of the Pittsburgh study are important, it still leaves a huge pool of children who have something behind their eardrums for a prolonged period of time. What is the story with the current understanding of tympanostomy tubes? Gonzalez et al. (*Laryngoscope* 96:1330, 1986) studied 65 children in a blinded, prospective, randomized study designed to determine the efficacy of tympanostomy tubes, antibiotic prophylaxis, and placebo. Five of 22 children in the tympanostomy group had recurrent ear infections, compared with 12 of 20 in the placebo group. There were eight treatment failures in the 21 children who were given prophylactic sulfisoxazole (500 mg orally twice daily for those under age 5 years, and 1.0 gm twice daily for older children). These authors concluded that tympanostomy tube insertion may be warranted and is at least as effective as prophylactic antibiotics.

Maybe we should be doing what some others are doing in Great Britain. Curley (*Clin. Otolaryngol.* 11:1, 1986) did a study that was designed to answer numerous questions. For example, how long does a tube remain in place and remain functional? It was found that the average time until a tube was blocked was 8 months and 8.6 months until it fell out. How likely is it for an individual child to require repeated admission for tube placement? The answer to this was that the average number of admissions per child was 1.6. Does an earlier age at first admission for tube placement imply an increased likelihood of further admissions? The answer was yes, especially in children aged 3–4 years. How frequently is a middle ear effusion diagnosed in an outpatient setting and yet not present at the time of surgery? The answer to this one was an astonishing 29% of all myringotomies revealing a dry middle ear. Was this disappearance of fluid affected by the waiting time or seasonal influences? You're absolutely correct. Children who had to wait for their surgery, especially during the summer rush season for elective tube placement (semielective), had a very high rate of spontaneous resolution. The British study also examined the frequency of complication rates with tube placement. Complications occurred in 4% of the overall group and included chronic perforation, retention of a tube requiring anesthesia for its removal, secondary inflammation resulting in polyps and granulation formation, and the loss of one tube into the middle ear!

Other workers have suggested that if, when you look inside the middle ear prior to tube placement, you see actively beading cilia, you may not need to place a tube at all (Wacker, D.F., et al.: *Otolaryngol. Head Neck Surg.* 95:434, 1986). Children who maintain middle ear ciliary function seem to be more likely to recover spontaneously on their own.

So if tympanostomy tubes don't work in all children, nor do antibiotics work, what about steroids? Recently, a lot of work has been done with steroid therapy in patients with chronic middle ear effusion. Lambert et al. (*Otolaryngol. Head Neck Surg.* 95:193, 1986) found no benefit after 2 months of pharmacologic doses of prednisone. Two years ago, two papers presented at the Ambulatory Pediatric Association Plenary Sessions described attempts to examine the role of prednisone in the resolution of middle ear fluid. One study, not particularly well controlled, seemed to show some benefit (Grose, K., et al.: *Am. J. Dis. Child.* 140:317, 1986). The other (Woodhead, J.C., et al.: *Am. J. Dis. Child.* 140:318, 1986) showed no benefit. The real question that we now face is what else can we try to treat with steroids. The answer to that question perhaps is obvious. Steroids should be administered to all cats. They will get fat and float better.—J.A. Stockman III, M.D.

Early Recurrences of Otitis Media: Reinfection or Relapse?

Susan A. Carlin, Colin D. Marchant, Paul A. Shurin, Candice E. Johnson, D. Murdell-Panek, and Stephen J. Barenkamp (Case Western Reserve Univ., Cleveland, Washington Univ., and St. Louis Children's Hosp.)
J. Pediatr. 110:20–25, January 1987   16–15

Recurrences of otitis media remain a therapeutic dilemma, particularly when they occur soon after antibiotic therapy. In a prospective study, 103 patients ranging in age from 2 months to 12 years were evaluated to identify risk factors for recurrences of otitis media occurring within 1 month of initial diagnosis and to determine if the second episode was caused by the same pathogen (relapse) or a new organism (reinfection). If the same bacterial species were recovered in both episodes, *Streptococcus pneumoniae* was serotyped and *Hemophilus influenzae* was classified by biotypes and by electrophoretic pattern of the outer membrane proteins.

Thirty-six patients (35%) had early recurrence of acute otitis media. Recurrences developed 11–34 days (median, 27 days) after initial antibiotic treatment was begun. Children who had early recurrences were more likely to have had three or more episodes of otitis media in the preceding 6 months compared with patients without recurrence. Tympanocentesis was peformed in 29 children. Thirteen had sterile middle ear exudates either initially or at the time of recurrence; of the other 16 patients, 12 (75%) had reinfection and 4 (25%) had relapse.

Unless initial therapy is ineffective or the patient is noncompliant, early recurrences of otitis media frequently represent reinfection with a new organism. This finding suggests that underlying susceptibility to middle ear infection is important in the development of recurrent otitis media. Tympanocentesis aids in choosing the appropriate antibiotic therapy.

▶ Recurrences of otitis media are particularly troublesome when they develop soon after antibiotic therapy. This study attempts to address several issues: Which patients are most likely to have recurrences? Is the second episode of otitis media caused by the same pathogen (relapse), or by a new bacterial species (reinfection)? When is a change in antimicrobial therapy indicated? The investigators found that early recurrences of acute otitis media are more often caused by a new organism. This finding suggests that an underlying suscepti- bility to middle ear infection is as important as anything else in the develop- ment of recurrent otitis media. If these data are correct, we as pediatricians should not assume that early recurrences are necessarily the result of failure of initial treatment. I, for one, wholeheartedly endorse the concept that tym- panocentesis is being used too little to help sort out these various problems. The most fascinating part about the report abstracted above is the fact that if you substitute urinary tract infection for otitis media, you come up with not that dissimilar a set of conclusions. You can also substitute "suprapubic aspi- ration" for "tympanocentesis." Maybe the pathophysiology of infections of the urinary tract and middle ear are not really all that different.

Perhaps the only thing that we are left with to fight off otitis media is the age-old concept of prolonged breast-feeding. Unfortunately, severe blows have recently been dealt to the concept that breast-feeding protects against infection. Leventhal, J.M. (*Pediatrics* 78:896, 1986) examined this problem. The initial crude results suggested that breast-feeding is protective. However, when the data were stratified by the severity of the child's condition at the time of presentation to the hospital, the apparent protective effect of breast- feeding was markedly diminished. It would appear that breast-feeding pro- tected young infants from being hospitalized but not from infections per se. Bauchner et al. (*JAMA* 256:887, 1986) carefully dissected 20 prior studies that suggested that breast-feeding helped to prevent infections in infancy. They suggested that most of the studies had major methodologic flaws that may have compromised their conclusions. For the few studies that met important methodologic standards and controlled for confounding variables, it was found that breast-feeding had, at most, only a minimal protective effect in industrial- ized countries.

This is a strange industrialized country that we live in. We have investigators who in a randomized controlled fashion go about showing that breast-feeding really isn't as good as it should be. Did you know that there were 7,110,427 gallons of calamine lotion sold in the United States in 1985? I've never seen a randomized, controlled, blinded study to determine if calamine lotion really works. I, for one, will speak out as loudly and as gloriously as possible in praising the benefits of breast milk. That is certainly better than being silent. Glory may be fleeting, but obscurity is forever. We should try to stay with therapies that are the least innocuous. Antibiotics, antihistamines, tympanostomy tubes, and steroids are not all that innocuous. Pubilius Syrus, some 2,000 years ago, made an appropriate observation: "There are some remedies worse than the disease."—J.A. Stockman III, M.D.

Acute Mastoiditis: Diagnosis and Complications

John W. Ogle and Brian A. Lauer (Univ. of Colorado)
Am. J. Dis. Child. 140:1178–1182, November 1986   16–16

Early antimicrobial therapy of acute otitis media is now standard practice and acute mastoiditis has become rare. However, the disease still may occur and complications are common. During 1983 and 1984, an unexpectedly large number of children were admitted to the hospitals of the University of Colorado with acute mastoiditis. A review was made of the hospital records of 30 patients younger than age 16 years with a discharge diagnosis of mastoiditis between 1973 and 1984. The age range was 3 months to 14 years, including 43% younger than age 2 years.

TABLE 1.—CLINICAL AND LABORATORY FEATURES ON ADMISSION IN 30
CHILDREN WITH ACUTE MASTOIDITIS

Features	No. (%) of Patients
Clinical (n=30)	
Abnormal tympanic membrane	30 (100)
Swelling over mastoid bone	26 (86)
Erythema over mastoid bone	19 (63)
History of fever	22 (73)
Fever (temperature>38 C on first hospital day)	20 (67)
Prior antibiotic treatment	12 (40)
Otorrhea	10 (33)
Laboratory	
White blood cell count elevated (15,000/cu mm[15.0x10^9/L])(n=28)	14 (50)
Erythrocyte sedimentation rate elevated (30 mm/hour)(n=13)	7 (54)

(Courtesy of Ogle, J.W., and Lauer, B.A.: Am. J. Dis. Child. 140:1178–1182, November 1986.)

TABLE 2.—ROENTGENOGRAPHIC FEATURES OF 30 CHILDREN
WITH ACUTE MASTOIDITIS

Roentgenologic Finding (n=25)	No. (%) of Patients
Clouding of mastoid	12 (48)
Osteitis	
Demineralization (hazy septae or loss of detail)	4 (16)
Gross bone destruction (coalescent mastoiditis)	3 (12)
Normal	6 (24)

(Courtesy of Ogle, J.W., and Lauer, B.A.: Am. J. Dis. Child. 140:1178–1182, November 1986.)

TABLE 3.—BACTERIA ISOLATED BY SITE FROM 30 CHILDREN WITH ACUTE MASTOIDITIS

Bacteria	No. of Patients	No. of Isolates by Site*						
		Blood (n=23)	CSF	Tympano-centesis (n=9)	Surgical Specimens (n=11)	Postauricular Aspirate (n=5)	External Auditory Canal (n=7)	CIE, Urine (n=6)
Streptococcus pneumoniae	7	0	0	3	2	0	2	0
Staphylococcus epidermidis	5	0	0	2	0	0	3	0
Hemophilus influenzae‡	3	1	0	1	1	0	0	1
Group A streptococcus§	3	0	0	1	2†	1	0	0
Anaerobes	3	0	2	0	1	1	0	0
Staphylococcus aureus¶	2	0	0	0	1	0	1	0
Pseudomonas aeruginosa‖	1	0	0	0	0	0	1	0
Total positive	...	1	2	7	7	2	7	1

*CSF = cerebrospinal fluid; CIE = counterimmunoelectrophoresis.
†One culture each mixed with S. epidermidis.
‡Hemophilus influenzae type b from blood and subdural effusion in 1 patient; H. influenzae type a from tympanocentesis in 1 patient; and H. influenzae type b antigen detected by urine CIE in 1 patient.
§Group A streptococcus from mastoid and postauricular aspirate in 1 patient.
‖Fusobacterium nucleatum from CSF in 1 patient; Bacteroides assacbrolyticus from postauricular aspirate in 1 patient; Bacteroides fragilis from CSF, mixed with nonhemolytic streptococcus, Candida albicans, and Morganella morganii from mastoid in 1 patient.
¶Staphylococcus aureus mixed with Streptococcus intermedius and S. epidermidis from mastoid in 1 patient; mixed with Escherichia coli and Klebsiella species from the external auditory canal in 1 patient.
(Courtesy of Ogle, J.W., and Lauer, B.A.: Am. J. Dis. Child. 140:1178–1182, November 1986.)

All children had abnormalities of the ipsilateral tympanic membrane, and 26 (87%) had swelling above or posterior to the ear (Table 1). Acute otitis media was present in 29 children and serous otitis media in 1. Post-auricular swelling was noted in 86% of the patients. Orally administered antibiotics had been given to 42% of the patients within 2 weeks prior to hospitalization, and 36% were being treated with antibiotics at the time of admission. Findings on mastoid radiographs included clouding (12) and osteitis (7); the other 6 radiographs were normal (Table 2). Bacteria were recovered from 13 patients (43%) from normally sterile sites (Table 3). All patients were treated intravenously with antibiotics upon hospitalization until their conditions improved, at which time treatment was continued with antibiotics orally for another 3–4 weeks.

Complications occurred in 13 children, including subperiosteal abscess (7), meningitis (4), osteitis (7), facial palsy (1), and subdural empyema and brain abscess (1). Surgical procedures were performed in 14 patients, including myringotomy (3), simple mastoidectomy (9), radical mastoidectomy (1), and radical mastoidectomy plus craniotomy (1). Most patients' conditions improved rapidly. Most children with acute mastoiditis who have no meningitis or subperiosteal abscesses should first be treated with antimicrobial therapy plus myringotomy before mastoidectomy is considered.

▶ The data of this study are remarkably similar to those of a study done in Sweden (Prellner, K., et al.: *Acta Otolaryngol.* 102:52, 1986). Most of this decline in the frequency of mastoiditis occurred with the introduction of antibiotics. For those who track the frequency of mastoiditis, it has an incidence of about 1% of that just 10 years ago. In Sweden they are still performing mastoidectomies fairly commonly but, as the previously referenced study showed, most children who are operated on for mastoiditis have sterile mastoid fluid because most have been treated for several hours or for a few days with antibiotics that seemed to be capable of sterilizing such fluid. In this day and age it would seem that mastoidectomy should be reserved for those children who are not responding quickly, or in whom it is obvious that the mastoids have been destroyed and fluctuation is present. Curiously, even though the incidence of mastoiditis has diminished, the rate of complications per individual case has not changed very much at all. Mastoiditis is still a bad actor and can lead to things like meningitis.

The only bad thing about the changing trends in mastoiditis is the fact that we have a whole new generation of ENT specialists coming up who may never have operated on a child for acute mastoiditis. Well, maybe that's not so bad after all.—J.A. Stockman III, M.D.

17 Endocrinology

Isolated Growth Hormone Deficiency After Cerebral Edema Complicating Diabetic Ketoacidosis
Richard J. Keller and Joseph I. Wolfsdorf (Joslin Diabetes Ctr. and Harvard Univ.)
N. Engl. J. Med. 316:857–859, Apr. 2, 1987   17–1

Severe cerebral edema developed in a child being treated for ketoacidosis. Although the patient survived, GH deficiency was found subsequently.

Girl, 4 years 8 months, had the classic features of diabetic ketoacidosis, with a blood glucose value of 513 mg/dl; she was treated with regular insulin and bicarbonate. After 5 hours she became unresponsive and cyanotic, with gasping respirations, and the intracranial pressure was elevated at 18–22 mm Hg. Computed tomography showed cerebral edema but no midline shift (Fig 17–1). The neurologic status improved with treatment for elevated intracranial pressure, but right hemiplegia and aphasia remained. Repeat CT after 3 weeks showed resolution of cerebral edema and changes of infarction in the left temporal, thalamic, and hypothalamic regions. The diabetes was well controlled a year after presentation, when CT showed diffuse brain atrophy.

Growth of only 2 cm/year through ages 5–7 years, and a bone age of 4.5 years at a chronologic age of 7.5 years, prompted neuroendocrine studies, which documented GH deficiency. Marked endogenous insulin deficiency was confirmed, despite the small insulin requirement. Thyroid function was normal, and prolactin and gonadotropin determinations gave normal results.

This patient had growth failure and decreasing insulin requirements after recovering from cerebral edema, and GH deficiency was documented. Hypothalamic and pituitary dysfunction may develop in survivors of cerebral edema complicating diabetic ketoacidosis, and possibly also in survivors of cerebral edema of other origin.

▶ Howard S. Traisman, M.D., Professor of Pediatrics, Northwestern University Medical School, comments.—J.A. Stockman III, M.D.
▶ This is an important clinical observation about a problem that plagues diabetologists. Concern regarding cerebral edema in diabetic ketoacidosis was reported by Young and Bradley from the Joslin Clinic (*N. Engl. J. Med.* 276:665–669, 1987). Many causes have been proposed for this unpredictable complication of diabetic ketoacidosis, but nothing has been substantiated. It has been proposed that cerebral edema is secondary to cerebral hypoxia. Injury to the cerebral capillary endothelium releases substances that rapidly cause brain cell edema is another etiologic hypothesis. Prevention of this deadly complication is essential, as therapy for cerebral edema is not that successful.

Cerebral edema becomes evident about 6–10 hours after treatment for diabetic ketoacidosis has been instituted. At this time, the blood glucose level is

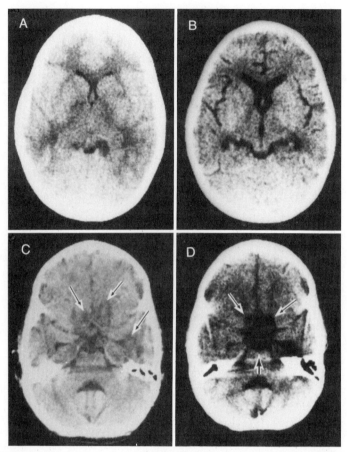

Fig 17–1.—Computed tomography scans of the head in a patient with isolated growth hormone deficiency after cerebral edema. **A,** view through the level of the lateral ventricles at the time of presentation. There is acute cerebral edema with small ventricular spaces. **B,** scan at the same level obtained 3 weeks after presentation shows resolution of the cerebral edema. The ventricular and subarachnoid spaces have become dilated. **C,** view through the level of the fourth ventricle and temporal horns 3 weeks after presentation demonstrates attenuated areas in the thalamic, hypothalamic, and left temporal areas *(arrows)*. **D,** scan obtained through the same level 1 year after presentation *(large arrow)* and wedge-shaped areas of infarction in the adjacent tissue *(small arrows)*. There is further evidence of cerebral atrophy. (Courtesy of Keller, R.J., and Wolfsdorf, J.I.: N. Engl. J. Med. 316:857–859, Apr. 2, 1987.)

approaching normal, satisfactory circulation has been established, and the patient's clinical status is improving. Headache, a sudden change in mental status, abnormal neurologic signs, and onset of coma are the stages in the development of cerebral edema. Unexplained fever as well as signs and symptoms of pulmonary edema may also signify this condition. Respiratory arrest occurs with brain stem herniation. There is a 90% mortality associated with this complication of diabetic ketoacidosis. If the patient survives, there may be severe neurologic damage. The child with diabetic ketoacidosis requires constant bedside nursing and house physician care. At the first symptom or sign of cerebral edema, mannitol should be administered and respirator care instituted with transfer to the intensive care unit. A CT scan should be performed. The CT scan can demonstrate not only increased intracranial pressure and change of ventricular size, but also thromboses and subarachnoid hemorrhage.

Avoidance of rapid and large-volume fluid replacement therapy is the best prevention. Initial fluid therapy of 20 cc of normal saline per kg during the first hour is recommended. This can be repeated if no substantial clinical improvement occurs. Ten cc of albumin or plasma expanders per kg may be used if there is evidence of hypoperfusion. Half of the replacement fluid should be given within the first 8 hours and the remaining deficit should be replaced in the next 36–48 hours. The maximum infusion should not exceed 200 cc/sq m/ hour or 4,000 cc/sq m/24 hours. Hypotonic fluids should not be used. A constant insulin infusion is recommended for patients with all but mild diabetic ketoacidosis.—H.S. Traisman, M.D.

Detection of Congenital Hypopituitary Hypothyroidism: Ten-Year Experience in the Northwest Regional Screening Program
Cheryl E. Hanna, Patricia L. Krainz, Michael R. Skeels, Richard S. Miyahira, David E. Sesser, and Stephen H. LaFranchi (Oregon Health Science Univ. and the Oregon State Public Health Lab., Portland)
J. Pediatr. 109:959–964, December 1986   17–2

The optimal strategy in screening for congenital hypothyroidism remains controversial. The primary thyroxine (T_4) test with supplemental thyrotropin (TSH) determinations can detect hypopituitary hypothyroidism as well as primary TSH screening can. The Northwest Regional Screening Program uses the primary T_4-supplemental TSH method in the detection of hypopituitary hypothyroidism. The results of its 10-year experience were evaluated to determine whether the detection of hypopituitary hypothyroidism is a justified advantage of the primary T_4-supplemental TSH strategy and to determine whether all such infants could be detected by this screening approach.

Of the 850,431 infants screened, 192 had primary hypothyroidism, for an overall frequency of 1:4,429. Nineteen infants were diagnosed as having hypopituitary hypothyroidism: eight were detected by the screening program, for a frequency of 1:106,304, and seven were detected on recognition of clinical features before a screening sample was obtained or pending test results. The other four infants were identified only in retrospect despite clinical features of hypopituitarism and a low serum T_4 level and a TSH concentration below assay sensitivity on at least one screening sample. Therefore, among the 12 infants for whom a screening sample was obtained prior to starting thyroid hormone therapy, eight (67%) were detected by the screening program. Clinical features suggestive of hypopituitarism, evident in 16 of the 19 patients, included hypoglycemia, hyperbilirubinemia, microgenitalia, diabetes insipidus, midface hypoplasia, cleft lip or palate, and abnormalities of vision. The most accurate assessment of total cases came from Oregon where all infants with congenital hypopituitarism were referred to the center; the frequency was 1:29,000. Newborn screening using T_4 with supplemental TSH determinations is a useful adjunct to recognition of clinical features in detecting infants with hypopituitary hypothyroidism.

▶ It's really fun sitting on the sidelines watching the debate about the best way to screen for congenital hypothyroidism. I've come to the conclusion that there are no answers, only cross references. Let's talk about some of these cross references.

The optimal strategy in screening for congenital hypothyroidism certainly remains controversial. Most screening programs in the United States and Canada use a primary T_4 testing supplemented by a TSH determination in those infants whose T_4 level is below a selected cutoff point. Most European and Japanese programs use primary TSH testing. One argument presented in support of the primary T_4-supplemental TSH strategy is the ability to detect infants with hypothalamic-pituitary dysfunction causing hypothyroidism. The program described in the abstract detected hypopituitary hypothyroidism at a rate of 1:106,304.

If you think everything is OK among the mavens who believe in primary T_4-supplemental TSH testing, recognize the fact that there are pitfalls. Hypopituitary hypothyroidism is often mild and screening T_4 values are not absolutely low, often falling between the third and tenth percentiles. Thus, some infants with primary hypopituitarism would be missed. However, most of these infants have clinical features related to hypopituitarism in the newborn period. This differs from congenital primary hypothyroidism in which most infants have no symptoms whatsoever. One should look for signs of neonatal hypoglycemia, persistent jaundice, microphallus, or evidence of a syndrome known to be associated with hypopituitarism, e.g., optic nerve hypoplasia, CNS abnormalities, midline facial defects, or aplasia of the pituitary gland. The presence of associated malformations and neonatal complications is well described (Fernhoff, P.M., et al.: *Lancet* 1:490, 1987). The latter investigators showed that when infants are born with congenital malformations there is often a delay in recognition that certain types of malformations are associated with congenital hypothyroidism. For example, in the Fernhoff report, infants with hypothyroidism but no congenital malformations were screened much earlier (average, 4 days vs. 13 days) and treated earlier (average, 19 days vs. 32 days). A word to the wise should be sufficient relative to all this for our neonatologist friends.

The argument continues to rage as to whether or not children with congenital hypothyroidism who are promptly given thyroid replacement achieve normal intellectual levels. Yes, says the New England Congenital Hypothyroidism Collaborative Study. The study reported at the Society for Pediatric Research meetings last spring showed that there was no significant difference in IQ or on school achievement test scores if infants were given therapy promptly after neonatal screening detection. On the other side of the fence is the report of Rovet et al. (*J. Pediatr.* 110:700, 1987). The latter investigators, looking at the Canadian data, found that if infants are divided into two groups—those with delayed bone age at the time of treatment with thyroid hormone and those with normal bone age—intellectual impairment can be demonstrated, particularly perceptual-motor, visuospatial, and with regard to language. The group that had a delayed bone age showed this phenomenon. This lends some credence to the concern that the effects of intrauterine hypothyroidism may not be reversible in some children despite very prompt postnatal treatment. Also see the article of Holtzman et al. (*Pediatrics* 78:553, 1986). These investigators tell us why infants with congenital hypothyroidism are missed by our screening programs. Most of these misses result from laboratory procedure problems.

Obviously, what we need is a test that can be performed on the mother to detect the carriage of an infant affected with congenital hypothyroidism. To date, there has been no valid test for such a problem except in women known to have preexisting thyroid disorders themselves. As an interesting aside, Professor Tato and colleagues (*Lancet* 1:803, 1987) found no infants with congenital hypothyroidism in northeast Italy between May and October of 1986 when pregnant women were taking extra iodine after the Chernobyl incident. They speculated that giving pregnant women iodized salt could be important in preventing the presence of congenital hypothyroidism. What an intriguing idea! What a way to have to come up with this fascinating approach—a nuclear accident! The Chernobyl accident is proof positive that nothing is as inevitable as a mistake whose time has come.

By now you're probably tired reading this long-winded commentary. What you've read is nothing more than a variation on the old story of what is the best way to deal with the problem of congenital hypothyroidism. It doesn't seem to matter whether the facts indicate one thing or another; they always seem to be interpreted whatever way a particular investigative group wants. Frank Lloyd Wright probably had the right idea when he said, "If your facts are wrong but your logic is perfect, then your conclusions are inevitably false. Therefore by making mistakes in your logic, you have at least a random chance of coming to a correct conclusion." How apt this is to the thyroid controversy.—J.A. Stockman III, M.D.

Reversibility of Severe Hypothyroidism With Supplementary Iodine in Patients With Endemic Cretinism

Jean B. Vanderpas, Maria T. Rivera-Vanderpas, Pierre Bourdoux, Kapata Luvivila, Raphael Lagasse, Noémi Perlmutter-Cremer, François Delange, Leo Lanoie, André M. Ermans, and Claude H. Thilly (Free Univ. of Brussels and Saint-Pierre Univ. Hosp., Brussels, Institut de Recherche Scientifique, Kinshasa, Zaire, and Communauté Evangelique de l'Ubangi-Mongala, Karawa, Zaire)
N. Engl. J. Med. 315:791–795, Sept. 25, 1986   17–3

The reversibility of thyroid dysfunction in children with endemic cretinism treated with supplemental iodine is unknown. To address this question, 51 patients with cretinism, aged 14 years or younger, were randomly assigned to receive 0.5 ml of iodized oil intramuscularly or no treatment. Patients were further subdivided into younger (less than 4 years) and older (4–14 years) groups. All patients had severe hypothyroidism initially, with a geometric mean serum thyrotropin level of 223 μU/ml and a mean initial serum level of thyroxine of 1.0 μg/dl. Thyroid function was reassessed for 5 months after treatment.

Within 1 month after iodine supplementation, significantly more younger patients (13 of 14) had thyrotropin values of less than 20 μU/ml than older patients (1 of 9) had. At 5 months after treatment, thyroid hormone levels were within the euthyroid range in all of the younger patients but only in some of the older ones (2 of 14 children, thyrotropin; 8 of 14, thyroxine; and 9 of 13, triiodothyronine). In the untreated group, three of the nine younger children but none of the older children regained normal thyroid function despite the persistence of a very low supply of iodine.

Correction of iodine deficiency results in a biochemical euthyroid state in all younger children with cretinism but only in certain older children, suggesting that the thyroid may be irreversibly impaired in some older patients with cretinism. This age-dependent reversibility of severe hypothyroidism with iodine supplementation supports the hypothesis that a progressive loss of functional capacity of the thyroid occurs in some patients with cretinism. In addition, spontaneous recovery of normal thyroid function can occur in younger cretins.

▶ Endemic cretinism constitutes the principal public health problem associated with iodine deficiency. This syndrome has two clinical presentations. Neurologic cretinism is characterized by mental deficiency, spastic diplegia, an ataxic gait, abnormal hearing, and strabismus; it is not necessarily associated with either stunted growth or hypothyroidism. Myxedematous cretinism is characterized by various levels of mental deficiency, stunted growth, and overt hypothyroidism; neurologic signs are discrete or absent. The distribution of the two forms varies substantially according to the endemic area, and mixed forms also are encountered. In countries such as Zaire, the mixed endemic form of cretinism is the most common. The pathogenesis is poorly understood. Hypothyroidism is established in early life, and the clinical picture is similar to that of sporadic cretinism.

The disorder can be prevented by administration of slowly absorbable iodine to women during their last 3 months of pregnancy; the success of this procedure suggests that the thyroid gland is intact in hypothyroid fetuses. In contrast, adults with cretinism have severe alterations of the thyroid gland; iodine uptake and the iodine pool are markedly lower than in normal adults. The study abstracted above shows that early diagnosis and introduction of iodine into a child's diet is likely to reverse abnormal thyroid function. Waiting until a child is older, however, may result in permanent, presumably structural, changes in the thyroid gland that may be associated with permanent hypothyroidism, even in the presence of adequate amounts of iodine.

Endemic cretinism still occurs even in the United States, although it is a rare phenomenon. One must be careful about the use of iodine in a pregnant woman, however, if one is trying to maintain thyroid function in the fetus. Recently, a 6-week-old girl was described who had transient congenital hypothyroidism. The hypothyroidism appeared to result from the topical use of a solution of povidone iodine in a pregnant woman. The solution was used to help control furunculosis. The mother also was breast-feeding this infant. The amount of iodine absorbed through the skin remarkably shut off thyroxine production. Unfortunately, povidone iodine is a common topical antiseptic and is not always considered by mothers to be a drug; in some instances we may miss hypothyroidism resulting from this cause as opposed to congenital hypothyroidism. The former cause, of course, is transient (Danziger, Y., et al.: *Arch. Dis. Child.* 62:296, 1987).

If you make a diagnosis of hypothyroidism in a child, think of two other well-established associations: the presence of hypercalcemia and acquired von Willebrand's disease. Children with congenital hypothyroidism may have elevated serum calcium concentrations before and during treatment with thyroid hormones. This phenomenon occurs only occasionally in children and is rare in adults. Hypersensitivity to vitamin D has been proposed as a possible cause or as an aggravating factor of the hypercalcemia in children with hypothyroidism. In any event, at least one study to date suggests that we should be following serum calcium levels when attempting to manage children with congenital hypothyroidism (Tau, C., et al.: *J. Pediatr.* 109:808, 1986).

As far as von Willebrand's disease is concerned, several individuals have now been described who at the time of presentation for treatment of hypothyroidism also had bleeding manifestations. Their coagulation profiles were entirely consistent with von Willebrand's disease. Each of the patients had a prolonged bleeding time in the presence of normal platelet function, low coagulant assays for factor VIII, and abnormal von Willebrand's factor antigen assays. Treatment with thyroid hormone rapidly corrected the coagulation disorders (Smith, S.R., et al.: *Lancet* 1:1314, 1987).

Before leaving the topic of hypothyroidism, it never hurts to emphasize that children with Down's syndrome have a very high rate of congenital or acquired hypothyroidism. The congenital form usually results from athyroidism or from dyshormonogenesis. The acquired form may be caused by lymphocytic thyroiditis or by dysplasia, or by the coexistence of both conditions (Radetti, G., et al.: *Helv. Paediatr. Acta* 41:377, 1986). It is increasingly important to detect these problems in children with Down's syndrome because the average life expectancy of such children who have no cardiac abnormalities is approaching that of the general population.—J.A. Stockman III, M.D.

Comparison of Dose Frequency of Human Growth Hormone in Treatment of Organic and Idiopathic Hypopituitarism

Wayne V. Moore, Selna Kaplan, Salvatore Raiti, and The National Hormone and Pituitary Program (NHPP), Growth Hormone Committee (Univ. of Kansas, Univ. of California at San Francisco, and Univ. of Maryland)
J. Pediatr. 110:144–148, January 1987   17–4

The optimal dosage and schedule of administration of human growth hormone (hGH) for the treatment of short stature associated with GH deficiency remains to be established. The effects on the growth rate of two weekly injections of pituitary hGH and three weekly injections for a total dose of 0.24 international units of hGH per kg were compared during the first and second years of therapy in children with idiopathic and organic hypopituitarism. Crossovers in the dosage schedule were made at 6, 12, and 18 months after the start.

In the first 6 months, patients with organic hypopituitarism had significantly increased growth rates with either two or three weekly injections. However, the growth rate was significantly decreased in patients switched from three times weekly dosing to biweekly dosing compared with a nonsignificant growth change in those switched from biweekly to three times weekly dosing. In contrast, patients with idiopathic hypopituitarism in either dosage regimen did not have significant growth changes during the first 6 months of therapy. After the first crossover, patients who switched from three times weekly to twice weekly injections had a significant decrease in growth rate, whereas those who switched to three times weekly doses retained their initial growth rates. There was no advantage to therapy three times weekly during the second year of therapy in either group. The additional increment in height after 1 year of three weekly injections was approximately 1–2 cm/year greater than in the group given biweekly therapy. However, this increment should be weighed against the pain, cost, and inconvenience of the three times per week dosing as compared with biweekly therapy.

These data indicate that the three injections of hGH weekly are more effective in the first 6 months of therapy in patients with organic hypopituitarism and during the second 6 months in patients with idiopathic hypopituitarism. Three weekly injections of hGH are recommended in the first year for the treatment of GH deficiency, followed by biweekly injections should long-term therapy be indicated. Neither of these therapy regimens, however, represents optimal management. Other schedules of treatment should be evaluated for an optimal dosage and dose schedule for hGH therapy for GH deficiency.

▶ Dr. Joseph M. Gertner, Program Director, Pediatric Clinical Research Center, The New York Hospital-Cornell Medical Center, comments.—J.A. Stockman III, M.D.

▶ In the past few years, genetic engineering has promised to make useful but scarce therapeutic agents widely available. Human GH was the first, and remains the only, approved agent for which this promise has been fulfilled. By remarkable coincidence, trials of recombinant GH had reached their final stages when, in 1985, the sparse supply of GH extracted from human pituitaries was interrupted by the discovery of a handful of patients with Creutzfeld-Jacob disease, all long-term recipients of the hormone (Brown, P., et al.: *N. Engl. J. Med.* 313:728–731, 1985). The extracted hormone is no longer available in the United States, but two recombinant products, methionyl hGH (Protropin, Genentech) and natural GH (Humatrope, Eli Lilly), are now approved for prescription.

Whereas the price of recombinant GH remains high, the reality is that we have moved from an age of GH famine to one of feast. The ready availability of GH, and the presumption that its price will fall considerably as production costs are amortized, force pediatricians to make new choices and consider hitherto unavailable options. Major questions to be addressed include the following: (1) What are the relative merits of methionyl and methionyl-free GH? (2) What are the optimal dose, frequency, and route of administration of GH? (3) What is "GH deficiency," and can the growth of nondeficient children be improved with GH? (4) What is the potential usefulness of GH for conditions other than short stature? The latter question will not receive further consideration in this review.

1.—*The relative merits of methionyl and methionyl-free GH.* Methionyl GH has an extra amino acid (methionine) at the "N terminal" end of the GH molecule. Growth hormone was produced in this way for technical reasons. The ability to synthesize a methionine-free (identical to natural human GH) recombinant product came later after methionyl GH had already received extensive clinical trials. The perceived advantage of the methionine-free form is that, being identical with natural GH, it might be less likely to induce anti-GH antibodies in the recipient. However, current data suggest that the incidence of antibodies of measurable binding capacity is about the same (less than 3%) to Protropin as to Humatrope. At this stage we can regard the two products as therapeutically equivalent.

2.—*Optimal dose, frequency, and route of administration.* The dose of GH formerly provided to deficient patients by the National Hormone and Pituitary Program (NHPP) was 0.1 unit per kg three times weekly intramuscularly. This dose was chosen because it was the minimum effective dose and was, in essence, forced on prescribers of GH by the severe shortage of extracted GH. Data from the initial large trials of Protropin (Kaplan, S.L., et al.: *Lancet* 1:697–700, 1986) and from a small trial using high doses of extracted GH (Gertner, J.M., et al., 1987, personal communication) suggest that improved growth rates can be attained when doses two to three times higher than old NHPP standard (i.e., 0.6–0.9 unit per kg per week) are used. The long-term efficacy of any increase in dose, and the ultimate safety of these higher doses, remain to be determined.

Questions concerning the best route and frequency of GH administration have been reexamined. Growth hormone can be safely and effectively given subcutaneously, and we have demonstrated the effectiveness of giving GH by continuous subcutaneous infusion using a battery-powered syringe pump. Clinical trials of daily versus three times weekly administration are now in progress. No conclusion can yet be drawn as to the optimal frequency of administration (see the preceding abstract), but there is a growing consensus that subcutaneous injection is just as effective as intramuscular injection and is more acceptable to the patient.

3.—*What is "GH deficiency," and can the growth of nondeficient children be improved with GH?* Poorly growing children who fail to attain serum GH levels above 7 ng/ml after provocative stimuli (e.g., insulin hypoglycemia) may be regarded as "classically" GH deficient. They usually respond well to GH replacement. Recent publications have confirmed observations from the 60s that some short children not "classically" GH deficient may have accelerated growth with GH therapy. It remains very much an open question as to how we can predict which nondeficient children will show such responses, however. It has been suggested (Spiliotis, B.E., et al.: *JAMA* 251:2223–2330, 1984) that reduced spontaneous GH secretion, especially at night, may indicate a type of "physiologic" GH deficiency, even in children who respond normally to pharmacologic tests for GH release. However, these sleep studies are tedious to perform and, while the theory underlying them sounds logical, it has not yet been shown that 24-hour or nighttime GH sampling can help us to decide who should receive treatment.

Attitudes and practice regarding GH therapy are changing rapidly. Many pharmacologic, physiologic, and ethical issues remain to be resolved as we struggle for the answers as to who should be treated, how, and, not least, why.—J.M. Gertner, M.D.

Addison Disease in Children: Associated Anomalies
G. Kalifa, B. Silberman, J.L. Chaussain, C. Diebler, and J. Bennet (Hôpital Saint-Vincent de Paul, Paris)
Ann. Radiol. 29:327–332, 1986   17–5

Addison's disease, or adrenal insufficiency, in children is characterized by a distinct clinical and biologic pattern; it is frequently associated with other primary or secondary adrenal abnormalities of hereditary origin. A retrospective review was made of the case reports of all children with Addison's disease who were treated between 1972 and 1985.

The series included 56 children, 47 boys (85%) and 9 girls aged 12 days to 16 years, in whom Addison's disease was diagnosed on the basis of elevated ACTH levels and the absence of the plasma cortisol response to tetracosactide stimulation. Five infants less than 8 months old had congenital Addison's disease. Of 56 children, 25 had associated adrenoleukodystrophy, 13 had autoimmune adrenal insufficiency, 5 had congenital Addison achalasia-alacrimation syndrome, 8 had congenital adrenal hypoplasia, and 5 had unclassified disorders. Most of the patients had associated mineralocorticoid and glucocorticoid deficits.

Addison's disease was diagnosed on the basis of presenting symptoms of adrenal insufficiency in only 30 of 56 patients. In the others the diagnosis was reached by a systematic search of family histories. A hereditary link was found in 50% of the children. Of eight patients with congenital adrenal hypoplasia, four had early osteoporosis that did not respond to treatment. None of these children had abnormal calcium or phosphorus metabolism. Adrenoleukodystrophy represented the largest group of associated disorders. There was no relationship between CT findings and the clinical condition. A diagnosis of autoimmune Addison's disease was made on the basis of testing for human leukocyte antigen antibodies.

Because of the high incidence of associated disorders found in boys with Addison's disease, CT examinations, upper gastrointestinal tract x-ray studies, and skeletal studies should be done routinely in these patients. Boys with achalasia and leukodystrophy should be examined for the presence of asymptomatic Addison's disease.

▶ Orville C. Green, M.D., Professor of Pediatrics, Northwestern University

Medical School, and Director of Endocrinology, Children's Memorial Hospital, Chicago, comments.—J.A. Stockman III, M.D.

▶ This paper appears in a radiologic journal, was written by radiologists, and consequently is slanted toward technical studies in that specialty. The authors lump all of the etiologic causes of adrenal problems seen by them into one bag and recommend a series of radiologic studies (CT, gastrointestinal series, and skeletal evaluations) as routine procedures in all forms of adrenal disease. Clinicians dealing with problems of adrenal disease in children are more likely to divide the classification into etiologic causes before ordering a series of expensive radiologic investigations as routine procedures. The radiologic bias is evident in the etiologic list, with 45% of these conditions caused by adrenoleukodystrophy and 9% caused by the syndrome of adrenal insufficiency, achalasia, and alacrima (AAA syndrome). The incidence of adrenal insufficiency in most pediatric clinics is primarily attributed to two disorders: congenital virilizing adrenal hyperplasia and acquired autoimmune disease.

All textbooks stress the autoimmune basis for acquired disease and the fact that such children may also have other autoimmune disorders, if not at presentation, possibly in the future. Follow-up medical evaluations must always involve detailed system review and a careful physical examination. Scattergun laboratory and radiologic evaluations seem unwarranted, even in the rare families subject to adrenoleukodystrophy. if there were some form of therapy for the neurologic deterioration that occurs in that disease, frequent CT scans might be of value, but in the absence of such therapy the disease will manifest itself clinically without repeated costly interventions. In agreement with this report, it is certainly true that every child with alacrima must be carefully examined for adrenal and esophageal disease; these are treatable. These children are usually first seen by an ophthalmologist.

Most endocrinologists today reserve the term "Addison's disease" for deficiencies of all adrenal zones (glucocorticoid, mineralocorticoid, and androgen). Patients with adrenoleukodystrophy and AAA syndrome may only have glucocorticoid deficiencies when first seen. Any patient with the separate or combined unexplained problem of pigmentation, hypoglycemia, recurrent vomiting, or circulatory collapse with illness must be suspect for adrenal disease. In most cases, the pediatrician will find the neonatal cause to be congenital in origin (adrenal hyperplasia, adrenal hypoplasia, or adrenal hemorrhage) and the later onset to be autoimmune in origin. It is helpful to be reminded by radiologists that such patients may also have the rarer forms associated with adrenoleukodystrophy and AAA syndrome, but this reviewer believes the clinician will detect such patients without subjecting all of those with adrenal disorders to multiple routine radiologic studies.

In the Endocrine Clinic of The Children's Memorial Hospital of Chicago, the frequency of adrenal insufficiency during a 23-year period is as follows: Salt-losing form of congenital virilizing adrenal hyperplasia, 52 patients; acquired autoimmune disease, 18; adrenal hypoplasia, 2; adrenoleukodystrophy, 3; and AAA syndrome, 1, for a total of 76 patients. Of the 18 patients with acquired autoimmune disease, 5 had hypothyroidism alone, 1 had diabetes mellitus alone, 2 had hypothyroidism plus diabetes mellitus, and 1 had vitiligo.—O.C. Green, M.D.

Treatment of Growth-Hormone Deficiency With Growth-Hormone-Releasing Hormone

R.J.M. Ross, C. Rodda, S. Tsagarakis, P.S.W. Davies, A. Grossman, L.H. Rees, M.A. Preece, M.O. Savage, and G.M. Besser (St. Bartholomew's Hosp. and Inst. of Child Health, London)
Lancet 1:5–8, Jan. 3, 1987   17–6

Most GH-deficient children have a hypothalamic defect in GH release and will show a GH response after the administration of GH-releasing hormone (GHRH). Eight pre-pubertal GH-deficient children were treated with twice-daily subcutaneous injections of the GHRH analogue, GHRH (1-29) NH2. Doses were 250 µg and 500 µg for children weighing less than and more than 20 kg, respectively. Treatment lasted for 6–12 months in 14 patients and 18 months in 1. Fifteen patients previously received human GH (hGH).

Height velocity increased in 12 children after GHRH treatment. In eight of these children, height velocity increased by more than 2 cm/year (range, 2.7–11.2 cm/year) during the first 6 months of treatment. These children have now been treated for 6–18 months and their increase in height velocity has been maintained. Of the patients previously treated with hGH, height velocity during GHRH treatment correlated well with height velocity while they were taking hGH. However, for unknown reasons, four of these patients had growth deceleration with GHRH. When the peak pretreatment serum GH response to intravenously administered GHRH was more than 30 mU/ml, the response to GHRH was good; a lower peak did not preclude a growth response, however. There was no evidence of a desensitization or consistent priming effect of GHRH therapy on either growth or serum GH responses to GHRH. Anti-GHRH antibodies developed in 14 patients but had no effect on the growth or GH responses to GHRH. Except for slight stinging at the site of injection, adverse side effects were not noted.

The twice-daily administration of GHRH (1-29) NH2 subcutaneously is as effective as conventional hGH in the treatment of certain GH-deficient children. Other methods of administration need to be evaluated.

▶ Alan D. Rogol, M.D., Ph.D., Professor of Pediatrics and Pharmacology, University of Virginia School of Medicine, Charlottesville, comments.—J.A. Stockman III, M.D.

▶ The study of Ross and co-workers treating GH-deficient children uses the precept that many (most) GH-deficient children have hypothalamic dysfunction rather than a deficit of pituitary somatotropes. Thus, replacement therapy with GHRH (or an active analogue, in this case) represents a more physiologic approach to hormonal replacement.

Is this form of therapy as efficacious and safe as the standard therapy, i.e., hGH given intramuscularly or subcutaneously three times a week? At present, this question is moot because of the problem of Creutzfeldt-Jakob disease in young adults with hypopituitarism previously treated with human cadaveric GH. However, previous data and those being gathered at present with several preparations of recombinant hGH indicate that growth rates of 8–12 cm/year are attainable in children with hypopituitarism.

The children in this study represent a mixture of patients with hypopituitarism of several etiologies, many of whom had been treated with GH in the recent past. They were divided arbitrarily into "responders" and "nonresponders." The growth rates of the responders were within the lower range of those expected with GH, especially since many had been taking long-term therapy and it is well known that the growth rate decelerates with increasing duration of therapy. However, a large percentage of children did not respond with accelerated or "catch-up" growth. Does it mean that this pharmacologic agent will be useful only in highly selected children?

Our own ongoing studies published only in part (*N. Engl. J. Med.* 312:4–9, 1985, and *Clin. Endocrinol.* 25:35–44, 1986) indicated that unselected, previously untreated GH-deficient children will attain markedly accelerated growth rates given GHRH every 3 hours for 12 or 24 hours, or given subcutaneous injections twice a day at a dose of 8–16 μg/kg/day. Are there pertinent differences between our study and that of Ross and co-workers that might account for the lesser number of patients and degree of response in the latter study? Although no single factor defines the differences in these studies, there may be subtle ones because of cranial irradiation in some of the patients in the Ross study (however, some were responders and some did not respond) and because many had been treated recently with GH and probably were still in the "catch-down" phase of their growth.

What then may be concluded about this newly described growth factor? We can say that (1) it is safe and efficacious in most GH-deficient patients, and (2) a dose of at least 8 μg/kg/day is required in most patients, although other factors may preclude efficacy within that dose range.

The ultimate role of this agent and its agonist analogues in the treatment of GH deficiency is presently being determined. The optimal preparation, dose, route, and frequency of administration have yet to be determined. However, there are theoretical reasons for believing that a sustained release preparation of GHRH may be effective in restoring intermittent pulsatile GH secretion (the physiologic mode) and accelerated linear growth in GH-deficient children.— A.D. Rogol, M.D., Ph.D.

Methionyl Human Growth Hormone and Oxandrolone in Turner Syndrome: Preliminary Results of a Prospective Randomized Trial

Ron G. Rosenfeld, Raymond L. Hintz, Ann J. Johanson, Jo Anne Brasel, Stephen Burstein, Steven D. Chernausek, Teresa Clabots, James Frane, Ronald W. Gotlin, Joyce Kuntze, Barbara M. Lippe, Patrick C. Mahoney, Wayne V. Moore, Maria I. New, Paul Saenger, Elizabeth Stoner, and Virginia Sybert (Stanford Univ., and other medical centers in the United States)
J. Pediatr. 109:936–943, December 1986   17–7

Because of the inevitable reduced adult height of patients with Turner's syndrome, numerous studies have assessed the potential therapeutic value of androgens, estrogens, and human GH (hGH) in these patients. Seventy girls with Turner's syndrome, ranging in age from 4 to 12 years (mean, 9.3 years), were randomly assigned to one of four study groups: (1) control, no treatment; (2) methionyl hGH, 0.125 mg/kg intramuscularly three times per week; (3) oxandrolone, 0.125 mg/kg/day orally; or (4) a combination of methionyl-hGH and oxandrolone. Baseline growth rates averaged 4.3 cm/year, and all were within 2 SD of the mean growth velocity for age in girls with Turner's syndrome.

Sixty-seven girls remained in the study for a minimum of 1 year. Twelve-month cumulative growth rates and growth velocity in all treatment groups were significantly greater than baseline growth rates and the rate of the control group. The mean growth rates and growth velocity (in SD for age in girls with Turner's syndrome) were 6.6 cm/year ($+2.3$ SD) for hGH, 7.9 cm/year ($+3.7$ SD) for oxandrolone, and 9.8 cm/year ($+5.4$ SD) for combination therapy, compared with 3.8 cm/year (-0.1 SD) for the control group. The groups receiving methionyl hGH and combination therapy had significantly elevated levels of plasma somatomedin-C. Oxandrolone, either alone or in combination, did not stimulate elevation in plasma somatomedin-C levels. The mean bone age was advanced 1.0 year by methionyl hGH, 1.3 years by oxandrolone, and 1.6 years by combination therapy. However, median increments in height age:bone age ratios ranged from 1.0 to 1.1 for treatment groups, compared with 0.8 for controls. In addition, the predicted adult height with the Bayley-Pinneau method was significantly increased in all treatment groups, with a 2.5-cm increase for either oxandrolone or methionyl hGH and 3.2 cm for combination therapy. Except for mild clitoral enlargement and accelerated skeletal maturation in patients given oxandrolone, no other serious side effects were noted. Both hGH and oxandrolone, alone or in combination, can stimulate short-term skeletal growth and possibly increase final adult height.

▶ Although considerable variability in the phenotypic expression of Turner's syndrome exists, the overwhelming majority of patients have short stature as adults. Because of the virtual inevitability of reduced adult height, numerous studies have been performed to assess the potential value of treatment with androgens, estrogens, and hGH. Most of these studies have been small in scale, uncontrolled, and generally retrospective. The Rosenfeld study, however, does meet the criteria for an adequately designed investigation and does show that children with Turner's syndrome can have acceleration of their growth with the use of GH. Now that the biosynthethic hormone is widely available, the amounts required for treatment of children with Turner's syndrome are now feasibly available. Ross et al. (*J. Clin. Endocrinol. Metab.* 63:1028, 1986) have also shown that biosynthethic GH increases growth rates in children with Turner's syndrome. They have also worked out the doses required. The amount used, 0.15 unit/kg three times weekly, is feasible given the availability of biosynthetic hormone. The amounts required are quite a bit in excess of what would be used for primary GH deficiency.

To date, no one knows exactly how tall girls with Turner's syndrome will be with the use of GH. Unlike other situations in which there may be abuses of biosynthetic GH use, Turner's syndrome seems to be a legitimate disorder that should be treated in an attempt to achieve as near maximal growth as possible. We do, however, need to learn more about the side effects of these larger doses of GH. Raiti et al. (*J. Pediatr.* 109:944, 1986) also have shown the same results in the management of Turner's syndrome with biosynthetic GH.

Biosynthethic GH is expensive. The dollar cost for treatment of primary GH deficiency is on the order of $10,000 to $20,000 yearly for the product alone. It is possible that one can get more punch for the money by adding to the GH therapy a simple antihistamine, cyproheptadine. Cyproheptadine, an antihistamine with serotonin antagonist activity, has a well-documented stimulatory effect on appetite. Theoretically, a sustained increase in caloric intake should enhance the growth stimulatory actions of GH, particularly in children in whom weight gain is suboptimal. Furthermore, an enhanced caloric intake might counteract the waning effects of GH after the first year of treatment that may be secondary to depletion of the subcutaneous fat stores initially present in most patients with GH deficiency.

Kaplowitz et al. (*J. Pediatr.* 110:140, 1987) have shown precisely this. In a preliminary report they found that weight gain induced by cyproheptadine results in improved linear growth in patients receiving GH, and that this drug may be useful in optimizing the response to GH therapy. Aside from mild, usually transient drowsiness, the use of this drug has been associated with no significant side effects. It would be nice if the data of this latter report hold up so that we can perhaps minimize the amount of GH that needs to be used. Right now, some investigators are using extraordinary amounts of GH for various forms of dwarfism, Turner's syndrome, and so on, in a kind of overkill, similar to Patty Reagan's wedding. The number of guests at that wedding was 134. The number of secret service agents and other peace keepers present was 180. That truly was overkill, or certainly some exclusive wedding!—J.A. Stockman III, M.D.

Treatment of Precocious Puberty in the McCune-Albright Syndrome With the Aromatase Inhibitor Testolactone

Penelope P. Feuillan, Carol M. Foster, Ora H. Pescovitz, Karen D. Hench, Thomas Shawker, Andrew Dwyer, James D. Malley, Kevin Barnes, D. Lynn Loriaux, and Gordon B. Cutler, Jr. (Natl. Inst. of Child Health and Human Development and Dept. of Radiology and Div. of Computer Res. and Technology, NIH, Bethesda, Mott Children's Hosp., Ann Arbor, and Univ. of Minnesota)
N. Engl. J. Med. 315:1115–1119, Oct. 30, 1986   17–8

The McCune-Albright syndrome, or fibrous dysplasia of bone with precocious puberty and café au lait pigmentation, is characterized by marked fluctuations in plasma estrogen levels. Aromatase inhibitors, which block the final step in estrogen synthesis, might reduce ovarian estradiol secretion in these patients. Testolactone, an aromatase inhibitor, was used to treat five girls with McCune-Albright syndrome after success was obtained in a pilot case. All five patients had lesions of fibrous dysplasia, and all but one had areas of café au lait pigmentation.

Testolactone was given in doses up to 40 mg/kg daily and was withheld temporarily from four patients after a 2-month trial. The mean plasma estradiol level fell from 163 pg/ml to 32 pg/ml during testolactone therapy and rose again when treatment was stopped. Estrone levels followed a similar pattern. Ovarian volume decreased during treatment. Follicle-stimulating hormone levels increased significantly. Growth rates declined during treatment with testolactone, and the mean rate of bone maturation decreased from 2 to 1.4 bone-age years per chronologic year. Menstrual bleeding decreased in frequency. One patient had transient diarrhea during treatment. Testolactone therapy had favorable effects in these girls with McCune-Albright syndrome, and the drug was well tolerated.

▶ Conventional therapy for central precocious puberty has been limited to the progestational agent medroxyprogesterone acetate, or the progestational antiandrogen, cyproterone acetate. These agents have not been uniformly successful in halting the progression of the secondary sexual changes and have had little or no effect on the rapid bone growth and early epiphyseal fusion that lead to the adult short stature associated with precocious puberty. These drugs also cause significant side effects, e.g., cushingoid features, adrenal suppression, and chromosomal breakage. Thus, enter stage left, the aromatase inhibitor, testolactone. Aromatase inhibitors block the last step in estrogen biosynthesis and have been used for more than 20 years to treat women with estrogen-dependent breast cancer. Most importantly, testolactone has no demonstrated important side effects. The McCune-Albright syndrome was first recognized 50 years ago as an association of fibrous dysplasia of bone, café au lait pigmentation, and precocious puberty. In these patients, plasma estrogen levels may fluctuate dramatically at intervals of 4–6 weeks. Sequential pelvic ultrasound has demonstrated the growth and disappearance of large ovarian cysts that parallel the rise and fall of plasma estrogens. Thus, the McCune-Albright syndrome would be a perfect model in which to use a drug such as testolactone to prevent the onset of precocious puberty. Indeed, as the abstract indicates, this drug is effective in the management of the precocious puberty that is associated with this syndrome.

Administration of long-acting analogues of LHRH inhibits the release of LH and FSH. Short-term administration of LHRH suppresses gonadotropins and sex steroids in children with central precocious puberty. Thus, this is another means of treatment for central precocious puberty (Comite, F., et al.: *JAMA* 255:2613, 1986). In the latter report, this drug was used for more than 4 years in a group of children to delay the onset of precocious puberty. No significant side effects were noted whatsoever.

Ketoconazole may also be a worthwhile agent in the management of certain children with precocious puberty. This, of course, is an antifungal agent. It induces inhibition of androgen production, predominantly through inhibition of the C_{17-20} lyase step in testosterone biosynthesis. Ketoconazole, therefore, is useful in the control of precocious sexual puberty in boys with gonadotropin-independent precocious puberty, so-called testotoxicosis (Holland, F.J., et al.: *J. Clin. Endocrinol. Metab.* 64:328, 1987; Root, A.W., et al.: *J. Pediatr.* 109:1012, 1986). Perhaps soon we will see one or more of these drugs used in combination to help attack the precocious puberty in the Kabuki makeup syndrome (mental retardation, postnatal dwarfism, peculiar facies, skeletal anomalies, and precocious puberty) (Kuroki, Y., et al.: *J. Pediatr.* 110:750, 1987).

If you are interested in reading more about these problems, see the excellent editorial comment in *The Lancet* (1:1179, 1987). Analogues of LHRH may well be the wave of the future in contraception methods. Ovarian function, spermatogenesis, and the production of sex steroid hormones are dependent on appropriate stimulation from the anterior pituitary gland hormones, i.e., LH and FSH. These hormones in turn are controlled by the decapeptide LHRH, which is released from the hypothalamus in pulses every 1–2 hours in amounts controlled by feedback of the sex steroid hormones. The relatively recent development of LHRH analogues has produced ways of "switching off" the pituitary access. Studies from Sweden, West Germany, and the United States have shown that LHRH analogues such as buserelin effectively shut off the CNS axis and are potent contraceptive agents. The main problem with these drugs is that they suppress estrogen production and can cause hot flashes, vaginal dryness, and alter bone mineral metabolism. Theoretically, such agents should also work in men, but the findings to date suggest that complete azoospermia for effective male contraception does not occur. The man is off the hook again.

To conclude this commentary, if there is one absolute indication for the use of drugs to prevent precocious puberty, it would be the Barbie doll. The Barbie doll was introduced by the Mattel Toy Company in 1959. The Barbie doll was the brain child of the company's founders, Ruth and Elliott Handler, who noticed in the Eisenhower years that their daughter Barbie preferred teenage cut-out dolls to the then rampant burpers and cooers. The idea behind the Barbie doll was to make young children want to grow up to be fashionable adults. Success was indeed found. It has been estimated that laid end-to-end, the number of existing Barbie dolls would orbit the Earth four times around. The reason for mentioning the use of agents to prevent precocious puberty is based on the recently disclosed information about what Barbie's measurements would be if she were life sized. They are fairly dramatic (39–23–33). No wonder the dolls have a difficult time standing up straight without falling over.—J.A. Stockman III, M.D.

Growth Hormone Secretion in Patients With Constitutional Delay of Growth and Pubertal Development

Roberto Lanes, Lottys Bohorquez, Vianey Leal, Guadalope Hernández, Marietta Borges, Evelyn Hurtado, and Gustavo Moncada (Hosp. Central "Dr. Carlos Arvelo," Caracas)
J. Pediatr. 109:781–783, November 1986   17–9

Constitutional growth delay (CGD) is a frequent cause of short stature, and children with CGD usually have normal growth rates, with a growth curve parallel to but below the fifth percentile. These children have marked retardation of skeletal age that approximates that of height age, delayed sexual maturation, tend eventually to attain normal adult height, and are commonly believed to have no endocrine or medical abnormalities. However, several reports have suggested that patients with CGD may have decreased GH responses to provocative stimuli before puberty and diminished spontaneous GH secretion during sleep. Whether children with CGD have decreased GH secretion was investigated.

Growth hormone concentrations were measured after stimulation with clonidine and during frequent overnight sampling. Somatomedin C concentrations were determined in 20 prepubertal children with GCD and their GH responses were compared with those of 10 prepubertal control children. There was no significant difference in mean 9-hour overnight GH concentrations between groups (4.5 ng/ml in the CGD group and 4.4 ng/ml in the control group). The mean total GH output (258 units vs. 222 units), total number of nocturnal GH pulses (3.6 vs. 3.3), peak GH response during nocturnal sampling (13 ng/ml vs. 13.2 mg/ml), and basal somatomedin C concentration did not differ in children with growth delay and controls. Prepubertal patients with constitutional delay of growth and puberty secrete GH normally and do not seem to have any abnormality in GH regulation.

▶ This report may put one more nail in the coffin of those who fiddle around with children with constitutional delay of growth. These investigators showed no evidence of defective GH responses to provocative stimulation.

An international workshop on advances in research on human GH (hGH) was sponsored by the National Institutes of Child Health and Human Development in late 1986 (Kolata, G.: *Science* 234:22, 1986). The participants all agreed that companies are tooling up to produce huge quantities of hGH using recombinant DNA technology. They also believe that these companies are not planning to market the drug solely for treatment of pituitary dwarfs, because there aren't that many to treat. Their concern for the short term was that many affluent parents of constitutionally short children will have them treated with GH. Another abuse would be the use of GH to obviate dieting as a method of weight reduction. Another misuse clearly will be the black market for it among athletes. Some have speculated that GH may even retard aging, improve wrinkles, and redistribute fat deposits in older people. Some drug!

I suppose we're lucky that some common sense is being advised with respect to the potential indiscriminate administration of GH. In a review of GH treatment and a decision to treat or not treat, Bercu makes the following statement: "The pediatrician can play a critical role in the early identification of children with growth problems, thereby giving the pediatric endocrinologist an opportunity to help the child (most important) grow to a height as close as possible to that of his or her peers and, ultimately, come closer to achieving his or her genetic potential. As pediatric endocrinologists, we strongly and vehemently discourage the indiscriminate use of growth hormone in all short children, regardless of cost. We further condemn the use of growth hormone as a treatment to achieve weight loss, and in athletes, body builders, and weight lifters, in whom growth is not even the desired end point. The decision to treat the short child is best left to the pediatric endocrinologist, as the individual most experienced in problems of growth and sexual development." The latter comments are articulated in more detail in a commentary by Dr. Robert Blizzard that appeared in the *AAP News* (vol. II, No. 10, October, 1986).

It seems obvious that we have a lot to learn about what the potential side effects are of the biosynthethic GH. To date, the side effects appear to be fairly minimal, but we are learning more. For example, there may be suppression of immune function in GH-deficient children during treatment with hGH. Rapaport et al. (*J. Pediatr.* 109:434, 1986) showed a decline of percent T cells and of helper T cells/suppressor ratios in some children being treated with hGH. As you might suspect, this brought about an immediate response from Genentech in the form of a letter to the editor. Genentech was the first licensed manufacturer of biosynthethic GH. If you want to read the retort to the immune story, see Ammann (*J. Pediatr.* 110:663, 1987). The Genentech people correctly note that no one has ever demonstrated any increased susceptibility to infection with the use of biosynthethic GH.

There are at least minor problems with these products. For example, hypoglycemia may develop after their administration (Press, M., et al.: *Lancet* 1:1002, 1987). A slipped capital femoral epiphysis may be a rare complication, and blood lipid levels may increase, but whether this increase is of clinical significance is not known. Also, in diabetic patients, glucose control may deteriorate. Whether these complications represent just the tip of the iceberg or the entire iceberg is not yet known.

One way around the administration of hGH for children with constitutional growth delay may be the administration of clonidine. Clonidine is a potent stimulator of the release of hypothalamic GH-releasing hormone (GHRH). This neuropeptide specifically stimulates GH release. Administration of GHRH to children with short stature of the constitutional delay of growth variety does result in a sizable GH response. This indicates the presence of functioning pituitary somatotrophs and the existence in these children of impaired hypothalamic GHRH synthesis and/or release. Clonidine is an α-adrenergic antagonist that is capable of effecting GHRH release and has now been shown to accelerate growth in children with constitutional growth delay (Pintor, C., et al.: *Lancet* 1:1226, 1987). There may be a wide temptation now to use clonidine for constitutional short stature. It can be given orally in a twice-daily dosage form. No side effects were noted during many months of therapy. Because by definition constitutional delay of growth affects about 2.5% of all children and adolescents, it might be worthwhile putting money in the stock of clonidine manufacturers, at least amounts equal to those put in by manufacturers of biosynthetic GH. Right now it is difficult to tell which company one should invest in, in any event. For example, when the Food and Drug Administration (FDA) approved the marketing of Protropin, a recombinant DNA GH developed by Genentech, the company thought it had the market cornered. Sales totalled approximately $14 million in 1986 and the curve looked like it was going to go through the ceiling. However, on March 8, 1987, the FDA approved Eli Lilly's Humatrope, an hGH product with 101 amino acid residuals. Some have speculated that Humatrope may be superior to Protropin, which has one extra amino acid-amethionyl group that produces antibody responses in approximately 30% of recipients. Genentech has countered stating that this 30% has been reduced to 8% after changes in the manufacturing process. Clinical stud-

458 / Pediatrics

ies to date have shown no apparent side effects from the antibody response. The upshot of all this is that Genentech instituted a law suit against the FDA based on the Orphan Drug Act that approved Protropin as an orphan drug, which, in theory, should give it 7 years without competition. The FDA approved the new Lilly drug on the grounds that it is a different product because it contains one fewer amino acids than Protropin. It should be nice sitting outside the boxing ring and watching this bout between two heavy hitters.

If you're indeed thinking about investing in stock in these products, remember this author's rules: Never invest in anything that eats, and never bet on a loser because you think his luck is bound to change. Those two rules should serve you well.—J.A. Stockman III, M.D.

Growth Failure and Growth-Hormone Deficiency After Treatment for Acute Lymphoblastic Leukaemia
Judy A. Kirk, Michael M. Stevens, Margaret A. Menser, Arnold Tink, Palany Raghupathy, Christopher T. Cowell, Mary Bergin, Robert H. Vines, and Martin Silink (The Children's Hosp., Camperdown, New South Wales)
Lancet 1:190–193, Jan. 24, 1987   17–10

Studies on the effect of therapy on the growth of children with acute lymphoblastic leukemia (ALL) have been conflicting, suggesting both normal and abnormal growth patterns and endocrine function. In the authors' experience, after treatment with combined chemotherapy and 24 Gy cranial radiation, with maintenance chemotherapy intrathecally, most long-term survivors have suboptimal growth.

The present study (1976–1982) was undertaken to evaluate growth and to determine the frequency of GH deficiency in 137 children with ALL who had received therapy with a modified LSA$_2$L$_2$ protocol that included cyclophosphamide, vincristine, prednisone, methotrexate, daunorubicin, cytarabine, thioguanine, L-asparaginase, lomustine, and hydroxyurea in an induction, consolidation, and maintenance regimen. Also, prophylactic radiation (24 Gy) was administered to the entire cranial cavity during the second month of treatment. It was delivered to the midline in 15 fractions during a 3-week period by telecobalt therapy with an 80-cm skin-to-source distance. Six doses of methotrexate, 12 mg/sq m, were given intrathecally during radiotherapy; and two doses, 6.25 mg/sq m, were administered every 10 weeks during maintenance therapy. In 1980, the intrathecal methotrexate dose was changed to a standard 12-mg dose for patients aged 3 years and older, 10 mg for those aged 2–3 years, and 8 mg for those aged less than 2 years. Six doses were given during CNS prophylaxis, with one dose every 10 weeks during maintenance therapy. By 1985, 83 patients were in continuous complete remission 3–9.5 years after diagnosis. Seventy-seven patients were available for follow-up.

The patients' growth slowed and they crossed height percentiles toward the end of treatment or afterward. The mean height expressed as a Z score was 0.16 at diagnosis; 2 years later it was −0.30; 4 years later, −0.71; and 6 years later, −1.37. Height for age had fallen by more than 1 SD of the population mean in 32% of survivors. Younger children and those tall for age at diagnosis were more severely affected. The GH response to standard provocation tests was measured in 46 patients; 30 had partial or complete GH deficiency. The mean pulsatile GH secretion was low in 34 tested patients.

Cranial irradiation is probably the most important causative factor in the development of GH deficiency in survivors of ALL. It is hoped that advances in ALL treatment, in particular as they relate to CNS prophylaxis, will produce fewer late adverse effects.

▶ Growth hormone failure is a particularly troublesome complication of the treatment of ALL. It is also frequently associated with panhypopituitarism manifested initially by hypothyroidism. Clayton also used GH therapy for individuals who had received CNS irradiation. The GH seems to work extremely well, but the postirradiation GH deficiency reported in the Clayton study appeared to be permanent (Clayton, P.E.: *Arch. Dis. Child.* 62:222, 1987). There has also been concern that administration of GH could cause relapse of irradiated brain tumors. Growth hormone can stimulate more than bone in terms of growth. However, a study from Manchester, England, has shown that GH administration to children with brain tumors does not increase the relapse frequency (Clayton, P.E., et al.: *Lancet* 2:711, 1987).—J.A. Stockman III, M.D.

Early Growth Predicts Timing of Puberty in Boys: Results of a 14-Year Nutrition and Growth Study

James L. Mills, Patricia H. Shiono, Leona R. Shapiro, Patricia B. Crawford, and George G. Rhoads (Natl. Inst. of Child Health and Human Development, NIH, Bethesda, and Univ. of California at Berkeley)
J. Pediatr. 109:543–547, September 1986   17–11

Investigators have long been interested in the relationship of nutrition, early growth, and onset of puberty. It is well established that malnutrition may delay puberty and that exogenous obesity may accelerate it. Studies of children in the latter part of the first decade of life suggest that height and weight are related to onset of puberty. However, it has been difficult to determine the relationship between puberty and weight, height, and adiposity in early life because of the need for a longitudinal study of normally nourished children of documented dietary and anthropometric status. An attempt was made to provide this information. Diet and growth were studied prospectively in 78 boys aged 6 months to 14 years. All were well nourished and not grossly obese. Pubertal development was assessed at age 14 years, and results were then correlated with diet and early growth.

No nutrients were significantly correlated with stage of pubertal development. However, boys with more advanced pubic hair development and longer penile length had been markedly heavier at ages 6 months, 2 years, and 4 years. Muscle mass, as determined by the cross-sectional area of the upper arm, had been substantially greater in the early maturers at the same ages. Although the more sexually mature boys had also been taller and had larger skinfolds at virtually all measurements from age 6 months to age 4 years, the differences were less marked. In an adequately nourished male population, body size in the first years of life is significantly correlated with the timing of puberty.

▶ Could it be that our mothers were correct when they made us finish our plates every night when we were boys? The findings of this study confirm earlier reports that boys who were significantly heavier at 6 months to 4 years of age turn out to be those who mature through pubescence earlier. The same is true of sexually mature boys who also were taller and had larger skinfolds at virtually all measurements from 6 months to 4 years of age. In case you think this is a new finding, or relatively new, Boas reported almost 100 years ago that children who were tall before puberty were likely to enter puberty earlier than children who were short (*Science* 5:570, 1897). The findings of the report abstracted above support the concept that genetic influences, perhaps hormonally mediated, dictate the timing of growth and puberty. Anabolic hormones such as GH or insulin could produce the increase in muscle mass seen in this study. The particularly strong relationship between early weight, lean body mass, and pubic hair development raises the possibility that an adrenal factor may be responsible.

These hypotheses require further investigation, along with the hypothesis that force feeding by some mothers to fatten up their sons may also be responsible. You could always tell these boys from the rest of us. If you were at a drive-in movie, they would be the ones coming out of the snack bar with a whole tray full of food for themselves. We had a saying for what they were up to—we called it "grazing in the car." Perhaps early grazers do have a selective advantage to premature, or at least slightly early, maturation.—J.A. Stockman III, M.D.

Calcium-Regulating Hormones and Minerals From Birth to 18 Months of Age: A Cross-Sectional Study. I. Effects of Sex, Race, Age, Season, and Diet on Vitamin D Status

P. Lichtenstein, B.L. Specker, R.C. Tsang, F. Mimouni, and C. Gormley (Univ. of Cincinnati and Children's Hosp. Res. Found., Cincinnati)
Pediatrics 77:883–890, June 1986   17–12

There is a lack of adequate normative data on bone metabolism and vitamin D physiology in infants younger than 18 months of age. A cross-sectional, prospective study of 198 infants was undertaken to obtain comprehensive normative data on vitamin D status in such infants, particularly with regard to the influence of sex, race, age, season, and diet (cow's milk vs. human milk).

Sex did not affect any of the vitamin D metabolites measured. Black infants had significantly higher serum levels of 1,25 dihydroxyvitamin D $[1,25(OH)_2D]$ than white infants had. Serum $1,25(OH)_2D$ concentrations did not change during the first 18 months of life, but serum vitamin D-binding protein concentrations increased slightly with age. Serum concen-

TABLE 1.—Diet Effects on Serum Concentrations of Vitamin D Metabolites in Infants Younger Than 6 Months of Age*

Vitamin D Metabolite	Human Milk		Formula		P Value
25-Hydroxyvitamin D (ng/mL)	29 ± 3	(43)	54 ± 2	(79)	<.001†
1,25-Dihydroxyvitamin D (pg/mL)	54 ± 3	(42)	65 ± 3	(73)	.01‡
24,25-Dihydroxyvitamin D (ng/mL)	1.72 ± 0.22 (41)		3.95 ± 0.18 (67)		<.001†
Vitamin D-binding protein (μg/mL)	307 ± 10	(34)	346 ± 8	(61)	.003†

*Results are means ± SEM, with numbers of infants in parentheses. P values are based on t test.
†Difference between diet groups remained significant in analysis of covariance.
‡Insignificant by analysis of covariance.
(Courtesy of Lichtenstein, P., et al.: Pediatrics 77:883–890, June 1986.)

TABLE 2.—Factors Related to Different Vitamin D Indices

Vitamin D Index	Race	Age	Season	Diet
25-Hydroxyvitamin D	No	No	Yes, lower in winter	Yes, lower in human milk-fed
1,25-Dihydroxyvitamin D	Yes, lower in whites	No	Yes, lower in summer	No
24,25-Dihydroxyvitamin D	No	No	Yes, lower in winter	Yes, lower in human milk-fed
Vitamin D-binding protein	No	Yes, increase with age	Yes, lower in summer	Yes, lower in human milk-fed

(Courtesy of Lichtenstein, P., et al.: Pediatrics 77:883–890, June 1986.)

trations of 25-hydroxyvitamin D (25-OHD) and 24,25-dihydroxy vitamin D [24,25-$(OH)_2D$] were significantly lower, whereas 1,25-dihydroxyvitamin D and vitamin D-binding protein concentrations were significantly higher in winter as compared with summer. Bottle-fed infants had significantly higher serum concentrations of all vitamin D metabolites than breast-fed infants had. However, after taking into account the confounding variables of season and age, only serum 25-OHD, 24,25$(OH)_2D$, and vitamin D-binding protein concentrations were significantly higher in bottle-fed infants (Table 1).

Normative values for vitamin D metabolites in infants younger than 18 months can be affected significantly by race, age, season, and diet (Table 2). These factors should be considered in assessing the vitamin D status of infants.

18 The Musculoskeletal System

Routine Analysis of Synovial Fluid Cells Is of Value in the Differential Diagnosis of Arthritis in Children
Ilkka Kunnamo and Pirkko Pelkonen (Univ. of Helsinki and Aurora Hosp., Helsinki)
J. Rheumatol. 13:1076–1080, December 1986   18–1

The value of routine synovial fluid cell analysis and chemical determinations in the differential diagnosis of arthritis in children was examined. The results of synovial fluid total white blood cell counts, white blood cell differential counts, and total protein, glucose, and lactate determinations were studied in joint aspirations of 129 children, including 91 with juvenile rheumatoid arthritis (JRA), 13 with septic arthritis, 12 with enteroarthritis, 12 with acute transient arthritis, and 1 with bacillus Calmette-Guerin arthritis.

All patients with septic arthritis, five with polyarticular onset JRA, one with systemic-onset JRA, one with enteroarthritis, and two with acute transient arthritis had total white blood cell counts of more than 40,000/cu mm. Polymorphonuclear cells were dominant in smears obtained from patients with polyarticular and systemic-onset JRA, enteroarthritis, and septic arthritis, but mononuclear cells were dominant in patients with oligoarticular JRA (Fig 18–1). No significant differences were seen in the total protein, glucose, and lactate levels in the synovial fluid in the various diagnostic groups. Although a final diagnosis of arthritis in children is based on clinical, serologic, and bacteriologic findings, analyzing synovial fluid cells is of value in the differential diagnosis.

▶ Dr. Balu H. Athreya, Director, the Pediatric Rheumatology Center, Children's Seashore House and the Children's Hospital of Philadelphia, comments.—J.A. Stockman III, M.D.

▶ Rapid diagnosis of acute monarticular arthritis is not always simple, particularly when you see a patient who has received antibiotics for suspected sepsis at some other site in the body, e.g., the ears or throat. Any diagnostic test that is easy to perform, rapid, and reliable will be most welcome, but determining the total and differential count of cells in the synovial fluid is *not* that magic test.

The conclusion of the authors that a synovial fluid cell count of more than 40,000/cu mm is sensitive and specific for septic arthritis cannot be made based on their reported results for the following reasons: (1) This was a *retrospective* study; (2) joints were aspirated at different times after onset of arthritis; (3) the authors probably included all patients with noninfectious arthritis but

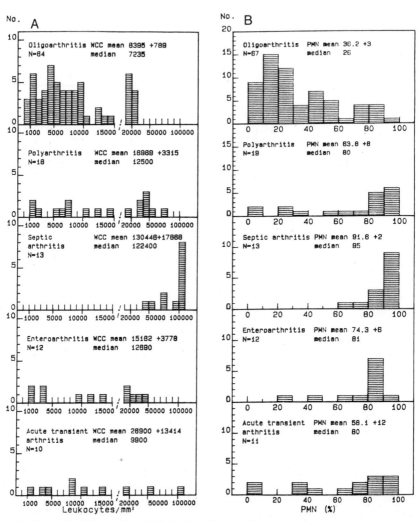

Fig 18–1.—Distribution of synovial fluid white cell counts (A) and proportions of polymorphonuclear (PMN) cells (B) in the various groups of patients studied. Mean ± SEM and median are given. The number of patients does not represent the total number because both measurements were not recorded for all patients. The two patients with systemic-onset JRA are not included. (Courtesy of Kunnamo, I., and Pelkonen, P.: J. Rheumatol. 13:1076–1080, December 1986.)

only 13 patients with septic arthritis. With such a population, how can one calculate sensitivity and specificity values? Further, the authors themselves point out, "High white cell counts can occur in nonseptic arthritis and low ones in septic arthritis."

The major area where one needs help is in differentiating monarticular arthritis caused by JRA, ankylosing spondylitis, and reactive arthritis from septic arthritis. Patients with septic arthritis often look ill or toxic with systemic features, usually have more severe pain in the joint, the range of motion is severely restricted with pain on even minimal motion of the joint passively, and may also have another focus of infection. When there is any doubt, given one or more of these findings, one should obtain synovial fluid for analysis.

The synovial fluid cell count can be useful, but without the help of clinical details it cannot truly differentiate between various categories of joint inflammation. True, cell counts of more than 50,000 are rarely seen in conditions other than septic arthritis. But one can observe such counts in gout (adult disease) and in an acutely inflamed joint in JRA. Also, a differential count with more than 90% polymorphs is rarely seen in conditions other than septic arthritis, although it may be seen on occasion in patients with JRA. In addition, all of these findings may be present in Lyme disease. Low polymorph counts do not rule out septic arthritis either, particularly if a child has been exposed to antibiotics. The last-mentioned situation is an especially difficult one—differentiating partially treated septic arthritis from JRA.

Here is where many of the tests come in, including synovial fluid analysis for sugar, lactate, lysozyme, and acid phosphatase, and counterimmunoelectrophoresis of the fluid. The latter study is specific, but is useful only for certain organisms. All other tests reflect the intensity of the inflammation, not its etiology. Therefore, none of the tests can truly differentiate "infectious" inflammation from "immune complex" inflammation.

It is finally clinical judgment, not laboratory tests, that must guide us. As Sidney Gellis once said, "If you are one of those who likes every little piece to fall into place, you should be in carpentry."—B.H. Athreya, M.D.

Serum-Sickness-Like Disease Is a Common Cause of Acute Arthritis in Children
I. Kunnamo, P. Kallio, P. Pelkonen, and M. Viander (Univ. of Helsinki, Aurora Hosp., Helsinki, and Univ. of Turku, Finland)
Acta Paediatr. Scand. 75:964–969, November 1986   18–2

Childhood arthritis caused by hypersensitivity has been reported. During a prospective incidence of arthritis in 283 children, 15 had self-limited serum sickness-like symptoms. The median age of the children was 6.4 years. Clinical symptoms included urticaria or erythema and mostly polyarticular arthritis. The average duration of joint symptoms was 5.9 days. The joints most commonly affected were the ankles, the metacarpophalangeal joints of the hands, the wrists, and the knees.

A preceding infection was reported in 12 patients, and 12 had received drugs. Four observations suggested that hypersensitivity to drugs was the major cause of the symptoms: (1) Nine patients received penicillin; (2) the time interval (mean, 12.8 days) between onset of antibiotic therapy and the beginning of serum sickness-like symptoms was remarkably similar in most patients; (3) the syndrome was significantly associated with antibiotic therapy rather than infection; and (4) the symptoms recurred in 4 of 15 patients when penicillin was reinstituted. Circulating immune complexes were detected in 12 patients. However, specific immunoglobulin IgE antibodies to penicillin were detected in only three, and IgM and IgG antibodies to penicillin were negative in all of the patients. The estimated annual incidence of this disease was 4.7/100,000 children younger than age 16 years.

Serum sickness-like disease is a common cause of arthritis in children. The presence of urticaria and/or erythema, a typical history, arthritis, and its transient course should help in the differential diagnosis of arthritis in children.

▶ In the recent literature there are actually few reports of children with arthritis caused by hypersensitivity reactions. The single most common identified agents were antibiotics, particularly penicillin. The average lag time between penicillin administration and the onset of serum sickness-associated arthritis was 2 weeks and could be more than 30 days. As the abstract notes, results of the usual tests that one performs looking for evidence of penicillin hypersensitivity were remarkably negative. One has to be careful about making a diagnosis of serum sickness purely on a clinical basis (joint involvement with or without fever and with or without urticaria), because in certain viral infections these symptoms are part of the presentation. For example, infectious hepatitis, infectious mononucleosis, and some Coxsackie infections are well known to be associated with such symptoms. Obviously, Henoch-Schönlein purpura can present in very much the same way if there is no purpura present initially.

One wonders why we still use the term serum sickness. Essentially few use serum injections these days. Perhaps this should be called urticaria with arthritis syndrome, or better yet, simply hypersensitivity arthritis. Please pay attention to the signs and symptoms described in this article. The transient nature of serum sickness may be the reason why this has lately escaped the attention of many care providers. The recognition of serum sickness by means of the clinical appearance and typical history in a patient with joint symptoms helps in making the differential diagnosis and helps to avoid unnecessary laboratory examinations. I would also note that it helps to relieve a parent's mind to know that their child does not have juvenile rheumatoid arthritis with all of its implications. A lot of parents easily get their own joints bent out of shape when that dignosis is applied mistakenly.—J.A. Stockman III, M.D.

Clinical Signs and Laboratory Tests in the Differential Diagnosis of Arthritis in Children
Ilkka Kunnamo, Pentti Kallio, Pirkko Pelkonen, and Tapani Hovi (Univ. of Helsinki and Aurora Hosp., Helsinki)
Am. J. Dis. Child. 141:34–40, January 1987   18–3

The spectrum of arthritis in children differs from that in adults. Early diagnosis is often difficult, and some forms of arthritis may require long periods of observation before a definite diagnosis can be established. Analysis was made of the clinical signs and results of laboratory tests in 278 children with clinically confirmed arthritis who were part of an epidemiologically representative series. Univariate analysis and multivariate logis-

TABLE 1.—Duration of Joint Symptoms

No. of Patients, Duration of Symptoms

Diagnostic Group	<2 wk	2-6 wk	>6 wk	Total
Juvenile arthritis	0	0	55	55
Enteroarthritis	2	2	9	13
Septic arthritis	7	11	0	18
Transient synovitis of the hip	122	8	1	131
Schönlein-Henoch purpura	9	0	0	9
Serum sickness	14	1	0	15
Acute transient arthritis	31	4	2	37
Total (% of All Patients)	**185** (67)	**26** (9)	**67** (24)	**278** (100)

(Courtesy of Kunnamo, I., et al.: Am. J. Dis. Child. 141:34–40, January 1987.)

TABLE 2.—Joint Involvement at Presentation

No. of Joints Involved

Diagnostic Group	1	2-4	≥5	Total
Juvenile arthritis	36	18	1	55
Enteroarthritis	6	6	1	13
Septic arthritis	18	0	0	18
Transient synovitis of the hip	126	5	0	131
Schönlein-Henoch purpura	1	7	1	9
Serum sickness	1	7	7	15
Acute transient arthritis	26	10	1	37
Total (% of All Patients)	**214** (77)	**53** (19)	**11** (4)	**278** (100)

(Courtesy of Kunnamo, I., et al.: Am. J. Dis. Child. 141:34–40, January 1987.)

tic regression analysis were used to find independent predictive factors for diagnosing septic arthritis, juvenile arthritis, and enteroarthritis.

Children in the study were younger than age 16 years, and diagnosis was based on joint swelling or limitation of motion with heat, pain, or tenderness. Diagnoses included juvenile arthritis in 55 children, enteroarthritis in 13, septic arthritis in 18, transient synovitis of the hip in 131, Schönlein-Henoch purpura in 9, serum sickness in 15, and acute transient arthritis in 37. Also included in the study were 25 children with arthralgia but no objective arthritis, 13 with orthopedic disease, and 4 with other diseases.

Juvenile arthritis, septic arthritis and transient synovitis of the hip were most common in children aged less than 1 to 3 years; transient synovitis was most common in those aged 4–6 and 7–9 years, and juvenile arthritis and transient synovitis were most common in those aged 10–12 years. In 185 patients (67%) the duration of symptoms was less than 2 weeks (Table 1). In 214 patients (77%) only one joint was involved (Table 2). At presentation a high fever was observed in 32 patients (12%) and skin symptoms were seen in 38 (14%) (Table 3). Laboratory tests were classified

TABLE 3.—Fever and Skin Symptoms at Presentation

	No. of Patients	
Diagnostic Group	Temperature >38.5°C	Skin Symptoms
Juvenile arthritis (n = 55)	1	3
Enteroarthritis (n = 13)	3	1
Septic arthritis (n = 18)	14	0
Transient synovitis of the hip (n = 131)	5	3
Schönlein-Henoch purpura (n = 9)	0	8
Serum sickness (n = 15)	1	14
Acute transient arthritis (n = 37)	8	9
Total (% of All Patients) (n = 278)	**32** (12)	**38** (14)

(Courtesy of Kunnamo, I., et al.: Am. J. Dis. Child. 141:34–40, January 1987.)

TABLE 4.—Diagnostic Tests in Assessment of Arthritis in Children

Category	Application	Test
A	All children with joint symptoms	C-reactive protein, erythrocyte sedimentation rate, complete blood cell count, platelet count, urinalysis, bacterial culture of throat smear
B	Arthritis lasting longer than 2 wk	Antinuclear antibodies, serum immunoglobulins, *Yersinia* antibodies, *Salmonella* antibodies, stool bacterial culture
C	Special indications (see text)	Rheumatoid factor, antistreptolysin O, viral antibodies, *Chlamydia* antibodies

(Courtesy of Kunnamo, I., et al.: Am. J. Dis. Child. 141:34–40, January 1987.)

into three categories, A, B, and C, according to their value in the assessment of arthritis in children. Tests in category A are indicated for all children with joint symptoms, those in category B are indicated for patients with prolonged symptoms and in those suspected of enteroarthritis, and category C tests are complementary tests for special indications (Table 4). This diagnostic scheme may be helpful in reaching the correct primary diagnosis of arthritis in children.

The Impact of Childhood Rheumatic Diseases on the Family

Marie C. McCormick, Margaret M. Stemmler, and Balu H. Athreya (Children's Hosp. of Philadelphia and Univ. of Pennsylvania)
Arthritis Rheum. 29:872–879, July 1986 18–4

As in many chronic illnesses in children, much of the burden of providing health care and economic and psychosocial support for children with rheumatic disease falls on the parents. To learn more about the impact of these conditions on the family, telephone interviews were conducted with 138 families of children with rheumatic diseases to determine factors affecting maternal perceptions of the impact of childhood rheumatic diseases. The mother was the respondent in 93.5% of cases.

Stepwise multivariate analysis indicated that the most important predictor of high family impact was the child's limited ability to perform activities of daily living. Other important predictors were the mother's educational level, male sex of the child, the mother's perception of the child's health, the degree of medical care use, and low annual family income. The medical care use and out-of-pocket expenditures were high and resulted in proportionately higher impact scores for the family. In addition, the high impact scores of medical care use reflected the severity of illness among patients who relied on the hospital clinic for health care. Families who are most vulnerable to the stress of having a child with a rheumatic disease are those whose medical care requirements are disporportionate to the resources available to provide the care.

▶ The impact of rheumatic diseases on families is not a minor league problem. Juvenile rheumatoid arthritis, the most common of the rheumatic diseases, reportedly affects about 10 children in every 10,000, or between 13,000 and 63,000 children in the United States. The actual number is probably even significantly higher than this. Part of the difficulty with this disorder, from a family's point of view, is the uncertainty concerning the long-term outcome. We're just beginning to see what some of those data really are.

Scott et al. (*Lancet* 1:1108, 1987) looked at the long-term outcome of treatment of rheumatoid arthritis after 20 years. Most of their patients were adults, but there were a fair number of younger individuals in this series as well. Fortunately, early age of onset was associated with a good prognosis. Rheumatoid factor seropositivity at presentation was a poor prognostic factor. For young adults and middle-aged adults with rheumatoid arthritis the outlook is probably nowhere nearly as good as for children. By 20 years from the time of diagnosis, 35% of the patients had died. Mortality was most often attributed to complications associated with rheumatoid arthritis. Even though adults tend to have functional improvement in the first decade after diagnosis, there is a slippage in this during the subsequent 10 years, so that at 20 years from the time of diagnosis for those who survived, 19% were severely disabled. These data support the notion that juvenile rheumatoid arthritis and adult rheumatoid arthritis are probably two different diseases, but they can be very difficult to distinguish in the older pediatric age group.

If you look at adolescents, arthritis makes up a fairly large component of chronic disease. Siegel (*JAMA* 257:3396, 1987) has done us all a service by providing a very comprehensive overview on adolescents and chronic disease. The leading chronic disease categories in terms of prevalence in children aged from infancy to 20 years in the United States were (in 1980) as follows: asthma (38/1,000), visual impairment (30/1,000), mental retardation (25/1,000), hearing impairment (10/1,000), congenital heart disease (7/1,000), cerebral palsy (2.5/1,000), and arthritis (2.2/1,000). After that were at least 30 other diagnostic categories associated with a much lower prevalence rate. From these numbers it can be seen that the cost for chronic care in the United States is staggering. It has been estimated at more than 2.9 billion dollars. The magnitude of the problem of chronic care is such that approximately 36% of total hospital days for all children in the United States younger than age 15 years was for chronic disorders.

Anyone involved with care of the chronically disabled child realizes the ineffectiveness with which this problem is being addressed in terms of program support on a national level. I have seen, as I am sure many of you have, parents who literally cannot move from one state to another for fear that they no longer will have the means to obtain care for their disabled child. Our children are a national resource, not one to be bargained with on a state's rights basis.—J.A. Stockman III, M.D.

Utility of Rheumatoid Factor in the Diagnosis of Juvenile Rheumatoid Arthritis

Andrew H. Eichenfield, Balu H. Athreya, Robert A. Doughty, and Randall D. Cebul (Children's Seashore House and Children's Hosp. of Philadelphia)
Pediatrics 78:480–484, September 1986   18–5

Children with musculoskeletal symptoms and undiagnosed fever are often screened for IgM rheumatoid factor at the request of their general physicians to rule out juvenile rheumatoid arthritis. A study was conducted to determine whether rheumatoid factor testing is useful in making a diagnosis of rheumatoid arthritis in the young patient.

The symptoms, diagnosis, or both, in 437 young patients in whom rheumatoid factor assays were performed were categorized as being of the musculoskeletal system or of an "autoimmune" nature. Rheumatoid factor was assayed by the latex particle agglutination method, and titers of 1:80 or more were considered to be positive tests.

Of 11 patients who had positive tests for rheumatoid factor, 5 had juvenile rheumatoid arthritis. Of the 426 with negative tests, 100 had juvenile rheumatoid arthritis (table). In the outpatient setting the positive predictive values were 0.5% to 0.7%, and the marginal benefits were 0.3% to 0.4%. Both indices increased significantly when the tests were conducted on the recommendation of a physician in a pediatric rheumatology center.

Rheumatoid factor testing was incapable of establishing or ruling out a diagnosis of juvenile rheumatoid arthritis. Rheumatoid factor testing should be performed only in older children with polyarticular arthritis.

▶ Carol G. Ragsdale, M.D., Assistant Professor, Division of Pediatric Rheu-

CONTINGENCY TABLE*

Rheumatoid Factor	Juvenile Rheumatoid Arthritis	
	Positive	Negative
Positive	5	6
Negative	100	326

*Sensitivity = 5/105 (4.8%); specificity = 326/332 (98%).
(Courtesy of Eichenfield, A.H., et al.: Pediatrics 78:480–484, September 1986.)

matology, C.S. Mott Children's Hospital, Ann Arbor, comments.—J.A. Stockman III, M.D.

▶ Rheumatoid factors are often found in chronic inflammatory states and not exclusively in rheumatic conditions. In children, rheumatoid factors occur more frequently in association with systemic lupus erythematosus or systemic vasculitides than with juvenile rheumatoid arthritis (JRA), and occasionally in chronic infections or malignancies. Healthy children do not have positive tests for rheumatoid factor if performed by reliable examiners. So, if appropriate exclusions are made, a positive test for rheumatoid factor can reinforce suspicion of a chronic inflammatory or rheumatic disease.

The test for rheumatoid factor in a child with JRA does have prognostic value in identifying a disease with a high disabling potential. In addition, when the diagnosis is known and rheumatoid factor is present, the titer for rheumatoid factor, over time, may indicate disease activity and aid the clinician in recommending gold, reducing the steroid dosage, or determining whether fever means flare or infection.

A variety of rheumatoid factor assay kits are used in clinical laboratories and their results vary greatly in reliability. They depend on human training and vision to detect agglutination; technical factors, inexperience, and presbyopia all contribute to the variability observed when standard sera are surveyed in diverse laboratories. Many rheumatoid factor assays are included in packages ordered as "arthritis profiles," which may also report antinuclear antibodies (ANAs) the erythrocyte sedimentation rate, or even B27 positivity. These profiles increase the risk of obtaining a "false positive" result because of inexperience or technical unreliability. False positive tests for rheumatoid factor or ANA are now most commonly responsible when healthy children are referred for consultation.

The rheumatoid factor test, correctly performed and interpreted, is informative and helpful, but rheumatoid factor assays don't make diagnoses, and laboratory studies cannot substitute for thoughtful clinical problem solving.—C.G. Ragsdale, M.D.

Fluoride Treatment in Corticosteroid Induced Osteoporosis
F. Rejou, R. Dumas, C. Belon, P.J. Meunier, and C. Edouard (Hôpital Saint-Charles, Montpellier, and Faculté Alexis Carrel, Lyon, France)
Arch. Dis. Child. 61:1230–1231, December 1986   18–6

Sodium fluoride is currently used to treat idiopathic osteoporosis in aging adults. Its role in the treatment of corticosteroid-induced osteoporosis in two children was reviewed.

Two children, aged 7 years and 10 years, had dermatomyositis and were treated with high doses of prednisone and alfacalcidol. Severe osteoporosis with multiple vertebral fractures occurred in both patients. Administration of sodium fluoride, 1 mg/kg/day, supplemented with calcium, resulted in clinical improvement and absence of new vertebral fractures despite relapsing dermatomyositis in one child. Histomorphometric data on bone biopsy specimens after a year of fluoride treatment showed inconsistent improvement: The trabecular bone volume was unchanged, and the calcification rate was increased in one child.

Fluoride treatment, in conjunction with calcium and vitamin D therapy, should be an integral part of the curative treatment of corticosteroid-induced osteoporosis.

▶ If fluoride is working so well in corticosteroid-induced osteoporosis, perhaps we should be using it in other forms of osteopenia, e.g., that produced by aluminum intoxication (see Chapter 10, The Genitourinary Tract). If nothing else, it will help one's smile.—J.A. Stockman III, M.D.

Clinical Prediction of Cervical Spine Injuries in Children: Radiographic Abnormalities
Ingrid Rachesky, W. Thomas Boyce, Burris Duncan, John Bjelland, and Barbara Sibley (Univ. of Arizona)
Am. J. Dis. Child. 141:199–201, February 1987   18–7

The consequences of overlooking a cervical spine injury are potentially very serious, thus even the remote possibility of injury to the cervical vertebrae may often require cervical spine radiographs. To determine the incidence of cervical spine injuries in children and the factors that would identify those at high risk for such injuries, 2,133 cervical spine radiographs of children younger than 18 years were reviewed retrospectively.

· Twenty-five children (1.2%) had confirmed evidence of cervical spine injury on x-ray films. The mean age was 13.4 years, and the male to female ratio was 4:1. Vehicular accidents and sports and playground injuries together accounted for nearly three fourths of all confirmed injuries. Analysis of historical and physical examination variables indicated that clinical assessment consisting of either a complaint of neck pain or involvement in a vehicular accident with head trauma would have correctly identified all 25 children with cervical spine injury. If this clinical marker was used prospectively, the number of cervical spine radiographs ordered would have been reduced by 32%. This would also translate to a one third reduction in the cost and radiation exposure associated with cervical spine radiographs.

The presence of a history of neck pain or vehicular accident with head trauma will correctly identify all children with cervical spine injuries. The clinical usefulness of this marker, however, should be confirmed by other studies before it is accepted as a recommendation.

▶ The authors of this study concluded with the following comments: "Perhaps critical reviews of the use of common radiographic procedures will ultimately result in a more efficient and parsimonious approach to their utilization in the course of clinical diagnosis." As interesting and as relatively important as the findings of this report are, I am not so certain that one should be too parsimonious in a request for a cervical spine film. Although neck pain and a history of head trauma correctly predicted all 2.9% of cervical films that were abnormal, we don't know how many children might have otherwise been missed because no films were obtained at all. That may seem a weak argument, but I, for one, would like to see a much larger series before refusing to check off the box that says cervical spine films just on the basis of a negative history of cervical pain or head injury. Maybe they are right, maybe they are wrong, but the error should be on the side of too many false negative films. Perhaps a 97% false negative rate is too high, but I would imagine that there were reasonably legitimate concerns that warranted so many films being done.

This report is limited by being a retrospective study, and all possible clinical markers could never have been recorded in the emergency room chart. Will someone go back now and propose a prospective study as the next logical step in evaluating the clinical utility of cervical spine films, please?

While on the topic of the neck, there are a few interesting things that have popped up over the last year or so. One is the recognition that atlanto-occipital instability, although a rare condition, does occur in children. A series of children with this problem were seen at the Alfred I. duPont Institute in Wilmington. Two of four patients classically had prior trauma. A third child, a 10-year-old boy, had been in an automobile accident more than 2 years previously. After the accident he had intermittent periods of headaches and neck pain. Physical examination found evidence of proximal muscle weakness in both the upper and lower extremities. Cervical films in extension showed atlanto-occipital instability that required fusion. A fourth patient was a 14-year-old boy who had no history of trauma, only neck pain. He experienced severe spasm of the neck muscles that led to hospitalization for cervical traction. A diagnosis ultimately was made of this same problem and required fusion.

The reason for mentioning these cases of instability is based on the fact that a plain set of cervical radiographs certainly may not disclose such abnormalities. None of these children, by the way, had Down's syndrome. The predominant problem with Down's syndrome, as has been discussed on multiple occasions in the YEAR BOOK and by the Committee on Sports Medicine of the American Academy of Pediatrics, is that of atlantoaxial instability. It's interesting to note that with all the information that has become available about this interrelationship with Down's syndrome, a new variant on this problem has arisen, i.e., atlanto-occipital instability in Down's syndrome. The first reports of atlanto-occipital instability in children with Down's syndrome were made by Rosenbaum et al. (*AJR* 146:1269, 1986). Obviously, atlanto-occipital instability in Down's syndrome patients is rare compared with the 10% to 20% of individuals with that syndrome who have atlantoaxial instability, but this too must be carefully looked for at the time of radiographic screening. As you are aware, the Academy has stated that ". . . some physicians may prefer to screen all of their patients with Down syndrome at the age of 5 or 6 years. A distance of greater than 4.5 mm between the anterior arch of C1 and the odontoid, or an abnormal odontoid, are adequate reasons to restrict participation in sports involving possible trauma to the head and neck." Simply add to that caution the business about atlanto-occipital instability and all bases should be covered.

Perhaps that's not even a correct statement. Pueschel et al. have gone one step beyond the plain radiograph (*J. Pediatr.* 110:515, 1987). These investigators indicate that no single assessment technique provides a definitive answer concerning the identification of early neurologic signs in children with Down's syndrome in asymptomatic atlantoaxial instability. In other words, once a film is obtained that shows this instability, one really should not stop there. Some children may be at higher risk than others for the development of subluxation, and some children may already have neurologic impairment that is below the threshold of detection on a routine neurologic examination. These authors suggest that a combined approach, after x-ray examination of the lateral cervical spine in neutral, flexion, and extension, should include CT scans, detailed neurologic examinations, and somatosensory evoked response latency measures if useful information concerning risk status is going to be obtained. Those patients with Down's syndrome and early signs of neurologic symptoms then should have further evaluation; if indicated, surgical intervention to prevent injury to the spine should follow.

After the article abstracted above appeared, there was another study in the *Annals of Emergency Medicine* (Jaffe, D.M., et al.: 16:270, 1987) that addressed the same issue of how to develop a clinical approach to the early management of cervical spine injuries in children with trauma. The conclusion was drawn that one should immobilize and obtain cervical spine radiographs on every child who has one or more of the following eight findings: neck pain, neck tenderness, abnormal reflexes or changes in strength and sensation, history of neck trauma, limitation of neck mobility, and abnormal mental status. The sensitivity of this algorithmic approach was 98%, meaning that only 2% of children might be missed using such an approach. The specificity was an amazingly high 54%.

Obviously, there is wide variation in how cervical injuries are approached. The previous editor of the YEAR BOOK OF PEDIATRICS, an individual whose opinions and comments I not only respect but practically revere, has said in his weekly reviews that he would "choose to order a CT scan for any infant or child suspected of having injured his cervical spine." For once I have to differ. If the plain films of the neck are entirely negative (done in all the appropriate positions, and so forth), and if there is no evidence of retropharyngeal soft tissue swelling, I would not think CT is needed every time one thinks of getting a cervical x-ray study. A CT is extremely useful if the plain films are negative, but there is widening of the retropharyngeal space (Apple, J.S., et al.: *Pediatr. Radiol.* 17:45, 1987). Sorry, Dr. G., you'll have to fight this one out with Mr. T. if you really want to prove your point.—J.A. Stockman III, M.D.

Ultrasound Screening for Hip Abnormalities: Preliminary Findings in 1001 Neonates
Laurence Berman and Leslie Klenerman (Northwick Park Hosp. and Clinical Res. Ctr., Harrow, England)
Br. Med. J. 293:719–722, Sept. 20, 1986   18–8

Current neonatal clinical screening methods have proved somewhat flawed in detecting the incidence of hip dislocation in infancy; in some cases, the practice of splinting hips has proved unnecessary, because the hips would have developed normally if left alone. Ultrasound testing is a viable alternative to conventional screening methods, and early ultrasound research by Graf led to his classification of four main types of infant hip, classifications that call for various treatment protocols. A study was undertaken to compare conventional and ultrasound screening in detecting hip instability in 1,001 neonates.

Fourteen of 17 infants with hip instability detected by conventional methods were not splinted as a result of ultrasound findings. The hips developed normally. Two infants with no clinical signs were shown by ultrasound to have severe hip abnormalities. These results indicate that ultrasound can detect dysplastic hips that standard evaluation methods do not detect. Ultrasound imaging may also help to avoid the overtreatment that appears to occur in current practice.

▶ H. Theodore Harcke, M.D., Director of Medical Imaging, Alfred I. duPont Institute, Wilmington, Delaware, comments.—J.A. Stockman III, M.D.

▶ Ultrasound is now being used in both the United States and Europe to evaluate infants for congenital hip dislocation and/or dysplasia (CDH). In addition to the abstracted article, I am aware of nine additional papers and an atlas on the subject of infant hip ultrasound that were published in 1986. The growing popularity of hip sonography is based on its greater sensitivity and the fact that it has no ionizing radiation. For initial evaluation of the infant hip and to monitor treatment, sonography can be used in place of an x-ray study (Harcke, H.T.: *Semin. Ultrasound, CT, and MR* 7:331–338, 1986).

At present, only a few centers have physicians and/or ultrasound technologists skilled in performing hip sonography. The equipment used, however, is the same as that used for other commonly performed ultrasound studies (e.g., those of the infant brain, abdominal organs, and fetal gestation), so that virtually every hospital has the potential to do infant hip studies. With real-time equipment, one is able to see the cartilaginous components of the hip not visible on conventional radiographs and to assess stability by observing the hip during the performance of stress maneuvers. The technique is effective up until about 1 year of age.

Hip screening of infants using ultrasound has been performed successfully by others in Europe in addition to Berman and Klenerman (Graf, R.: *Ultrasound Annual 1985,* pp. 177–186, 1985, and Zieger, M.: *Pediatr. Radiol.* 16:488–492, 1986). In the United States, infant hip screening by physical examination is not expected to be replaced by mass screening with ultrasound because of the cost and resources that would be required. Referral of infants for hip ultrasound in lieu of x-ray will be based on abnormal or questionable findings on physical examination or high risk (breech delivery, foot deformity, torticollis, parent or sibling with CDH). The advantages of sonography over radiography are becoming more widely appreciated as experience with the technique increases and reports in the literature proliferate. Pediatricians and orthopedists may wish to urge their colleagues in radiology to learn the technique so that x-ray exposure of infants can be curtailed. Those of us who do hip sonography look forward to the time when the method becomes as routine in pediatric care as sonography of the brain and abdominal organs.—H.T. Harcke, M.D.

Hip Joint Instability in Breech Pregnancy

Marie Luterkort, P.-H. Persson, Staffan Polberger, and Ingrid Bjerre (Univ. of Lund, Malmö, Sweden)
Acta Paediatr. Scand. 75:860–863, 1986   18–9

It is thought that the etiology of hip instability in the newborn is multifactorial, involving genetic, hormonal, and mechanical factors. Experimental studies on animals and observations among certain ethnic groups have established that environmental mechanical factors are important in the development of hip instability. Breech presentation increases the risk of this condition, probably because of mechanical factors affecting the fetus in utero or during delivery. In particular, delivery in frank breech presentation, where the legs of the newborn are extended, has been linked to hip instability. Fetuses in breech presentation were investigated with repeated ultrasound examinations to follow the subsequent occurrence of hip instability in relation to the intrauterine attitude of the fetus.

Ultrasound studies were used to follow 222 consecutive fetuses in breech position in gestational week 33; repeat examinations were done in weeks 35 and 38. Ninety-one fetuses persisted in breech presentation until delivery; cephalic version occurred in the rest. The frequencies of hip instability were 21% in the breech delivery group and 1.5% in the vertex delivery group. At each ultrasound examination the position of the fetal legs was established. The intrauterine fetal attitude was classified as extended when the fetus had extended knees and maximally flexed hips at all ultrasound examinations. This was observed in 30 breech-delivered fetuses, in 47% of whom hip instability developed. Only 8% of the breech-born infants with flexed legs in utero had hip instability. Instability of the hip would appear to be a consequence of intrauterine attitude rather than of breech delivery per se.

▶ This very interesting report clearly demonstrates that position in utero may be associated with dislocation of the hips. Heretofore, it was thought that the actual delivery in breech presentation was responsible for hip joint instability. This is an important distinction, because in this day and age few breech presentations are allowed to come to vaginal delivery. This author certainly does not recommend routine ultrasound in every pregnancy at 33 weeks' gestation. However, if such studies are performed around this time and breech presentation with legs extended is found, then the risk for loose hips will be almost 50%. As much as I admire this study, my cross-filing reference found another report (Pizer, B.L., et al.: *Arch. Dis. Child.* 61:908, 1986) that also studied 222 consecutive fetuses with ultrasound at 33 weeks' gestation and found 47% with hip instability as well. I would suspect that my filing system has picked up the same series reported in the Scandinavian literature and now in the British literature. I should warn these investigators that it's not nice to fool Mother Nature, and one would hope that the same series does not crop up again in the American literature.

There has been a great deal written in the past year about techniques that may be useful in screening for detection of congenital dislocation of the hip.

An especially good article appeared in the *Archives of Diseases of Childhood* (Special Report: *Arch. Dis. Child.* 61:921, 1986). What will be interesting in the future is to learn whether ultrasound will ultimately replace physical examination in the detection of congenital dislocations. One might envision the time when it actually could be more swift, more cost effective, and less time-consuming simply to put an ultrasound transducer against the hip than to go through all of the physical maneuvers necessary to make a diagnosis of congenital dislocation of the hip. I emphasize the word "might." For the time being at least, we will continue to go on using our clinical acumen as the best tool of diagnosis.

One can add to the list of clinical tools a couple of maneuvers reported recently by Stone et al. (*Lancet* 1:954, 1987). These investigators describe a two-part clinical test based on the attenuation of sound transmission across the hip. Its use is not restricted to the early weeks of life. The two maneuvers are these: (1) The comparative sound transmission test is performed with the patient supine and hips extended. The examiner then listens with a stethoscope diaphragm over the symphysis pubis while a vibrating 256-Hz medical tuning fork is applied to each patella in turn. The procedure can be reversed, listening over the patella with applying a tuning fork to the symphysis. Any difference in the volume of sound transmitted is sought, this difference being most apparent as the sound fades. Dislocation is characterized by a reduction in sound on the affected side. (2) This is known as the comparative flexion/extension test. The procedure described in the first test is repeated on each hip to compare the difference in sound transmission when the hip is moved from extension to 90 degrees of flexion. In a normal hip, the sound volume is generally reduced with hip flexion, although in a dislocated hip it increases with flexion. Whereas the comparative sound transmission test depends on a normal hip for comparison, the flexion extension test does not. I have not yet had the opportunity to try out these two tests, but they seem quite nifty, perhaps just too good to believe in the diagnosis of loose hips. Perhaps you could put the tuning fork under the chin and a stethoscope on the forehead and find out who has a loose tongue. Colonel Oliver North claimed he wasn't a loose cannon on deck; maybe you could put a tuning fork on the cannon and a stethoscope on the deck and find out. Clearly, there are many ramifications to this *Lancet* article!—J.A. Stockman III, M.D.

Instability of the Patellofemoral Joint in Down Syndrome
Thomas W. Dugdale and Thomas S. Renshaw (Newington Children's Hosp., Newington, Conn.)
J. Bone Joint Surg. [Am.] 68-A:405–413, March 1986   18–10

Previous studies of patellofemoral instability in Down's syndrome patients did not include a classification of the degree of instability or a description of the method used to assess instability. These issues were examined in institutionalized Down's syndrome patients and in a group of noninstitutionalized outpatients with Down's syndrome.

The study population was comprised of 210 patients, 132 males (62.9%)

and 78 females (37.1%), ranging in age from 15 to 67 years (median, 36 years) and 151 noninstitutionalized Down's syndrome outpatients. All were examined for patellofemoral instability of both knees, which was classified on a 5-point system. According to this system, the patella was dislocatable or dislocated in 35 knees (8.3%) in the institutionalized group and in 12 knees (4.0%) in the noninstitutionalized group. Although this interfered with walking in some patients, only three were completely unable to walk. None of the 210 institutionalized patients and only 3 of the noninstitutionalized patients used an orthosis. One of these patients was a 10-year-old girl with bilateral grade 5 instability and a fixed 20-degree knee-flexion contracture, but wearing an orthosis did not stabilize the dislocated patella. Corrective surgery was performed on eight knees in one institutionalized patient and in four noninstitutionalized patients with patellofemoral instability; four knees had satisfactory results. Instability of the patellofemoral joint in patients with Down's syndrome is common, but is rarely disabling, because almost all patients in this study were able to walk.

▶ We've already noted the problem of atlantoaxial instability and atlanto-occipital instability in children with Down's syndrome. Now we see a report of instability of the patellofemoral joint. Children with Down's syndrome also have a higher risk for scoliosis, congenital hip dysplasia, metatarsus vasas, and pes planus. These orthopedic problems are becoming more apparent now that life expectancy in Down's syndrome patients is increasing. Baird et al. (*J. Pediatr.* 110:849, 1987) have shown us that for patients with Down's syndrome without congenital heart anomalies, survival to age 1 year is 91%; to age 5 years, 87.2%; to age 10 years, 84.9%; to age 20 years, 81.9%, and to age 30 years, 79.2%. If a child is born with congenital heart anomalies, these percentages drop to about two thirds of the above values. The long-term outlook for individuals with Down's syndrome may not be as promising, because in many of these patients an Alzheimer's type illness develops. Recent work that has focused on isolation of the gene for β-amyloid protein, which is found as deposits in the brains of individuals with Alzheimer's disease and in older individuals with Down's syndrome, suggests an intriguing theory. One research group studying the genetics of Alzheimer's disease used DNA probes to carry out linkage analysis in familial Alzheimer's disease and found that the gene conferring susceptibility maps not only to chromosome 21, but to a region that carries the amyloid protein gene. This tends to connect more tightly the already established suspicion that there is a relationship between Down's syndrome and Alzheimer's disease (*Lancet* 2:1011, 1987). Is the deposition of amyloid protein in Down's syndrome a result of the effect of an extra copy of chromosome 21? An intriguing hypothesis, and also a long way from the topic of the above abstract, so this commentary now ends.—J.A. Stockman III, M.D.

The Syndrome of Inappropriate Antidiuretic-Hormone Secretion Following Spinal Fusion

Gordon R. Bell, Alan R. Gurd, James P. Orlowski, and Jack T. Andrish (Cleveland Clinic Found.)
J. Bone Joint Surg. [Am.] 68-A:720–724, June 1986   18–11

Healthy adolescents who undergo spinal fusion often have a striking reduction in postoperative urinary output despite the absence of hypovolemia, possibly as a result of inappropriate antidiuretic hormone secretion. To verify this hypothesis, serum sodium, serum osmolality, urine sodium, urine osmolality, and serum antidiuretic hormone concentrations were determined in ten adolescent or preadolescent patients who underwent spinal fusion for idiopathic scoliosis or spondylolisthesis.

In most of the patients a rapid, pronounced rise in the serum antidiuretic hormone concentration occurred within a few hours postoperatively, in seven reaching levels 10–100 times more than the preoperative level. Values gradually returned to normal by the third postoperative day. This resulted in a reduced urinary output, which was maximum on the day of operation and rose gradually to normal during the next 3 days. The fluid intake on the day of operation (average, 5,962 ml) exceeded the urinary output (average, 1,121 ml) by a ratio of almost 7 to 1. There was increased renal resorption of water, resulting in expansion of body fluid as evidenced by decreased serum sodium and serum osmolality. Urine sodium and urine osmolality were increased at the same time.

The syndrome of inappropriate antidiuretic hormone secretion and its associated low urinary output postoperatively is common after spinal fusion. Management consists of restriction of fluids rather than fluid replacement.

Scoliosis and Fractures in Young Ballet Dancers: Relation to Delayed Menarche and Secondary Amenorrhea
Michelle P. Warren, J. Brooks-Gunn, Linda H. Hamilton, L. Fiske Warren, and William G. Hamilton (Columbia College of Physicians and Surgeons and St. Luke's-Roosevelt Hosp., New York)
N. Engl. J. Med. 314:1348–1353, May 22, 1986   18–12

Prolonged hypoestrogenism is a complication of dieting, weight loss, and physical training in young women. A high incidence of delayed menarche, secondary amenorrhea, and irregular menstrual periods has been demonstrated in young ballet dancers. Because the secretion of gonadal steroids, particularly estrogen, has important physiologic effects on bone, a study was designed to examine the incidence of skeletal aberrations in ballet dancers who may have alterations in estrogen secretion during an important phase of their growth and development. Included in the study were 75 female dancers in four highly competitive professional ballet companies of national standing. The mean age was 24 years.

The prevalence of scoliosis was 24% and rose with increased age at menarche. Fifteen of 18 dancers (83%) with scoliosis had had a delayed menarche (14 years or older), as compared with 31 of 57 dancers (54%)

without scoliosis. Dancers with scoliosis had a slightly higher prevalence of secondary amenorrhea (44% vs. 31%), the mean duration of their amenorrhea was longer (11 months vs. 4 months), and they scored higher on a questionnaire that assessed anorectic behavior. The incidence of fractures (61%, or 46 of 75 dancers) rose with increasing age at menarche. Most (69%) were stress fractures and occurrence had a strong correlation with increased age at menarche. The incidence of secondary amenorrhea was twice as high among dancers with stress fractures and the duration was longer. In seven of ten dancers in whom endocrine studies were carried out the amenorrheic intervals were marked by prolonged hypoestrogenism. These data suggest that a delay in menarche and prolonged intervals of amenorrhea that reflect prolonged hypoestrogenism may predispose ballet dancers to the development of scoliosis and to stress fractures.

▶ The problem of scoliosis continues to plague both the pediatrician and the orthopedist. The article abstracted above received wide national, indeed international, attention when it appeared. It seemed clearly to demonstrate relationships between delayed menarche, secondary amenorrhea, scoliosis, and ballet dancing. One of the working assumptions in all of this was that the vigorous exercise of ballet dancing predisposed the relatively young girl to hypoestrogenism (an otherwise well-described phenomenon in very athletic girls). One could additionally postulate that this would result in delayed skeletal maturation, prolonging the period during which girls would be at risk for the development of progressive scoliosis. We all know that curves cease to continue to evolve once skeletal maturation has occurred. Chances are the story is even much more complex than that, as we have noted in earlier YEAR BOOKS.

There is a well-described association of hypomastia and the mitral valve prolapse syndrome. The latter syndrome, among its fuller expressions, can include not only mitral valve prolapse, but also hypocholesterolemia, pectus excavatum, and a tall, thin body build (the so-called ballerina-type body build). Rosenberg et al. (*N. Engl. J. Med.* 315:1417, 1986) postulate that this represents defective development in the sixth week of gestation. It is at this time that the centers of chondrification begin to form in the vertebra. The mesenchymal components of the breast and mitral valve are also actively developing during this period. One, therefore, could weave a thin web linking scoliosis or straight back, mitral valve prolapse, and perhaps even hypomastia. It should also be noted that many patients with a mitral valve prolapse syndrome also have a variant of von Willebrand's disease. That's a little harder to fit into this embryologic development theory, but maybe there is a clue that relates to this as well.

A curious episode was recently described that possibly suggests a relationship between the artificial sweetener aspartame and panic attacks in a patient with mitral valve prolapse. A 33-year-old woman had reproducible panic attacks when consuming excessive amounts of aspartame-sweetened soft drinks. She also had mitral valve prolapse. It was suggested that mitral valve prolapse and panic symptoms are both common and may overlap, but patients with mitral valve prolapse may be predisposed to panic symptoms under the influence of agents such as aspartame that are known to have potential effects on brain amines. It was also suggested that, although there was no evidence that aspartame is harmful in usual amounts, perhaps patients with mitral valve prolapse should be cautioned against immoderate use of this substance (Drake, M., et al.: *Lancet* 2:631, 1986). To present the full side of this, please note that products containing aspartame are consumed by more than 100 million people in the United States alone. The NutraSweet Company appropriately suggests that untoward events are going to occur in some of these individuals after ingestion of aspartame, and that the type of temporal relationship noted in the referenced article does not prove that the two events are related. The NutraSweet Company, which manufactures aspartame, will provide any physician who believes that there may be a causal relationship between a patient's symptoms and the consumption of aspartame with aspartame and a placebo capsule so that the symptoms can be evaluated scientifically (Moser, R.H., NutraSweet Company, Skokie, Illinois 60076).

One of the most interesting theories I think yet to come along to help explain why scoliosis develops in some girls appeared in *Spine* (11:405, 1986). Investigators in Stockholm, Sweden speculated that a differential rate of rib length growth on one side of the chest as opposed to the other could result in scoliosis. They also theorized that, because asymmetric development of the breast is fairly common, it is possible that the increased vascularity with a slightly larger breast on one side could result in an increased length of the underlying ribs, leading to scoliosis (I'm not making this up). So what they did was to study thermal emission from the skin of girls with scoliosis and normal girls. They claim to have found substantial evidence that unilateral stimulation of rib growth caused by greater vascularity of the left breast and the underlying costosternal junctions may be an initiating factor in the development of right convex thoracic idiopathic scoliosis in adolescent girls.

This seems a bit farfetched, but it certainly could raise interesting therapeutic potentials. If an early curve is detected, why not put a heating pad on the opposite chest several hours a day, or perhaps apply ice to the culprit side? If you follow this to its logical conclusion, someone might even recommend reduction mammoplasty. I for one would like to see the results of the Swedish study repeated and then analyzed critically. It was an interesting observation, however.

(Quiz: Can you guess the number of toe shoes that the New York City Ballet orders for its principal dancer, Suzanne Farrell, each season? The answer is 350.)—J.A. Stockman III, M.D.

Long-Term Effects on Personality Development in Patients With Adolescent Idiopathic Scoliosis: Influence of Type of Treatment
Kerstin Fällström, Thomas Cochran, and Alf Nachemson (Univ. of Göteborg, Sweden)
Spine 11:756–758, September 1986   18–13

All individuals experience an identity crisis during adolescence. During this period, an illness that changes a person's external appearance as well as demands a treatment that limits his social flexibility can alter that person's identity formation. A specific psychological interview was conducted in 157 patients treated surgically and/or with a Milwaukee brace to determine the long-term effects of treatment on personality development in adolescent idiopathic scoliosis. Total brace-wearing times were comparable in both groups: 6–9 months postoperatively followed by gradual weaning over a 12-month period (mean, 17 months) for the 92 surgical patients and 18 months full time followed by gradual weaning for 8 months (mean, 26 months) for brace-treated patients. The semistructured interview evaluated reactions concerning the treatment phase, attitudes and reactions to treatment, attitudes toward hospital staff, and body image concepts at an average of 9 years after treatment.

When informed about the diagnosis, brace-treated patients more often said that they experienced more fear and anxiety than the surgical patients reported. Nearly all patients initially reacted negatively to brace treatment in both groups; nevertheless, more surgical patients gradually accepted the brace than did brace-treated patients. More brace-treated patients had negative attitudes toward the hospital staff. End results were equal in both groups, 33-degree curvature in the brace-treated group and 36-degree curvature in the surgically treated patients. However, 50% of the brace-treated patients had definite signs of negative body image concept and only 8% had a definitely positive body image, compared with 33% and 27%, respectively, in the surgical patients. There was no correlation between later increase of the curvature or residual rib deformity and negative body image. These findings indicate that psychological disturbances caused by brace treatment can have a considerable negative impact on an individual's long-term personality development.

▶ If it is a particular brand of beer that has made Milwaukee famous, it is the scoliotic brace that has made it infamous. What we see from this report is that most girls who are treated with Milwaukee braces view them as an instrument of physical and psychological torture. It is precisely because of the unpopularity of full-time bracing that other methods of treating scoliosis are being pursued actively, hence the upsurge in the use of electrical stimulation. This is not to say that Milwaukee braces do not have demonstrable efficacy. They certainly do for most patients who use them. It just seems like a lot to ask of a person at a particularly vulnerable period of time in his or her life.

Green (J. Bone Joint Surg. 68a:738, 1986) made an interesting observation. He noted that fewer than 15% of girls with scoliosis were fully compliant with the standard 24-hour Milwaukee brace regimen. He wondered if those who were not as compliant had as good a result as those who were fully compliant. In fact, what he showed was very little difference between part-time use of the Milwaukee brace and full-time use. The difference was sufficiently insignificant that this author suggested that allowing girls to go without the brace for 8 hours or so was probably permissible, assuming adequate follow-up. At least this may be a step in the right direction.

Another step in the right direction was taken by Robb et al. (Acta Orthop. Scand. 57:220, 1986), who removed the myth that patients with idiopathic scoliosis have a high incidence of abnormal EEGs. Studies done in the later

1970s and early 1980s reported that about 30% of children with this condition have abnormal EEGs. Not so, say Robb et al. They found no difference between study patients and controls with respect to abnormal EEGs.—J.A. Stockman III, M.D.

Extremity Injuries in Children: Predictive Value of Clinical Findings
Frederick P. Rivara, Ruth Ann Parish, and Beth A. Mueller (Univ. of Washington and Harborview Med. Ctr., Seattle)
Pediatrics 78:803–807, November 1986   18–14

Injuries are one of the major health problems in the United States today, and children and young adults sustain a disproportionate share of the total number of these injuries. Most of the injuries in children and adolescents treated in emergency rooms are to the extremities. A study was conducted to assess the worth of radiography in evaluation of extremity trauma in 189 children (64% boys) and to identify the criteria or clinical indicators having high sensitivity for extremity fractures.

The children were 1–15 years of age. All were treated during a 10-month period for a total of 209 extremity injuries. The most common cause of injury was sports (29%), followed by falls (21%), pedestrian-motor vehicle collisions (11%), and bicycle-related incidents (9%). The most common mechanisms of injury were falls (35%), blunt trauma (31%), twisting or hyperextension (15%), and crushing (13%). Data were analyzed separately for upper and lower extremity injuries.

Upper extremity injuries accounted for 116 (55.5%) of the total number. The presence of gross deformity and point tenderness of the upper ex-

TABLE 1.—DISTRIBUTION OF CLINICAL AND DEMOGRAPHIC INDICATORS FOR CHILDREN WITH UPPER EXTREMITY INJURIES AND RELATIVE RISK OF FRACTURES IF ATTRIBUTE PRESENT*

Attribute	No. (%) of Children With Attribute				Risk of Fracture If Attribute Present	95% Confidence Interval
	No Fracture (n = 57)		Fracture (n = 59)			
Male	33	58	40	68	1.5	0.7–3.3
Nonwhite	27	48	32	54	1.3	0.6–2.7
Age (yr)						
<5	13	23	7	12	1.0	
5–9	9	16	13	22	2.7	0.8–9.4
10–15	35	61	39	66	2.1	0.7–5.7
Clinical indicators						
Swelling[a]	32	57	37	64	1.3	0.6–2.8
Pain[a]	54	96	58	100		
Point tenderness[b]	15	27	41	72	7.0	3.2–15.6
Ecchymosis[a]	15	27	8	14	0.4	0.2–1.1
Crepitance[c]	0	0	5	9		
Gross deformity[c]	2	4	22	37	16.1	4.7–54.9
Decreased range of motion[b]	23	41	34	59	2.0	0.9–4.3
Pain on motion[b]	40	71	48	84	2.1	0.9–5.3
Decreased sensation[b]	8	14	5	9	0.6	0.2–1.9

*Missing values are indicated as follows: [a]two missing values, [b]three missing values, [c]one missing value.
(Courtesy of Rivara, F.P., et al.: Pediatrics 78:803–807, November 1986.)

TABLE 2.—DISTRIBUTION OF CLINICAL AND DEMOGRAPHIC INDICATORS FOR CHILDREN
WITH LOWER EXTREMITY INJURIES AND RELATIVE RISK OF FRACTURES IF ATTRIBUTE PRESENT[*]

Attribute	No. (%) of Children With Attribute				Risk of Fracture If Attribute Present	95% Confidence Interval
	No Fracture (n = 57)		Fracture (n = 59)			
Male	34	58	27	79	2.8	1.1–7.4
Nonwhite	32	54	14	41	0.6	0.3–1.4
Age (yr)						
<5	6	10	4	12	1.0	
5–9	16	27	3	9	0.3	0.1–1.6
10–14	37	63	26	79	1.1	0.3–4.1
Clinical indicators						
Swelling[a]	33	57	22	67	1.5	0.6–3.7
Pain[b]	55	100	33	100		
Point tenderness[c]	25	46	22	69	2.6	1.1–6.6
Ecchymosis[d]	10	18	8	24	1.5	0.5–4.3
Crepitance[d]	0	0	3	9		
Gross deformity[a]	0	0	9	27		
Decreased range of motion[d]	14	24	15	47	2.8	1.1–6.9
Pain on motion[c]	36	66	31	97	16.4	3.4–84.4
Decreased sensation[e]	3	6	3	10	1.8	0.3–9.5
Pain on weight bearing[f]	37	71	29	94	5.9	1.4–24.5

[*]Missing values are indicated as follows: [a]Two missing values, [b]five missing values, [c]six missing values, [d]three missing values, [e]eight missing values, [f]ten missing values.
(Courtesy of Rivara, F.P., et al.: Pediatrics 78:803–807, November 1986.)

tremities correctly identified 81% of the fractures (sensitivity) and 82% of the children without fractures (specificity), whereas in only 59 of 116 injuries (51%) was the x-ray film positive for fracture or dislocation (Table 1). Gross deformity and pain on motion were the best predictors of lower extremity fractures, in that 97% of children with lower extremity fractures were identified correctly. However, only 34 of 93 lower extremity x-ray films (37%) were positive for fracture (Table 2). Physical examination is predictive of fracture in extremity injuries of children; in the absence of specific physical findings, the probability of a fracture being found radiographically is low.

▶ A lot of people had trouble with this report when it appeared. The results seem to be just too clear-cut. I asked Dr. James J. Conway, Chief, Division of Nuclear Medicine at Children's Memorial Hospital, and Professor of Radiology at Northwestern University Medical School, for his thoughts on this.—J.A. Stockman III, M.D.

▶ I have read with interest the article entitled "Extremities Injuries in Children: Predictive Value of Clinical Findings." I am concerned that the information would be applied to all children when the mean age of the population was 11.1 years (SE ± 0.285). This indicates to me a specific population group of predominantly older children. Elastic and plastic injuries are much more common in younger groups and are not associated with deformity or crepitance but are principally manifested by pain or limitation of motion of the injured part. We recently reported a series of 30 patients, who presented primarily with pain or limitation of motion, all of whom had normal findings on x-ray studies, but gross abnormalities seen on bone scintigraphy. Frequently, the history of trauma was minor or obscure. Importantly, x-ray films are obtained in the younger population to exclude other abnormalities such as infection (osteomyelitis, septic arthritis) or neoplasms (neuroblastoma, histiocytosis-X). The x-ray studies and bone scintigraphy are warranted not only for medical/legal purposes but also for social service management (child abuse). I am sure that if this study were extended to infants and younger children that the discriminators noted in the study would fail just as the discriminators for adult skull fracture do not apply to children. I think that their report should be retitled, "Extremity Injuries in Adolescence."—J.J. Conway, M.D.

Sports-Related Injuries in Children: A Study of Their Characteristics, Frequency, and Severity, With Comparison to Other Types of Accidental Injuries
Anne Tursz and Monique Crost (Institut National de la Santé et de la Recherche Médicale, Paris)
Am. J. Sports Med. 14:294–299, July–August, 1986   18–15

Sports accidents in children have not been studied extensively in France. In an effort to do so, data were collected on all accidents involving children aged from birth to 15 years treated in a French health care unit in 1981–1982. The frequency, type of lesion, and level of medical consumption were compared with other types of accidental injuries.

Of the 7,182 accidents, 789 (11%) were sports related with 76% resulting from out-of-school sports activities. Also, 62% of the injuries were sustained by boys, and 53% were incurred by children 12 years of age and older. Out-of-school sports accidents were more frequent among boys, but boys and girls had similar injury rates in association with school physical education. Sports areas were the most frequent places of accident among children older than 11 years. Compared with other types of accidents, sports injuries resulted in the highest rate of upper limb injuries (43%). The fracture rate was 22%. Usually, the injuries were sustained by falling, and the child was injured without contacting other players or sports equipment. Sports-related injuries were usually benign; the most common lesions were contusions. Yet, 11% of the children were hospitalized and 20% required several hospitalizations for the same accident. In addition, the time elapsed between the accident and the end of the last hospital stay was significantly longer than with other kinds of accidents, possibly as a result of a higher rate of epiphyseal fractures (10%) and internal fixation (17%). Twelve percent of inpatient children experienced angulation or shortening of a limb or limited joint mobility.

Sports-related injuries in children are frequent in France. These injuries are usually mild, but caution is required because of musculoskeletal sequelae. Preventive measures should be directed toward teaching and training children rather than toward changing sports equipment.

▶ Now I know what it means to be a sport: It means you get hurt.—J.A. Stockman III, M.D.

Digital Ischemia in Baseball Players

Makoto Sugawara, Toshihiko Ogino, Akio Minami, and Seiichi Ishii (Hokkaido Univ. and Sapporo Med. College, Japan)
Am. J. Sports Med. 14:329–334, July–August 1986   18–16

Throwing injuries to the shoulder and elbow in baseball players have been studied widely, but digital ischemia associated with the repetitive impact of catching a ball has received less attention. The incidence of digital ischemia among baseball players was studied.

A questionnaire was mailed to 578 baseball players who belonged to baseball clubs in junior high schools (207), high schools (299), and colleges (72). None of the 207 junior high school students, 66 of 299 high school students (22.1%), and 29 of 72 college students (40.3%) reported digital ischemia. The incidence of digital ischemia in the ring, middle, and little fingers and in the thumb was low; but 58 of 66 high school students (87.9%) and all 29 college students had digital ischemia of the index finger. The incidence of digital ischemia was higher among first basemen and catchers than among players of other positions. The incidence of digital ischemia was also related to the frequency of practice sessions and the number of years played.

Eight right-handed, male baseball players aged 16–26 years had digital ischemia in the left index finger of the gloved hand as a result of repetitive ball impact. Symptoms included coldness (8), numbness (4), cyanosis (3), nail deformities (2), and a positive digital Allen's test (4). Angiography was performed in four of eight players. All angiograms showed segmental occlusion and narrowing of the digital arteries of the left index finger. Thermography was performed in five of eight players. All thermograms showed a cool area on the index finger. Digital ischemia in baseball players is not rare; rather, it has been overlooked in the past.

▶ I'm willing to bet that you think I included this article on sports-related injuries just to continue my diatribe against exercise. You are right. Let me summarize for you some of the past year's information related to exercise activities and injury.

Backpacking can cause a suprascapular neuropathy; swimming goggles can damage the supraorbital nerve; surfing can cause a neuropathy of the lower legs; and playing the flute (loosely defined as a sport) can damage the first common digital nerve (*N. Engl. J. Med.* 316:555, 1987). Huffy bike riding can cause hematuria (*N. Engl. J. Med.* 315:768, 1986), as can power walking (also known as doing the goose step) (*JAMA* 257:1332, 1987). Shooting firearms can expose one to enormous quantities of lead (JAMA 257:803, 1987). And, as noted in the abstract above, baseball playing can cause digital ischemia. It was mentioned in last year's YEAR BOOK that jogging can cause hematuria and blood loss in the stool. Then there's jogger's leukocytosis (*N. Engl. J. Med.* 316:223, 1987). The latter wouldn't be too bad except for the fact that there is also an associated marked increase of neutrophil degranulation and activation during jogging. If that isn't enough to turn you off from running, read the report of "Fatal Rhabdomyolysis in a Marathon Runner" (*Lancet* 2:857, 1987) or heel pain in child athletes (*J. Pediatr. Orthop.* 7:34, 1987). And how about the cluster of spinal injuries that occurred with the introduction of water slides (*Am. J. Public Health* 76:284:1986). Finally, there was an article entitled "Body Builders' Psychosis" (*Lancet* 1:863, 1987—I think we all knew this anyway).

The underlying theme in much of this injury-prone saga is the fact that we Americans tend to go overboard a bit. This is not a new phenomenon. For example, more than 100 years ago it was noted that it was that more people had been killed or maimed on July 4 since establishment of this country's independence than were hurt by the British forces attempting to shut off the present noisy celebrations (JAMA 9:48, 1887). That is certainly true 100 years later.

Fear not, I think we're beginning to see the light. Perhaps all this physical activity is not all it's cracked up to be, and maybe things are changing. Recall, for example, that a few months back a report appeared in *The New England Journal of Medicine* (314:605, 1986) suggesting that exercise was associated with an increase in longevity in a group of 1,936 Harvard alumni. This study purported to show that by the age of 80, alumni spending 2,000 or more kcal per week could expect an additional 2.15 years of survival. Now, just what do the statisticians say about this study? A careful review of *The New England Journal of Medicine* article demonstrates that the total exercise time needed to reach a level of 2,000 kcal per week for 52 weeks a year for the 60 years from graduation to the age of 80 would be 1.18 to 2.37 years. Thus, to gain two extra years of survival you would have to exercise for approximately 2 years' worth of time. That's not even a fair trade. Not only is it not a fair trade, it's a heck of a waste of food to generate that many kcal (Jacoby, D.B.: *N. Engl. J. Med.* 315:399, 1986).

If that doesn't convince you, read the Letter to the Editor of *Lancet* (2:1207, 1987) entitled "Joggers Grow Old." In a careful scientific study performed in Switzerland examining the most important Swiss running event, the Morat-Fribourg race, it was noted that there was a distinct shift to the right in the age distribution of runners between 1982 and 1986. This was clearly suggestive of a uniform cohort aging effect and may indeed suggest a declining rate of jogging among young people. If the authors of this article will permit, I will close this commentary with their words: "It seems, to put our conclusions in terms of the epidemiology of a contagious disease, that jogging has already lost much of its 'contagiousness' and that it is tending towards 'chronification' among the affected. Jogging will turn out to be a self-limited epidemic." Would that the last member of our noble species not be a subspecies called "Homo sapien helveticus jogger."—J.A. Stockman III, M.D.

19 Gastroenterology

Foreign Bodies of the Gastrointestinal Tract
Richard R. Bloom, Phillip H. Nakano, Stephen W. Gray, and John E. Skanda-
lakis (The Piedmont Hosp. and Emory Univ., Atlanta)
Am. Surg. 52:618–621, November 1986   19–1

Emergency room staff frequently are called upon to treat patients with foreign bodies lodged in the gastrointestinal tract. Approximately 1,500 persons die each year after ingestion or placement of a foreign body. Data were reviewed concerning the case histories of 60 patients with foreign bodies in the alimentary tract. The patient charts were screened for age, length of hospital stay, type of foreign body, and site.

Of the 60 foreign objects, 41 were lodged in the esophagus, 7 in the stomach, and 10 in the small intestine, appendix, colon, or rectum; and

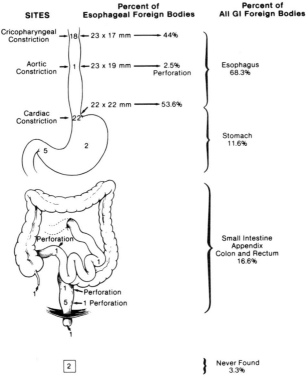

Fig 19–1.—Distribution of 60 foreign bodies. By far the greatest number lodged at the upper and lower constrictions of the esophagus.

(Courtesy of Bloom, R.R., et al.: Am. Surg. 52:618–621, November 1986.)

2 were never found (Fig 19–1). Barium swallow with esophagography was the most common diagnostic tool for determining the site of objects lodged in the esophagus. Most objects were removed by esophagoscopy. One of the foreign bodies caused perforation, requiring a two-layer closure. Five of the seven objects lodged in the stomach were bezoars that were dislodged or removed by upper endoscopy with the help, in four cases, of active enzymes. Presenting symptoms were nausea, vomiting, pain, diarrhea, and weight loss.

The small intestine was the involved site after a nail and a toothpick had been swallowed. The latter perforated the intestine, causing symptoms of peritonitis. The object in the appendix was found by incidental appendectomy during hysterectomy. A fishbone in the sigmoid colon caused perforation and peritonitis. Five objects found in the rectum had been inserted via the anus. In one case, rectal perforation and peritonitis led to adult respiratory distress syndrome.

The four perforations (one in the esophagus, one in the terminal ileum, and two in the colon) all resulted in longer hospital stays, and in two instances peritonitis developed. There was no association between denture wearing, age, or alcoholism and the incidence of a foreign body lodged in the alimentary tract.

▶ There is no telling at all what people will put in their gastrointestinal tracts. When a foreign body becomes lodged in the esophagus, appropriate management depends on the nature of the swallowed object. As may be seen from this study, esophageal foreign bodies are the most common. Prompt endoscopic removal is recommended for a sharp-edged or pointed foreign body because of its potential for esophageal wall penetration and perforation. Likewise, small disk batteries such as those used in electronic watches and calculators should be withdrawn without delay to prevent caustic erosion and perforation of the esophagus. However, if the foreign body has a smooth surface and is nontoxic, one may justify delaying extraction because most blunt objects will pass spontaneously without incident.

To hasten passage into the stomach, a number of noninvasive pharmacologic and mechanical measures have been advocated, including glucagon to relieve lower esophageal sphincter spasm, sublingual nitroglycerin to eliminate more widespread smooth muscle spasm, and carbon dioxide gas to distend the esophagus and push impacted food beyond fixed strictures. When noninvasive methods fail to dislodge a blunt object, extraction is required. Currently, most foreign bodies are removed with instruments passed through an endoscope or with a Foley catheter balloon inflated distal to the impaction and withdrawn under fluoroscopic control. A recently introduced method for removing blunt foreign bodies from the esophagus was described by Shaffer et al. (AJR 147:1010, 1986). With this technique, foreign bodies are removed with a wire basket under fluoroscopic guidance. The procedure is particularly useful for removing soft food masses and hard spherical objects (e.g., fruit pits) that have become impacted above the esophageal stricture.

Even food can get stuck in the gastrointestinal tract. There are three foods, however, that are not likely to do so. Do you know the three foods that Americans hate most in order of least preference? They are tofu, liver, and yogurt. Believe it or not, a survey uncovered that little tidbit (*The Harper's Index Book,* New York, Henry Colt Inc., 1987).—J.A. Stockman III, M.D.

Gastroesophageal Reflux in Children: Clinical Profile, Course, and Outcome With Active Therapy in 126 Cases
R.W. Shepherd, J. Wren, S. Evans, M. Lander, and T.H. Ong (Royal Children's Hosp. and Univ. of Queensland, Brisbane)
Clin. Pediatr. (Phila.) 26:55–60, February 1987   19–2

Gastroesophageal reflux (GER) can result in serious morbidity and even mortality in children. The clinical profile, course, and outcome in 126 infants and children with GER were reviewed. The median age at diagnosis was 2.5 months. Follow-up ranged from 1.5 years to 3.5 years.

Most patients had overt regurgitation, rumination, or both (table). Feeding problems in children younger than age 1 year and maternal distress were common, and in four children were associated with child abuse. Cineroentgenography, gastric scintiscans, and pH tests were useful only to confirm the presence or absence of GER. Peptic esophagitis was observed in 34 of 62 patients who underwent endoscopy. All patients initially received medical management consisting of positional therapy in the prone position, thickening of feeds, antacids, and in some cases bethanechol or metoclopromide, augmented by cimetidine in patients with proved esophagitis. Most patients (81%) were symptom free by age 18 months, 17% underwent fundoplication with good results, and 2% had persistent symptoms beyond age 2 years (Fig 19–2). There were no deaths. Primary in-

---

CLINICAL FEATURES OF GER IN 126 INFANTS AND CHILDREN

	No.	%
Repeated regurgitation/rumination	124	98.4
Feeding problems/dysphagia	65	51.6
"Colic," excessive crying, irritability	56	44.5
Sleep disturbance	36	28.6
Minor hematemesis	23	18.3
Sutcliffe–Sandifer syndrome	10	7.9
Respiratory symptoms (total 49%)		
Recurrent cough/wheeze (XR normal)	23	18.3
Apnea, cyanosis (>1 episode)	18	14.3
Recurrent aspiration (chest XR changes)	12	9.5
Failure to thrive (inadequate weight gain/loss)	23	18.3
Weight < 3rd percentile	11	8.7
Weight < 10th percentile	45	35.7
Weight < 50th percentile	107	84.9
Neurologic deficit	6	4.7
Child abuse	4	3.2

(Courtesy of Shepherd, R.W., et al.: Clin. Pediatr. [Phila.] 26:55–60, February 1987.)

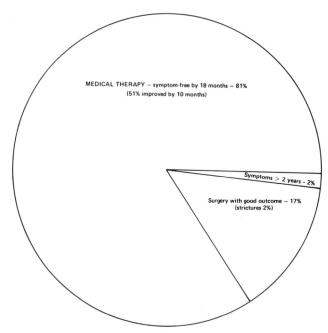

MEDICAL THERAPY — symptom-free by 18 months — 81%
(51% improved by 10 months)

Symptoms > 2 years - 2%

Surgery with good outcome — 17%
(strictures 2%)

Fig 19–2.—Outcome of 126 infants and children with GER. (Courtesy of Shepherd, R.W., et al.: Clin. Pediatr. [Phila.] 26:55–60, February 1987.)

dications for operation included recurrent apnea-aspiration in 6%, refractory esophagitis or stricture in 5%, and failed medical management in 7%. Esophagitis was a significant indicator of prognosis.

Gastroesophageal reflux remains a cause of considerable morbidity in children. Children with GER should be treated initially with medical measures, which will result in a favorable response in most. The importance of early endoscopy in selected patients with "pathologic" GER is emphasized, as abnormal findings indicate the need for aggressive treatment.

▶ I made a silent promise last year that there would be no articles included in the 1988 YEAR BOOK OF PEDIATRICS that dealt with GER. The reason for this was that many, myself included, were suffering from reflux just seeing the number of articles that were saying the same old thing over and over again. This past year, however, was a banner one in that it has seen the rise and fall of various treatment modalities. For example, does thickening of infant feedings improve the clinical status of children with GER? As always, the answer is, "It depends." Orenstein et al. (*J. Pediatr.* 110:181, 1987), using technetium scintigraphy, found that thickened and unthickened feedings were followed by similar amounts of GER. Nonetheless, little critters that have been fed thickened formulas tended to spend less time crying and more time sleeping as a consequence of the formula modification. Bailey et al. (*J. Pediatr.* 110:187, 1987), using esophageal pH monitoring, found no significant difference in the percentage of time with reflux after thickened as opposed to unthickened feedings. In fact, infants put into the prone position with a head elevation of 30 degrees had a remarkably increased amount of esophageal reflux time with thickened feedings.

This whole business with esophageal reflux, although stressing our patience (as well as our patients), is no laughing matter. Wald et al. (*Clin. Pediatr.* 25:541, 1986) described 22 patients previously given the diagnosis of GER in infancy who were now at an average age of 14 years. When they were examined for pulmonary function, a marked degree of abnormality was found even more than a decade later. The typical finding was that of reactive airway disease, maldistribution of ventilation, and airway obstruction. There was no problem with restricted lung volumes.

This past year has also seen a further understanding of the complications of the Nissen fundoplication procedure. In one series (Dedinsky, G.K., et al.: *Am. J. Surg.* 153:177, 1987) 16% of the patients undergoing this procedure had significant complications, including herniation or breakdown at the suture sites, postoperative bowel obstruction, strictures, and intra-abdominal abscesses and fistulas. The postoperative mortality rate was about 1%. Despite this bad news, fundoplication successfully controlled symptoms of reflux in 92% of the children. An additional strike against milk thickening was reported by Vadenplas et al. (*Clin. Pediatr.* 26:66, 1987). These individuals found that milk-thickening agents, although seemingly effective for treatment of GER in individual cases, can lead to occult GER episodes of long duration, possibly increasing the risk for esophagitis or respiratory dysfunction.

So what can be said about all of this? Who knows? An editorial on the sad story related to thickened feedings appeared in the *Journal of Pediatrics* (Ulshen, M.H.: *J. Pediatr.* 110:254, 1987). This editorial was entitled "Treatment of esophageal reflux: Is nothing sacred?" The answer is, Obviously not. Having just purchased a new *Webster's Unabridged Dictionary,* I looked up the word sacred to see how it might apply in this instance. Clearly, esophageal reflux has never been "held as being sacred, belonging to a god, related to a religion, entitled to the highest respect or reverence," and is certainly not in a class "not to be profaned, violated, or made common." If there is anything sacred about thickened feedings and GER it is that thickened feedings are usually made by adding cereal to a milk formula. Therefore, the closest thickened feedings come to holiness is the classification of a "sacred cow." For now I suppose we'll have to be satisfied with the fact that, even though "beefing up" a feeding doesn't decrease reflux, at least we have more contented children as a result.—J.A. Stockman III, M.D.

Spectrum of Biliary Disease in Childhood

Maria Frexes, Wallace W. Neblett, III, and George W. Holcomb, Jr. (Vanderbilt Univ.)

South. Med. J. 79:1342–1349, November 1986   19–3

Obstructive biliary disease in childhood is uncommon. However, it should be considered when an infant or child presents with jaundice, abdominal pain, or an abdominal mass. A review was made of the records

BILIARY TRACT DISORDERS OF CHILDHOOD	
Type of Disorder	*No. Patients*
Congenital (12)	
Stenosis of extrahepatic bile ducts	3
Caroli's disease	1
Choledochal cyst	5
Primary neoplasm	1
Miscellaneous	2
Acquired (75)	
Neonatal cholestatic syndromes	
Biliary atresia	20
Biliary hypoplasia	5
Neonatal hepatitis	5
Calculous disease	
Cholelithiasis	36
Choledocholithiasis	2*
Fibrosing pancreatitis	3
Sclerosing cholangitis	2
Secondary neoplasm	3
Total	87

*One patient with a primary hepatic duct stone had gallstones 4 years previously.
(Courtesy of Frexes, M., et al.: South. Med. J. 79:1342–1349, November 1986.)

of all children treated for biliary disease during a 15-year period at Vanderbilt University Children's Hospital.

The series included 87 children aged 18 years or younger, including 12 (14%) who had congenital obstructive biliary disorders and 75 with acquired disorders (table). Congenital obstructive biliary disorders included stenosis of the common bile duct and common hepatic duct in three, choledochal cyst in five, and congenital septate biliary tree, congenital teratoma of the common bile duct and common hepatic duct, isolated atresia, and Caroli's disease in one patient each. Acquired obstructive biliary disorders included neonatal cholestatic syndromes in 30, calculous disease in 37, fibrosing pancreatitis in 3, sclerosing cholangitis in 2, and secondary neoplasm in 3.

Operations were performed in 11 of 12 patients with congenital disorders. One patient died of unrelated causes, and one was lost to follow-up. The ten remaining patients were doing well at postoperative follow-up. The outcome in children with acquired obstructive biliary disorders was much less favorable, with an especially low survival rate among those with biliary atresia and neoplastic conditions.

Primary Sclerosing Cholangitis in Children
Martin Classen, Hermann Götze, Hans-Joachim Richter, and Steffen Bender (Univ. of Essen and J.W. Goethe Univ., Frankfurt/Main, West Germany)
J. Pediatr. Gastroenterol. Nutr. 6:197–202, March–April 1987   19–4

Primary sclerosing cholangitis is a rare disease of unknown origin that is characterized by inflammatory obliterating fibrosis of the biliary tract. Only ten detailed case reports have been presented in the literature. Eight children were seen with primary sclerosing cholangitis, all of whom were treated over a 13-year period at two pediatric centers in West Germany. The five boys and three girls ranged in age from 4 to 13 years; six had concomitant inflammatory bowel disease. All eight presented initially with unspecific symptoms (e.g., abdominal pain and fever), but signs of liver disease were rare. Admission laboratory data showed mildly elevated levels of transaminases and alkaline phosphatase, markedly elevated IgG levels in seven, an elevated erythrocyte sedimentation rate, and the presence of anti-nuclear antibodies in four. None had hyperbilirubinemia or abnormal serologic findings for hepatitis A, hepatitis B, or Epstein-Barr virus infection. However, needle liver biopsy provided highly characteristic histologic data in all eight patients, including portal tracts considerably expanded by edema and chronic inflammation, a finding that was diagnostic of nonsuppurative cholangitis and nonsuppurative fibrosing pericholangitis. None of the patients was treated because no specific therapy is available for primary sclerosing cholangitis. Patients with concomitant inflammmatory bowel disease were treated with salazosulfapyridine. As bile duct surgery increases the risk of liver transplantation and the rate of ascending cholangitis, these procedures should be avoided in children with primary sclerosing cholangitis who may ultimately require liver transplantation when their disease advances to a life-threatening stage.

▶ Why we have not been seeing more cases of primary sclerosing cholangitis baffles many people. It could well be because in many such patients the disease follows a mild course, with only minimal progression in most patients. Just as likely an explanation might be the lack of awareness of this disease among pediatricians. The vast majority of patients described so far in the literature are patients who have concomitant inflammatory bowel disease. The onset of liver involvement is associated with nonspecific symptoms, e.g., abdominal pain and fever. On physical examination signs of liver disease are rare. What this study tells us, if nothing else, is that every patient with a diagnosis of inflammatory bowel disease must be followed with routine liver function studies. One must be very astute, however, to recognize the subtle abnormalities that can be seen on liver function studies. All patients have minimal to slight elevations of aspartate aminotransferase and alanine aminotransferase. The alkaline phosphatase level is elevated in most patients at the time of initial diagnosis. However, chemical hyperbilirubinemia is usually not present early on. The most uniform finding is an elevation of gammaglobulins. Some patients may have antinuclear antibodies. The histology is that of periportal tract inflammation with edema. The diagnosis can also be suspected on cholangiography performed by means of endoscopic retrograde cannulation of the biliary tract. Ductal stenosis, ectasia, and decreased arborization of the biliary tree are seen.

The natural history of primary sclerosing cholangitis in children is not known. Adults with this disorder survive somewhere between 5 and 7 years. Management of the inflammatory bowel disease does not seem to have much effect on what goes on with the liver. In patients with ulcerative colitis who have colectomy, the liver problem seems to follow an independent course. There is no specific therapy for primary sclerosing cholangitis so far. As the abstract notes, as little as possible monkeying around with the biliary tract should be done. This is to minimize the complication rate if the patient must ultimately come to liver transplantation. Primary sclerosing cholangitis is different from primary biliary cirrhosis. The latter is a disorder affecting young adults (but can be seen in children), and 90% to 95% of these patients are women. If you'd like to read an excellent review of primary biliary cirrhosis see the article by Kaplan (*N. Engl. J. Med.* 316:521, 1987).

It is possible that there is some overlap between the pathogenesis of these two disorders, and perhaps we in pediatrics could be a little more imaginative in terms of therapy, taking clues from the adult disorder. For example, trials of cyclosporine are currently underway as part of the treatment of primary biliary cirrhosis. In the latter disorder it has also been suggested that some of the hepatic lesions could result in part from the intrahepatic accumulation of potentially toxic endogenous bile acids. Currently, there are reports of the possible value of using ursodeoxycholic acid. This bile acid can be fed to patients in the hope of preventing hepatic damage and cholestasis by offsetting the presence of more toxic bile acids (Poupon, R., et al.: *Lancet* 1:834, 1987).

I think we'll be hearing more and more about primary sclerosing cholangitis in children. The fact that we are recognizing more of it is a good sign, at least in terms of learning to follow its natural history. We should keep our eyes open whenever we see inflammatory bowel disease. As can be seen in Abstract 19–3, there are numerous other causes of acquired biliary obstruction. These must all be ruled out based on age or other clinical findings.—J.A. Stockman III, M.D.

Endoscopic Retrograde Cholangiopancreatography in Children

Mark Allendorph, Steven L. Werlin, Joseph E. Geenen, Walter J. Hogan, Rama P. Venu, Edward T. Stewart, and Ellen L. Blank (Med. College of Wisconsin, Milwaukee Children's Hosp., and St. Luke's Hosp., Racine, Wis.)
J. Pediatr. 110:206–211, February 1987   19–5

Endoscopic retrograde cholangiopancreatography (ERCP) is widely used in the diagnosis and treatment of pancreaticobiliary tract disease in adults; its use in children with similar problems has been limited. Suspected pancreaticobiliary disorders in 39 children and adolescents aged 6 months to 18 years (mean, 12.5 years) were evaluated with ERCP using standard adult and pediatric side-viewing endoscopes. The study was performed under general anesthesia in 18 patients, and intravenous sedation was used in 21. In addition, ERCP manometric study of the sphincter of Oddi, endoscopic sphincterotomy, or balloon extraction of common bile duct stones was performed in selected patients.

Overall, ERCP was successful in 92% of the patients, identified structural abnormalities in 19, and provided valuable anatomical information for selection and planning of operative or endoscopic management in 14. Of the 21 patients with pancreatic disorders, 10 had abnormal ERCP findings that included pancreas divisum, communicating pancreatic pseudocyst and chronic pancreatitis, choledocochal cyst, and choledochocele. Biliary tract disorders were suspected in 11 patients, and 5 had abnormalities, e.g., common duct stone, sclerosing cholangitis, and choledochal cyst. Three of seven patients with biliary-type abdominal pain were helped by either an endoscopic or operative procedure. Mild pancreatitis developed in four patients and responded to supportive, short-term therapy.

This procedure is safe and valuable diagnostically and as therapy in children suspected of pancreaticobiliary tract disease. Indications and contraindications are similar, for the most part, to those established for adults.

▶ Although ERCP is used for a variety of diagnostic purposes these days, I find it to be most helpful as part of the diagnostic approach to patients with pancreatic disorders and biliary tract disease. The most puzzling problem we tend to run across is that of the child with recurrent abdominal pain who may or may not have chronic pancreatitis, but you can't document it because of failure to see significant rises in the pancreatic enzyme levels. In some of these patients ERCP is helpful because it shows narrowing of the drainage of the pancreas caused by inflammation. Of course, ERCP should always be done in conjunction with other diagnostic modalities, e.g., abdominal ultrasound. The study still may be negative in patients with chronic pancreatitis and then you're left pretty much on your own to decide how to make the diagnosis in a child who has recurrent abdominal pain.

A different approach could be the use of evocative tests that assist in the diagnosis of chronic relapsing pancreatitis in children. Buntain et al. (*Am. J. Surg.* 152:628, 1986) described the concomitant use of morphine, which tends to contract the sphincter of Oddi, and prostigmine, which increases pancreatic secretions. The idea here is to measure serial amylase levels and show that they go up in patients who have chronic relapsing pancreatitis. Normal children do not have this elevation. I suppose the latter may be a good test, although I was always trained not to use narcotics in children or adults with inflammation of the pancreas because the drug may produce enough obstruction to make the pancreatitis worse. I suppose I will have to trust the surgeons who report the beneficial use of these evocative tests. It will not be a blind trust, however. I trust everybody, but I still cut the cards.—J.A. Stockman III, M.D.

Evaluation of the Pediatric Patient for Liver Transplantation
Basil J. Zitelli, J. Jeffrey Malatack, J. Carlton Gartner, Jr., Andrew H. Urbach, Laurel Williams, Joanne W. Miller, and Beverly Kirkpatrick (Univ. of Pittsburgh)
Pediatrics 78:559–565, October 1986   19–6

Since liver transplantation has become an acceptable therapeutic modality for patients with end-stage liver disease, physicians at increasing numbers of institutions are beginning to perform this procedure. Clinical

TABLE 1.—High-Risk Conditions for
Pediatric Liver Transplantation

Contraindications
Primary extrahepatic unresectable malignancy
Malignancy metastatic to the liver
Progressive or terminal nonhepatic disease uncorrect-
able by liver transplantation
Inability of parents (or patient) to understand or ac-
cept the procedure
High-Risk Conditions
Massive arteriovenous shunting with profound cy-
anosis (Pao$_2$ < 50 mm Hg)
Positive hepatitis B surface antigen
Stage III or IV coma
Portal vein thrombosis
Intraabdominal abscess
Multiple intraabdominal operations
Weight <5 kg

(Courtesy of Zitelli, B.J., et al.: Pediatrics 78:559–565,
October 1986.)

evaluation is a crucial part of any liver transplantation program. A review
was made of a 3-year experience, which may serve as a model for evaluating
and accepting pediatric patients for liver transplantation.

During a 36-month period, 209 children aged 7.5 months to 18 years
were evaluated for liver transplantation at the Children's Hospital of Pittsburgh. The purpose of the evaluation was to confirm or establish the
diagnosis through review of clinical records, biopsy specimens, and laboratory data, assess the severity, progression, and complications of the
liver disease, as well as anatomical suitability for liver transplantation, do
a psychosocial profile of the family and child to anticipate support and

TABLE 2.—Indications and Outcome of Evaluations

	No. of Patients Receiving Transplants (Deaths After Transplantation)	No. of Deaths While Awaiting Transplantation	No. of Candidates Not Active	Total*
Biliary atresia†	38 (10)	25	9	104
Biliary hypoplasia	9 (3)	1	5	21
Metabolic disorders				
α$_1$-antitrypsin deficiency	14 (2)	5	6	29
Wilson disease	1 (0)	2	1	4
Tyrosinemia‡	2 (0)	0	1	3
Sea blue histiocyte syndrome‡	1 (0)	0	0	1
Familial hypercholesterolemia§	1 (0)	0	0	1
Glycogen storage disease I	1 (0)	0	0	1
Glycogen storage disease IV	0	1	0	1
Wolman disease	0	0	1	1
Neonatal hepatitis	3 (0)	2	3	8
Hepatitis	4 (2)	2	0	9
Familial cholestasis	7 (2)	0	0	8
Miscellaneous	4 (2)	3	8	18

*The number of patients on the active waiting list is represented by the difference between the total and the sum of
the other three columns.
†Includes one auxiliary transplant.
‡Patients had hepatocellular carcinoma also.
§Combined heart/liver transplantation.
(Courtesy of Zitelli, B.J., et al.: Pediatrics 78:559–565, October 1986.)

coping mechanisms, and educate the family and the child, if old enough, about the transplantation procedure.

Of 209 patients evaluated, 174 were found suitable for liver transplantation. However, 41 (24%) of these 174 died prior to surgery because a suitable organ could not be found, including 15 who died within 30 days of evaluation. One patient was lost to follow-up. The other 34 patients (16%) were not considered suitable candidates for transplantation because high-risk conditions precluded their eligibility (Table 1). In all 85 (41%) of the evaluated patients underwent liver transplantations; 64 (75%) survived for a minimum of 12 months (Table 2). The mean waiting period for a transplant increased from 80.3 days to 232 days during the study period. In view of the tragic loss of 41 patients who died prior to transplantation because a suitable organ could not be located in time, pediatricians should be willing to take a more active role in seeking organ donations.

Reyes Syndrome: Salicylate Metabolism, Viral Antibody Levels, and Other Factors in Surviving Patients and Unaffected Family Members

Anita B. Chu, Lata S. Nerurkar, Norma Witzel, Brian D. Andresen, Michael Alexander, Ellen S. Kang, Pim Brouwers, Paul Fedio, Young Jack Lee, and John L. Sever (Natl. Inst. of Health, Bethesda, Ohio State Univ., and Univ. of Tennessee)
Am. J. Dis. Child. 140:1009–1012, October 1986   19–7

Five patients were studied to determine various etiologic factors in Reye's syndrome. Salicylate metabolism was measured to study the link between aspirin and Reye's syndrome, immunologic assays were conducted to evaluate the role of antecedent viral infections, genetic tests were made to search for evidence of association with human leukocyte antigens (HLAs), and neuropsychological consequences were investigated.

Five survivors of Reye's syndrome aged 8–15 years and their families were studied 3–10 years after the acute disease. Three of the patients had no exposure to salicylates before the disease developed. Salicylate metabolism was evaluated by measuring serum salicylate concentrations after single oral doses of aspirin. Blood samples were tested for influenza A and influenza B, varicella, herpes simplex, cytomegalovirus, and Epstein-Barr virus. Three families underwent HLA typing. Tests of intelligence, memory, attention, learning, perception, concept formation and shifting, and verbal fluency were given to four former Reye's syndrome patients and their unaffected siblings.

The patients with Reye's syndrome had lower serum salicylate concentrations than their siblings and parents. They had higher antibody titers for influenza A and varicella than found in their families (table). There was no association between Reye's syndrome and HLA antigen subtype. No residual neuropsychological impairments were detected by any of the tests.

Unlike the findings in other studies, no association was found for Reye's

VIRAL ANTIBODY TITERS, MONONUCLEAR CELL STUDIES, AND LYMPHOCYTE STIMULATION*

| | Serum Viral Antibody Titers | | | | | | | Mononuclear Cells, % Positive† | | | | | Lymphocyte Stimulation‡ | | | | | | | | |
| | | | | | | | | | | | | | Mitogens | | | Viral Antigens | | | | | |
	VZV	Flu A	Flu B	HSV-1	HSV-2	CMV	EBV-VCA	OKT3	OKT4	OKT8	OKIa	OKT4:OKT8	PHA	Con A	PWM	VZV	Flu A	Flu B	HSV-1	HSV-2	CMV
Family 1																					
Father	1024	32	32	1024	64	4	320	66.31	41.24	25.48	14.53	1.6	89.8	39.6	43.1	14.9	2.4	10.0	2.5	2.0	1.0
Mother	1024	16	4	512	32	4	640	73.27	57.44	20.50	15.53	2.8	97.7	49.4	57.6	9.3	4.9	15.8	9.8	7.6	1.3
Sibling	1024	4	4	64	4	4	5	44.09	28.10	12.60	15.53	2.2	125.9	74.7	70.0	7.1	2.3	5.8	0.9	1.0	1.1
Patient 1a	2048	32	4	32	4	4	160	53.95	31.65	14.14	10.82	2.2	168.3	66.0	70.6	4.1	9.8	7.8	1.4	1.1	1.3
Patient 1b	2048	32	8	64	4	64	320	57.78	27.47	25.67	11.85	1.1	129.8	70.6	49.6	4.8	2.6	4.0	0.8	1.4	1.1
Family 2																					
Father	512	4	4	4	4	4	160	76.71	50.69	24.96	11.03	2.0	73.4	41.7	39.5	4.9	13.6	12.3	0.9	2.0	1.2
Mother	1024	16	16	16	4	512	1280	64.58	38.44	29.63	14.14	1.3	171.9	65.6	98.1	38.6	11.4	24.0	1.3	0.9	2.2
Sibling	2048	32	16	256	2	4	640	59.89	29.79	25.85	12.81	1.2	79.7	23.9	35.0	3.5	3.4	2.7	0.7	3.0	0.8
Patient 2	2048	64	4	32	4	8	160	66.71	44.31	21.60	10.28	2.1	146.4	54.1	64.9	11.2	7.3	2.9	0.9	2.0	1.0
Family 3																					
Father	128	4	4	512	4	128	160	64.69	46.39	17.26	14.51	2.7	99.3	61.5	39.2	3.6	2.4	2.1	0.4	0.9	1.4
Mother	256	8	8	256	2	128	160	71.99	43.61	24.58	11.63	1.8	96.5	45.9	47.6	2.2	1.7	5.3	0.7	4.0	1.0
Sibling	256	8	8	128	4	4	5	65.59	41.72	16.73	10.17	2.5	80.2	56.8	39.7	3.1	2.2	3.5	0.4	2.5	1.5
Patient 3	1024	16	4	1024	2	128	320	67.55	35.58	20.04	10.24	1.8	65.3	35.4	31.2	1.6	2.2	2.7	0.7	2.1	1.1
Family 4																					
Father	64	16	8	128	8	32	320	70.93	43.91	26.43	...	1.7	...	...	...						
Mother	1024	16	8	32	16	128	320	70.39	29.63	38.81	...	0.8	...	...	...						
Sibling	256	4	4	32	4	32	320	70.15	35.76	28.24	...	1.3	...	...	...						
Patient 4	1024	128	16	1024	2	4	640	62.08	34.32	32.10	...	1.1	...	...	...						

*VZV: varicella; Flu: influenza; HSV-1 and -2: herpes simplex virus types 1 and 2; CMV: cytomegalovirus; EBV-VCA: Epstein-Barr viral capsid antigen; Con A: concanavilin A; PWM: pokeweed mitogen.

†OKT3 reacts with all T cells; OKT4, with helper T cell subset; OKT8, with suppressor T cell subset; OKIa, with Ia-positive mononuclear cells.

‡Measured by stimulation index as (CPM in stimulated cells)/(CPM in unstimulated cells). Family 4 was not studied.

(Courtesy of Chu, A.B., et al.: Am. J. Dis. Child. 140:1009–1012, October 1986.)

syndrome and salicylate ingestion; in fact, salicylate concentrations were lower in the patients than in controls. High titers to varicella and influenza A in the patients suggest some association between Reye's syndrome and viral infections, a finding consistent with earlier reports.

▶ The aspirin story and Reye's syndrome appear to be aging with grace and with beauty. Every report to date, good or bad, seems to be in support of the concept that salicylate ingestion increases the risk of the occurrence of Reye's syndrome. The above report suggests that patients who recover from Reye's syndrome do not have any difficulty in metabolizing salicylates. In fact, they may even have an accelerated metabolism. This in no way, however, negates the possibility that salicylates are culpable in the etiology of Reye's syndrome. Britain, which had long lagged behind the United States in dealing with the aspirin issue, now has moved to the forefront. The Committee on Safety of Medicine (the British government's drug regulatory body) now is urging health professionals to advise families that "aspirin is not, on the evidence now available, a suitable medicine for children with minor illnesses." The pharmaceutical industry in Britain has voluntarily undertaken to inform the public about the risk of giving aspirin to children; in addition, pediatric aspirin products will be withdrawn, and adult aspirin labels will be changed to warn against giving aspirin to children (*Lancet* 1:1396, 1986; *Br. Med. J.* 292:1543, 1986).

In the past 8 years there has been a remarkable decline in the number of patients with Reye's syndrome. Some have attributed this to a decrease in aspirin use in the United States (Arrowsmith, J.B., et al.: *Pediatrics* 79:858, 1987). Indeed, a survey of aspirin use and Reye's syndrome awareness among parents (Morris, L.A.: *Am. J. Public Health* 76:1422, 1986) supports the concept that the message is getting through to parents that aspirin is a bad actor. Only 12% of the total sample surveyed said that they would give their children aspirin if the child were to contract flu or chicken pox. Slightly more than 50% of the parents were aware of the specific contraindication against aspirin use, and 40% could spontaneously recall the name Reye's syndrome. This still leaves room for further education, but it is a remarkable achievement on the part of our public health agencies with respect to dissemination of this information. All this was occurring at a time when aspirin manufacturers were applying direct pressure on the Office of Management and Budget to delay public warnings or package labeling, and these same groups openly threatened a lawsuit if the American Academy of Pediatrics published any formal warnings. If, indeed, the salicylate/Reye's syndrome story is accurate, the reduction in the use of salicylates now has resulted in the inability to do much in the way of collaborative studies of Reye's syndrome because there were so few cases in the last several years of this disorder relative to the previous 5-year period.

Before leaving the subject of Reye's syndrome, it is worthwhile mentioning a few other pieces of information that have appeared recently. You may have heard about the potential for insecticides, particularly the spruce budworm control insecticide, being associated with Reye's syndrome. A careful epidemiologic study now shows no association between Reye's syndrome and spruce budworm spraying (Wood, R.B., et al.: *Am. J. Epidemiol.* 124:671, 1986). We can now get back to budworm spraying. An additional bit of information regarding the etiology of Reye's syndrome appeared in *The Lancet* (Larrick, J.W.: *Lancet* 2:132, 1986). Evidence was presented to support the hypothesis that salicylates release a necrosis factor that can contribute to the pathogenesis of Reye's syndrome. Actually, this necrosis factor is released by macrophages and can be activated in this process by viral infection as well.

The past year has also raised issues as to whether or not liver biopsies are in fact needed as part of the evaluation for Reye's syndrome. This issue, I thought, was dead in terms of its utility in the diagnosis of Reye's syndrome. The Japanese, however, still recommend liver biopsy as part of the workup of children (Kumura, A., et al.: *J. Pediatr. Gastroenterol. Nutr.* 6:153, 1987). Internists also are still recommending liver biopsy for Reye's syndrome in adults (Meythaler, J.M.: *Arch. Intern. Med.* 147:61, 1987). You will recall from previous discussions in the YEAR BOOK that Beckwith et al. have clearly shown that the histologic changes seen in Reye's syndrome are not pathognomonic of this disorder and can be present in association with several other entities. Here in the United States we tend to make the diagnosis on purely clinical grounds without this invasive test. I believe we are doing it correctly and that the issue of liver biopsy is indeed a deceased one. I don't know what it takes to remove established or well-ingrained approaches, but the issue of liver biopsy obviously is a standing one in other countries. These countries should recognize that just because something is standing doesn't mean that it's not dead.—J.A. Stockman III, M.D.

Peritoneal Lavage in Pediatric Patients Sustaining Blunt Abdominal Trauma: A Reappraisal

Randall W. Powell, Johnny B. Green, M. Gage Ochsner, Scott W. Barttelbort, Steven R. Shackford, and Michael J. Sise (U.S. Naval Hosp., San Diego, Univ. of California at San Diego, and Univ. of South Alabama, Mobile)</p>

J. Trauma 27:6–10, January 1987   19–8

The efficacy of peritoneal lavage among pediatric patients who sustain blunt abdominal trauma has been reported in several prospective studies. A reappraisal of this procedure was undertaken in a retrospective review of information on 128 children aged from less than 1 month to 18 months who underwent diagnostic peritoneal lavage after sustaining blunt abdominal trauma. Emergency celiotomy was performed on the basis of qualitative colorimetric analysis of the lavage fluid.

There were 78 negative and 50 positive lavages. No patient who had negative lavage required celiotomy. Of the 41 patients who underwent exploratory celiotomy after a positive lavage, 12 sustained injuries that did not require operation, illustrating the main weakness of peritoneal lavage, which is its oversensitivity in the face of a minor injury.

Peritoneal lavage is an excellent method of screening patients with possible abdominal injuries. However, in hemodynamically stable patients, a strongly positive lavage no longer mandates immediate exploratory celiotomy. Further diagnostic tests (e.g., abdominal CT to document the site and extent of injury) are warranted in these patients.

▶ Dr. Marleta Reynolds, Assistant Professor of Surgery, Northwestern University Medical School, and member of the Department of Surgery, Children's Memorial Hospital, Chicago, comments.—J.A. Stockman III, M.D.

▶ Dr. Powell and his colleagues have collected important data concerning peritoneal lavage in the evaluation of children with blunt abdominal trauma. They have shown that peritoneal lavage is an accurate diagnostic tool to identify intra-abdominal injury. The authors have also answered the crucial question: "Is lavage useful in determining which patient needs emergency laparotomy?" They conclude that a positive lavage is no longer an absolute indication for laparotomy and recommend that further studies be done to identify the site and extent of injury and the decision to proceed with laparotomy be made on clinical findings.

Did the 78 patients who had a negative lavage have an unnecessary invasive procedure? In my opinion, yes. Furthermore, 12 of their patients underwent unnecessary laparotomies. Because the authors recommend noninvasive studies and clinical evaluation to determine the need for laparotomy, why not avoid the lavage altogether? When clinical findings suggest intra-abdominal injury, appropriate roentgenographic or CT studies could be obtained. Laparotomy should be reserved for those patients whose clinical findings indicate the need.—M. Reynolds, M.D.

Patterns of Liver Injury in Childhood: CT Analysis
H. Philip Stalker, Robert A. Kaufman, and Richard Towbin (Univ. of Cincinnati and Children's Hosp. Med. Ctr., Cincinnati)
AJR 147:1199–1205, December 1986   19–9

Blunt abdominal trauma in childhood frequently results in injury to solid organs, often the spleen and liver. Although the appearance of hepatic trauma on CT scans has been described in both children and adults, there has been no systematic evaluation of these injuries or of the possibility of encountering a given type of injury. Between August 1981 and September 1985, 216 consecutive hemodynamically stable children with blunt abdominal injury and clinically suspected solid organ damage were evaluated by abdominal CT. Liver injury was diagnosed in 48 children, 29 boys and 19 girls aged 1–16 years.

No type of injury was more likely to occur in a given age group. The ratio of boys to girls was about the same for each type of injury. Table 1 lists the injuries by anatomical location. In 17 children, multiple hepatic segments were injured, and four injuries involved more than one hepatic lobe. The right lobe of the liver was damaged four times more often than the left and 20 times more often than the caudate lobe. Caudate injury occurred only with multilobar trauma. The posterior segment of the right lobe, the most vulnerable segment, was injured in 65% of all patients. Tables 2 and 3 categorize the injuries as simple vs. complex and superficial vs. deep. Although simple lesions were three times more common than complex lesions in the right lobe, the two types occurred with almost equal

TABLE 1.—ANATOMICAL DISTRIBUTION OF
INJURIES IN 48 CHILDREN

Site	No. of Patients (%)
Right lobe:	
Posterior segment	31 (65)
Dome	15 (31)
Anterior segment	10 (21)
Total*	40 (83)
Left lobe:	
Medial segment	7 (15)
Lateral segment	5 (10)
Total*	11 (23)
Caudate	2 (4)

*Numbers in columns add up to more than totals, and totals do not add up to 48 because some children were injured in more than one side.
(Courtesy of Stalker, H.P., et al.: AJR 147:1199–1205, December 1986.)

frequency in the left lobe. The frequencies of superficial and deep lesions in the right and left lobes were significantly different, with right-sided injuries twice as likely to be superficial and left-sided injuries three times as likely to be deep. Most deep injuries were perihilar. Retroperitoneal blood collections were observed around the adrenal gland in a distribution not reported previously. Injuries to the hepatic dome were most characteristic and were often associated with injuries to the lung base, kidney, ribs, and pneumothorax.

Categorization of hepatic injury by the anatomical segment(s) involved enables recognition of characteristic injury patterns. These are the right

TABLE 2.—CHARACTERIZATION OF INJURIES IN
48 CHILDREN: SIMPLE VS. COMPLEX

Type of Injury	No. of Patients (%)
Simple:	
Right lobe	30 (63)
Left lobe	6 (13)
Total*	35 (73)
Complex:	
Right lobe	10 (21)
Left lobe	5 (10)
Total*	13 (27)

*Some of the 48 children were injured in both the right and left lobes, thus numbers add up to more than totals.
(Courtesy of Stalker, H.P., et al: AJR 147:1199–1205, December 1986.)

TABLE 3.—CHARACTERIZATION OF INJURIES IN
48 CHILDREN: SUPERFICIAL VS. DEEP

Type of Injury	No. of Patients (%)
Superficial:	
Right lobe	26 (54)
Left lobe	3 (6)
Total*	28 (58)
Deep:	
Right lobe	14 (29)
Left lobe	8 (17)
Total*	20 (42)

*Some of the 48 children were injured in both the right and left lobes, thus numbers add up to more than totals.
(Courtesy of Stalker, H.P., et al.: AJR 147:1199–1205, December 1986.)

lobe and left lobe injuries. In the present study, caudate injuries were never isolated and followed the pattern of the associated right lobe or left lobe injury. Most common is the right hepatic lobe injury, present in four of every five patients with liver trauma. This preponderance has been noted by other workers and is attributed to the fact that the right lobe constitutes most of the volume of the liver. The present study has extended this observation, noting that the posterior segment of the right lobe is involved in nearly two thirds of all hepatic injuries. This may be because the posterior segment is surrounded by relatively "fixed" structures (e.g., the ribs and spine) against which it may impact during blunt abdominal trauma. Also, fixation of the liver by the coronary ligaments in this region may increase the effect of acceleration-deceleration injuries locally.

▶ Blunt abdominal trauma has become a leading cause of mortality in children (Cooney, D.R.: *Surg. Clin. North Am.* 61:1165, 1981). Although the most severely injured children do not arrive at the hospital alive, correct diagnosis and treatment at the hospital can still prevent a significant percentage of deaths. What this study shows us is that the CT scan can tell us whether or not the liver is injured by a hematoma or laceration, what the segmental distribution of bleeding is, and its relationship to major vessels. It can aid in the decision concerning conservative (nonsurgical) as opposed to surgical treatment. It also provides information about injury to other organs, e.g., the kidneys and pancreas. In the past year, two other groups of investigators have reported similar CT findings and have demonstrated the value of CT scanning as part of the evaluation of blunt abdominal trauma (Vock, P., et al.: *J. Pediatr. Surg.* 21:413, 1986; Oldham, K.T., et al.: *Surgery* 100:542, 1986). The information derived from all of these studies is somewhat analogous to where we were a short while ago with splenic injuries. Computed tomography now allows us to decide whether we can "sit on" liver trauma as opposed to calling for immediate surgery.

If a decision is made to operate on an injured liver, and if there is no contraindication to removal of the appendix, it might be a good idea to recommend this procedure as frequently as possible; most surgeons do. The reason for mentioning this is the fact that prophylactic appendectomy, if you're in the abdomen for other reasons, may spare a girl the risk of subsequent tubal infertility. Mueller et al. (*N. Engl. J. Med.* 315:1506, 1986) have shown that the risk of infertility is almost five times higher among women who have a history of ruptured appendix. Because the baseline rate of infertility in the United States is already fairly high, these numbers, therefore, are staggering. This adds credence to the old dictum, when in doubt, cut it out.—J.A. Stockman III, M.D.

Protracted Diarrhoea of Infancy: Evidence in Support of an Autoimmune Variant

Rita Mirakian, Anne Richardson, Peter J. Milla, John A. Walker-Smith, Joseph Unsworth, Martin O. Savage, and Gian Franco Bottazzo (Middlesex Hosp., Inst. of Child Health, and Queen Elizabeth Hosp. for Children, London)
Br. Med. J. 293:1132–1136, Nov. 1, 1986   19–10

Circulating autoantibodies to gut enterocytes have been noted in isolated reports of young children with protracted diarrhea of infancy. Prompted by these reports, 25 children ranging in age from 1 month to 1 year at onset of symptoms were investigated for unexplained protracted diarrhea.

Circulating enterocyte autoantibodies were detected by indirect immunofluorescence in 14 patients. The intensity of the immunofluorescence was more accentuated on the apical border of the mature enterocytes. Enterocyte autoantibodies were predominantly of the IgG class in 13 patients, but 11 were also positive for IgM and IgA. Five of 14 positive sera were able to fix complement. Absorption studies of sera positive for autoantibodies with an IgA-coupled immunoabsorbent did not modify the intensity of the staining, indicating that these antibodies were not directed against secretory IgA. In addition, 6 of 14 patients with autoantibodies had overt clinical autoimmune disorders, and 13 of 14 had other organ or nonorgan-specific autoantibodies; these were found in members of their families as well. In contrast, similar specificities were not detected in 50 control children with nongastroenterologic disorders. Follow-up studies showed that high titers of autoantibodies with complement-fixing ability indicated a poorer prognosis despite the use of immunosuppressive drugs. Spontaneous remissions were observed only in patients without enterocyte antibodies, even with less aggressive therapy. Despite the rare occurrence of autoimmune disease in childhood, the data suggest the existence of an autoimmune variant of protracted diarrhea of infancy.

▶ Three cheers for these investigators. All of us have run across the problem of the infant who presents with diarrhea that then becomes protracted and ultimately is unable to be assigned a specific cause. This protracted diarrhea of infancy has been the bane of the existence of many a pediatrician or gastroen-terologist. Now we learn that protracted diarrhea of infancy may be an autoim-mune disorder. Not only may it be an autoimmune disorder, there may be a test in hand to diagnose this. The test is a serum test for autoantibodies against the enterocytes. Sure, this test will be criticized in the sense that if autoantibodies against enterocytes are present we don't know if it is a chicken or an egg phenomenon. By that it is meant that perhaps damage to the enter-ocyte from any cause might elicit an autoantibody against the enterocyte, as opposed to the autoantibody being the primary cause of the problem. I sup-pose time will sort this out. In any event, from the evidence of this report, it is tempting to conclude that an autoimmune form of enteropathy may well account for about half the cases of protracted diarrhea for which previously no cause could be found. These investigators also note that follow-up studies may be of some importance. Regular testing for these antibodies does have prog-nostic implications. Persistently low titers of antibody or declining titers are associated with an improved clinical status of the infant. In contrast, high titers and complement fixing of the autoantibodies at presentation and during follow-up indicate a poorer prognosis and worse outcome.

If these data are believable, the approach certainly is better than doing serial small bowel biopsies. Goldgar et al. (*Gastroenterology* 90:257, 1986) found a total lack of correlation of small bowel biopsies in the clinical course of patients with intractable diarrhea of infancy. Also, before throwing in the towel and resorting to total parenteral nutrition in refractory intractable diarrhea of in-fancy, read the report of Orenstein et al. (*J. Pediatr.* 109:277, 1986). They noted that among 13 infants randomly allocated to treatment with continuous enteral nutrition with elemental formula versus those who received total par-enteral nutrition, no difference could be seen in terms of correction of malnu-trition. The enteral feeding program, however, was associated with a more rapid resolution of diarrhea and caused many fewer other complications.

Before leaving the poopy part of this chapter, a few fast facts seem to be in order. First off, the attenuated rotavirus vaccine is passing all of its clinical trials (Hanlon, P., et al.: *Lancet* 1:1342, 1987; Editorial Comment: *JAMA* 258:12, 1987; Maldonado, Y., et al.: *J. Pediatr.* 109:931, 1986). This is ob-viously good news and it comes none too soon, especially when we are seeing reports suggesting that breast-feeding is no longer thought to reduce the risk of rotavirus enteritis (Duffy, L.C., et al.: *Am. J. Dis. Child.* 140:1164, 1986).

On to a different infectious agent: *Yersinia enterocolitica.* Major outbreaks of *Yersinia* infection are now being reported in various parts of the world concom-itant with the ingestion of poorly cooked or raw pork (Tauxe, R.V., et al.: *Lancet* 1:1129, 1987). No wonder little piggies are called swine.

On to another infection: *Campylobacter pyloridis.* This curious bacteria has really come of age in the past 2 years. There is an unequivocal association between infection with *C. pyloridis* and severe inflammation of the pylorus of the stomach and of the first part of the small bowel. This little bug can cause severe peptic ulcer disease and bleeding (Drumm, B., et al.: *N. Engl. J. Med.* 316:1557, 1987; Czinn, S.J., et al.: *J. Pediatr.* 110:569, 1987; McNulty,

C.A.M., et al.: *Br. Med. J.* 293:645, 1986). At a time when we're learning a lot more about *C. pyloridis,* we are also seeing a new test that may be helpful in making the diagnosis of this infection. This organism is a very potent urea-splitting organism. If you give 13C-urea to an individual who is infected, the urea will be broken down by the urease activity of the *Campylobacter* organism. This will release $13CO_2$, which will be exhaled. The test itself is a pretty straightforward one, similar to the breath hyrogen analysis test, but it is called the 13C-urea breath test—a pretty nifty test at that (Graham, D.Y., et al.: *Lancet* 1:1174, 1987).

And yet another organism: the Snow Mountain agent. This is one more agent that has been added to the growing list of organisms that can cause acute gastroenteritis in children. Guest et al. (*Pediatrics* 79:559, 1987) described a 1984 outbreak of vomiting and diarrhea that affected one third of 1,800 students at a New York City high school. The infection was caused by this recently identified agent known as the Snow Mountain agent.

On to another infectious agent: *Salmonella.* This past year has been a really hot one with respect to *Salmonella.* Chloramphenicol-resistant *Salmonella* has been traced to hamburgers, including those sold by fast-food restaurants. The hamburger was made from the meat of cows, some of which were dairy cows rather than the usual steers raised in feed lots (Spika, J.S.: *N. Engl. J. Med.* 316:565, 1987). The poor old dairy cow, after having been worn out by milk giving, is frequently sent to slaughter and the meat used for ground beef. *Salmonella* is resistant to chloramphenicol in many instances. Although treatment with chloramphenicol in animals used for food production has never been legal in the United States, it seems fairly clear that some farmers do use it, and relatively indiscriminately at that. Chloramphenicol is licensed for canine use, but the Food and Drug Administration (FDA) estimated in 1981 that less than 1% of more than 28,989 kg of oral veterinary solutions of chloramphenicol sold in the United States were used for the intended species approved by the FDA. Perhaps the only thing we can do to protect ourselves is to stop asking, "Where's the beef?" and start ordering from the salad bar. Before leaving the topic of *Salmonella,* realize that you are better off flying coach than first class. Passengers flying in first class on airlines are 15 times more likely to get *Salmonella* than those sitting in the coach section (Tauxe, R.V., et al.: *Am. J. Epidemiol.* 125:150, 1987). This is another candidate for Ripley's Believe It or Not. Lastly, recognize that vacuum cleaners are very efficient collectors and distributors of *Salmonella* (Haddock, R.L.: *Lancet* 2:637, 1986). Hoover would roll over in his grave if he heard that one.

Finally, be wary of that pet store puppy. The Centers for Disease Control surveyed a sample of 14 pet shops in the Atlanta area to see whether or not the puppies that were being sold were infectious. Fifty-two percent were found to have at least one intestinal parasite, the most common of which was *Giardia.* The next most prevalent organism was *Toxocara canis,* found in 12% of animals. No wonder dogs are so expensive to take care of. In the United States it is estimated that the cost of raising a medium-sized dog through age 11 years is $5,902.

(Quiz: Rank in order the most popular name for American dogs. The answer is Rover, Spot, and Max.)—J.A. Stockman III, M.D.

Ontogenic Development of Gastrointestinal Motility: IV. Duodenal Contractions in Preterm Infants

Frank H. Morriss, Jr., Marylynn Moore, Norman W. Weisbrodt, and M. Stewart West (Univ. of Texas at Houston)

Pediatrics 78:1106–1113, December 1986   19–11

Although the developmental physiology of the lung, circulation, retina, and brain during the perinatal period has been studied widely, the developmental physiology of gastrointestinal tract motility has not been examined in depth. Duodenal motility was studied in healthy preterm infants and assessment made of the effects of antenatal corticosteroid administration and certain types of CNS abnormality on duodenal motility.

The series included 27 healthy preterm infants of 26–42 weeks' gestational age at birth whose mothers were not treated ante partum with β-methasone, 11 healthy preterm infants of 27–32 weeks' gestational age whose mothers were treated with β-methasone within 24 hours before the infants were born, and 7 infants of 31–40 weeks' gestational age with acquired structural CNS abnormalities or severe perinatal asphyxia. All infants were studied with an indwelling intraluminal manometry system to measure the duodenal contraction rate and peak intraluminal pressure during the first week before enteral feeding was begun.

In normal infants, the duodenal contraction rate was low before 29

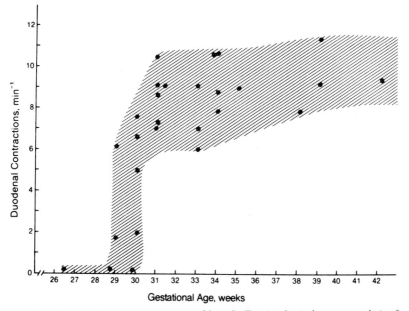

Fig 19–3.—Duodenal contraction rate measured by indwelling intraluminal manometry during first postnatal week in 27 healthy infants of 26–42 weeks' gestational age before start of enteral feeding. Increase in rate is significant function of gestational age ($P = .015$) from 26 to 32 weeks and is associated with an increase in contractions per burst that occurs during this postconceptual interval.

(Courtesy of Morriss, F.H., Jr., et al.: Pediatrics 78:1106–1113, December 1986.)

weeks' postconceptual age, but it abruptly increased between 29 weeks and 32 weeks after conception (Fig 19–3). Administration of β-methasone during 26–29 weeks after conception had a pronounced maturational effect on duodenal motility. Children with congenital CNS abnormalities or those who sustained asphyxial insult had fasting duodenal contraction rates less than half those in normal infants of similar gestational age.

Neonatal duodenal motility undergoes marked maturational changes between 29 and 32 weeks after conception. These changes may be induced before 29 weeks by maternal corticosteroid administration. An intact CNS appears to be essential to normal maturational changes of duodenal motility.

▶ These are amazing results and this is a gem of a little study. The fact that the prenatal administration of steroids to a pregnant woman can potentially mature the motility of the small bowel of a preterm infant is amazing. How all this comes about is obviously not known, unlike the lung maturation story. It would be interesting to see if other aspects of gastrointestinal tract function are "maturable" with steroids. For example, immunoglobulin-producing cells are normally absent from the gastrointestinal tract mucosa at birth. Secretory IgA plays a very significant role in the defense mechanism of the gastrointestinal tract. Is it conceivable that prenatal steroid administration could accelerate the production of mucosal immunoglobulins? Stay tuned, we should be hearing more about these possibilities.

Before moving on to the next abstract, this commentator cannot fail but to note the status of the rivalry between "Pampers" and "Huggies." Kimberly-Clarke Corporation began to move ahead with "Huggies" because of the unique features that "Huggies" have (elastic gathers at the leg that prevent leakage to some extent). Then came the counterattack by Procter and Gamble with "Ultra Pampers," diapers containing polyacrylate granules that sop up more than 100 times their weight in liquid. The counterattack by Kimberly-Clarke is with "Huggies Super Trim," which also contain superabsorbents. I guess there's a lot at stake here. Last year disposable diapers generated a $3 billion market in the United States. To show you what a large number that is, that's approximately ten times the third of a billion dollar budget that Coca Cola sets aside for advertising. It's a strange world.—J.A. Stockman III, M.D.

Type I Procollagen as a Biochemical Marker of Growth in Children With Inflammatory Bowel Disease
Jeffrey S. Hyams, Dennis E. Carey, Alan M. Leichtner, and Burton D. Goldberg (Hartford Hosp., Conn., Univ. of Connecticut, Farmington, Newington Children's Hosp., Conn., and Univ.. of Wisconsin at Madison)
J. Pediatr. 109:619–624, October 1986   19–12

Growth failure and delayed pubertal development are major complications of inflammatory bowel disease in childhood. These complications affect up to 30% of persons with Crohn's disease and up to 10% of those with ulcerative colitis. Although physicians who care for children with inflammatory bowel disease have evaluated the effects of disease activity and therapy on growth over intervals of months or longer, there is no reliable biochemical marker for assessing growth over shorter, more current intervals. Because linear growth requires new bone, which in turn requires synthesis of type I collagen, it is hypothesized that a peptide derived from the procollagen precursor (pColl-I-C) may reflect growth of new bone and may be a reliable biochemical marker for evaluating growth over the short term.

To examine the relationship between pColl-I-C concentrations and growth in a large group of children with inflammatory bowel disease and in children with functional bowel disease, a radioimmunoassay technique was used to measure the levels of pColl-I-C in sera from 69 children with functional bowel disease (control population), in 18 children with ulcerative colitis, and in 35 children with Crohn's disease. Sexually mature, fully grown adolescents from all three patient groups had mean concentrations of pColl-I-C that were similar to those previously reported for adults. However, children with functional bowel disease and normal growth had markedly higher concentrations than did fully grown adolescents. In patients who had inflammatory bowel disease there was a significant relationship between velocity of growth and concentration of pColl-I-C. Lower concentrations of pColl-I-C were observed in patients who received daily prednisone therapy, compared with those who received alternate-day therapy or those who did not take the drug.

Concentrations of pColl-I-C reflect growth activity in children. It is likely that repeated determinations may permit rapid assessment of the effects of various therapeutic modalities on growth in children with inflammatory bowel disease.

▶ Robert J. Winter, M.D., Associate Professor of Pediatrics, Northwestern University Medical School, and member of the Division of Pediatric Endocrinology, Children's Memorial Hospital, Chicago, comments.—J.A. Stockman III, M.D.

▶ As any anxious parent of a short child knows, growth is a slow, normally methodical process not well suited to close scrutiny over short (weeks) intervals. Indeed, most growth specialists measure children no less frequently than every 3 months, recognizing as they do so the great number of variables affecting that measurement. Not only is technique of measurement crucial, but factors such as time of day (we and our patients "shrink" during the day because of vertebral column compression), seasonal growth, presence or absence of socks, and type of hairstyle may influence the observed interval growth. A 3-month growth of 1.27 cm (0.5 in.) amounts to a normal childhood rate of 5.08 cm/year. A quarterly measurement error of 5.0 mm (0.2 in.) distorts the annual rate by 2.0 cm. One's entire diagnostic and therapeutic approach may be greatly altered by the growth rate of 3.0 cm/year resulting from such an error.

One solution to this measurement accuracy issue, developed at the National Institutes of Health earlier in this decade (*J. Clin. Endocrinol. Metab.* 58:717,

1984), is an ulnar length measuring device. This consists of a condylograph that locates the recess between the styloid process of the ulna and the os triquetrum. By fixing the forearm firmly in place on the apparatus, ulnar growth in increments of 0.183 mm can be measured accurately in intervals as short as 2–3 weeks. However, reproducibility is much better than availability.

This paper by Hyams et al. offers a newer solution to the quest for a widely available measure of short-term growth rates. If the sensitivity (will it become a tool for accurate, longitudinal monitoring of growth rate?), specificity (collagen is involved in a great many processes in addition to linear growth), and applicability and availability to the clinical laboratory can all be confirmed with further testing over a diverse population of growth disorders, the management of those disorders may be drastically altered and improved.—R.J. Winter, M.D.

Myocarditis in Children With Inflammatory Bowel Disease
Christina Frid, Björn Bjarke, and Margareta Eriksson (Karolinska Inst., and St. Göran's Children's Hosp., Stockholm)
J. Pediatr. Gastroenterol. Nutr. 5:964–965, November–December 1986 19–13

Myocarditis is a rare extracolonic manifestation in patients with inflammatory bowel disease. During a 10-year period, two such patients were observed among 106 treated at St. Goran's Children's Hospital. Twenty-three others have been described in the literature.

Boys, 11 years and 19 years, were relatively free of gastrointestinal tract symptoms at the time of diagnosis of myocarditis. One had ulcerative colitis at age 12 years, and in the other Crohn's disease was not correctly diagnosed until 3 years after initial presentation. Fatigue and dyspnea were the presenting complaints. One boy had severe heart failure, arrhythmia, and bilateral pleural effusions, and in the other ST segment depression was observed on the ECG. Both responded to steroid therapy without sequelae despite fulminant illness in one.

Of the 23 patients reported in the literature, all but three were adults and most had ulcerocolitis. Nineteen had active disease at the time that myocarditis developed. All recovered, although relapses of myocarditis occurred.

Myocarditis in children with inflammatory bowel disease may be more common than thought previously. Despite a fulminant course in some cases, the prognosis is usually good, provided that the underlying bowel disease is treated correctly.

Prospective Study of Colitis in Infancy and Early Childhood
S.K.F. Chong, A.J. Blackshaw, B.C. Morson, C.B. Williams, and J.A. Walker-Smith (King's College Hosp., St. Bartholomew's Hosp., and St. Mark's Hosp., London)
J. Pediatr. Gastroenterol. Nutr. 5:352–358, May–June 1986   19–14

Most infants and children with bloody diarrhea have acute, self-limited illnesses caused by a pathogen that can be identified by stool culture.

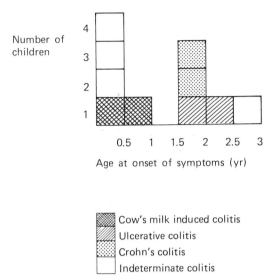

Number of children

Age at onset of symptoms (yr)

Cow's milk induced colitis
Ulcerative colitis
Crohn's colitis
Indeterminate colitis

Fig 19–4.—Age at onset of colitis in ten children seen at St. Bartholomew's Hospital. (Courtesy of Chong, S.K.F., et al.: J. Pediatr. Gastroenterol. Nutr. 5:352–358, May–June 1986.)

However, a small number of children have chronic bloody diarrhea for which no cause can be identified. Colonoscopy and biopsy findings in ten children with chronic bloody diarrhea were reviewed.

The children were aged 3 years or younger and had endoscopic and histologic evidence of colitis, which was shown not to be of an infective type by stool culture and serologic tests. The types of colitis identified by endoscopic and histologic examinations were ulcerative (two patients), cow's milk induced (two), indeterminate (four), and Crohn's disease (two). Age at onset tended to be extremely early for indeterminate and cow's milk-induced colitis and later for ulcerative and Crohn's colitis (Fig 19–4).

Six months after treatment with sulfasalazine, prednisolone, or both, the children with ulcerative colitis and Crohn's disease were asymptomatic. Once cow's milk was removed from the maternal diet, the two breast-fed infants with allergic colitis experienced resolution of the condition. Of the four children with indeterminate colitis, one was cured, two continued with sulfasalazine therapy with minimal symptoms, and one underwent subtotal colectomy. Histopathologic examination uncovered features of intestinal Behçet's disease.

Colitis in young children is a heterogeneous group of conditions. Among these ten children with symptoms of colitis, colonoscopy and repeated mucosal biopsy permitted diagnosis in six. Precise diagnosis of the type of colitis is necessary for establishment of the correct diet regimen and drug therapy.

▶ In the past, total colonoscopy has not been possible in infancy and early childhood, and the relative importance of chronic inflammatory bowel disease has not been clear at this early age. Food allergy in the etiology of colitis and rectal bleeding has been recognized for some time as a cause of sporadic problems in infancy, but food allergy certainly cannot account for all cases in early childhood of such clinical signs and symptoms. What the authors have done is to show that with all the current technologies available to the gastroenterologist, a diagnosis of inflammatory bowel disease is certainly possible even in very early childhood. They show us that the syndrome of colitis in infancy and early childhood presents as a homogeneous clinical entity with bloody diarrhea as a hallmark. They also tell us that food-allergic colitis, most often called cow's milk-induced colitis, remains a major cause of infantile colitis. However, a diagnosis of Crohn's disease or ulcerative colitis is still possible even in children 1, 2, or 3 years of age. Establishment of an accurate diagnosis is necessary, because the specific management of inflammatory bowel disease is very different from the management used for other causes of bloody diarrhea. The latter statement goes without saying.

What becomes of these children with inflammatory bowel disease, and how should they be best managed in the long haul? The underlying issue here is the risk of colon cancer with ulcerative colitis. Most gastroenterologists and current textbooks recommend that patients who have widespread ulcerative colitis for a period of 7–10 years should be entered into a surveillance program designed to detect colonic dysplasia (precancer). This involves frequent colonoscopies and multiple mucosal biopsies. How correct are these recommendations? A critical review of all studies to date was recently presented by Collins et al. (*N. Engl. J. Med.* 316:1654, 1987). This *New England Journal of Medicine* report really shakes the foundation of our understanding about the risk of cancer in this disease. The authors conclude that only the following statements are justified:

1. The premises on which the argument for surveillance is based are not well established.

2. There is no compelling evidence that surveillance is beneficial.

3. Being enrolled in a surveillance program does not guarantee that lethal cancers will not develop.

4. If some patients benefit, it is not clear that this justifies the large cost of surveillance.

Indeed, the authors point out that each cancer found or prevented costs about $200,000 in detection. Thus, patients with long-standing, extensive, ulcerative colitis who are not sick enough to require colectomy face a dilemma because of their increased risk of colon cancer. Three options are available: The first is to ignore the risk. This is a logical approach if the risk is slight, as is suggested by some studies, and may be the preferred approach in patients in whom colitis develops when they are older because they have fewer years at risk. The second option is prophylactic colectomy 8–10 years after the onset of colitis; this eliminates the risk of colon cancer and is logical if the risk is very high, as has been suggested by some other studies. However, the morbidity and mortality associated with colectomy, especially among adolescents, and the adaptation to ileostomy are not minor problems. Nonetheless, this may be the preferred approach in patients with onset of colitis at a young age because the cumulative life-time risk will be large and colonoscopic surveillance cannot be depended on to remove the risk of cancer. The third option is colonoscopic surveillance with colectomy if dysplasia is found, but the costs of this are enormous and compliance may be poor. What seems obvious from all this is the recognition that a good solution to the increased risk of colon cancer in patients with long-standing ulcerative colitis is not at hand, and we are fooling ourselves by whatever we use as an approach to this problem.

I would suspect that most patients faced with all of this evidence will throw up their hands and simply ask their doctor what his or her opinion is about the best way to go about minimizing the risk of colonic cancer. It is curious how we Americans choose doctors and place our trust in them. As an example of this, when a large number of people were asked to rank what TV doctors they would go to if they existed, they ranked in order: Marcus Welby, Hawkeye Pierce, and Donald Westphall. I have to admit they are hard acts to beat.—J.A. Stockman III, M.D.

Childhood Celiac Disease: A Long-Term Analysis of Relapses in 91 Patients

David H. Shmerling and Johan Franckx (The Children's Hosp., Zürich)
J. Pediatr. Gastroenterol. Nutr. 5:565–569, July–August 1986   19–15

Celiac disease is an enteropathy caused by sensitivity to dietary gluten, resulting in flattening of the intestinal villi and subsequent malabsorption. Of the 314 infants and children in whom the diagnosis of celiac disease was established by the presence of a flat proximal small bowel mucosa in untreated patients and an unequivocal response and remission on a gluten-free diet, 91 underwent one or more interruptions of their disease. These interruptions were documented with repeated small bowel mucosal biopsies and evaluated to determine the permanence of the mucosal reaction to gluten in celiac disease. Most (68%) of the challenges were initiated by the patients themselves.

The patients were classified according to the results of their last intestinal biopsy. Group A consisted of 71 (81.4%) patients who had flat mucosa after 0.25–14.67 years of not following a gluten diet. Group B (11 patients, 12%) had progressive deterioration of mucosa without it becoming flat within 0.5–6.67 years after interruption of the gluten-free diet. Group C (6 patients, 6.6%) had normal mucosa after 2.24–6.92 years without the gluten-free diet. Three patients were still under study, being without the diet for less than 2 years. The median age at diagnosis was similar in all three groups. The median duration of following a gluten-free diet was significantly shorter in group A patients (15.67 years) than in group B patients (4.59 years). The duration of gluten challenge was significantly shorter in group A patients than in group C patients. Of the 24 patients who underwent a planned gluten challenge and were biopsied at regular intervals, 21 (87.5%) had mucosal relapse within 2 years after the beginning of challenge.

Only a minority of patients with celiac disease will not have mucosal relapse after interruption of the gluten-free diet, and another 12% will deteriorate very slowly. These findings indicate that routine gluten challenges in all patients with celiac disease are not justifiable.

Antibodies to Gliadin by ELISA as a Screening Test for Childhood Celiac Disease

M.-R. Ståhlberg, E. Savilahti, and M. Viander (Univ. of Turku and Univ. of Helsinki)

J. Pediatr. Gastroenterol. Nutr. 5:726–729, September–October 1986   19–16

Enzyme-linked immunosorbent assay (ELISA) for IgA and IgG antigliadin antibodies (AGA) might be a useful screening test for pediatric patients suspected of having celiac disease. Thirty-one children with celiac disease were studied. Eleven had severe villous atrophy initially and relapse later followed gluten challenge after a gluten-free diet had been instituted. The other 20 children had normal biopsy findings at reevaluation when taking a gluten-free diet. The mean age at initial biopsy, when AGA were estimated, was 5.5 years. The control group included 278 children with a mean age of 6 years who had normal small bowel mucosa.

One study patient had selective IgA deficiency. The IgA-AGA test was positive in 27 of the other 30 patients, and the IgG-AGA test was positive in 29 of all 31. The IgA-AGA test was positive in 37 of 271 control children without selective IgA deficiency, and the IgG-AGA test was positive in 93 of all 278 (table). The IgA-AGA test was 90% sensitive and 86% specific for celiac disease. The IgG-AGA test was 94% sensitive and 67% specific.

The ELISA test for AGA appears to be a useful screening measure for determining which patients suspected of having celiac disease should undergo intestinal biopsy. It is technically simpler than the indirect immunofluorescence test for reticulin antibody.

▶ Dr. John Lloyd-Still, Professor of Pediatrics, Northwestern University Medical School, and Chief, Division of Gastroenterology, Children's Memorial Hospital, Chicago, comments.—J.A. Stockman III, M.D.

▶ The last comments on celiac disease (1980 YEAR BOOK) related to the xylose absorption test. The past few years have seen a profusion of studies attempting to screen for celiac disease by immunologic techniques using AGAs (IgA and IgG class) and antireticulum antibody (IgA class). The results remain controversial (*Gastroenterology* 89:217, 1985). These tests all have high sensitivity for celiac disease, but specificity is usually low and they probably offer little

ELISA-AGA IN PATIENTS WITH CELIAC DISEASE
AND IN CONTROLS

	IgA-AGA Positive*	IgG-AGA Positive†
Celiac disease (n = 31)	27/30	29/31
Controls (n = 278)	37/271	93/278

*χ^2 = 94.035; df = 1; P <.001.
†χ^2 = 42.157; df = 1; P <.001.
(Courtesy of Ståhlberg, M.-R., et al.: J. Pediatr. Gastroenterol. Nutr. 5:726–729, September–October 1986.)

advantage over the current screening tests of absorption (xylose and/or serum carotene). However, progress is occurring in molecular biology. There is a striking association between celiac disease and human leukocyte antigen (HLA)-B8, HLA-DR3, and/or HLA-DR7 and HLA-DC3. Nonetheless, fewer than 0.2% of individuals with those serologic HLA specificities have celiac disease, and the disease is not always concordant among monozygotic twins.

Kagnoff et al. (*J. Exp. Med.* 160:1544, 1984) examined protein sequences sharing amino acid homologies with A-gliadin and found that there is a region of sequence homology with human adenovirus type 12, an adenovirus usually isolated from the intestinal tract. The authors suggested that an encounter of the immune system with antigenic determinants produced during intestinal viral infection may be important in the pathogenesis of this disease, and there is some support for this hypothesis (Karagiannis, J.A., et al: *Lancet* 1:884, 1987). Recently, a molecular marker that distinguishes the celiac disease HLA-D region haplotype from a serologically identical haplotype in unaffected controls was reported (Howell, M.D., et al: *J. Exp. Med.* 164:333, 1986). Using a specific probe and restriction endonuclease, a polymorphic 4.0-kb fragment was detected which in DQw2 individuals was associated with a 40-fold increased relative risk for the development of celiac disease.

The paper from Zurich is impressive for its numbers (the incidence of this disease has decreased in most countries) and length of follow-up. The findings show that 87.5% of patients challenged with gluten ultimately relapse, but whether the remaining 12.5% really had celiac disease cannot be proven by this paper. Surprisingly, 68% of the challenges were initiated by the patients themselves (I thought Swiss patients usually followed doctor's orders.). However, most gastroenterologists would disagree with the suggestion that rechallenge with gluten was unnecessary. The golden rule in the management of celiac disease remains the ESPGAN criteria (McNeish, A.S., et al.: *Arch. Dis. Child.* 54:783, 1979). What we still need is a reliable test of rechallenge that eliminates repeated intestinal biopsies.

One reason for poor dietary control during adolescence and adulthood may be alcohol consumption. Guidance in this area was discussed (Cole, S.B., et al.: *Ann. Rev. Nutr.* 5:241, 1985). Gluten is not present in distilled spirits. Thus rye whiskey, scotch whiskey, and other cereal-derived spirits can be consumed. Similarly, brandy and wine made from fruit should cause no problem. Beer and ale are produced from barley, and their approval in the diet differs among medical centers (most rigidly exclude beer), although the authors stated that there was a lack of clinical evidence that beer and ale activate disease.—J. Lloyd-Still, M.D.

Acetylcholinesterase Activity in Rectal Biopsies: An Assessment of its Diagnostic Value in Hirschsprung's Disease
F.E. Wells and G.M. Addison (Booth Hall Children's Hosp., Manchester, England)
J. Pediatr. Gastroenterol. Nutr. 5:912–919, November–December 1986 19–17

The diagnosis of Hirschsprung's disease relies mainly on the absence of ganglion cells in the myenteric and submucosal plexuses on serial section of the rectal biopsy. The role of biochemical measurement of acetylcholinesterase (AChE) activity in homogenized rectal tissue remains to be established because of the frequent false negative and a few false positive findings associated with its use. In 392 patients suspected of having Hirschsprung's disease, AChE activity was measured in rectal suction biopsies to determine the specificity, sensitivity, and predictive value of this measurement in the diagnosis.

Acetylcholinesterase activity did not differ significantly among patients with or without Hirschsprung's disease. There was considerable overlap in the AChE activity and AChE% for the two groups. There were 4 false positive and 13 false negative results. Sample instability was a significant source of error. Analysis of duplicate biopsies and false negative results showed that tissue inhomogeneity or incorrect siting of the biopsy appeared to be likely causes of error.

Two criteria had been suggested previously in choosing the optimum diagnostic decision level: AChE activity and AChE%. Examination of a range of decision levels indicated an optimal choice of AChE activity of more than 10 rate units and AChE% of not less than 60%. At a prevalence of 10%, this decision level resulted in a sensitivity of 64.9%, specificity of 98.7%, predictive value of positive 85.7%, and predictive value of negative 96.3%. Using this criterion, four false negatives could have been avoided, but five additional false positive results would have been produced at the same time. Of the four false positive results, three would have remained unequivocal.

Although there remains a considerable overlap between rectal biopsy AChE activity in those with and without Hirschsprung's disease, AChE activity of more than 10 rate units and an AChE% of not less than 60% are the suggested criteria for the diagnosis. The diagnostic value of AChE measurement in rectal biopsies in patients with Hirschsprung's disease remains doubtful.

▶ At this point in time, I am very willing to throw up my hands and leave the entire issue of how to make a diagnosis of Hirschsprung's disease to the surgeon. This, that, or another recommendation has been put forth in terms of more accurate ways to make the diagnosis. Nonetheless, most of these do not hold up over the years. The study reported suggests that AChE activity in rectal biopsies is of limited diagnostic value. Add to this the report that the barium enema is not a very specific screening procedure for Hirschsprung's disease (Taxman, T.L., et al.: *Am. J. Dis. Child.* 140:881, 1986) and you suddenly come to the realization that maybe there is no such thing as Hirschsprung's disease.

We all wish that someone would come up with the perfect diagnostic test. Maybe, just maybe, monoclonal antibodies are part of the answer. There has been developed a monoclonal antineurofilament antibody that can be used to stain resected areas of large bowel to determine whether or not neurofilamentous structures are present (Kluck, P., et al.: *Am. J. Clin. Pathol.* 86:490, 1986). One place where monoclonal antibody staining is helpful is in that small group of about 20% of patients who undergo resection for Hirschsprung's disease but who have persistent constipation afterward. The Kluck study illustrates that, with monoclonal antibody staining, you can show that there is a zone of disorganized ganglia present in the resected margins of children who have postoperative constipation. This apparently is not detectable with routine light microscopy.

I suppose that we will be forced to bear with additional techniques or tests for Hirschsprung's disease. For every new test that comes along, we should have expunged from the medical literature all the old ones that were so valueless. That at least would conform to the Oliver North method of approaching a problem. That approach is characterized by "try the very best you can but if you fail, destroy all evidence that you ever even tried.—J.A. Stockman III, M.D.

Constipation and Meconium Ileus Equivalent in Patients With Cystic Fibrosis

Steven Rubinstein, Richard Moss, and Norman Lewiston (Children's Hosp. at Stanford and Stanford Univ.)
Pediatrics 78:473–478, September 1986   19–18

In patients with cystic fibrosis, constipation and meconium ileus equivalent (distal intestinal obstruction syndrome) become management problems. Such patients do not respond to laxatives and tend to have refractory constipation, with or without obstruction, if treatment is inadequate. The authors conducted a retrospective study of cystic fibrosis patients to determine the prevalence of acute bowel problems.

The records of 168 patients with cystic fibrosis were reviewed for episodes of abdominal cramping and decreased stool frequency, which responded to laxatives. Meconium ileus equivalent was characterized by postneonatal partial or total bowel obstruction unresponsive to laxatives. Symptoms and signs of bowel obstruction were severe abdominal pain and

---

CLINICAL FEATURES OF MECONIUM ILEUS
EQUIVALENT

Abdominal pain: diffuse or localized
Change in stooling patterns common but not invariable
Recent history of increased fluid loss from respiratory infection, exercise, or warm weather
Recent adjustment in pancreatic enzyme dosage
Right lower quadrant mass
Copious quantities of fecal material on abdominal radiographs with or without air-fluid levels
Neuhauser's sign on abdominal radiographs
Unresponsiveness to conventional oral laxative treatment
Other abdominal pathology ruled out

(Courtesy of Rubinstein, S., et al.: Pediatrics 78:473–478, September 1986.)

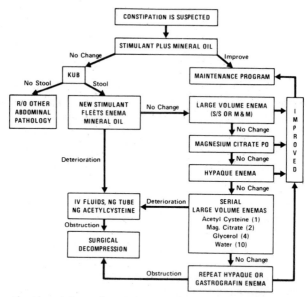

Fig 19–5.—Algorithm of therapy for constipation and meconium ileus equivalent in patients with cystic fibrosis. Large-volume enemas are up to 2.5 L in adults and 30 ml/kg in children. *S/S,* soapsuds enema; *M&M,* milk and molasses; *R/O,* rule out; *PO,* oral; *IV,* intravenous; *NG,* nasogastric; *mag,* magnesium; and *KUB,* kidney, ureter, bladder roentgenogram.
(Courtesy of Rubinstein, S., et al.: Pediatrics 78:473–478, September 1986.)

air-fluid interfaces or other signs of intestinal obstruction on roentgenograms (table).

Boy, 9 years, who had vomiting, poor appetite, and abdominal cramping for 3 days, was found to have diffuse tenderness in the right upper quadrant. Abdominal x-ray films showed a diffuse granular stool, but no air-fluid levels. The condition was unresponsive to administration of two Fleet enemas and Agoral twice daily. A 1-L soapsuds enema was successful. Agoral and oral magnesium citrate treatment, every 6–8 hours, led to full catharsis within 24 hours. Maintenance therapy included administration of Agoral and psyllium. Enzymatic supplementation and a high-fiber diet were encouraged.

Constipation occurs more often in patients older than age 30 years (73%) than in patients younger than age 5 years (14%). Meconium ileus equivalent is also more frequent in older than in younger patients. If fluids, high-bulk diets, exercise, Docusate, bulk laxatives and pancreatic enzymes are not helpful the following therapy is recommended: Oral doses of magnesium citrate, Hypaque enema, or serial large-volume enemas should be tried in that order. If deterioration occurs, the nasogastric administration of acetylcysteine, pancreatin, or a balanced intestinal lavage solution should be tried. Obstruction is treated by surgical decompression (Fig 19–5). Once improvement occurs, maintenance therapy should be instituted.

▶ Constipation may be one of the most critical problems in the management of certain individuals with cystic fibrosis. Intestinal obstruction from fecal impaction or meconium ileus equivalent, also known as the distal intestinal obstruction syndrome, develops in a small but important percentage of patients with cystic fibrosis. These patients usually do not respond to standard laxative therapy. Without adequate treatment, true obstruction can occur. When meconium ileus equivalent does happen, its management should be vigorous. O'Halloran et al. (*Arch. Dis. Child.* 61:1128, 1986) have shown that oral Gastrografin in the relief of acute meconium ileus is successful in more than 80% of patients. If a single dose doesn't work, a second dose 24 hours later usually produces prompt results in the remainder of children. These authors suggest that Gastrografin is more acceptable to children than are the usual other measures including enemas, MucoMist, laxatives, and manipulations of pancreatic enzyme supplements. We hope that no one will come up with some per rectum suctioning technique to deal with the problem of cystic fibrosis and meconium ileus equivalent. The large bowel in these patients is too prone to prolapse to permit that.

While on the topic of negative pressure situations, be careful about using airplane and cruise line toilets. Wynne (*JAMA* 257:1177, 1987) alerts us to this risk. Dr. Wynne had the occasion to assist in the treatment of a 70-year-old, slightly obese woman who flushed the toilet she was sitting on in a cruise liner. The suction created caused the prolapsing of several feet of small intestine. These types of toilets work on a vacuum system, although this is the first reported case of such a bizarre complication. Nonetheless, it will be a long time before I occupy one of those kinds of seats again.—J.A. Stockman III, M.D.

Review Articles of Interest to the Pediatrician

The Newborn:

Benitz, W.E., et al.: The pharmacology of neonatal resuscitation and cardiopulmonary intensive care. *West. J. Med.* 144:704, 1986.

Blisard, K.S., et al.: Neonatal hemochromatosis. *Hum. Pathol.* 17:376, 1986.

Elhassani, S.B.: Neonatal poisoning: Causes, manifestations, prevention, and management. *South Med. J.* 79:1535, 1986.

Girard, J.: Gluconeogenesis in late fetal and early neonatal life. *Biol. Neonate* 50:237, 1986.

Goodman, S.I.: Inherited metabolic disease in the newborn: Approach to diagnosis and treatment. *Adv. Pediatr.* 33:197, 1986.

Karp, W.E., et al.: Vitamin E in neonatology. *Adv. Pediatr.* 33:127, 1986.

Pearson, H.A.: A neonatal program for sickle cell anemia. *Adv. Pediatr.* 33:381, 1986.

Seppanen, U.: Perinatal postmortem radiography. *Acta Radiol.* 27:481, 1986.

Shepard, T.H.: Human teratogenicity. *Adv. Pediatr.* 33:225, 1986.

Warshaw, J.B.: Intrauterine growth retardation. *PIR* 8:107, 1986.

Infectious Disease and Immunity:

Guerrant, R.L., et al.: Acute infectious diarrhea. *Pediatr. Infect. Dis.* 5:353, 458, 1986.

Heiner, D.C.: Management of IgG subclass deficiencies. *Pediatr. Infect. Dis.* 6:235, 1987.

Israele, V, et al.: Periorbital and orbital cellulitis. *Pediatr. Infect. Dis.* 6:404, 1987.

Jackson, K., et al.: Periorbital cellulitis. *Head Neck Surg.* 9:227, 1987.

Jarvis, W.R.: Epidemiology of pediatric nosocomial infections. *Pediatr. Infect. Dis.* 6:344, 1987.

Klein, J.O., et al.: Report of the task force on diagnosis and management of meningitis. *Pediatrics* 78:(5) suppl, 1986.

Ochs, H.D.: Immunoglobulin therapy for pediatric AIDS patients. *Pediatr. Infect. Dis.* 6:509, 1987.

Onorato, I.M., et al.: Laboratory diagnosis of pertussis: The state of the art. *Pediatr. Infect. Dis.* 6:145, 1987.

Radetsky, M., et al.: Identification of streptococcal pharyngitis in the office laboratory. *Pediatr. Infect. Dis.* 6:556, 1987.

Ransome, O.J., et al.: Urinary tract infection in childhood. *S. Afr. Med. J.* 70:417, 1986.

Simon, M.W., et al.: The amoebic meningoencephalitides. *Pediatr. Infect. Dis.* 5:562, 1986.

Viscidi, R.P., et al.: Molecular diagnosis of infectious diseases by nucleic acid hybridization. *Molecular and Cellular Probes* 1:3, 1987.

Wilfert, C.M., et al.: *Chlamydia trachomatis* infections of infants and children. *Adv. Pediatr.* 33:49, 1986.

Nutrition and Metabolism:

Barness, L.A.: History of infant feeding practices. *Am. J. Clin. Nutr.* 46:168, 1987.

Bell, E.F.: History of vitamin E in infant nutrition. *Am. J. Clin. Nutr.* 46:183, 1987.

Brown, R., et al.: Total nutrient admixture: A review. *J. Parenter. Enteral. Nutr.* 10:650, 1986.

Burton, B.K.: Inborn errors of metabolism: The clinical diagnosis in early infancy. *Pediatrics* 79:359, 1987.

Fomon, S.J.: Reflections on infant feeding in the 1970s and 1980s. *Am. J. Clin. Nutr.* 46:171, 1987.

Gahl, W.A.: Cystinosis coming of age. *Adv. Pediatr.* 33:95, 1986.

Kaufman, S.S. et al.: Nutritional support for the infant with extrahepatic biliary atresia. *J. Pediatr.* 110:679, 1987.

Khattab, A.E.K.: Oral rehydration therapy. *Pediatr. Rev. Comm.* 1:31, 1987.

Koldovsky, O., et al.: Hormones in milk. *J. Pediatr. Gastroenterol. Nutr.* 6:172, 1987.

Kossoy, A.F., et al.: Renal tubular acidosis in infancy. *South. Med. J.* 79:1256, 1986.

Muenzer, J.: Mucopolysaccharidoses. *Adv. Pediatr.* 33:269, 1986.

Phelp, D.L.: Current perspectives on vitamin E in infant nutrition. *Am. J. Clin. Nutr.* 46:187, 1987.

Reeves, J.D.: Iron supplementation in infancy. *PIR* 8:177, 1986.

Robinson, R.O.: Differential diagnosis of Reye's syndrome. *Dev. Med. Child Neurol.* 29:110, 1987.

Salusky, I.B., et al.: Nutritional factors and progression of chronic renal failure. *Adv. Pediatr.* 33:149, 1986.

Santosham, M., et al.: Oral rehydration therapy and dietary therapy for acute childhood diarrhea. *PIR* 8:273, 1987.

Specker, B.L., et al.: Vitamin D in infancy and childhood: Factors determining vitamin D status. *Adv. Pediatr.* 33:1, 1986.

Zeisel, S.H.: Dietary influences on neurotransmission. *Adv. Pediatr.* 33:23, 1986.

Allergy and Dermatology:

Newhouse, M.T., et al.: Control of asthma by aerosols. *N. Engl. J. Med.* 315:870, 1986.

Schur, P.H.: IgG subclasses-a review. *Ann. Allergy* 58:89, 1987.

Walker-Smith, J.A.: Milk intolerance in children. *Clin. Allergy* 16:183, 1986.

Weinberger, M.: Pharmacologic management of asthma. *J. Adolesc. Health Care* 8:74, 1987.

Weston, W.L.: Blistering diseases in children. *Postgrad. Med.* 80:241, 1986.

Miscellaneous Topics:

Kirkpatrick, J.A., Jr.: Imaging procedure in pediatrics. *Adv. Pediatr.* 33:77, 1986.

Burton, B.K.: Alpha-fetoprotein screening. *Adv. Pediatr.* 33:181, 1986.

Brody, A.S., et al.: Magnetic resonance imaging. *PIR* 8:87, 1986.

Chadley, A.E.: Fragile X syndrome. *J. Pediatr.* 110:821, 1987.

Fryers, T.: Survival in Down's syndrome. *J. Ment. Defic. Res.* 30:101, 1986.

Gusella, J.F.: Recombinant DNA techniques in the diagnosis of inherited disorders. *J. Clin. Invest.* 77:1723, 1986.

Hunt, C.E., et al.: Sudden infant death syndrome: 1987 perspective. *J. Pediatr.* 110:669, 1987.

Ledley, F.D.: Somatic gene therapy for human disease. *J. Pediatr.* 110:1, 1987.

Levy, J., et al.: Pulmonary hemosiderosis. *Pediatr. Pulmonol.* 2:385, 1986.

Light, D.W.: Corporate medicine for profit. *Sci. Am.* 255:(6)38, 1986.

Neurology and Psychiatry:

Breningstall, G.N.: Neurologic syndromes in hyperammonemic disorders. *Pediatr. Neurol.* 2:253, 1986.

Cooper, P.J., et al.: The nature of bulimia nervosa. *Pediatr. Rev. Comm.* 1:217, 1987.

Evans, O.B.: Guillain-Barré syndrome in children. *PIR* 8:69, 1986.

Fryer, A.E., et al.: Tuberous sclerosis—a clinical appraisal. *Pediatr. Rev. Comm.* 1:239, 1987.

Gerring, J.P.: Psychiatric sequelae of severe closed head injury. *PIR* 8:115, 1986.

Golden, G.S.: Tic disorders in childhood. *PIR* 8:229, 1987.

Healy, A.: Mental retardation *PIR* 9:15, 1987.

Hecht, F.: Advances in medical genetics: Huntington disease.

Olness, K.N., et al.: Recurrent headaches in children: diagnosis and treatment. *PIR* 8:307, 1987.

Parkes, J.D.: The parasomnias. *Lancet* 2:1021, 1986.

Prazer, G.: Conversion reactions in adolescents. *PIR* 8:279, 1987.

Shapiro, A.K., et al.: Pimozide treatment of tic and Tourette disorders. *Pediatrics* 79:1032, 1987.

Stumpf, D.A.: Acute ataxia. *PIR* 8:303, 1987.

Vining, E.P.G., et al.: Management of nonfebrile seizures. *PIR* 185, 1986.

Child Development:

Becker, P.G.: Counseling families with twins: Birth to 3 years of age. *PIR* 8:81, 1986.

Chagoya, L., et al.: Children who lie: A review of the literature. *Can. J. Psychiatry* 31:665, 1986.

Chamberlin, R.W.: Developmental assessment and early intervention programs for young children: lessons learned from longitudinal research *PIR* 8:237, 1987.

Green, M.: Behavioral and developmental components of child health promotion: How can they be accomplished? *PIR* 8:133, 1986.

Green, M.: Vulnerable child syndrome and its variants. *PIR* 8:75, 1986.

Kales, A., et al.: Sleep disorders: Insomnia, sleepwalking, night terrors, nightmares, and enuresis. *Ann. Intern. Med.* 106:582, 1987.

Parry, T.S.: Behavioral problems in toddlers. *Aust. Fam. Physician* 15:1038, 1986.

Palfrey, J.S., et al.: School placement. *PIR* 8:261, 1986.

Schmitt, B.D.: School refusal. *PIR* 8:99, 1986.

Adolescent Medicine:

Block, R.W.: The maladroit adolescent: Learning disorders and attentional deficits. *Adv. Pediatr.* 33:303, 1976.

D'Angelo, L.: Infectious disease problems in adolescents. *J. Adolesc. Health Care* 7:65S, 1986.

Greydanus, D.E.: Depression in adolescence. *J. Adolesc. Health Care* 7:109S, 1986.

Horowitz, D.A.: Physical examination of sexually abused children and adolescents. *PIR* 9:25, 1987.

Moscicki, A. et al.: Normal reproductive development in the adolescent female. *J. Adolesc. Health Care* 7:41S, 1986.

Prazer, G.: Conversion reactions in adolescents. *PIR* 8:279, 1987.

Rifkin, A., et al.: Psychotropic medication in adolescents: A review. *J. Clin. Psychiatry* 47:400, 1986.

Slap, G.B.: Normal physiological and psychosocial growth in the adolescent. *J. Adolesc. Health Care* 7:13S, 1986.

Therapeutics and Toxicology:

deLemos, R.A., et al.: Animal models for drug evaluation. *Pediatrics* 79:275, 1987.
Faber, M.M.: A review of efforts to protect children from injury in car crashes. *Fam. Comm. Health* 9:25, 1986.
Jones, K.L.: Fetal alcohol syndrome. *PIR* 8:122, 1986.
Hall, A.H., et al.: Mushroom poisoning: Identification, diagnosis, and treatment. *PIR* 8:291, 1987.
Shepard, T.H.: Human teratogenicity. *Adv. Pediatr.* 33:225, 1986.
Weinhouse, E., et al.: Digoxin toxicity in childhood. *Pediatr. Rev. Comm.* 1:67, 1987.

The Genitourinary Tract:

Fayez, J.A.: Advances in the diagnosis and treatment of menstrual disorders. Part I: Precocious puberty, delayed menarche, and primary amenorrhea. *Female Patient* 11:35, 1986.
Hamburger, E.K.: Urinary tract infections in infants and children. Guidelines for averting permanent damage. *Postgrad. Med.* 80:235, 1986.
Ransome, O.J., Thomson, P.D.: Urinary tract infection in childhood. *S. Afr. Med. J.* 70:417, 1986.
Drachman, D.B.: Present and future treatment of myasthenia gravis. *N. Engl. J. Med.* 316:743, 1987.
Scriver, C.R.: Cystinuria. *N. Engl. J. Med.* 315:1155, 1986.
Field, L.G., Springate, J.E., Fildes, R.D.: Acute renal failure. I. Pathophysiology and diagnosis. *J. Pediatr.* 109:401, 1986.
Fildes, R.D., Springate, J.E., Field, L.G.: Acute renal failure. II. Management of suspected and established disease. *J. Pediatr.* 109:567, 1986.
Committee on Adolescents: Sexuality, contraception and the media. *Pediatrics* 78:535, 1986.
Blau, E.B.: Hematuria in children. Is it cause for alarm? *Postgrad. Med.* 79:65, 1986.
Pinsonneault, O., Goldstein, D.P.: Gynecologic disorders in adolescence. Part I: Pain syndromes. *Female Patient* 11:26, 1986.
Kales, A., Soldatos, C.R., Kales, K.D.: Sleep disorders: Insomnia, sleep walking, night terrors, nightmares, and enuresis. *Ann. Intern. Med.* 106:582, 1987.
Sherwood, L.M.: Vitamin D parathyroid hormone and renal failure. *N. Engl. J. Med.* 316:1601, 1987.
Editorial comment: Erythropoietin. *Lancet* 1:781, 1987.
Harrison, M.R.: Organ procurement for children: The anencephalic fetus as a donor. *Lancet* 1:1383, 1986.
Editorial comment: Hydronephrosis, renal obstruction, and renography. *Lancet* 1:1301, 1987.

The Respiratory Tract:

Editorial comment: Oral snuff: A preventable carcinogenic hazard. *Lancet* 2:198, 1986.
Ricer, R.E.: Smokeless tobacco use: A dangerous habit. *Postgrad. Med.* 81:89, 1987.
Martin, R.J., Miller, M.J., Claro, W.A.: Pathogenesis of apnea in preterm infants. *J. Pediatr.* 109:733, 1986.
Denbert, M.L., Keith, J.F.: Evaluating the potential pediatric scuba diver. *Am. J. Dis. Child.* 140:1135, 1986.

Editorial comment: Current state of theophylline in asthma. *Arch. Dis. Child.* 61:1046, 1986.

Editorial comment: Multidrug resistant tuberculosis—North Carolina. *JAMA* 257:743, 1987.

Sloan, L.E.G.: Policy statement: Screening for cystic fibrosis. *Aust. Paediatr. J.* 22:264, 1986.

Rubio, T.T.: Infection in patients with cystic fibrosis. *Am. J. Med.* 81:73, 1986.

Committee on Adolescence: Tobacco use by children and adolescents. *Pediatrics* 79:479, 1987.

Committee on Fetus and Newborn: Use and abuse of the apgar score. *Pediatrics* 78:1148, 1986.

Frank, L., Sosenko, I.R.S.: Development of lung antioxidant enzyme system in late gestation: Possible implications for the prematurely born infant. *J. Pediatr.* 110:9, 1987.

Editorial comment: Smoking prevalence and cessation in selected states—1981–1983 and 1985—The behavioral risk factor surveys. *JAMA* 257:160, 1987.

Editorial comment: Anti-oestrogenic effect of cigarette smoking. *Lancet* 2:1433, 1986.

Editorial comment: Laws ban minors tobacco purchases, but enforcement is another matter. *JAMA* 257:3323, 1987.

Editorial comment: Smokeless tobacco use in the United States—Behavioral risk factors surveillance system, 1986. *JAMA* 258:24, 1987.

Leventhal, H., Glynn, K., Fleming, R.: Is smoking decision an "informed choice?": Effect of smoking risk factors on smoking beliefs. *JAMA* 257:3373, 1987.

Perry, C.L., Silvis, G.L.: Smoking prevention: Behavioral prescriptions for the pediatrician. *Pediatrics* 79:790, 1987.

DiFranza, J.R., Norwood, B.D., Garner, D.W., et al.: Legislative efforts to protect children from tobacco. *JAMA* 257:3387, 1987.

Editorial comment: Diagnosis of cystic fibrosis in premature infants. *Lancet* 1:24, 1987.

Editorial comment: Alpha$_1$-antitrypsin deficiency and prenatal diagnosis. *Lancet* 1:421, 1987.

The Heart and Blood Vessels:

Bisano, A.L.: Acute rheumatic fever: Forgotten but not gone. *N. Engl. J. Med.* 316:476, 1987.

Mason, J.W.: Amiodarone. *N. Engl. J. Med.* 316:455, 1987.

Moynihan, E.J.: Kawasaki disease: A novel feline virus transmitted by fleas. *Lancet* 1:195, 1987.

Moak, J.P., Smith, R.T., Garson, A.: Newer antiarrhythmic drugs in children. *Am. Heart J.* 113:179, 1987.

MacDonald, J.T.: Childhood migraine: Differential diagnosis and treatment. *Postgrad.* 80:301, 1986.

Parenzan, L.: Surgical treatment of tetrology of Fallot. *Ala. J. Med. Sci.* 23:151, 1986.

Garson, A.: Medical legal problems in the management of cardiac arrhythmias in children. *Pediatrics* 79:84, 1987.

Casscells, W.: Heart transplantation: Recent policy developments. *N. Engl. J. Med.* 315:1365, 1986.

Corrigan, J.J.: Kawasaki disease in the plight of the platelet. *Am. J. Dis. Child.* 140:1223, 1986.

Greenwood, R.D.: Mitral valve prolapse in children. *Postgrad. Med.* 80:257, 1986.

Silove, E.D.: Pharmacologic manipulation of the ductus arteriosus. *Arch. Dis. Child.* 61:827, 1986.

Feigen, R.D., Barron, K.S.: Treatment of Kawasaki syndrome. *N. Engl. J. Med.* 315:388, 1986.

Editorial comment: Looks like SVT. *Lancet* 2:612, 1986.

Campbell, R.M., Hammon, J.W., Acth, D.S., et al.: Surgical treatment of pediatric cardiac arrhythmia. *J. Pediatr.* 110:501, 1987.

Haddy, F.J.: Endogenous digitalis-like factor or factors. *N. Engl. J. Med.* 316:621, 1987.

Allen, H.: Is cardiac transplantation in children an experimental procedure? *Am. J. Dis. Child.* 140:1105, 1986.

Keen, G.: Spinal cord damage in operations for coarctation of the aorta: Aetiology, practice and prospects. *Thorax* 42:11, 1987.

diGroot, A.C., Nater, J.P., Herxheimer, A.: Minoxidil: Hope for the bald? *Lancet* 1:1019, 1987.

Task Force on Blood Pressure Control in Children: Report of the Second Task Force on Blood Pressure Control in Children—1987. *Pediatrics* 79:1, 1987.

Stehbens, W.E.: An appraisal of the epidemic rise of coronary artery disease and its decline. *Lancet* 1:606, 1987.

Nader, P.R., Taras, H.L., Sallis, J.F., et al.: Adult heart disease prevention in childhood colon: A national survey of pediatrician's practices and attitudes. *Pediatrics* 79:843, 1987.

McNamara, D.G.: Can (should) the pediatrician wage preventive medicine war against coronary heart disease? *Am. J. Dis. Child.* 140:985, 1986.

Committee on Nutrition: Prudent life-style for children: Dietary fat and cholesterol. *Pediatrics* 78:521, 1986.

Hirsh, J.: Hyperreactive platelets and complications of coronary artery disease. *N. Engl. J. Med.* 1543, 1987.

The Blood:

Erslev, A.: Erythropoietin coming of age. *N. Engl. J. Med.* 316:101, 1987.

Wheeler, J.G., et al.: Buffy coat transfusions in neonates with sepsis and neutrophil storage pool depletion. *Pediatrics* 79:422, 1987.

Mascola, L.: Semen donors as the source of sexually transmitted disease in artificially inseminated women: The saga unfolds. *JAMA* 257:1093, 1987.

Kaplan, D.L., Wofsy, C.B., Volberding, P.A.: Treatment of patients with acquired immunodeficiency syndrome and associated manifestations. *JAMA* 257:1367, 1987.

Editorial comment: Autologous and aged blood donors. *JAMA* 257:1220, 1987.

Editorial comment: Update: Acquired immunodeficiency syndrome—United States. *JAMA* 257:433, 1987.

Harrington, W.J.: Are platelet-antibody tests worthwhile? *N. Engl. J. Med.* 316:211, 1987.

Editorial comment: Positive HTLV-III/LAV antibody test for sexually active female members of social-sexual clubs. *JAMA* 257:293, 1987.

Balistreri, W.F., Farrell, M.K., Bove, K.E.: Lessons from the E-Fero tragedy. *Pediatrics* 78:503, 1986.

Editorial comment: Immunization of children infected with human T-lymphocyte virus type III/lymphadenopathy-associated virus. *JAMA* 256:2477, 1986.

Schrier, S.L.: Why does the thalassemic red cell die? *Blood Cells* 12:91, 1986.

Francis, D.P., Chin, J.: The prevention of acquired immunodeficiency syndrome in the United States. *JAMA* 257:1357, 1987.

Matthews, G.W., Neslund, V.S.: The initial impact of AIDS on public health law in the United States—1986. *JAMA* 257:344, 1987.

Fisher, M.G.: Transfusion-associated acquired immunodeficiency syndrome—what is the risk? *Pediatrics* 79:157, 1987.

Hilgartner, M.W.: AIDS in the transfused patient. *Am. J. Dis. Child.* 141:194, 1987.

Editorial comment: Pain relief in sickle cell crisis. *Lancet* 2:320, 1986.

Editorial comment: Penicillin prophylaxis for babies with sickle cell disease. *Lancet* 2:1432, 1986.

Chapple, J.C., Dale, R., Evans, B.G.: The new genetics: Will it pay its way? *Lancet* 1:1189, 1987.

Ledley, F.D.: Somatic gene therapy for human disease: Background and prospects. *J. Pediatr.* 110:1, 1987.

Oncology:

Editorial comment: Growth factors in malignancy. *Lancet* 2:317, 1986.

Editorial comment: Should all patients with retinoblastoma be screened for chromosome deletions? *Lancet* 1:544, 1987.

Gershon, A.A.: Live attenuated varicella vaccine. *J. Pediatr.* 110:154, 1987.

Plotkin, S.A.: Varicella vaccine: A point of decision. *Pediatrics* 78:705, 1986.

Editorial comment: Gene amplification in malignancy. *Lancet* 1:839, 1987.

McWilliams, N.D.: Screening for neuroblastoma in North America. *Pediatrics* 79:1048, 1987.

Editorial comment: Oncogene amplification may indicate breast cancer prognosis. *JAMA* 258:19, 1987.

Editorial comment: First anti-oncogene discovered; linked to the development of retinoblastoma. *JAMA* 257:152, 1987.

Samaan, N.A., Schultz, P.N., Yang, K.P.P., et al.: Endocrine complications after radiotherapy for tumors of the head and neck. *J. Lab. Clin. Med.* 109:364, 1987.

Brecher, M.L.: Treatment of acute lymphoid leukemia in children: Current regimens and future prospects. *N.Y. State J. Med.* April, 1986 p. 188.

Bell, B.A., Whitehead, V.M.: Chemotherapy of acute lymphatic leukemia. *Dev. Pharmacol. Ther.* 9:145, 1986.

Pastan, I., Gottesman, M.: Multiple-drug resistance in human cancer. *N. Engl. J. Med.* 316:1388, 1987.

Butturini, A., Rivera, G.K., Bortin, M.M., et al.: Which treatment for childhood acute lymphoblastic leukemia in second remission? *Lancet* 1:429, 1987.

Rosenberg, S.A.: Autologous bone marrow transplantation in non-Hodgkins lymphoma. *N. Engl. J. Med.* 316:1541, 1987.

Ophthalmology:

Biglan, A.W., Brown, D.R., MacPherson, T.A.: Update on retinopathy of prematurity. *Sem. Perinatol.* 10:187, 1986.

Editorial comment: Ophthalmologists discuss methods to help physicians see what patients can't. *JAMA* 257:1025, 1987.

Avery, G.B., Glass, P.: Light and retinopathy of prematurity: What is prudent for 1986? *Pediatrics* 78:520, 1986.

Editorial comment: As the number of contact lens users increases, research seeks to determine risk factors, how best to prevent potential eye infections. *JAMA* 258:17, 1987.

Stehr-Green, J.K., Bailey, T.M., Brandt, F.H., et al.: Acanthamoeba keratitis in soft contact lens wearers: A case-controlled study. *JAMA* 258:57, 1987.

Palmer, E.A.: How safe are ocular drugs in pediatrics? *Ophthalmology* 93:1038, 1986.

Dentistry and Otolaryngology:

Editorial comment: Screening for hearing impairment in the newborn. *Lancet* 2:1429, 1986.

Eimas, P.D., Kavanagh, J.F.: Otitis media, hearing loss, and child development: A NICHD conference summary. *Public Health Rep.* 101:289, 1986.

McDonald, T.J.: Twenty questions about middle-ear fluid and ventilation tubes. *Postgrad. Med.* 81:239, 1987.

Committee on Early Childhood, Adoption, and Dependent Care: Oral and dental aspects of child abuse and neglect. *Pediatrics* 78:537, 1986.

Editorial comment: Anesthesia for tonsillectomy. *Lancet* 2:1357, 1987.

Myer, C., Cotton, R.T.: Salivary gland disease in children: A review. Part I: Acquired non-neoplastic disease. *Clin. Pediatr.* 25:314, 1986.

Myer, C., Cotton, R.T.: Salivary gland disease in children: A review. Part II: Congenital lesions and neoplastic disease. *Clin. Pediatr.* 25:353, 1986.

Boraz, R.A.: A dental protocol for the pediatric cardiac transplant patient. *J. Dent. Child.* 27:382, 1986.

Black, R.: Tonsillectomy and adenoidectomy: A review. *Aust. Fam. Physician* 15:714, 1986.

Goepferd, S.J.: Infant oral health: A rationale. *J. Dent. Child.* 53:257, 1986.

Tsamtsouris, A., Stack, A., Padamsee, M.: Dental education of expectant parents. *J. Pedodont.* 10:309, 1986.

Editorial comment: Management of contacts of children in day care with invasive *Haemophilus influenzae* type b disease. *Pediatrics* 78:939, 1986.

Committee on School Health: Impedance Bridge (tympanometer) as a screening device in schools. *Pediatrics* 79:472, 1987.

Toye, F.J., Weinstein, J.D.: Clinical experience in percutaneous tracheostomy and cricothyroidotomy in 100 patients. *J. Trauma* 26:1034, 1986.

Endocrinology:

White, P.C., New, M.I., Dupont, B.: Congenital adrenal hypoplasia. Part I. *N. Engl. J. Med.* 316:1519, 1987.

White, P.C., New, M.I., Dupont, B.: Congenital adrenal hypoplasia. Part II. *N. Engl. J. Med.* 316:1580, 1987.

Baker, F.W.: Assessment of growth problems in adolescents. *Can. Fam. Physician* 32:2417, 1986.

Greene, D.A., Lattimer, S.A., Sima, A.A.: Sorbitol, phosphoinositides, and sodium-potassium-ATPase in the pathogenesis of diabetic complications. *N. Engl. J. Med.* 316:599, 1987.

Wilkin, T., Armitage, M.: Markers for insulin dependent diabetes: Towards early detection. *Br. Med. J.* 293:1323, 1986.

Knudtzon, J.: Growth hormone therapy of short stature. *Acta. Paediatr. Scand.* 75:353, 1986.

Lippe, B.: Neurotransmitter administration and manipulation of growth. *J. Pediatr.* 109:829, 1986.

Litt, I.F.: Amenorrhea in the adolescent athlete. *Postgrad. Med.* 80:245, 1986.

Stelling, M.W.: Stepwise evaluation of the short child: With comments on the status of growth hormone therapy. *Postgrad. Med.* 79:185, 1986.

Dunger, D.D., Ahmed, L.: Evaluation of short stature in childhood. *Practitioner* 230:775, 1986.

Rimoin, D.L., Borochowitz, Z., Horton, W.A.: Short stature-physiology and pathology. *West. J. Med.* 144:710, 1986.

Wood, F.C., Bierman, E.L.: Is diet the cornerstone in the management of diabetes? *N. Engl. J. Med.* 315:1224, 1986.

Pope, R.M.: Recent advances in thyroid disease. *Practitioner* 230:820, 1986.

Howlett, T.: Corticosteroid therapy. *Practitioner* 230:813, 1986.

Editorial comment: Pancreatic transplantation in diabetes. *Lancet* 1:1015, 1987.

Editorial comment: Vitamin D: New perspectives. *Lancet* 1:1122, 1987.

Editorial comment: Synthetic human calcitonin approved. *JAMA* 257:155, 1987.

Editorial comment: LHRH analogues for contraception. *Lancet* 1:1179, 1987.

Bercu, B.B.: Growth hormone treatment and the short child: To treat or not to treat? *J. Pediatr.* 110:991, 1987.

Blizzard, R.M.: Discretionary use of growth hormone advised. *AAP News* 2:1, 1986 (October).

Reichlin, S.: Secretion of somatostatin and its physiologic function. *J. Lab. Clin. Med.* 109:320, 1987.

Volpe, R.: Immunoregulation in autoimmune thyroid disease. *N. Engl. J. Med.* 316:44, 1987.

The Musculoskeletal System:

Editorial comment: Alzheimer's disease, Down syndrome and chromosome 21. *Lancet* 1:1011, 1987.

Baker, C.: Epidemiology of trauma: The civilian perspective. *Ann. Emerg. Med.* 15:1389, 1986.

Rosser, W., Feldman, W., McGrath, P.: Common skeletal problems in children and adolescents. *Can. Fam. Physician* 33:641, 1987.

Wiley, J.J.: In-toeing and out-toeing in children. *Can. Fam. Physician* 33:637, 1987.

Kallio, P., Ryoppy, S., Kunnamo, I.: Transient synovitis and Perthes' disease. *J. Bone Joint Surg.* 68-b:808, 1986.

Schlesinger, I., Waugh, T.: Slipped capital femoral epiphysis, unsolved adolescent hip disorder. *Orthopaed. Rev.* 16:33, 1987.

Luckstead, E.F.: Pediatric team physicians. *Pediatrics* 78:941, 1986.

Cohen, M.D.: Clinical utility of magnetic resonance imaging in pediatrics. *Am. J. Dis. Child.* 140:947, 1986.

Gibb, W.R.G., Lees, A.J.: The restless legs syndrome. *Postgrad. Med. J.* 62:329, 1986.

Allen, C.E.: Childhood bicycle injuries: What can we do? *Am. J. Dis. Child.* 141:135, 1987.

Cowart, V.: Physician-competitors advice to colleagues: Steroid users respond to education, rehabilitation. *JAMA* 257:427, 1987.

Ward, A.: Born to jog: Exercise programs for preschoolers. *Phys. Sportsmed.* 14:163, 1986.

Lawton, L.J.: Injuries associated with all-terrain vehicles. *Can. Fam. Physician* 33:717, 1987.

Williams, A.F., Lund, A.K.: Seatbelt use laws and occupant crash protection in the United States. *AJPH* 76:1438, 1986.

Sheps, S.B., Evans, G.D.: Epidemiology of school injuries: A two year experience in a municipal health department. *Pediatrics* 79:69, 1987.

Foege, W.H.: Highway violence and public health. *N. Engl. J. Med.* 316:1407, 1987.

Cowart, V.: National concern about drug abuse brings athletes under unusual scrutiny. *JAMA* 256:2457, 1986.

Committee on Accident and Poison Prevention: All terrain vehicles: 2-, 3-, 4-wheeled, unlicensed motorized vehicles. *Pediatrics* 79:306, 1987.

Siegel, D.M.: Adolescents and chronic illness. *JAMA* 257:3396, 1987.

Editorial comment. Screening for the detection of congenital dislocation of the hip. *Arch. Dis. Child.* 61:921, 1986.

Gastroenterology:

Hewson, P., Oberklaid, F., Menahem, S.: Infant colic, distress, and crying. *Clin. Pediatr.* 26:69, 1987.

Fromm, D.: Endoscopic coagulation for gastrointestinal bleeding. *N. Engl. J. Med.* 316:1652, 1987.

Editorial comment: Gilbert's syndrome—More questions than answers. *Lancet* 1:1071, 1987.

Beaudet, A.L.: Gaucher's disease. *N. Engl. J. Med.* 316:619, 1987.

Harrison, M.R.: Organ procurement for children: The anencephalic fetus as a donor. *Lancet* 1:1383, 1986.

Mowat, A.P.: Liver transplantation—A role for pediatricians. *Arch. Dis. Child.* 62:325, 1987.

Monson, T.P.: Pediatric viral gastroenteritis. *Am. Fam. Pract.* 34:95, 1986.

Wald, A.: Fecal incontinence: Effective non-surgical treatments. *Postgrad. Med.* 80:123, 1986.

Flye, M.W., Jendrisak: Liver transplantation in the child. *World J. Surg.* 10:432, 1986.

Rollins, B.J.: Hepatic veno-occlusive disease. *Am. J. Med.* 81:297, 1986.

Editorial comment: Man, dogs, and hydatid disease. *Lancet* 1:21, 1987.

Collins, R.H., Feldman, M., Fordtran, J.S.: Colon cancer, dysplasia and surveillance in patients with ulcerative colitis: A critical review. *N. Engl. J. Med.* 316:1654, 1987.

Meythaler, J.M., Varma, R.R.: Reye's syndrome in adults: Diagnostic considerations. *Arch. Intern. Med.* 147:61, 1987.

Kauffman, R.E., Roberts, R.J.: Aspirin use and Reye's syndrome. *Pediatrics* 79:1049, 1987.

Arrowsmith, J.B., Kennedy, D.L., Kuritsky, J.N., et al.: National patterns of aspirin use in Reye syndrome reporting, United States, 1982–1985. *Pediatrics* 79:858, 1987.

Editorial comment: A sound approach to the diagnosis of acute appendicitis. *Lancet* 1:198, 1987.

Raymond, C.A.: Experimental rotavirus vaccine passes first test: Eventual goal: Immunize newborns against most prevalent cause of life-threatening diarrhea. *JAMA* 258:12, 1987.

Lilly, J.R., Hall, R.J.: Liver transplantation and Kasai operation in the first year of life: Therapeutic dilemma in biliary atresia. *J. Pediatr.* 112:561, 1987.

Kaplan, M.M.: Primary biliary cirrhosis. *N. Engl. J. Med.* 316:521, 1987.

Subject Index

A

Abdomen
  trauma, blunt, peritoneal lavage after, 502
Abuse
  child, and recurrent apnea, 180
Accidents
  road, epidemiology of, 186
Acetylcholinesterase
  in rectal biopsy, 517
Acidosis
  lactic, ocular findings in, 399
Acyclovir
  news about, Special Article, Chapter 4, 141
Addison disease
  associated anomalies, 448
Adenoids
  lymphoma, non-Hodgkin's, 363
Adenosine
  deaminase deficiency, treatment, 115
Adenovirus
  enteric, in gastroenteritis, 106
Adolescence
  with diabetes, poor glycemic control during, 236
  erythroblastopenia during, transient, 341
  scoliosis during, and personality development, 481
  suicide during, heterogeneity of, 239
  thrombosis during, deep vein, 357
  thyroid carcinoma during, 376
Adolescent
  -physician views of teen health information concerns, 233
Age
  calcium-regulating hormones and minerals and, 135
  sickle cell disease and red cell counts, 347
  vitamin D status and, 460
AIDS
  calcification of basal ganglia in, 99
  congenital, heart involvement in, 312
  maternal HTLV-III/LAV, outcome of children, 97
Airway
  reactivity and pupillary responses in asthma, 401
Alcohol
  fetal alcohol syndrome, follow-up studies, 214
Allergic
  urticaria, cimetidine in, 175

Allergy
  atopic, cost-effectiveness of neonatal IgE-screening, 162
  milk, manifestations of, 144
Amenorrhea
  secondary, in young ballet dancers, 479
Amikacin
  in septicemia in newborn, 74
Amiodarone
  in arrhythmia, 304
Amoxicillin
  in otitis media with effusion, 432
Amyloidosis
  systemic, complicating cystic fibrosis, 293
Anemia
  hemolytic, autoimmune, gammaglobulin for, 340
  in prematurity, vitamin E supplement to prevent, 335
  screening with capillary microhematocrit for, 337
  sickle cell, prenatal diagnosis by DNA analysis, 345
Anomalies
  associated with Addison disease, 448
Anorexia nervosa
  long-term follow-up, 216
Antibiotics
  Hemophilus influenzae type B meningitis and, 70
Antibody(ies)
  anti-SS-a, in maternal systemic lupus erythematosus, 34
  to gliadin in screening of celiac disease, 516
  maternal, against fetal cardiac antigens in heart block, 305
  viral, in Reye's syndrome, 499
Antidiuretic hormone
  inappropriate secretion syndrome after spinal fusion, 478
Antigen(s)
  fetal cardiac, in heart block, 305
Antihistamine
  in otitis media with effusion, 432
Antioxidant
  bilirubin as, possible physiological importance, 20
Anti-SS-a antibodies
  in maternal systemic lupus erythematosus, 34
Antithrombin
  III deficiency causing cerebral thromboembolism, 207
Aortic
  dilation, dissection and rupture in Turner syndrome, 325

Author Index

A

Aaron, N.H., 68
Abraham, C., 340
Abuchowski, A., 115
Ackerman, B.A., 125
Adams, F.H., 301
Addante, R.R., 414
Addison, G.M., 517
Aladjem, M., 147, 264
Albert, D., 357
Alexander, M., 499
Allee, L.M., 408
Allendorph, M., 496
Al-Mateen, M., 210
Alpert, J.J., 192
Ames, B.N., 20
Amiel, S.A., 236
Amir, N., 76
Amylon, M., 369
Anderson, H.R., 152
Anderson, L.R., 64
Andresen, B.D., 499
Andrish, J.T., 478
Angelucci, E., 343
Angle, C.R., 295
Antonarakis, S.E., 353
Arce, J., 313
Aricò, M., 97
Armon, M.E., 25
Arnheim, N., 345
Aronis, S., 353
Arsenault, L., 186
Arts, W.F.M., 207
Arvin, A.M., 28, 30, 32
Athreya, B.H., 93, 468, 470
Au, D.S., 28, 30
Aureli, G., 343
Austin, R.D., 168
Axelsson, I., 122
Azzini, M., 97

B

Bäckdahl, M., 376
Bahakim, H., 52
Bailey, R., 228
Baker, M.D., 248
Balun, J.E., 121
Bamji, M., 15
Banejeh, S., 199
Baranak, C.C., 420
Barenkamp, S.J., 434
Barnes, K., 453
Baronciani, D., 343
Barrett, M.J., 245
Barriga, F., 428
Barsoum-Homsy, M., 397
Barthels, M., 270
Barton, C.W., 325
Barttelbort, S.W., 502
Bass, M., 181

Bauchner, H., 84
Bauer, S., 274
Beattie, J.T., 267
Becker, L.E., 372
Beer, S., 147
Beiser, A.S., 112
Beitchman, J.H., 230
Bell, E.F., 335
Bell, G.R., 478
Belman, A.L., 99
Belon, C., 471
Benach, J.L., 93
Bender, S., 494
Benediktsson, B., 122
Bennet, J., 448
Benson, J.W.T., 40
Bergin, M., 458
Berkowitz, C.D., 228
Berman, L., 474
Berthier, A., 356
Besser, G.M., 450
Betts, R.F., 104
Bhat, M., 408
Biggar, W.D., 69
Bjarke, B., 512
Bjelland, J., 472
Bjerre, I., 475
Black, R.E., 119
Blackshaw, A.J., 512
Blackstone, E.H., 308
Blair, G.K., 283
Blanchette, V.S., 335
Bland, J.M.,152
Blank, E.L., 496
Block, J., 219
Block, J.H., 219
Bloom, B.A., 208
Bloom, R.R., 489
Bloss, R.S., 252
Blossom, P., 104
Bluestone, C.D., 408
Boddy, S.-A.M., 276
Bogle, S., 43
Bohorquez, L., 455
Borges, M., 455
Bottazzo, G.F., 506
Boucek, M.M., 66
Bourdoux, P., 442
Bowerman, J.G., 168
Boyce, W.T., 472
Boyd, J.H., 74
Boyett, J.M., 369
Brandenburg, K., 166
Brann, B.S., IV, 13
Brasel, J.A., 451
Brasfield, D.M., 81
Breederveld, C., 207
Bregman, D., 245
Brem, A.S., 209
Brenchley, P.E.C., 267
Bricker, J.T., 252
Bro, P.V., 378
Brochstein, J.A., 312
Brodehl, J., 270
Brom, A.G., 323

Brooks-Gunn, J., 479
Brouwers, P., 499
Brown, E.J., 335
Brown, F.E., 414
Brown, K.H., 119
Brown, Q., 389
Brown, V.A., 353
Brunell, P.A., 111
Brunham, R.C., 51
Brunot, V., 314
Brunson, S.C., 238
Bubis, S.C., 83
Buchanan, G., 369
Buchanan, G.R., 350, 360
Buchi, K.F., 35
Buckley, A., 57
Buckley, R.H., 115
Bucknall, C.A., 304
Buis, T., 323
Burke, B.A., 293
Burlington, D.B., 245
Burns, J.C., 112, 113
Burstein, S., 451
Bussel, J.B., 340
Butler, J., 65
Buttery, C.M.G., 111
Butzirus, S.M., 215
Byloos, J., 287

C

Calhoun, J.H., 398
Callaghan, J., 209
Camitta, B., 369
Campbell, A.N., 372
Campbell, J.R., 45
Campbell, T.J., 45
Carey, D.E., 510
Carlin, S.A., 434
Carlsen, N.L.T., 378
Carpenter, M.W., 13
Carr, R.F., 411
Carstensen, L.L., 243
Caselli, D., 97
Casey, C.S., 345
Cass, A.S., 208
Cassell, G., 81
Castaneda, A.R., 321
Castillo, P., 227
Castillo-Duran, C., 132
Cates, K.L., 72
Catlin, E.A., 13
Cayazzo, M., 127
Cebul, R.D., 470
Chabut, S., 147
Chamaret, S., 356
Champion, H.R., 187
Chan, H.S.L., 372
Chan, L., 108
Chanatry, J., 64
Chaussain, J.L., 448
Chen, Y., 256
Chernausek, S.D., 451